Safety Pharmacology

Safety Pharmacology

Editor: Atlas Holmes

AMERICAN
MEDICAL PUBLISHERS
www.americanmedicalpublishers.com

AMERICAN
MEDICAL PUBLISHERS
www.americanmedicalpublishers.com

Cataloging-in-Publication Data

Safety pharmacology / edited by Atlas Holmes.
p. cm.
Includes bibliographical references and index.
ISBN 979-8-88740-445-5
1. Pharmacology. 2. Drugs--Physiological effect. 3. Chemotherapy--Safety measures.
4. Drugs--Standards. I. Holmes, Atlas.
RM103 .S24 2023
615.5--dc23

American Medical Publishers,
41 Flatbush Avenue,
1st Floor, New York,
NY 11217, USA

ISBN 979-8-88740-445-5 (Hardback)

Contents

Preface

I am honored to present to you this unique book which encompasses the most up-to-date data in the field. I was extremely pleased to get this opportunity of editing the work of experts from across the globe. I have also written papers in this field and researched the various aspects revolving around the progress of the discipline. I have tried to unify my knowledge along with that of stalwarts from every corner of the world, to produce a text which not only benefits the readers but also facilitates the growth of the field.

Safety pharmacology deals with the detection and analysis of the potential adverse pharmacodynamic and pharmacological effects of new chemical entities (NCEs) on physiological processes, apart from the desired therapeutic effects. Such adverse effects of NCEs can be dangerous, especially in people who have damaged or reduced organ system functions. Safety pharmacology is vital throughout the process of drug discovery and development. There are three main goals of non-clinical safety pharmacology evaluations. First goal is to protect phase I clinical trial volunteers from acute drug side effects; second goal is to protect patients (including patients in phase II and III clinical trials), and last goal is to reduce the risk of failure during drug development and post-marketing phase due to undesirable pharmacodynamic effects. It is a fast-growing area of study in pharmacology and requires regulatory guidance. This book is a valuable compilation of topics, ranging from the basic to the most complex advancements in safety pharmacology. It explores all the important aspects of this field in the present day scenario. This book will serve as a valuable reference source for students and researchers.

Finally, I would like to thank all the contributing authors for their valuable time and contributions. This book would not have been possible without their efforts. I would also like to thank my friends and family for their constant support.

Editor

1

In Silico Assessment of Efficacy and Safety of I_{Kur} Inhibitors in Chronic Atrial Fibrillation: Role of Kinetics and State-Dependence of Drug Binding

Nicholas Ellinwood[1], *Dobromir Dobrev*[2], *Stefano Morotti*[1]*, *and Eleonora Grandi*[1]

[1] *Department of Pharmacology, University of California, Davis, Davis, CA, United States,*

[2] *West German Heart and Vascular Center, Institute of Pharmacology, University Duisburg-Essen, Essen, Germany*

Correspondence:
Stefano Morotti
smorotti@gmail.com

Current pharmacological therapy against atrial fibrillation (AF), the most common cardiac arrhythmia, is limited by moderate efficacy and adverse side effects including ventricular proarrhythmia and organ toxicity. One way to circumvent the former is to target ion channels that are predominantly expressed in atria vs. ventricles, such as $K_V1.5$, carrying the ultra-rapid delayed-rectifier K^+ current (I_{Kur}). Recently, we used an *in silico* strategy to define optimal $K_V1.5$-targeting drug characteristics, including kinetics and state-dependent binding, that maximize AF-selectivity in human atrial cardiomyocytes in normal sinus rhythm (nSR). However, because of evidence for I_{Kur} being strongly diminished in long-standing persistent (chronic) AF (cAF), the therapeutic potential of drugs targeting I_{Kur} may be limited in cAF patients. Here, we sought to simulate the efficacy (and safety) of I_{Kur} inhibitors in cAF conditions. To this end, we utilized sensitivity analysis of our human atrial cardiomyocyte model to assess the importance of I_{Kur} for atrial cardiomyocyte electrophysiological properties, simulated hundreds of theoretical drugs to reveal those exhibiting anti-AF selectivity, and compared the results obtained in cAF with those in nSR. We found that despite being downregulated, I_{Kur} contributes more prominently to action potential (AP) and effective refractory period (ERP) duration in cAF vs. nSR, with ideal drugs improving atrial electrophysiology (e.g., ERP prolongation) more in cAF than in nSR. Notably, the trajectory of the AP during cAF is such that more I_{Kur} is available during the more depolarized plateau potential. Furthermore, I_{Kur} block in cAF has less cardiotoxic effects (e.g., AP duration not exceeding nSR values) and can increase Ca^{2+} transient amplitude thereby enhancing atrial contractility. We propose that *in silico* strategies such as that presented here should be combined with *in vitro* and *in vivo* assays to validate model predictions and facilitate the ongoing search for novel agents against AF.

Keywords: ultra-rapid delayed-rectifier K^+ current, atrial fibrillation, mathematical modeling, ion channel blockers

---

Abbreviations: AP, action potential; APD, AP duration; APD_{40}, APD to 40% repolarization; APD_{90}, APD to 90% repolarization; AF, atrial fibrillation; C, closed state; cAF, chronic AF; CaT, Ca^{2+} transient; CaT_{amp}, CaT amplitude; CL, cycle length; EAD, early afterdepolarization; E_m, membrane potential; ERP, effective refractory period; G_{Kur}, maximal conductance of the ultra-rapid delayed-rectifier K^+ current; I, inactivated state; I_{Kur}, ultra-rapid delayed-rectifier K^+ current; nSR, normal sinus rhythm; O, open state.

INTRODUCTION

Atrial fibrillation (AF) is characterized by rapid, irregular heart contractions following fast, disorganized electrical signals in the atria. AF is the most common cardiac arrhythmia, occurring in 1–2% of the general population and projected to increase dramatically in the coming decades (to 4% by 2050) with an aging westernized population (Andrade et al., 2014). The most effective current treatment for preventing recurrence of AF in the clinic is radiofrequency ablation. Pharmacological therapy against AF is limited by low efficacy and substantial adverse side effects including an increased risk of lethal ventricular tachyarrhythmias.

To maximize efficacy and minimize proarrhythmic risk, an AF-selective drug should exert potent effects on fibrillating atria without significantly impacting ventricular tissue function during normal sinus rhythm (nSR) (Ehrlich et al., 2008; Van Wagoner et al., 2015). A potential strategy to achieve this goal is to target ion channels that are predominantly expressed in atria vs. ventricles, such as $K_V1.5$, carrying the ultra-rapid delayed-rectifier K^+ current (I_{Kur}). Genetic mutations causing both loss- and gain-of-function of I_{Kur} have been associated with atrial arrhythmias in human (Olson et al., 2006; Christophersen et al., 2013; Colman et al., 2017). In a previous investigation, we used an *in silico* strategy to define optimal $K_V1.5$-targeting drug characteristics, including kinetics and state-dependent binding, that maximize AF-selectivity (i.e., fast pacing-rate selectivity) in human atrial cardiomyocytes (Ellinwood et al., 2017). Because this work was conducted in atrial cardiomyocytes under nSR conditions, the best-performing drug properties identified would have relevance for patients with paroxysmal AF that have not undergone extensive AF-related electrical remodeling (Grandi et al., 2012; Nattel and Dobrev, 2016).

Building on our previously established simulation framework, the major goal of this investigation was to determine the optimal drug characteristics of I_{Kur} inhibitors in long-standing persistent (chronic) AF (cAF) conditions. Although not a universal finding (Yue et al., 1997; Bosch et al., 1999; Grammer et al., 2000; Workman et al., 2001), previous reports showed that I_{Kur} is strongly diminished in cAF patients (Van Wagoner et al., 1997; Brandt et al., 2000; Van Wagoner and Nerbonne, 2000; Dobrev and Ravens, 2003; Christ et al., 2008; Caballero et al., 2010), making the therapeutic potential of inhibitors targeting this current uncertain (Ravens et al., 2013; Grandi and Maleckar, 2016). Indeed, evidence of anti-arrhythmic efficacy of $K_V1.5$ inhibitors in clinical trials is lacking (Ravens et al., 2013). However, recent studies have suggested an anti-arrhythmic potential of I_{Kur}-targeting drugs in cAF (Christ et al., 2008; Ford et al., 2013, 2016; Loose et al., 2014), as they can prolong action potential (AP) and effective refractory period (ERP) in atrial cardiomyocytes of cAF patients. Moreover, experimental evidence suggests that block of I_{Kur} enhances force of contraction of isolated human atrial trabeculae in cAF (Wettwer et al., 2004; Schotten et al., 2007). Our human atrial cardiomyocyte model confirmed that block of I_{Kur} results in prolongation and elevation of the AP plateau, which augments the Ca^{2+} transient (CaT) amplitude (CaT_{amp}), thereby eliciting a positive inotropic effect (Grandi et al., 2011). Thus, I_{Kur} might be a useful atrial-selective target to potentially prevent reentry and related atrial hypocontractility in cAF. We propose that our computational approach, combined with *in vivo* and *in vitro* validation, might be useful to facilitate the identification of atrial-selective anti-arrhythmic drugs against AF (Bers and Grandi, 2011; Grandi and Maleckar, 2016).

METHODS

Atrial AP Model and Simulations

APs and CaTs were simulated with the Grandi et al. model of the human atrial cardiomyocyte in nSR and cAF (Grandi et al., 2011; Morotti et al., 2016b). I_{Kur} gating was described by a 6-state Markov type model (**Figure 1A**) as in Ellinwood et al. (2017), and I_{Kur} maximal conductance (G_{Kur}) in cAF was reduced by 50% compared to nSR (Grandi et al., 2011).

Simulations were equilibrated for 300 beats at 1-Hz pacing or 900 beats at 3-Hz pacing. After the 300th or 900th beat, the time to 40 and 90% repolarization of the AP (APD_{40} and APD_{90}) were calculated, along with diastolic intracellular Ca^{2+} concentration ($[Ca^{2+}]_i$), CaT_{amp} and time to 50% CaT decay. The atrial ERP was determined using a standard S_1-S_2 premature stimulation protocol (Wang et al., 1996; Shinagawa et al., 2000; Christ et al., 2008; Zhao et al., 2009), where the S_1 basal stimulus (5 ms in duration) was applied to a steady-state human atrial cardiomyocyte model. As previously described (Ellinwood et al., 2017), ERP was determined by applying the premature S_2 stimulus (5 ms in duration, 2-fold the diastolic threshold of excitation) at progressively smaller S_1-S_2 intervals from 700 ms to refractoriness by decrements of 2 ms. The longest S_1-S_2 interval that failed to elicit an AP was taken as the local ERP (i.e., maximum upstroke velocity $\geq$5 V/s and AP with an amplitude $\geq$50% of the amplitude of the preceding AP elicited by S_1).

An irregular pacing protocol was run for 20 s, starting from steady-state conditions at the fixed 3-Hz pacing. The cycle length (CL) was allowed to vary randomly following a uniform distribution between 285.7 and 400 ms, corresponding to a minimum pacing frequency of 2.5 Hz and a maximum pacing frequency of 3.5 Hz, with a mean of 333.3 ms (corresponding to 3-Hz pacing). The time course of membrane potential (E_m), APD_{90}, and CL was tracked over the course of the simulation.

All simulations and analysis were performed in MATLAB (The MathWorks, Natick, MA, USA) using the stiff ordinary differential equation solver ode15s. The model code is available for download at the following webpages: https://somapp.ucdmc.ucdavis.edu/Pharmacology/bers/ and http://elegrandi.wixsite.com/grandilab/downloads.

Parameter Sensitivity Analysis

Parameter sensitivity analysis was performed with the population-based approach described in Sobie (2009), Morotti et al. (2017), and Morotti and Grandi (2017) to investigate the role of various currents and transporters in the regulation of AP duration (APD), ERP, and CaT characteristics. Two populations of 900 atrial cardiomyocyte models were generated by randomly

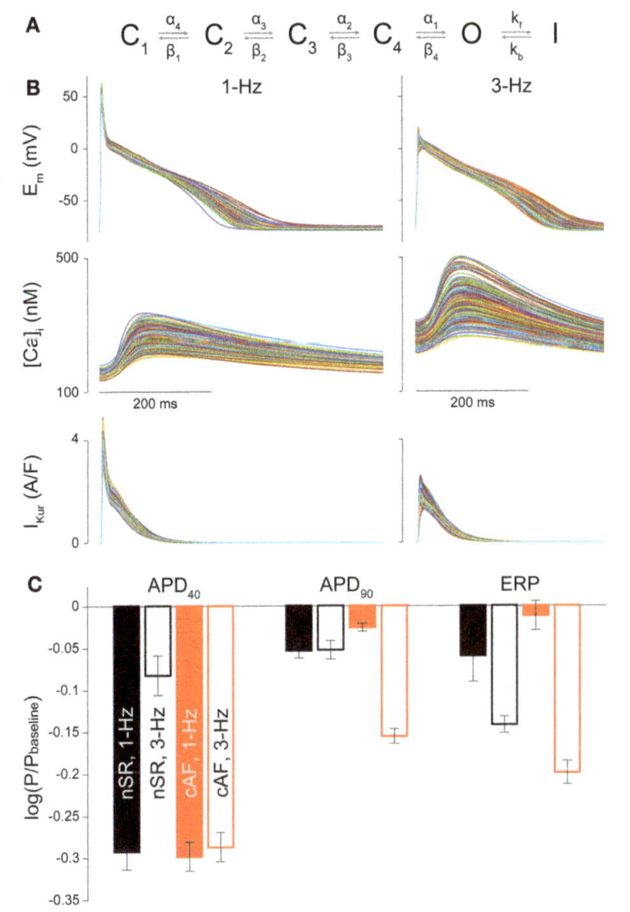

FIGURE 1 | Sensitivity of nSR and cAF cardiomyocyte electrophysiology to I_{Kur} changes. **(A)** Drug-free Markov model of I_{Kur} derived from Zhou et al. (2012). The model has 4 closed states (C_1, C_2, C_3, C_4), a conducting open state (O), and an inactivated state (I). Transition rates equations and parameters are those in Ellinwood et al. (2017). **(B)** AP, CaT, and I_{Kur} in a subset of 300 cAF cardiomyocyte model variants at 1-Hz and 3-Hz pacing rates. **(C)** Bar graphs show the average regression coefficients indicating how perturbations in G_{Kur} affect APD_{40}, APD_{90}, and ERP in nSR and cAF at 1-Hz and 3-Hz pacing rates. Error bars represent one standard deviation.

varying the values of 18 parameters (see list in the Supplementary Materials) in the baseline nSR and cAF models. Specifically, the default value of each conductance or maximal transport rate was independently varied with a log-normal distribution (with standard deviation of 0.1). Multivariable regression (non-linear iterative partial least squares method) on log-transformed values was performed for 30 random subsets of 300 model variants from the 900-variant population to correlate the variation in each parameter to the consequent effect on each output. In **Figure 1C** and Figures S1–S6 bars represent the mean regression coefficients and error bars represent one standard deviation.

K_V1.5 Drug-Binding Model

We utilized our recent I_{Kur} Markov formulation and approach to describe various drug-K_V1.5 channel binding schemes (**Figures 2A,F**; Ellinwood et al., 2017), as done by Lee et al. (2016). We previously showed that open state (O) blockers and open and inactivated state (O & I) blockers that target K_V1.5 display fast pacing-rate selectivity (Ellinwood et al., 2017). Thus, we focused on these two types of inhibitors when examining the relationship between electrophysiological parameters and drug-binding kinetics in cAF. We considered different theoretical drugs with variable forward (k_{on}) and reverse (k_{off}) drug-binding rates to the open and inactivated states of the K_V1.5 channel in the predicted physiological range of 0.01–100 s^{-1} (Lagrutta et al., 2006) using half-logarithmic increments resulting in nine transition rates for each drug state transition (0.01, 0.03, 0.1, 0.3, 1, 3, 10, 30, 100 s^{-1}). For a particular state of the channel, dissociation constants (K_d) for our drug scenarios were calculated as k_{off}/k_{on}, and affinity constants were calculated as k_{on}/k_{off}. To investigate the effects of these drug characteristics, for a given state-dependent binding inhibitor, we varied k_{on} and k_{off} together ($k_{on} = k_{off}$) or considered all permutations of the nine different rates of drug binding (producing a total of 81 different drug scenarios). For drugs that could bind to multiple states of the K_V1.5 channel, we also varied the relative affinity to open (K_O) vs. inactivated state (K_I). For O & I blockers, we included transitions between drug-bound states (orange transitions in **Figure 2F**) when specified. All drugs were simulated at the concentration causing a 50% reduction in peak I_{Kur} (i.e., IC_{50}). IC_{50} values were computed as described previously (Ellinwood et al., 2017), using a 200-ms down-ramp voltage-clamp protocol from +30 to −60 mV. After the application of a given [drug] (range: 1 nM−1 M), we allowed sufficient time for the degree of block to reach equilibrium. IC_{50} values were calculated at 1- and 3-Hz pacing rates as the [drug] causing a 50% reduction in peak I_{Kur} compared to drug-free conditions. We chose the down-ramp, as compared to a typical square pulse, because it more closely resembles the relative state occupancies of the closed states, open state, and inactivated state of the K_V1.5 channel during a physiological atrial AP, as we have shown in (Ellinwood et al., 2017).

RESULTS

Role of I_{Kur} in nSR and cAF Atrial Electrophysiology

We built 900 variations of our nSR and cAF human atrial cardiomyocyte models (Grandi et al., 2011) at 1- and 3-Hz pacing, and performed parameter sensitivity analysis on 30 random subsets of 300 model variants to determine how alterations in each maximum ionic conductance/transport rate differentially (in cAF vs. nSR) affect electrophysiological properties including APD_{40}, APD_{90}, ERP, CaT_{amp}, diastolic $[Ca^{2+}]_i$, and time to 50% CaT decay (Figures S1–S6). Simulated APs and CaTs in a representative group of 300 cAF cardiomyocyte model variants are shown in **Figure 1B**, and the average regression coefficients for G_{Kur} in nSR and cAF conditions at 1- and 3-Hz pacing are in **Figure 1C**. The values are negative because an increase in I_{Kur} shortens APD_{40}, APD_{90}, and ERP on average according to the regression algorithm. The analysis revealed that, while at a slow pacing rate APD_{90} and ERP

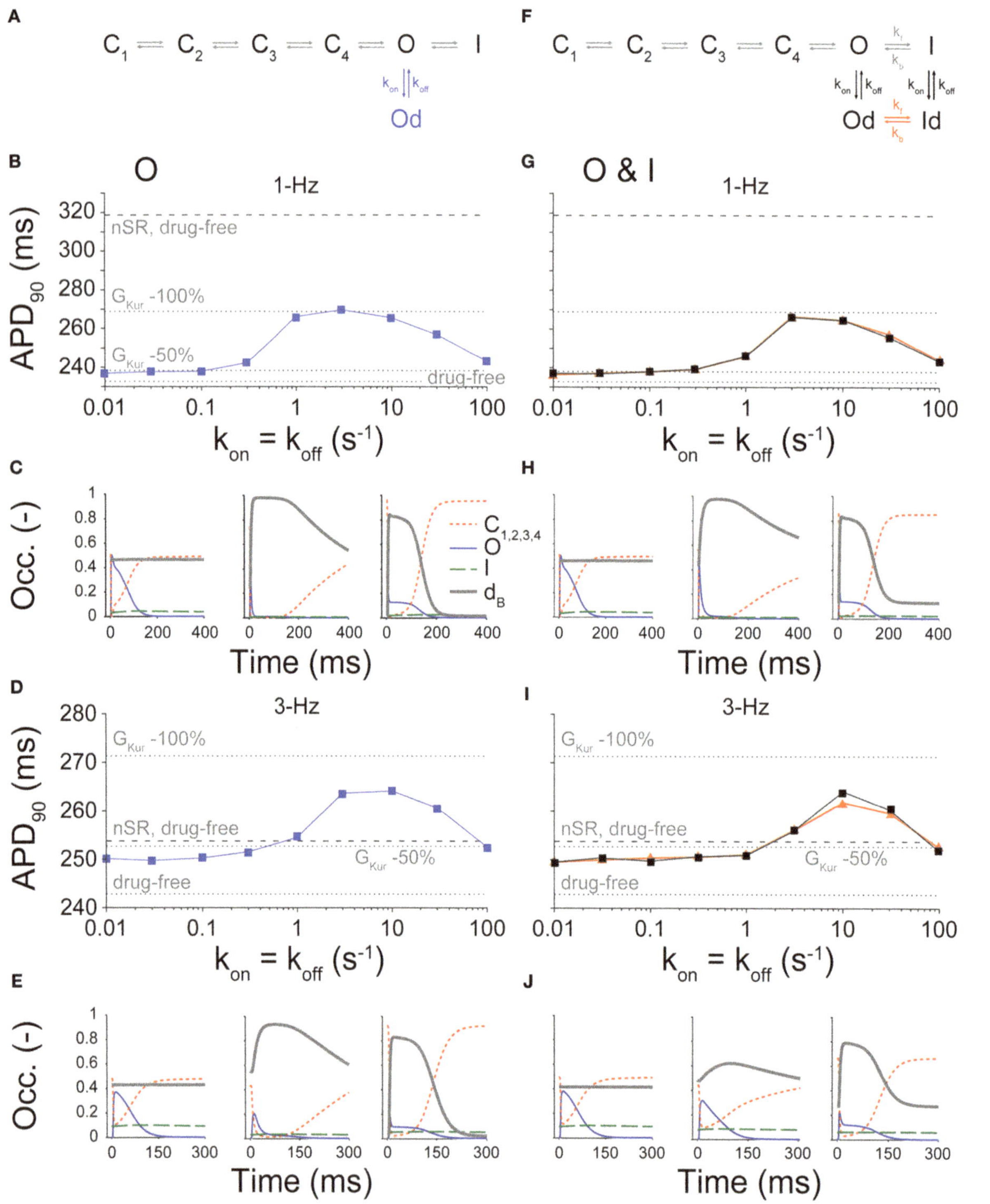

FIGURE 2 | Effect of state-dependence and kinetics of drug binding on APD_{90}. APD_{90} was determined for open (schematic in **A**, **B,** 1-Hz and **D**, 3-Hz pacing rate) and open and inactivated (schematic in **F**, **G** 1-Hz and **I**, 3-Hz pacing rate) state blockers given nine different rates of binding kinetics between 0.01 and 100 s^{-1} using half-logarithmic increments, whereby $k_{off} = k_{on}$, $K_d = 1\ \mu M$. For O & I blockers, we either allowed or prevented transitions between drug-bound states (orange vs. black traces in **G,I**). Simulations were also run in nSR and cAF drug-free conditions, and in cAF given a 50 and 100% reduction in G_{Kur} (dotted and dashed lines in **B**,**D**,**G**,**I**). Simulations were equilibrated for 300 beats at 1-Hz pacing or 900 beats at 3-Hz pacing using a [drug] equal to the IC_{50} value. **(C**,**E**,**H**,**J)** show the closed, open, inactivated and drug-bound (d_B, i.e., Od or Od+Id) state occupancies during an AP for three different drug-binding kinetics ($k_{off} = k_{on} = 0.01$, 3, and 100 s^{-1}).

are more sensitive to changes in G_{Kur}, APD_{40} is similarly sensitive in nSR and cAF (**Figure 1C**). At 3-Hz pacing, G_{Kur} impacts AP and ERP prolongation more in cAF vs. nSR despite the fact that G_{Kur} is smaller in cAF conditions. This points to I_{Kur} inhibition as a promising approach to counteract the abbreviated APD and ERP in cAF, while having a more moderate effect at physiological pacing rates. Therefore, we next ran simulations to reveal I_{Kur}-targeting drug properties that exhibit anti-AF selectivity and efficacy along with minimized proarrhythmic risk in cAF.

Effect of Conformational State Specificity and Binding/Unbinding Kinetics on Human Atrial Cardiomyocyte APD at Normal and Fast Pacing Rates in cAF Conditions

Figure 2 shows changes in APD caused by O and O & I inhibitors at varying drug-binding kinetics, whereby k_{on} is set equal to k_{off} (i.e., $K_d = 1\ \mu M$). These are compared to no block, 50, and 100% reduction in G_{Kur} in cAF conditions, as well as no block in nSR conditions. Similar to our findings in nSR (Ellinwood et al., 2017), both types of inhibitors display a biphasic relationship between APD and drug-binding kinetics at 1- and 3-Hz pacing. At 1-Hz pacing, APD in the presence of drug is comparable to a 50% reduction in G_{Kur} at slow and fast drug-binding kinetics (**Figures 2B,G**). Significant APD prolongation is only seen for intermediate drug-binding kinetics (0.3–30 s^{-1} for the open state blocker and 1–30 s^{-1} for the open and inactivated state blocker), and goes well beyond the little APD prolongation resulting from a constant 50% reduction in G_{Kur}. However, even the maximal APD prolongation produced by an O or O & I inhibitor in cAF is still ~50 ms less than the APD in nSR in drug-free conditions, which we interpret to suggest that such drugs would have limited toxicity at 1-Hz pacing rate.

At 3-Hz pacing, the two types of inhibitors cause stronger relative prolongation as compared to 1-Hz pacing across the same range of drug-binding kinetics (**Figures 2D,I**). Notably, all simulated drugs caused APD prolongation at 3-Hz pacing, but the maximal prolongation produced by these theoretical inhibitors did not match the APD prolongation caused by a 100% reduction in G_{Kur}. However, drugs with intermediate drug-binding kinetics (3–30 s^{-1} for the O blocker and 10–30 s^{-1} for the O & I blocker) did extend the APD at 3-Hz pacing above the APD in nSR conditions given no block of I_{Kur}. Thus, even though G_{Kur} is reduced by 50% in cAF as compared to nSR, **Figure 2** illustrates that I_{Kur} inhibitors can still prolong APD in cAF, particularly at 3-Hz pacing.

Figures 2C,II,E,J display the closed (red), open (blue), inactivated (green), and drug-bound (gray) state occupancies during the steady-state AP for the slowest (0.01 s^{-1}), intermediate (3 s^{-1}), and fastest (100 s^{-1}) drug-binding rates. In general, for the slowest drug-binding kinetics, the inhibitors do not bind readily during the AP, and the drug-bound state stays level below 0.4. At intermediate drug-binding kinetics, the inhibitors bind readily during the AP, thus significantly shrinking the open state occupancy. In addition, the off-rate of drug binding is slow enough to achieve maintenance in the drug-bound state during the AP. This allows for considerable AP prolongation, almost mimicking complete block of I_{Kur}. Finally, for the fastest drug-binding kinetics, the drugs again bind readily during the AP, but the off-rate of drug binding is so fast as to cause cycling between the drug-free open state and the drug-bound open state during a single AP. This results in prolongation of the drug-free open state occupancy later in the AP that limits AP prolongation. These results are consistent with our previous simulations in nSR. However, given the more positive plateau in the cAF cardiomyocyte AP, $K_V1.5$ channels stay open longer, and inactivate more markedly (especially at 3-Hz pacing) as compared to nSR (Figure S7).

Given not only the rapid, but irregular electrical activity seen with AF, we sought to determine how the kinetics of drug binding of I_{Kur} inhibitors affected the time course of E_m (**Figure 3B**) and APD_{90} (**Figure 3C**) in cAF cardiomyocytes with a randomly variable CL (**Figure 3A**). Results in drug-free conditions and for an O & I blocker (modeled as in **Figure 2F**, black) with $k_{on} = k_{off}$ ($K_d = 1\ \mu M$) in **Figure 3** again demonstrate a biphasic relationship between drug-binding kinetics and average APD_{90} (**Figure 3D**), as seen with constant pacing (**Figure 2I**). Thus, for all future simulations, we used a constant pacing interval that can more easily be standardized in a high-throughput drug-screening process.

Effect of Conformational State Specificity and Binding/Unbinding Kinetics on Human Atrial Cardiomyocyte ERP at Normal and Fast Pacing Rates in cAF Conditions

The desired effect of I_{Kur} inhibitors is prolongation of atrial ERP (Amos et al., 1996; Christ et al., 2008; Sanchez et al., 2012; Loose et al., 2014; Ford et al., 2016), particularly during fast pacing rates typifying AF. Thus, we assessed the effects of binding/unbinding kinetics on the ERP for O (**Figures 4A,B**) and O & I (**Figures 4C,D**) blockers. Simulations reveal a similar biphasic relationship between ERP and drug-binding kinetics at 1- and 3-Hz pacing for both types of inhibitors, which mirror the drugs' effects on APD (**Figure 2**).

At 1-Hz pacing, I_{Kur} inhibitors cause minimal ERP prolongation at slow drug-binding rates ($\leq$0.3 s^{-1} for O blockers and $\leq$1 s^{-1} for O & I blockers) and fast drug-binding rates (100 s^{-1}). Although substantial ERP changes are predicted at intermediate drug-binding rates (1–30 s^{-1} for O blockers and 3–30 s^{-1} for O & I blockers), ERP prolongation remains ~62 ms lower than the ERP in nSR given no block of I_{Kur} for both inhibitors.

At 3-Hz pacing, however, I_{Kur} inhibitors appear to be more effective at extending ERP than APD, which is a favorable drug property as previously demonstrated for Class I antiarrhythmic drugs which cause clinically relevant post-repolarization refractoriness. For all drug-binding kinetics, ERP prolongation is at least equivalent to that caused by a constant 50% reduction in G_{Kur} (**Figures 4B,D**). Notably, for intermediate drug-binding kinetics (3–30 s^{-1} for O inhibitors and 10–30 s^{-1} for O & I inhibitors), drug-induced ERP prolongation extends above the ERP in nSR in drug-free conditions, and the fastest drug-binding kinetics prolong the ERP to a point that closely

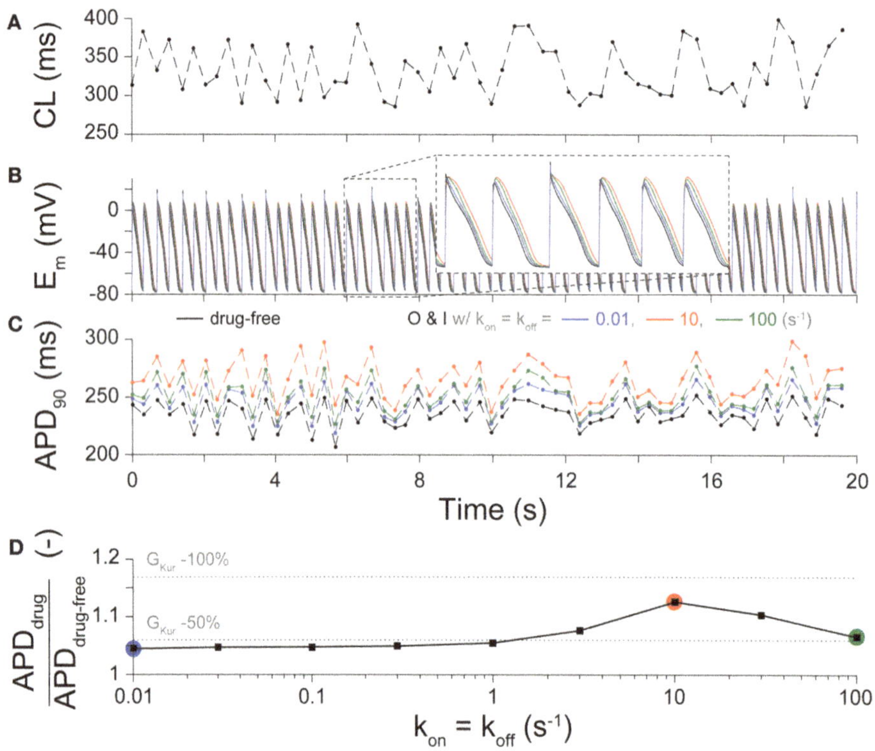

FIGURE 3 | Effect of drug-binding kinetics on APD during irregular pacing. **(A)** Beat-to-beat changes in CL during a 20-s irregular pacing protocol and the resultant time-course of **(B)** E_m, and **(C)** APD_{90} are shown in cAF cardiomyocytes in drug-free conditions (black), and for O & I blockers with slow (0.01 s^{-1}, blue), intermediate (10 s^{-1}, red), and fast (100 s^{-1}, green) drug-binding kinetics, given $k_{on} = k_{off}$. **(D)** summarizes the percent prolongation (mean APD_{90} after application of drug divided by mean APD_{90} in drug-free conditions during the simulation) for nine different rates of binding kinetics between 0.01 and 100 s^{-1} using half-logarithmic increments, whereby $k_{on} = k_{off}$, $K_d = 1\ \mu M$. These results are compared to 50, and 100% reduction in G_{Kur} (dotted lines) given the same irregular pacing protocol in **(A)**.

resembles that in nSR in drug-free conditions. These drugs showing substantial ERP prolongation at 3-Hz pacing in cAF (with APD at slow pacing rates being well below that in nSR, see **Figure 2**) might represent suitable compounds for AF-selective therapy.

Effects of Drug Binding/Unbinding Kinetics with Variable K_d on APD, ERP, and Ca^{2+} Handling

Figures 2, **3**, **4** show the results from drug scenarios where the on- and off-rate of drug binding are equal to one another ($k_{on} = k_{off}$, $K_d = 1\ \mu M$), but even closely related I_{Kur} inhibitors can have dissimilar K_d values (Lagrutta et al., 2006). Thus, we simulated all permutations of the nine different rates of drug binding (0.01 to 100 s^{-1}), yielding 81 different combinations of k_{on} and k_{off} for the O & I state inhibitors (assuming equal affinities for open and inactivated states) at 1- and 3-Hz pacing. We assessed the effects of these drugs (at their IC_{50} concentration) on APD, ERP, CaT_{amp}, and diastolic $[Ca^{2+}]_i$. **Figure 5** shows the output of the simulations for an O & I inhibitor (modeled as in **Figure 2F**, black) in the form of a heatmap, where the diagonals of the squares from the bottom left to the top right corner correspond to drug scenarios where $k_{on} = k_{off}$ ($K_d = 1\ \mu M$). Except for the drugs with the largest K_d values ($k_{off} >> k_{on}$), when k_{on} is held constant, APD, ERP, and Ca^{2+} handling are not very sensitive to changes in k_{off}. Thus, the effects of I_{Kur} inhibitors on atrial electrophysiology and Ca^{2+} handling are largely driven by k_{on} rates as compared to k_{off} rates.

In cAF conditions, ideal I_{Kur} inhibitors exhibiting AF-selectivity will prolong atrial refractoriness (ERP prolongation at 3-Hz pacing), have limited toxicity (minimal to no APD prolongation at 1-Hz pacing), and have a positive inotropic effect (an increase in CaT_{amp} at 1-Hz pacing). O & I inhibitors with a large K_d do not display any of the desired favorable drug properties including prolongation of ERP at 3-Hz pacing (**Figure 5B**) or increase in CaT_{amp} (**Figures 5C,D**), as their effects on APD, ERP, and Ca^{2+} handling are minimal, resembling drug-free conditions. Intermediate k_{on} rates (3–30 s^{-1} for 1-Hz pacing and 10–30 s^{-1} for 3-Hz pacing) cause the most significant increase in all the outputs displayed in **Figure 5**. For example, drugs with a k_{on} rate equal to 10 s^{-1} cause the greatest ERP prolongation at 3-Hz pacing (**Figure 5B**) and increase in CaT_{amp} and diastolic $[Ca^{2+}]_i$ (**Figures 5C,E**). Note, there is also significant APD prolongation at 1-Hz pacing when k_{on} is in the intermediate drug-binding range (**Figure 5A**), but none of the 81 permutations of the simulated open and inactivated state inhibitor cause the APD to get close to the APD in nSR at 1-Hz

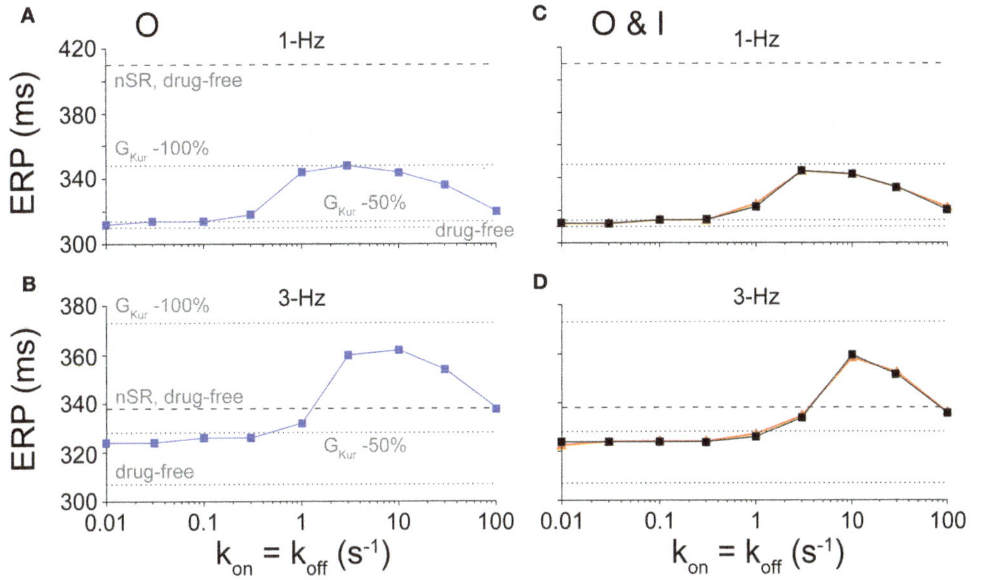

FIGURE 4 | Effect of state-dependence and kinetics of drug binding on ERP. ERP was determined for open (**A**, 1-Hz and **B**, 3-Hz pacing rate) and open and inactivated (**C**, 1-Hz and **D**, 3-Hz pacing rate) state blockers given nine different rates of binding kinetics between 0.01 and 100 s^{-1} using half-logarithmic increments, whereby $k_{off} = k_{on}$, $K_d = 1\ \mu M$. For O & I blockers, we either allowed or prevented transitions between drug-bound states (orange vs. black traces in **C,D**). Simulations were also run in nSR and cAF drug-free conditions, and in cAF given a 50 and 100% reduction in G_{Kur}.

pacing (320 ms). Thus, the APD prolongation seen in **Figure 5A** does not necessarily disqualify any of these theoretical drug candidates for AF therapy. Likewise, at 3-Hz pacing, the increase in CaT_{amp} and diastolic $[Ca^{2+}]_i$ mirrors the prolongation in APD and ERP at 3-Hz pacing (**Figures 5D,F**). While an excessive increase in diastolic $[Ca^{2+}]_i$ might be deleterious, we find it to remain well below the predicted value in the nSR human atrial cardiomyocyte model (~360 nM).

In our previous study in nSR (Ellinwood et al., 2017), we found that O & I inhibitors with the fastest drug-binding kinetics (30–100 s^{-1}) cause ERP prolongation at 3-Hz pacing and no APD prolongation at 1-Hz pacing. These same inhibitors display favorable fast pacing-rate selectivity in atrial cardiomyocytes from cAF according to our simulations shown in **Figures 5A,B**. However, if we are not as concerned with APD prolongation in cAF conditions at 1-Hz pacing, then drugs with a k_{on} rate in the intermediate drug-binding range (3–30 s^{-1}) would also be efficacious and perhaps more efficacious since they cause a positive inotropic effect at 1-Hz pacing (**Figures 5C,E**).

Effect of Relative State-Specific Drug Binding

Because many I_{Kur} inhibitors bind to multiple states of $K_V1.5$ with variable affinity (Bouchard and Fedida, 1995; Lagrutta et al., 2006; Ford et al., 2016), we allowed k_{on} for the open state ($k_{on,O}$), k_{off} for the open state ($k_{off,O}$), k_{on} for the inactivated state ($k_{on,I}$), and k_{off} for the inactivated state ($k_{off,I}$) to have any of the three binding rates (0.01, 3, and 100 s^{-1}), and varied them independently to yield 81 different drug combinations. We studied the effects of these I_{Kur} blockers in cAF conditions using a [drug] equal to their IC_{50} value at 1-Hz pacing for APD and 3-Hz pacing for ERP. Then, we compared the outputs of APD and ERP to no block, 50, and 100% reduction in G_{Kur} in cAF conditions (**Figure 6**, dotted lines), along with no block in nSR conditions (**Figure 6**, dashed lines).

Figures 6A,B display the relationship between APD (at 1-Hz pacing) and K_O/K_I. Data points in **Figure 6A** are separated by IC_{50} cutoffs of 0.1 μM, 10 μM, and 1 mM, and show that when $K_O/K_I < 1$, we almost always obtain maximal AP prolongation (this also corresponds to larger IC_{50} values). In **Figure 6B**, we separated the points according to the drug's $k_{off,O}$ rate (0.01, 3, or 100 s^{-1}), which revealed that when $K_O/K_I > 1$, we only obtain significant AP prolongation when $k_{off,O}$ is equal to 3 s^{-1} (i.e., the intermediate drug-binding rate). These results in the cAF-remodeled atrial cardiomyocyte correspond well with the results from our previous study of I_{Kur} inhibitors in nSR (Ellinwood et al., 2017). Nevertheless, none of the 81 simulated O & I inhibitors in **Figure 6** prolong the AP beyond the APD found in nSR at 1-Hz pacing.

Figures 6C,D present the relationship between APD at 1-Hz pacing and ERP at 3-Hz pacing for the O & I inhibitors with a variable K_O/K_I ratio. In **Figure 6C**, light gray symbols correspond to $K_O/K_I \leq 1$, and dark symbols correspond to $K_O/K_I > 1$). The O & I blockers displaying favorable pacing-rate selectivity, i.e., producing ERP prolongation at 3-Hz pacing while having moderate effect on APD (and ERP) at 1-Hz pacing, are the ones with $K_O/K_I > 1$, except if $k_{off,O}$ equals 3 s^{-1}. However, as none of the 81 simulated O & I inhibitors in **Figure 6** prolong the APD beyond that found in nSR at 1-Hz pacing, one could argue that none of the drugs is expected to cause harmful AP prolongation when AF is terminated. To try and enrich our metric, in **Figure 6D** we also categorize the drugs according to

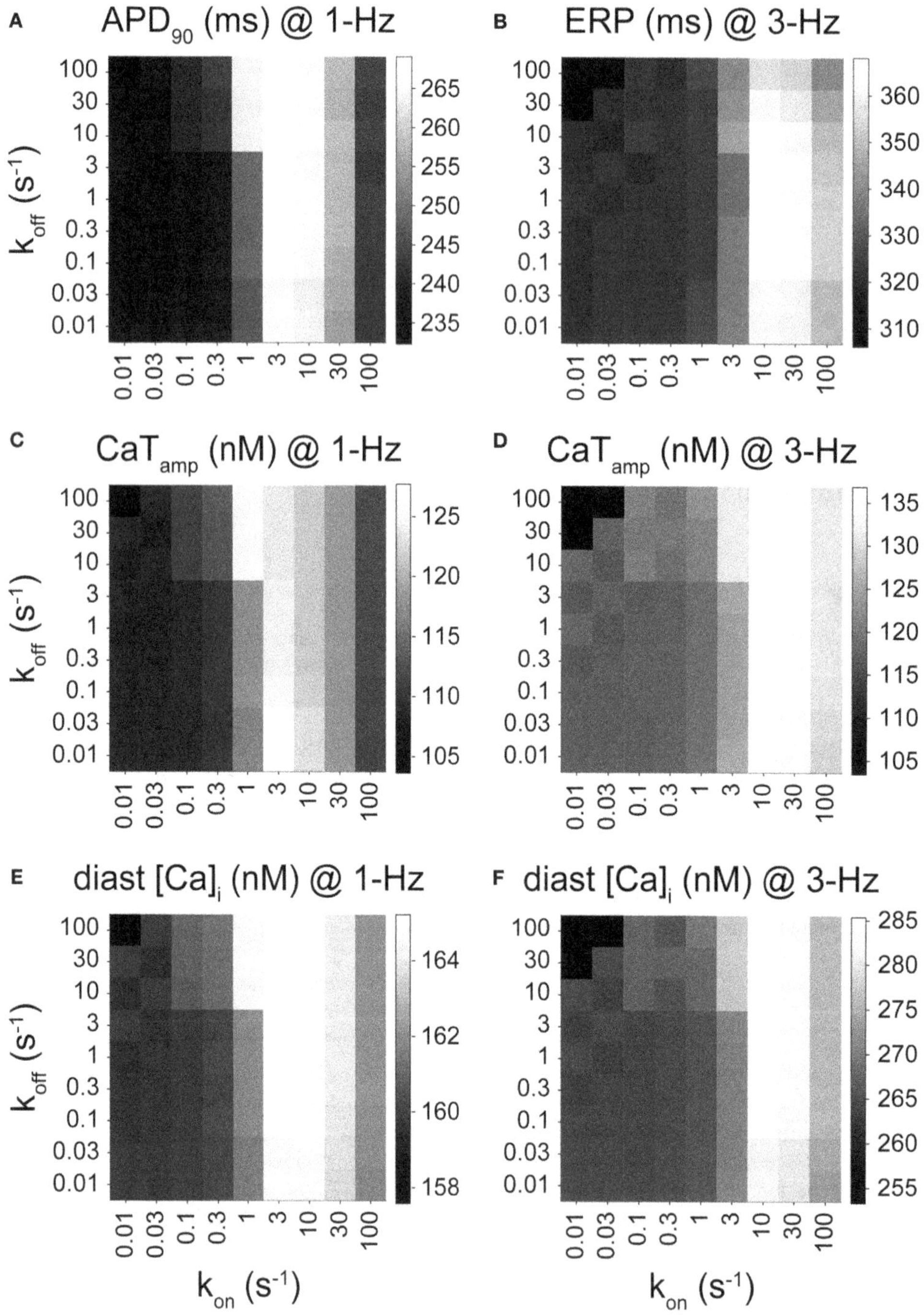

FIGURE 5 | Effect of drug-binding kinetics on APD_{90}, ERP, CaT_{amp}, and diastolic $[Ca^{2+}]_i$ for an open and inactivated state blocker. **(A)** APD_{90} (at 1 Hz), **(B)** ERP (at 3 Hz), **(C,D)** CaT_{amp} (at 1 and 3 Hz), and **(E,F)** diastolic $[Ca^{2+}]_i$ (at 1 and 3 Hz) are plotted for open and inactivated state blockers with varying binding kinetics, which were simulated via permutations of nine different drug-binding rates of (from 0.01 to 100 s^{-1}) while keeping $k_{on,O} = k_{on,I}$ and $k_{off,O} = k_{off,I}$. CaT_{amp} is 103.6, 109.4, and 120.4 nM at 1 Hz, and 103.4, 120.4, and 135.9 nM at 3 Hz for drug-free, 50 and 100% I_{Kur} block, respectively. Diastolic $[Ca^{2+}]_i$ is 157.6, 160.0, and 165.2 nM at 1 Hz, and 253.3, 266.9, and 286.9 nM at 3 Hz for drug-free, 50 and 100% I_{Kur} block, respectively.

percent increase in CaT_{amp}. The best-performing drugs will cause ERP prolongation at 3-Hz pacing in cAF (above nSR), and have a positive inotropic effect (**Figure 6D**, black). Corresponding with the results showcased in **Figure 5**, drugs with intermediate binding rates (e.g., $k_{off,O} = 3\ s^{-1}$) may thus be favorable given their stronger inotropic effect.

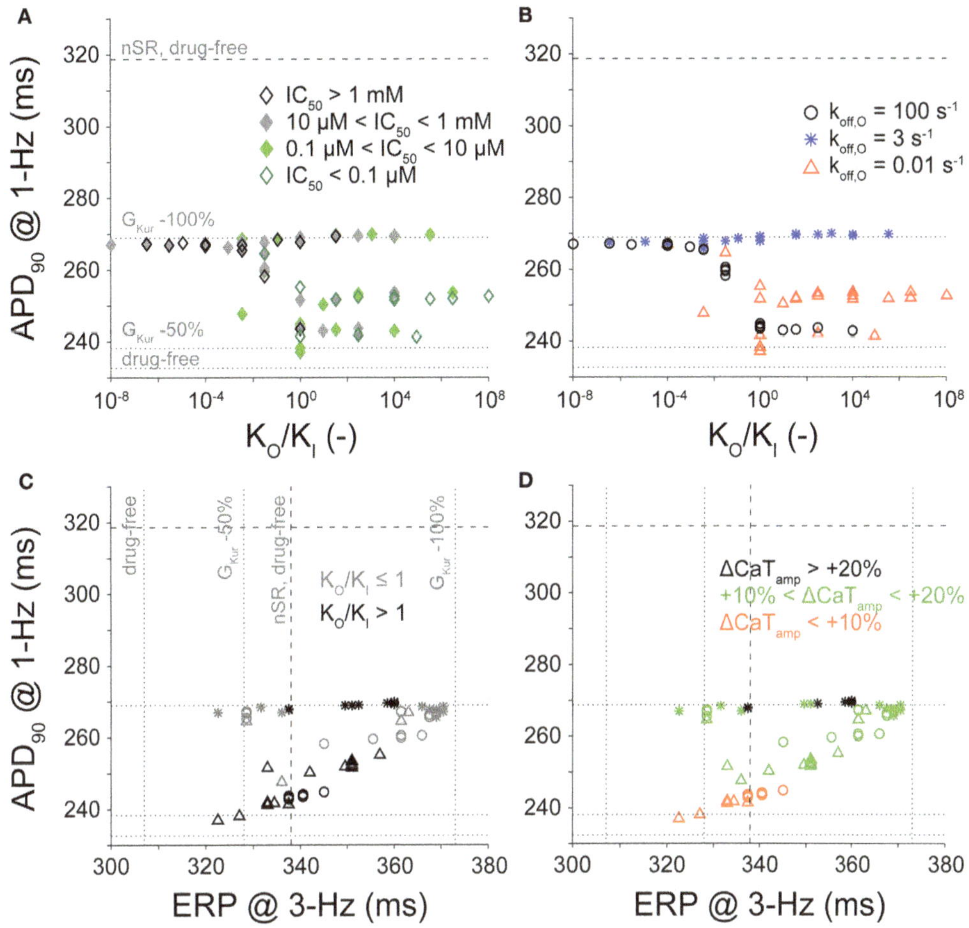

FIGURE 6 | Effect of conformational state affinity and drug-binding kinetics of an open and inactivated state blocker on APD_{90}, ERP, and Ca^{2+} handling. Open and inactivated state I_{Kur} blockers with varying affinities to the open and inactivated states were simulated via permutations of three different rates of binding kinetics (0.01, 3, and 100 s^{-1}). Simulations were equilibrated for 300 beats at 1-Hz pacing or 900 beats at 3-Hz pacing using a [drug] equal to the IC_{50} value. **(A,B)** report APD_{90} values (at 1 Hz) plotted as a function of the ratio of the open to the inactivated state affinity (K_O/K_I) used in each simulation. **(C,D)** report APD_{90} (at 1 Hz) and ERP values (at 3 Hz). Color code in **(A)** is for IC_{50} levels. Symbols in **(B,C,D)** indicate various $k_{off,O}$. Shades in **(C)** reflect either higher affinity to the open or the inactivated state. Color code in **(D)** corresponds to the variable degree of CaT_{amp} increase (at 1 Hz) induced by I_{Kur} block. Horizontal and vertical lines represent APD_{90} and ERP values obtained in cAF in drug-free conditions, and 50 and 100% reduction in G_{Kur} (dotted lines), and in nSR in drug-free conditions (dashed lines).

DISCUSSION

In this study, we sought to determine if I_{Kur} is a suitable anti-AF target despite it being downregulated in cAF patients, and, if so, what are the kinetic and state-dependent binding properties that maximize anti-AF efficacy and limit potential cardiotoxicity. Building off our previous study in nSR conditions (Ellinwood et al., 2017), we implemented an *in silico* assessment of I_{Kur} inhibitors in cAF atrial cardiomyocyte models, and identified metrics for delineating ideal $K_V1.5$ blockers against AF. Our results point to I_{Kur} inhibition as a valid strategy to prolong atrial refractoriness also generating a positive inotropic effect in cAF conditions. Although increasing force generation may not be a useful therapeutic goal at the high atrial rates seen during AF, it can be important to counteract atrial hypocontractility after cardioversion of AF to nSR. Interestingly, our simulations suggest that electrophysiological properties in cAF cardiomyocytes, such as shorter AP and more depolarized plateau potential, both might act to increase efficacy and dampen cardiotoxicity of potential $K_V1.5$-targeting drugs as compared to nSR (Ellinwood et al., 2017; **Figure 7**).

I_{Kur} Role in APD and ERP Regulation Is Preserved Despite Its Downregulation in cAF

Figure S7 shows the differences in the time courses of E_m, I_{Kur}, and closed, open, and inactivated state occupancies of $K_V1.5$ in cAF and nSR during the AP. Despite the reduced peak current, the channel stays open later in cAF (at both 1- and 3-Hz pacing) because of the more depolarized AP plateau. Thus, the consequences of I_{Kur} inhibition, including the extent of AP

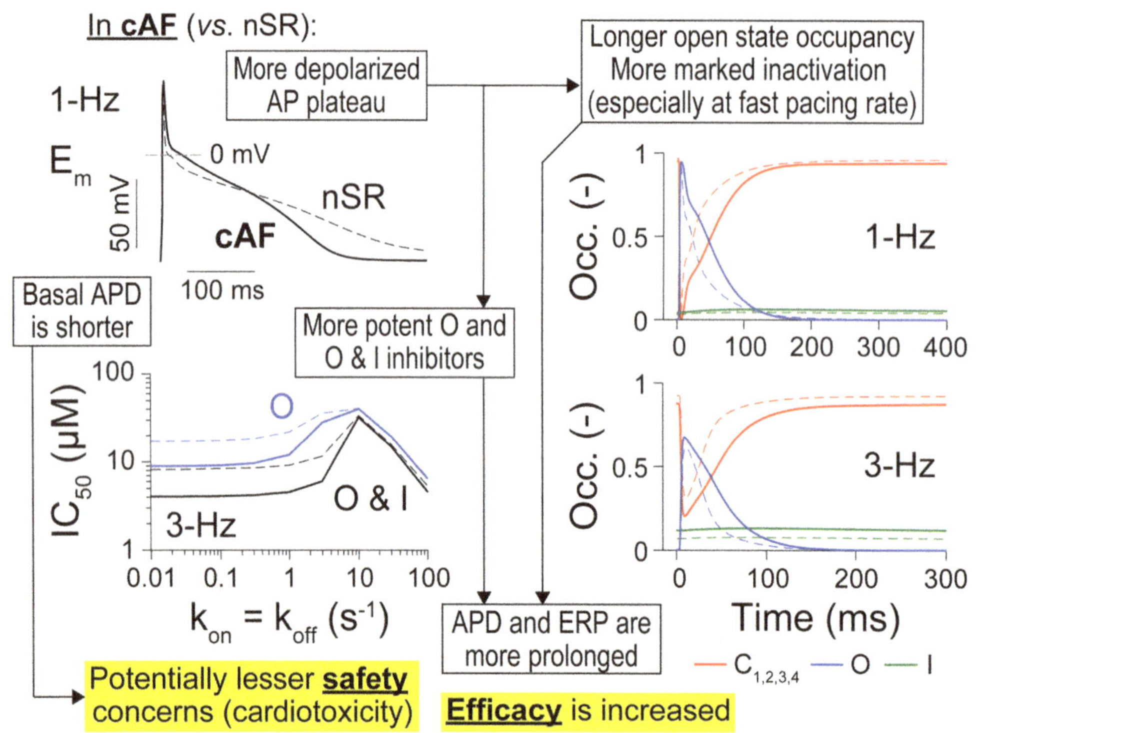

FIGURE 7 | Summary of main findings. Atrial cardiomyocytes in cAF (solid lines) vs. nSR (dotted lines) have different AP trajectories, including a shorter APD and more depolarized plateau (top left). The latter causes longer open state occupancy (right, blue solid vs. dashed lines) and stronger inactivation of the channel in cAF conditions (especially at fast pacing rates, right, green solid vs. dashed lines). I_{Kur} inhibitors appear also more potent in cAF vs. nSR (bottom left). These factors render APD and ERP more sensitive to inhibition by O and O & I inhibitors of $K_V1.5$, thus increasing efficacy of these drugs in cAF vs. nSR. Because basal APD is shorter in cAF, there are potentially less safety concerns due to drug-induced AP prolongation and subsequent afterdepolarization-driven proarrhythmia.

and ERP prolongation, depend not only on I_{Kur} magnitude (i.e., maximal conductance), but also on other fluxes affected by AF-induced remodeling, which affect E_m and thus E_m-dependent properties of I_{Kur} (**Figure 7**). For example, our group and others have hypothesized that the extent of AP and ERP prolongation due to I_{Kur} blockade depends on the AF-induced remodeling of other K^+ currents (Lagrutta et al., 2006; Morotti et al., 2016a; Aguilar et al., 2017; Colman et al., 2017), and relative strengths of I_{CaL} and I_{Kur} (Wettwer et al., 2004; Grandi and Maleckar, 2016). Our sensitivity analysis (**Figure 1C** and Figures S1–S6) revealed that APD_{90} and ERP are more sensitive to changes in G_{Kur} at fast vs. slow pacing rates. Aguilar et al. recently determined that the relative contribution of I_{Kur} to AP repolarization increases at higher frequencies because of reduced activation of the rapid delayed-rectifier current I_{Kr} (Aguilar et al., 2017). Our results concur with these findings, as our sensitivity analysis shows that APD_{90} and ERP are less sensitive to changes in G_{Kr} at 3-Hz pacing as compared to 1-Hz pacing in nSR conditions (Figures S2, S3). Most importantly, we also found that G_{Kur} impacted the duration of AP repolarization and refractoriness more in cAF vs. nSR (even though this parameter was halved in the cAF model) at 3-Hz, but not at 1-Hz pacing (i.e., fast pacing-rate selectivity). This is a favorable drug property to avoid harmful AP prolongation (which is also limited by the reduced basal APD) if AF is terminated. Similar to Aguilar et al. (2017), our results suggest that the APD- (and ERP)-prolonging effect of I_{Kur} block is not affected by I_{Kur} downregulation.

Enhanced Efficacy and Safety of I_{Kur} Inhibitors in cAF vs. nSR

We focused here on O and O & I blockers because we have previously shown that these inhibitors display fast pacing-rate selectivity in nSR (Ellinwood et al., 2017). This choice was also supported by the increased occupancy of open and inactivated states in cAF conditions (**Figure 7**). In our previous report in nSR (Ellinwood et al., 2017), we found that when $k_{on} = k_{off}$ (i) slow drug-binding kinetics caused minimal APD changes and modest ERP prolongation; (ii) intermediate drug-binding kinetics led to substantial AP and ERP prolongation; and (iii) fast drug-binding kinetics failed to produce substantial AP or ERP prolongation at normal pacing rate, but increased the ERP at 3-Hz pacing. While in cAF the overall biphasic relationship between APD/ERP and drug-binding kinetics was maintained (see **Figures 2–4**), notably, at 1-Hz pacing rate, even the maximal AP prolongation induced by I_{Kur} inhibition in cAF is not sufficient to reach the APD observed in nSR in drug-free conditions. This might indicate that there are less safety concerns for $K_V1.5$ block in cAF patients. At 3-Hz pacing, ERP prolongation is at least equivalent to that caused by a constant 50% reduction in G_{Kur}, and, for intermediate and fast drug-binding kinetics, the ERP is equal to or greater than the one obtained in nSR in drug-free conditions. These observations suggest that O and O & I inhibitors have a broader range of efficacy in cAF vs. nSR. We assessed whether closed state inhibitors, which displayed reverse-rate dependence in terms of potency (Ellinwood et al., 2017), may also be effective and safe anti-AF agents in cAF conditions (Figure S8). We found that these blockers prolong ERP at 3-Hz pacing (Figure S8G) while minimally prolonging the cAF AP at 1-Hz pacing at the fastest drug-binding kinetics ($\geq$30 s^{-1}, Figure S8B). However, they had a smaller maximal effect and kinetic range for prolonging the ERP at 3-Hz pacing beyond nSR conditions as compared to O and O & I blockers.

We enriched our metric for quantifying anti-AF efficacy and safety of I_{Kur} inhibitors by also accounting for changes in Ca^{2+}-handling parameters, namely CaT_{amp} and diastolic $[Ca^{2+}]_i$ (Tsujimae et al., 2008; Cavero and Holzgrefe, 2014; Lancaster and Sobie, 2016; Li et al., 2017), which provided additional detail to refine the search for best-performing drugs. In identifying the ideal drug characteristics, we looked for inhibitors that prolong ERP (especially at fast pacing rates), limit APD prolongation at slow pacing-rates, and improve atrial inotropy, i.e., increase CaT_{amp}. Increasing force generation might be a useful outcome after cardioversion to nSR.

When $K_O = K_I$, the best-performing O & I inhibitors were those with intermediate k_{on} rates (3–30 s^{-1}), because they prolonged ERP at 3-Hz pacing and increased CaT_{amp} and diastolic $[Ca^{2+}]_i$ at 1-Hz pacing (**Figure 5**). These inhibitors also prolonged the AP at 1-Hz pacing and increased CaT_{amp} and diastolic $[Ca^{2+}]_i$ at 3-Hz pacing—thus potentially predisposing to harmful AP prolongation and Ca^{2+} overload. However, we note that such cardiotoxicity is unlikely considering the fact that the maximum increases of APD and CaT_{amp} still remain far below the corresponding values obtained in nSR in drug-free conditions. In our previous study, we highlighted that the best-performing drugs in nSR were the O & I inhibitors with the fastest drug-binding kinetics (Ellinwood et al., 2017). While these drugs are still efficacious at prolonging ERP at 3-Hz pacing in cAF, they have limited effect on Ca^{2+} handling.

When K_I and K_O were varied, the relationships between APD at 1-Hz pacing and affinity ratio (K_O/K_I) are similar to those in nSR (**Figures 6A,B**; Ellinwood et al., 2017), except none of the 81 simulated O & I inhibitors prolonged the AP beyond the duration found in nSR in drug-free condition. Likewise, the relationship between APD at 1-Hz pacing and ERP at 3-Hz pacing is similar to nSR (**Figures 6C,D**; Ellinwood et al., 2017), but none of the drugs exhibit obvious toxicity. The same O & I inhibitors simulated in cAF conditions were more effective at prolonging ERP at 3-Hz pacing rates as compared to nSR conditions. Thus, on average, the same inhibitors in **Figure 6** exhibit less toxicity and greater efficacy in cAF vs. nSR.

In their simulation study, Aguilar et al. concluded that the ability of (simple pore) I_{Kur} block to terminate simulated AF was greatly attenuated by remodeling, because the block-induced AP prolongation was insufficient to counteract the strong effects of cAF-induced remodeling (Aguilar et al., 2017). Notably, here we show that depending on the drug-binding kinetics, certain I_{Kur} inhibitors can markedly counteract the effect of cAF-associated remodeling, and bring AP and ERP parameters close to nSR values, i.e., have a greater effect than simple pore blockers.

Limitations and Future Directions

We presented a theoretical study of the effects of I_{Kur} inhibitors in cAF, and compared our results to our previous study in nSR atrial cardiomyocytes. We acknowledge several limitations to the described approach, which provide opportunities for further extensions. First, we only considered direct drug effects on $K_V1.5$, and future analysis should consider multi-channel effects of I_{Kur} inhibitors (Ford and Milnes, 2008; Li et al., 2017), as this realistically occurs *in vivo* in the clinical setting. We only considered cardiotoxicity at the atrial level, assuming that the absence of I_{Kur} in ventricles prevents ventricular proarrhythmia. However, this might not be true for real I_{Kur} blockers with off-target effects. Here, we simulated I_{Kur} block at the cellular level with no contribution of structural tissue remodeling and defined I_{Kur} inhibitors' efficacy and toxicity by tracking only electrophysiological properties such as APD, ERP, CaT_{amp}, and diastolic $[Ca^{2+}]_i$. While this is an important first step in defining metrics for AF-selectivity, other arrhythmia indices and integration of such simulations into tissue and organ level models would improve our ability to discern best-performing drug characteristics of I_{Kur} inhibitors against AF. Since many antiarrhythmic drugs lose anti-AF efficacy with the progression of the arrhythmia, particularly in patients with atrial cardiomyopathy and comorbidities (Goette et al., 2016), I_{Kur} block might be less efficient against AF in the structurally remodeled atrium. Further studies including 2- and 3-dimensional tissue simulations are needed to address this clinically relevant issue. In addition, machine-learning methods have begun to be implemented to analyze AP metrics after the application of a drug and classify the risk (e.g., torsadogenic risk) of the candidate drug (Lancaster and Sobie, 2016). Such methods can also highlight which ion channels contribute most to such risk. Furthermore, this study revealed that the efficacy and toxicity of I_{Kur} inhibitors is modulated by the extent of atrial ionic remodeling, and likely by the relative expressions of many ion channels and transporters (Figures S1–S6). Thus, given the differences in AP properties and ion channel expression in patients with AF (Heijman et al., 2014), and differences in I_{Kur} remodeling in the right vs. the left atria (Dobrev and Ravens, 2003; Caballero et al., 2010), we hypothesize that certain subpopulations of nSR and cAF patients may be more responsive to therapy with I_{Kur} inhibitors, i.e., degree and heterogeneity of I_{Kur} remodeling in atrial tissue might impact safety and anti-AF efficacy of drugs. Future studies could identify which cell characteristics lead to more favorable responses to anti-I_{Kur} therapy utilizing sensitivity analysis and variations of nSR and cAF models similar to the methods discussed in **Figure 1** and in (Sobie, 2009; Lee et al., 2013; Cummins et al., 2014; Devenyi and Sobie, 2015; Morotti and Grandi, 2017). This information could be useful for a personalized (precision) medicine approach to AF treatment or helpful in suggesting potential combination therapies with I_{Kur} inhibitors.

Finally, advancements in high-throughput screening methods (Obergrussberger et al., 2016; Picones et al., 2016; Molokanova et al., 2017) provide functional drug screening capabilities that can be coupled with *in silico* investigations such as the one described here to help identify actual candidate compounds for *in vivo* testing. Such technologies can potentially be implemented to simultaneously screen many $K_V1.5$-selective compounds for the desired kinetics, state-dependence, and rate-dependence of I_{Kur} block. In addition, multi-parallel recordings from atrial-like cardiomyocytes from induced human pluripotent stem cells is also emerging as a preclinical model for evaluating drugs targeting atrial-specific ion channels, such as $K_V1.5$ (Devalla et al., 2015), particularly in combination with AP-clamp experiments. These could be coupled with *in silico* studies such as this one for delineating the ideal properties of AF-selective drugs and gaining a more comprehensive understanding of the arrhythmic risk of candidate compounds.

CONCLUSIONS

In this study, efficacy and cardiotoxicity on cAF atrial cardiomyocytes of theoretical I_{Kur} inhibitors were assessed *in silico*. We concluded that I_{Kur} is a promising anti-AF target, even if strongly downregulated in cAF condition. We confirmed that steady-state IC_{50} values are insufficient to predict how candidate compounds will interact with a dynamically changing electrophysiological substrate, thus emphasizing the importance of accounting for kinetic and state-dependent drug-binding properties. This approach could aid experimental and screening efforts to identify the complex net impact of I_{Kur} inhibition in different AF-remodeling conditions during the pre-clinical drug development process.

AUTHOR CONTRIBUTIONS

Designed simulation experiments: NE, SM, EG. Performed modeling and simulations: NE, SM. Wrote the manuscript: NE, DD, SM, EG.

ACKNOWLEDGMENTS

The authors would like to thank Dr. Lucía Romero Pérez, Polytechnic University of Valencia, for her critical reading of this manuscript. This work was supported by the National Institute of Health grant R01-HL131517 (to EG and DD), the American Heart Association grant 15SDG24910015 (EG), the Heart Rhythm Society post-doctoral fellowship 16OA9HRS (SM), the Bill Bertken Sudden Death Prevention Fund, and the National Center for Advancing Translational Sciences, National Institutes of Health, through grant number UL1 TR001860 and linked award TL1 TR001861 (NE).

REFERENCES

Aguilar, M., Feng, J., Vigmond, E., Comtois, P., and Nattel, S. (2017). Rate-dependent role of I_{Kur} in human atrial repolarization and atrial fibrillation maintenance. *Biophys. J.* 112, 1997–2010. doi: 10.1016/j.bpj.2017.03.022

Amos, G. J., Wettwer, E., Metzger, F., Li, Q., Himmel, H. M., and Ravens, U. (1996). Differences between outward currents of human atrial, and subepicardial ventricular myocytes. *J. Physiol.* 491, 31–50. doi: 10.1113/jphysiol.1996.sp021194

Andrade, J., Khairy, P., Dobrev, D., and Nattel, S. (2014). The clinical profile and pathophysiology of atrial fibrillation: relationships among clinical features, epidemiology, and mechanisms. *Circ. Res.* 114, 1453–1468. doi: 10.1161/CIRCRESAHA.114.303211

Bers, D. M., and Grandi, E. (2011). Human atrial fibrillation: insights from computational electrophysiological models. *Trends Cardiovasc. Med.* 21, 145–150. doi: 10.1016/j.tcm.2012.04.004

Bosch, R. F., Zeng, X.,Grammer, J. B., Popovic, K., Mewis, C., and Kuhlkamp, V. (1999). Ionic mechanisms of electrical remodeling in human atrial fibrillation. *Cardiovasc. Res.* 44, 121–131. doi: 10.1016/S0008-6363(99)00178-9

Bouchard, R., and Fedida, D. (1995). Closed- and open-state binding of 4-aminopyridine to the cloned human potassium channel Kv1.5. *J. Pharmacol. Exp. Ther.* 275, 864–876.

Brandt, M. C., Priebe, L., Bohle, T., Sudkamp, M., and Beuckelmann, D. J. (2000). The ultrarapid and the transient outward K^+ current in human atrial fibrillation. Their possible role in postoperative atrial fibrillation. *J. Mol. Cell Cardiol.* 32, 1885–1896. doi: 10.1006/jmcc.2000.1221

Caballero, R., de la Fuente M. G., Gomez, R., Barana, A., Amoros, I., Dolz-Gaiton, P., et al. (2010). In humans, chronic atrial fibrillation decreases the transient outward current and ultrarapid component of the delayed rectifier current differentially on each atria and increases the slow component of the delayed rectifier current in both. *J. Am. Coll. Cardiol.* 55, 2346–2354. doi: 10.1016/j.jacc.2010.02.028

Cavero, I., and Holzgrefe, H. (2014). Comprehensive *in vitro* proarrhythmia assay, a novel *in vitro*/*in silico* paradigm to detect ventricular proarrhythmic liability: a visionary 21st century initiative. *Expert Opin. Drug Saf.* 13, 745–758. doi: 10.1517/14740338.2014.915311

Christ, T., Wettwer, E., Voigt, N., Hala, O., Radicke, S., Matschke, K., et al. (2008). Pathology-specific effects of the $I_{Kur}/I_{to}/I_{K,ACh}$ blocker AVE0118 on ion channels in human chronic atrial fibrillation. *Br. J. Pharmacol.* 154, 1619–1630. doi: 10.1038/bjp.2008.209

Christophersen, I. E., Olesen, M. S., Liang, B., Andersen, M. N., Larsen, A. P., Nielsen J. B., et al. (2013). Genetic variation in KCNA5: impact on the atrial-specific potassium current I_{Kur} in patients with lone atrial fibrillation. *Eur. Heart J.* 34, 1517–1525. doi: 10.1093/eurheartj/ehs442

Colman, M. A., Ni, H., Liang, B., Schmitt, N., and Zhang, H. (2017). *In silico* assessment of genetic variation in KCNA5 reveals multiple mechanisms of human atrial arrhythmogenesis. *PLoS Comput. Biol.* 13:e1005587. doi: 10.1371/journal.pcbi.1005587

Cummins, M. A., Dalal, P. J., Bugana, M., Severi, S., and Sobie, E. A. (2014). Comprehensive analyses of ventricular myocyte models identify targets exhibiting favorable rate dependence. *PLoS Comput. Biol.* 10:e1003543. doi: 10.1371/journal.pcbi.1003543

Devalla, H. D., Schwach, V., Ford, J. W., Milnes, J. T., El-Haou, S., Jackson C., et al. (2015). Atrial-like cardiomyocytes from human pluripotent stem cells are a robust preclinical model for assessing atrial-selective pharmacology. *EMBO Mol. Med* 7, 394–410. doi: 10.15252/emmm.201404757

Devenyi, R. A., and Sobie, E. A. (2015). There and back again: iterating between population-based modeling and experiments reveals surprising regulation of calcium transients in rat cardiac myocytes. *J. Mol. Cell Cardiol.* 96, 38–48. doi: 10.1016/j.yjmcc.2015.07.016

Dobrev, D., and Ravens, U. (2003). Remodeling of cardiomyocyte ion channels in human atrial fibrillation. *Basic Res. Cardiol.* 98, 137–148. doi: 10.1007/s00395-003-0409-8

Ehrlich, J. R., Biliczki, P., Hohnloser, S. H., and Nattel, S. (2008). Atrial-selective approaches for the treatment of atrial fibrillation. *J. Am. Coll. Cardiol.* 51, 787–792. doi: 10.1016/j.jacc.2007.08.067

Ellinwood, N., Dobrev, D., Morotti, S., and Grandi, E. (2017). Revealing kinetics and state-dependent binding properties of I_{Kur}-targeting drugs that maximize atrial fibrillation selectivity *Chaos* 27:093918. doi: 10.1063/1.5000226

Ford, J. W., and Milnes, J. T., (2008). New drugs targeting the cardiac ultra-rapid delayed-rectifier current I_{Kur}: rationale, pharmacology and evidence for potential therapeutic value. *J. Cardiovasc. Pharmacol.* 52, 105–120. doi: 10.1097/FJC.0b013e3181719b0c

Ford, J., Milnes, J., El Haou, S., Wettwer, E., Loose, S., Matschke, K., et al. (2016). The positive frequency-dependent electrophysiological effects of the I_{Kur} inhibitor XEN-D0103 are desirable for the treatment of atrial fibrillation. *Heart Rhythm* 13, 555–564. doi: 10.1016/j.hrthm.2015.10.003

Ford, J., Milnes, J., Wettwer, E., Christ, T., Rogers, M., Sutton, K., et al. (2013). Human electrophysiological and pharmacological properties of XEN-D0101: a novel atrial-selective Kv1.5/I_{Kur} inhibitor. *J. Cardiovasc. Pharmacol* 61, 408–415. doi: 10.1097/FJC.0b013e31828780eb

Goette, A., Kalman, J. M., Aguinaga, L., Akar, J., Cabrera, J. A., Chen S. A., et al. (2016). EHRA/HRS/APHRS/SOLAECE expert consensus on atrial cardiomyopathies: definition, characterization, and clinical implication. *Europace* 18, 1455–1490. doi: 10.1093/europace/euw161

Grammer, J. B., Bosch, R. F., Kuhlkamp, V., and Seipel, L. (2000). Molecular remodeling of Kv4.3 potassium channels in human atrial fibrillation. *J. Cardiovasc. Electrophysiol.* 11, 626–633. doi: 10.1111/j.1540-8167.2000.tb00024.x

Grandi, E., and Maleckar, M. M. (2016). Anti-arrhythmic strategies for atrial fibrillation: the role of computational modeling in discovery, development, and optimization. *Pharmacol. Ther.* 168, 126–142. doi: 10.1016/j.pharmthera.2016.09.012

Grandi, E., Pandit, S. V., Voigt, N., Workman, A. J., Dobrev, D., Jalife, J., et al. (2011). Human atrial action potential and Ca^{2+} model: sinus rhythm and chronic atrial fibrillation. *Circ. Res.* 109, 1055–1066. doi: 10.1161/CIRCRESAHA.111.253955

Grandi, E., Workman, A. J., and Pandit, S. V. (2012). Altered excitation-contraction coupling in human chronic atrial fibrillation. *J. Atr. Fibrillation* 4:495. doi: 10.4022/jafib.495

Heijman, J., Voigt, N., Nattel, S., and Dobrev, D. (2014). Cellular and molecular electrophysiology of atrial fibrillation initiation, maintenance, and progression. *Circ. Res.* 114, 1483–1499. doi: 10.1161/CIRCRESAHA.114.302226

Lagrutta, A., Wang, J., Fermini, B., and Salata, J. J. (2006). Novel, potent inhibitors of human Kv1.5 K^+ channels and ultrarapidly activating delayed rectifier potassium current. *J. Pharmacol. Exp. Ther.* 317, 1054–1063. doi: 10.1124/jpet.106.101162

Lancaster, M. C., and Sobie, E. A. (2016). Improved prediction of drug-induced torsades de pointes through simulations of dynamics and machine learning algorithms. *Clin. Pharmacol. Ther.* 100, 371–379. doi: 10.1002/cpt.367

Lee, W., Mann, S. A., Windley,M. J., Imtiaz, M. S., Vandenberg, J. I., and Hill, A. P. (2016). *In silico* assessment of kinetics and state dependent binding properties of drugs causing acquired LQTS. *Prog. Biophys. Mol. Biol.* 120, 89–99. doi: 10.1016/j.pbiomolbio.2015.12.005

Lee, Y. S., Liu, O. Z., Hwang, H. S., Knollmann, B. C. and Sobie, E. A. (2013). Parameter sensitivity analysis of stochastic models provides insights into cardiac calcium sparks. *Biophys. J.* 104, 1142–1150. doi: 10.1016/j.bpj.2012.12.055

Li, Z., Dutta, S., Sheng, J., Tran, P. N., Wu, W., Chang, K. et al. (2017). Improving the *In silico* assessment of proarrhythmia risk by combining hERG (human ether-a-go-go-related gene) channel-drug binding kinetics and multichannel pharmacology. *Circ. Arrhythm. Electrophysiol.* 10:e004628. doi: 10.1161/CIRCEP.116.004628

Loose, S., Mueller, J., Wettwer, E., Knaut, M., Ford, J., Milnes, J., et al. (2014). Effects of I_{Kur} blocker MK-0448 on human right atrial action potentials from patients in sinus rhythm and in permanent atrial fibrillation. *Front. Pharmacol.* 5:26. doi: 10.3389/fphar.2014.00026

Molokanova, E., Mercola, M., and Savchenko, A. (2017). Bringing new dimensions to drug discovery screening: impact of cellular stimulation technologies. *Drug Discov. Today* 22, 1045–1055. doi: 10.1016/j.drudis.2017.01.015

Morotti, S., and Grandi, E. (2017). Logistic regression analysis of populations of electrophysiological models to assess proarrythmic risk. *MethodsX* 4, 25–34. doi: 10.1016/j.mex.2016.12.002

Morotti, S., Koivumäki, J. T., Maleckar, M. M., Chiamvimonvat, N., and Grandi, E. (2016a). Small-conductance Ca^{2+}-activated K^+ current in atrial fibrillation: both friend and foe. *Biophys. J.* 110:274a. doi: 10.1016/j.bpj.2015.11.1487

Morotti, S., McCulloch, A. D., Bers, D. M., Edwards, A. G., and Grandi, E. (2016b). Atrial-selective targeting of arrhythmogenic phase-3 early afterdepolarizations in human myocytes. *J. Mol. Cell Cardiol.* 96, 63–71. doi: 10.1016/j.yjmcc.2015.07.030

Morotti, S., Nieves-Cintron, M., Nystoriak, M. A., Navedo, M. F., and Grandi, E. (2017). Predominant contribution of L-type Cav1.2 channel stimulation to impaired intracellular calcium and cerebral artery vasoconstriction in diabetic hyperglycemia, *Channels* 11, 340–346. doi: 10.1080/19336950.2017.1293220

Nattel, S., and Dobrev, D. (2016). Electrophysiological and molecular mechanisms of paroxysmal atrial fibrillation. *Nat. Rev. Cardiol.* 13, 575–590. doi: 10.1038/nrcardio.2016.118

Obergrussberger, A., Bruggemann, A., Goetze, T. A., Rapedius, M., Haarmann, C., Rinke, I., et al. (2016). Automated patch clamp meets high-throughput screening: 384 cells recorded in parallel on a planar patch clamp module. *J. Lab. Autom.* 21, 779–793. doi: 10.1177/2211068215623209

Olson, T. M., Alekseev, A. E., Liu, X. K., Park, S., Zingman, L.V., Bienengraeber, M., et al. (2006). Kv1.5 channelopathy due to KCNA5 loss-of-function mutation causes human atrial fibrillation. *Hum. Mol. Genet.* 15, 2185–2191. doi: 10.1093/hmg/ddl143

Picones, A., Loza-Huerta, A., Segura-Chama, P., and Lara-Figueroa, C. O. (2016). Contribution of automated technologies to ion channel drug discovery. *Adv. Protein Chem. Struct. Biol.* 104, 357–378. doi: 10.1016/bs.apcsb.2016.01.002

Ravens, U., Poulet, C., Wettwer, E., and Knaut, M. (2013). Atrial selectivity of antiarrhythmic drugs *J. Physiol.* 591, 4087–4097. doi: 10.1113/jphysiol.2013.256115

Sanchez, C., Corrias, A., Bueno-Orovio, A., Davies, M., Swinton, J., Jacobson, I., et al. (2012). The Na^+/K^+ pump is an important modulator of refractoriness and rotor dynamics in human atrial tissue. *Am. J. Physiol. Heart Circ. Physiol.* 302, H1146–H1159. doi: 10.1152/ajpheart.00668.2011

Schotten, U., de Haan, S., Verheule, S., Harks, E. G., Frechen, D. Bodewig, E., et al. (2007). Blockade of atrial-specific K^+-currents increases atrial but not ventricular contractility by enhancing reverse mode Na^+/Ca^{2+}-exchange. *Cardiovasc. Res.* 73, 37–47. doi: 10.1016/j.cardiores.2006.11.024

Shinagawa, K., Mitamura, H., Takeshita, A., Sato, T., Kanki, H., Takatsuki, S., et al. (2000). Determination of refractory periods and conduction velocity during atrial fibrillation using atrial capture in dogs: direct assessment of the wavelength and its modulation by a sodium channel blocker, pilsicainide. *J. Am. Coll. Cardiol.* 35, 246–253. doi: 10.1016/S0735-1097(99)00488-X

Sobie, E. A. (2009). Parameter sensitivity analysis in electrophysiological models using multivariable regression. *Biophys. J.* 96, 1264–1274. doi: 10.1016/j.bpj.2008.10.056

Tsujimae, K., Murakami, S., and Kurachi, Y. (2008). *In silico* study on the effects of I_{Kur} block kinetics on prolongation of human action potential after atrial fibrillation-induced electrical remodeling. *Am. J. Physiol. Heart Circ. Physiol.* 294, H793–H800. doi: 10.1152/ajpheart.01229.2007

Van Wagoner, D. R., and Nerbonne, J. M. (2000). Molecular basis of electrical remodeling in atrial fibrillation. *J. Mol. Cell Cardiol.* 32, 1101–1117. doi: 10.1006/jmcc.2000.1147

Van Wagoner, D. R., Piccini, J. P., Albert, C. M., ,Anderson, M. E., Benjamin, E. J., Brundel, B. et al. (2015). Progress toward the prevention and treatment of atrial fibrillation: a summary of the heart rhythm society research forum on the treatment and prevention of atrial fibrillation, Washington, DC, December 9–10, 2013. *Heart Rhythm* 12, e5–e29. doi: 10.1016/j.hrthm.2014.11.011

Van Wagoner, D. R., Pond, A. L., McCarthy, P. M., Trimmer, J. S., and Nerbonne, J. M. (1997). Outward K^+ current densities and $K_V1.5$ expression are reduced in chronic human atrial fibrillation. *Circ. Res.* 80, 772–781. doi: 10.1161/01.RES.80.6.772

Wang, D., Shryock, J. C., and Belardinelli, L. (1996). Cellular basis for the negative dromotropic effect of adenosine on rabbit single atrioventricular nodal cells. *Circ. Res.* 78, 697–706. doi: 10.1161/01.RES.78.4.697

Wettwer, E., Hala, O., Christ, T., Heubach, J. F., Dobrev, D., Knaut, M., et al. (2004). Role of I_{Kur} in controlling action potential shape and contractility in the human atrium: influence of chronic atrial fibrillation. *Circulation* 110, 2299–2306. doi: 10.1161/01.CIR.0000145155.60288.71

Workman, A. J., Kane, K. A., and Rankin, A. C. (2001). The contribution of ionic currents to changes in refractoriness of human atrial myocytes associated with chronic atrial fibrillation. *Cardiovasc. Res.* 52, 226–235. doi: 10.1016/S0008-6363(01)00380-7

Yue, L., Feng, J., Gaspo, R., Li, G. R., Wang, Z., and Nattel, S. (1997). Ionic remodeling underlying action potential changes in a canine model of atrial fibrillation. *Circ. Res.* 81, 512–525. doi: 10.1161/01.RES.81.4.512

Zhao, Q., Tang, Y., Okello, E., Wang, X., and Huang, C. (2009). Changes in atrial effective refractory period and I_{KACh} after vagal stimulation plus rapid pacing in the pulmonary vein. *Rev. Esp. Cardiol* 62, 742–749. doi: 10.1016/S0300-8932(09)71687-2

Zhou, Q., Bett, G. C., and Rasmusson, R. L. (2012). Markov models of use-dependence and reverse use-dependence during the mouse cardiac action potential. *PLoS ONE* 7:e42295. doi: 10.1371/journal.pone.0042295

2

Uncertainty Quantification Reveals the Importance of Data Variability and Experimental Design Considerations for *In silico* Proarrhythmia Risk Assessment

Kelly C. Chang[1], Sara Dutta[1], Gary R. Mirams[2], Kylie A. Beattie[1], Jiansong Sheng[1], Phu N. Tran[1], Min Wu[1], Wendy W. Wu[1], Thomas Colatsky[3], David G. Strauss[1] and Zhihua Li[1]*

[1] Division of Applied Regulatory Science, Center for Drug Evaluation and Research, Office of Translational Sciences, Office of Clinical Pharmacology, Food and Drug Administration, Silver Spring, MD, United States, [2] Centre for Mathematical Medicine and Biology, School of Mathematical Sciences, University of Nottingham, Nottingham, United Kingdom, [3] Marshview Life Science Advisors, Seabrook Island, SC, United States

***Correspondence:**
Zhihua Li
Zhihua.Li@fda.hhs.gov

The Comprehensive *in vitro* Proarrhythmia Assay (CiPA) is a global initiative intended to improve drug proarrhythmia risk assessment using a new paradigm of mechanistic assays. Under the CiPA paradigm, the relative risk of drug-induced Torsade de Pointes (TdP) is assessed using an *in silico* model of the human ventricular action potential (AP) that integrates *in vitro* pharmacology data from multiple ion channels. Thus, modeling predictions of cardiac risk liability will depend critically on the variability in pharmacology data, and uncertainty quantification (UQ) must comprise an essential component of the *in silico* assay. This study explores UQ methods that may be incorporated into the CiPA framework. Recently, we proposed a promising *in silico* TdP risk metric (qNet), which is derived from AP simulations and allows separation of a set of CiPA training compounds into Low, Intermediate, and High TdP risk categories. The purpose of this study was to use UQ to evaluate the robustness of TdP risk separation by qNet. Uncertainty in the model parameters used to describe drug binding and ionic current block was estimated using the non-parametric bootstrap method and a Bayesian inference approach. Uncertainty was then propagated through AP simulations to quantify uncertainty in qNet for each drug. UQ revealed lower uncertainty and more accurate TdP risk stratification by qNet when simulations were run at concentrations below 5× the maximum therapeutic exposure (C_{max}). However, when drug effects were extrapolated above 10× C_{max}, UQ showed that qNet could no longer clearly separate drugs by TdP risk. This was because for most of the pharmacology data, the amount of current block measured was <60%, preventing reliable estimation of IC_{50}-values. The results of this study demonstrate that the accuracy of TdP risk prediction depends both on the intrinsic variability in ion channel pharmacology data as well as on experimental design considerations that preclude an accurate determination of drug IC_{50}-values *in vitro*. Thus, we demonstrate that UQ provides valuable information about *in silico* modeling predictions that can inform future proarrhythmic risk evaluation of drugs under the CiPA paradigm.

Keywords: uncertainty quantification, experimental variability, cardiac electrophysiology, action potential, Torsade de Pointes, ion channel, pharmacology, computational modeling

INTRODUCTION

Drugs that block cardiac ion channels encoded by the *human-ether-à-go-go Related Gene* (hERG) and consequently prolong the QT interval are associated with increased risk of Torsade de Pointes (TdP), a potentially lethal arrhythmia that caused several drugs to be withdrawn from market (Gintant et al., 2016). In 2005, the International Council on Harmonisation (ICH) S7B and E14 guidelines were established to address the issue of TdP liability for new drugs. As stated in these guidelines, their intent was to be used as a screening method to identify drugs that would require more intensive electrocardiographic monitoring of patients in late phase (e.g., phase 3) clinical trials. However, hERG block or QT prolongation does not necessarily correlate with TdP risk, and as a result of these guidelines, many novel compounds are screened out of development because of detected hERG block or QT prolongation without further evaluation of actual TdP risk. Additional insight into TdP risk for hERG-blocking and QT-prolonging drugs can be determined by also assessing whether drugs block inward currents such as, L-type calcium or late sodium (Duff et al., 1987; January and Riddle, 1989; Chézalviel-Guilbert et al., 1995; Guo et al., 2007). The Comprehensive *in vitro* Proarrhythmia Assay (CiPA) is a global initiative to revise the current guidelines with a new set of mechanistic assays that improve the specificity of the proarrhythmia screening process (Fermini et al., 2016).

The CiPA *in silico* assay will test new compounds for the potential to cause TdP by incorporating *in vitro* pharmacology data on multiple ion channels into a mathematical model of the cardiac action potential (AP). The AP model will be used to predict drug effects related to early afterdepolarizations (EADs), which are a known cellular trigger of TdP (Yan et al., 2001). Numerous studies have shown that when outward repolarizing currents such as, I_{Kr} (the current carried by hERG-encoded channels) are blocked in cardiac cells, the resulting imbalance of inward and outward currents prolongs the AP and can, at extreme levels, lead to inward current reactivation and EADs (January and Moscucci, 1992). However, EADs may not occur if a drug also significantly blocks inward currents, leading to a balanced block scenario where the AP is prolonged but inward currents cannot reactivate (Antzelevitch et al., 2004). Because it is difficult to know how much inward vs. outward current block is safe, or how dynamic effects might impact EAD propensity, the purpose of the CiPA *in silico* model will be to assess the integrated effects of multiple ion channel block on TdP risk. As with any model built on inherently variable experimental data, however, confidence in model predictions will depend on the level of uncertainty in model inputs (here, the drug-specific parameters) and the corresponding uncertainty in model outputs (Pathmanathan et al., 2015; Johnstone et al., 2016b). In order for CiPA to provide useful guidance to the drug development and regulatory process, it will be necessary to incorporate uncertainty quantification (UQ) into modeling predictions (Pathmanathan and Gray, 2013; Mirams et al., 2016).

The CiPA *in silico* ventricular AP model and a mechanism-based metric for TdP risk stratification have been trained on a designated set of 12 CiPA compounds with known TdP risk levels (High, Intermediate, or Low, see **Table 1**). These compounds were selected and categorized by a team of expert clinicians, safety pharmacologists, and electrophysiologists based on adverse event data and published reports (Colatsky et al., 2016). The current CiPA AP model was developed through a series of modifications to the O'Hara-Rudy (ORd) human ventricular AP model (O'Hara et al., 2011). Li et al. (2016) first developed a Markov model of the hERG channel that included temperature-sensitive gating, which was subsequently modified to recapitulate I_{Kr} from the original ORd model, with an added pharamacological component (Li et al., 2017). The hERG/I_{Kr} model was then incorporated into the ORd AP model to produce the I_{Kr}-dynamic ORd model. In the CiPAORdv1.0 model, we further optimized the I_{Kr}-dynamic ORd model by scaling ionic current conductances to better reflect changes in AP duration observed in human ventricular myocytes when ionic currents were blocked (referred to as the optimized I_{Kr}-dynamic ORd model in Dutta et al., 2017). With this model, we derived a new *in silico* biomarker for TdP risk, the qNet metric, which correlated well with *in silico* cell "distance" to EADs and thus provided a continuous marker for EAD susceptibility. Although we showed that the qNet metric could correctly stratify the 12 CiPA training drugs by known TdP risk, uncertainty in these modeling predictions was not evaluated.

In this study, methods for applying UQ to the CiPA *in silico* assay are presented. For the 12 CiPA training compounds, we examine the uncertainty in drug-specific kinetics parameters for drug binding and trapping in the I_{Kr}-dynamic model. In addition, we examine uncertainty in dose-response curve IC_{50} and Hill coefficients for the remaining six CiPA-selected ionic currents, as this can also be considerable (Elkins et al., 2013). We thereby characterize uncertainty in drug effects on ion channels due to variation in experiments, whatever the cause of this variation may be. We then sample from these probability distributions for the drug effects and run forward simulations to examine the subsequent uncertainty in qNet and TdP risk stratification.

TABLE 1 | TdP risk levels for the 12 CiPA training compounds.

Drug	CiPA TdP Risk
Dofetilide	High
Bepridil	High
Sotalol	High
Quinidine	High
Cisapride	Intermediate
Terfenadine	Intermediate
Ondansetron	Intermediate
Chlorpromazine	Intermediate
Verapamil	Low
Ranolazine	Low
Mexiletine	Low
Diltiazem	Low

MATERIALS AND METHODS

Human Ventricular Action Potential Model

The CiPAORdv1.0 model (the optimized model from Dutta et al., 2017) was used for all simulations in this study, in order to evaluate TdP risk for the set of 12 CiPA training compounds listed in **Table 1**. Parameter values for the model are listed in Tables S1, S2.

Multiple Ion Channel Pharmacology

Pharmacological effects of the 12 CiPA training compounds on ionic currents were modeled as in Li et al. (2017) and Dutta et al. (2017). The kinetics of hERG block were modeled with the I_{Kr} Markov model from Li et al. (2017), which was fit to voltage clamp data obtained at the U.S. Food and Drug Administration (FDA; parameters listed in **Table 2**). For six other ionic currents (L-type calcium, I_{CaL}; late sodium, I_{NaL}; fast sodium, I_{Na}; transient outward, I_{to}; slowly activating delayed rectifier, I_{Ks}; and inward rectifier, I_{K1}), drug effects were represented by a simple pore blocking model in which maximal current conductances were reduced according to the Hill equation. Hill equation parameters (**Table 3**) were fit to data from Crumb et al. (2016). Some of the data have been updated since publication and are available online (see section Software and Data).

Numerical Methods and Data Analysis

Model equations were written in C and compiled for use with version 3.3 of the R programming language (R Core Team, 2016) and version 1.14 of the deSolve package (Soetaert et al., 2010). Equations were integrated using the lsoda solver with relative and absolute error tolerances of 10^{-6} and other solver settings as default. For computationally intensive bootstrap simulations (see section Drug-hERG Binding Kinetics), a relative tolerance of 10^{-3} was used. Data analysis was performed in R, and figures were produced with version 2.2.0 of the ggplot2 package (Wickham, 2009).

Simulation Protocol for TdP Risk Evaluation

The CiPAORdv1.0 model was used to simulate APs at a cycle length (CL) of 2 s (stimulus amplitude $= -80\ \mu A/\mu F$, duration $= 0.5$ ms). The model was initialized from control (no drug) steady-state values (Table S3) and paced for 1,000 beats. Drugs were simulated at multiples of their maximum therapeutic concentrations (C_{max}, Table S4), ranging from 1 to 10× C_{max} (1× increments) and from 15 to 25× C_{max} (5× increments). At each concentration, TdP risk was evaluated using the metric qNet, defined as the net charge carried by six major currents (I_{Kr}, I_{CaL}, I_{NaL}, I_{to}, I_{Ks}, and I_{K1}) over an entire beat (Dutta et al., 2017). The qNet metric was computed by integrating the sum of the six currents from the start of the stimulus ($t = 0$ s) until the end of the beat ($t = 2$ s) using lsoda (see section Numerical Methods and Data Analysis).

Analysis was performed only on the last 250 beats of the pacing protocol to allow drug effects to reach quasi-steady state for simulations with beat-to-beat instability. Beats in which transmembrane potential (V_m) failed to depolarize above 0 mV were excluded from analysis, and simulations in which every beat failed to depolarize were excluded from TdP risk evaluation. The maximum slope during repolarization (dV/dt_{repol}) was defined as the maximum change in V_m (dV/dt) between 30 and 90% repolarization for beats that fully repolarized; as the maximum dV/dt between 30% repolarization and the end of the beat ($t = 2$ s) when V_m repolarized by 30% but not 90%; or as the maximum dV/dt between the AP peak and the end of the beat when V_m failed to repolarize by 30%. An EAD was defined to have occurred on any beat in which dV/dt_{repol} was greater than zero. Out of the last 250 beats, the beat with the steepest reactivation of the membrane potential (maximum dV/dt_{repol}) was used to calculate qNet, whether or not an EAD had occurred.

Uncertainty Characterization

Drug-hERG Binding Kinetics

In Li et al. (2017), time series measurements of the fractional hERG current in the presence of drug were obtained using a modified Milnes voltage clamp protocol (Milnes et al., 2010; Li et al., 2017). Because of the long duration of the protocol, each cell could only be tested at a single drug concentration, and the drug-hERG binding and trapping parameters (see **Table 2**) were fit to the fractional current traces measured during a voltage step to 0 mV, averaged across cells by concentration. Specifically, each dataset y consisted of a set of fractional current time series observations $x_{c,i}(t)$ ($c = 1, 2, \ldots, m$, where m is number of the concentrations tested; $i = 1, 2, \ldots, n_c$, where n_c is the number of cells tested at the cth concentration; and $x_{c,i}(t_j)$ were independent between concentrations). The mean drug response at the cth concentration was $\bar{x}_c(t) = \frac{1}{n_c}\sum_{i=1}^{n_c} x_{c,i}(t)$ (i.e., the average of fractional current traces across cells), and the overall mean response $\bar{y} = \left(\bar{x}_1(t), \bar{x}_2(t), \ldots, \bar{x}_m(t)\right)$ (i.e., the set of average fractional current traces at each concentration) was used to fit the optimal drug-hERG kinetics parameters ($\hat{\theta}(\bar{y})$). Parameters were fitted using the Covariance Matrix Adaptation Evolutionary Strategy (CMA-ES) (Hansen, 2006), with version 1.0-11 of the cmaes package (Trautmann et al., 2011). Details on the CMA-ES implementation can be found in the Supplemental Methods. Bounds for the dynamic drug-hERG binding parameters used to fit bootstrap samples can be found in Table S5.

TABLE 2 | Drug-hERG binding parameters for the 12 CiPA training compounds.

	$\log_{10}(K_{max})$	$\log_{10}(EC_{50}{}^{n})$	$\log_{10}(K_{max}/EC_{50}{}^{n})$
Dofetilide	1.5453 [0.9209, 6.8153]	2.3357 [1.7982, 7.5726]	−0.7905 [−1.0125, −0.6304]
Bepridil	6.7477 [5.4278, 7.1407]	8.1679 [6.803, 8.5243]	−1.4202 [−1.7124, −1.1736]
Sotalol	4.9831 [0.8193, 5.4306]	8.5861 [4.965, 8.9975]	−3.6029 [−4.5017, −3.1522]
Quinidine	2.4404 [1.1871, 6.4189]	4.731 [3.6678, 8.7601]	−2.2906 [−2.7484, −2.0986]
Cisapride	1.0095 [0.839, 1.6553]	1.6265 [1.4211, 2.2125]	−0.6171 [−0.9699, −0.4154]
Terfenadine	5.0095 [1.2953, 6.2265]	5.6123 [1.8881, 6.8917]	−0.6028 [−0.7791, −0.4311]
Ondansetron	5.2355 [1.5791, 6.3269]	7.718 [4.341, 8.7997]	−2.4825 [−2.7992, −2.2702]
Chlorpromazine	5.1984 [4.696, 6.5012]	7.6386 [7.0863, 8.9725]	−2.4402 [−2.7268, −2.2162]
Verapamil	6.2289 [1.5379, 6.803]	8.5258 [4.1385, 8.9922]	−2.2969 [−2.9551, −1.7767]
Ranolazine	1.723 [1.3627, 5.6536]	5.1553 [4.8122, 8.7298]	−3.4324 [−4.0139, −2.9363]
Mexiletine	1.1761 [1.0208, 1.497]	5.8591 [5.3159, 6.5914]	−4.683 [−5.5154, −3.9582]
Diltiazem	5.2613 [1.6549, 5.6663]	8.8246 [5.7087, 8.9997]	−3.5634 [−4.1562, −3.223]

	n	$\log_{10}(K_u)$	$V_{halftrap}$
Dofetilide	1.08 [0.9527, 1.467]	−4.7409 [−4.9767, −4.6633]	−1 [−26.01, −1]
Bepridil	0.9374 [0.8227, 1.074]	−3.7647 [−3.8713, −3.671]	−61.34 [−72.94, −18.36]
Sotalol	0.7513 [0.6594, 0.955]	−1.6527 [−2.0183, −0.4512]	−51.5 [−74.62, −7.756]
Quinidine	0.8488 [0.7775, 1.028]	−2.3869 [−2.3649, −1.7435]	−61.35 [−72.31, −5.445]
Cisapride	0.9615 [0.5928, 1.372]	−3.3808 [−3.4836, −3.2553]	−167.4 [−190.3, −156.5]
Terfenadine	0.6502 [0.5033, 0.7918]	−4.1086 [−4.2938, −4.0023]	−81.63 [−155, −73.87]
Ondansetron	0.891 [0.83, 1.002]	−1.6338 [−1.7335, −1.3971]	−82.2 [−88.69, −77.64]
Chlorpromazine	0.8871 [0.8006, 0.9916]	−1.3306 [−1.7312, −0.7396]	−14.45 [−66.29, −2.865]
Verapamil	1.043 [0.832, 1.317]	−3.088 [−3.1708, −2.6366]	−97.08 [−192, −85.3]
Ranolazine	0.9532 [0.8248, 1.106]	−1.6914 [−1.914, −0.0004]	−94.99 [−176.4, −81.16]
Mexiletine	1.139 [0.956, 1.34]	−1.1479 [−1.4011, −0.016]	−87.51 [−164.8, −77.68]
Diltiazem	0.9382 [0.8612, 1.086]	−0.5498 [−1.0751, 0]	−90.65 [−180.3, −81.18]

The optimal values are shown with 95% CIs obtained with bootstrapping. Units are as follows: K_{max} (unitless), K_u (ms^{-1}), EC_{50} (nM), n (unitless), and $V_{halftrap}$ (mV).

The non-parametric bootstrap method was used to characterize uncertainty in the fitted parameters (Efron and Tibshirani, 1986). Observations $x^*_{c,i}(t)$ were randomly drawn with replacement from $x_{c,i}(t)$ to obtain a bootstrap sample y^*_b of the same size as the original dataset, with an identical number of observations per concentration. A total of 2,000 bootstrap samples ($b = 1, 2, \ldots, 2000$) were generated using version 1.3-18 of the boot package (Davison and Hinkley, 1997; Canty and Ripley, 2016). The mean response $\bar{y}^*_b$ for each bootstrap sample was then computed in the same manner as $\bar{y}$ and used to refit the drug-hERG kinetics parameters ($\hat{\theta}(\bar{y}^*_b)$), yielding a joint sampling distribution of drug-hERG parameters.

Dose-Response Curves

For other ionic currents, uncertainty in dose-response curves was characterized using a Bayesian inference approach. Version 1.3.5 of the FME package was used to fit Hill equation parameters and to characterize uncertainty, using Markov-chain Monte Carlo (MCMC) simulation with the delayed rejection and adaptive Metropolis algorithm (Soetaert and Petzoldt, 2010). The percentage of ionic current block was assumed to be a normal random variable located at the Hill equation response curve with unknown variance σ^2. Log-transformed IC_{50}-values [$pIC_{50} = -\log_{10}(IC_{50}/c_0)$, where $c_0 = 10^9$ nM] were bounded to the range [−1, 19] for fitting and MCMC simulation (bounding IC_{50}-values between 10^{-10} and 10^{10} nM). Hill coefficients (h) were bounded to the range [0, 10]. Optimal IC_{50} and Hill coefficient (h)-values were fit using non-linear least squares (see **Table 3**). The joint probability distribution of IC_{50} and h was estimated using MCMC simulation. A uniform prior distribution was used for pIC_{50} and h. The error variance σ^2 was considered a nuisance parameter and was sampled as conjugate priors from an inverse gamma distribution during MCMC simulation. The proposal distribution was multivariate normal. A total of 2,000 MCMC samples (pIC_{50}, h) were saved for each drug-current combination to form a joint sampling distribution of Hill equation parameters (see Supplemental Methods for implementation details).

Credible Intervals

Variability of model inputs (parameters) or outputs (predicted responses) was summarized with 95% credible intervals (95% CIs, the 2.5–97.5% quantiles of the marginal distributions).

Uncertainty Propagation

Samples from the joint distribution of drug-hERG parameters and the joint distributions of Hill equation parameters for a

TABLE 3 | Hill equation parameters for the 12 CiPA training compounds.

		I_{CaL}	I_{K1}	I_{Ks}
Dofetilide	pIC_{50}	6.5845 [−0.7468, 7.9108]	6.4041 [−0.7384, 7.8736]	N/A
	h	1.163 [0.32, 9.622]	0.765 [0.2685, 9.658]	N/A
Cisapride	pIC_{50}	2.0331 [−0.8172, 6.4905]	4.5305 [−0.7411, 6.7042]	1.0906 [−0.767, 6.528]
	h	0.4261 [0.4063, 9.736]	0.5133 [0.2572, 9.63]	0.2921 [0.2409, 9.67]
Bepridil	pIC_{50}	5.5516 [5.2752, 5.71]	N/A	4.5432 [3.4422, 4.9682]
	h	0.6486 [0.4351, 0.9191]	N/A	0.7061 [0.3907, 1.142]
Verapamil	pIC_{50}	6.6951 [6.6029, 6.7891]	0.4574 [−0.8155, 5.7514]	N/A
	h	1.097 [0.861, 1.43]	0.2728 [0.2526, 9.655]	N/A
Terfenadine	pIC_{50}	6.1547 [6.0876, 6.2131]	N/A	3.3982 [0.0077, 5.9477]
	h	0.6601 [0.595, 0.7367]	N/A	0.543 [0.2777, 9.728]
Ranolazine	pIC_{50}	N/A	N/A	1.4418 [−0.624, 4.3335]
	h	N/A	N/A	0.5191 [0.3292, 8.066]
Sotalol	pIC_{50}	2.1511 [1.7907, 2.3628]	2.5157 [2.385, 2.5955]	2.3745 [2.0951, 2.507]
	h	0.8651 [0.5902, 1.259]	1.204 [0.9066, 1.611]	1.167 [0.7741, 1.698]
Mexiletine	pIC_{50}	4.4175 [3.9423, 4.6525]	N/A	N/A
	h	1.031 [0.6484, 1.576]	N/A	N/A
Quinidine	pIC_{50}	4.2874 [3.8501, 4.5293]	1.4024 [−0.7594, 5.0793]	5.3099 [5.2008, 5.3813]
	h	0.5892 [0.4384, 0.7362]	0.3468 [0.2715, 9.492]	1.363 [0.9565, 2.122]
Ondansetron	pIC_{50}	4.6469 [4.4138, 4.7937]	N/A	3.2443 [2.138, 3.9253]
	h	0.7526 [0.5478, 1.024]	N/A	0.6535 [0.3954, 1.238]
Diltiazem	pIC_{50}	6.9504 [6.7786, 7.1267]	N/A	N/A
	h	0.7142 [0.5344, 1.008]	N/A	N/A
Chlorpromazine	pIC_{50}	5.0866 [4.9108, 5.2128]	5.0329 [4.8446, 5.1718]	N/A
	h	0.8441 [0.6105, 1.189]	0.6878 [0.5226, 0.8822]	N/A
		I_{to}	I_{NaL}	I_{Na}
Dofetilide	pIC_{50}	7.7254 [6.8317, 7.9571]	3.1231 [−0.754, 7.8227]	6.4196 [−0.6142, 8.0307]
	h	0.7712 [0.3735, 1.147]	0.2597 [0.1543, 9.49]	0.892 [0.2235, 9.497]
Cisapride	pIC_{50}	3.6594 [−0.6456, 5.6778]	N/A	N/A
	h	0.243 [0.1166, 0.5656]	N/A	N/A
Bepridil	pIC_{50}	5.0658 [−0.5052, 5.3383]	5.7414 [5.6743, 5.8074]	5.5333 [5.3948, 5.6158]
	h	3.541 [0.4166, 9.499]	1.416 [1.133, 1.789]	1.164 [0.8083, 1.71]
Verapamil	pIC_{50}	4.8719 [1.1464, 5.5056]	5.1532 [−0.6313, 5.8804]	N/A
	h	0.8222 [0.2414, 1.793]	1.031 [0.222, 9.41]	N/A
Terfenadine	pIC_{50}	3.6198 [−0.0501, 5.1184]	4.6977 [2.6363, 5.8293]	5.3185 [4.8576, 6.0114]
	h	0.2559 [0.1246, 0.5777]	0.6011 [0.269, 3.232]	1.015 [0.6554, 9.176]
Ranolazine	pIC_{50}	N/A	5.1033 [4.9859, 5.2079]	4.1626 [3.2696, 4.5616]
	h	N/A	0.945 [0.7247, 1.256]	1.425 [0.6228, 9.116]
Sotalol	pIC_{50}	1.3651 [−0.3529, 2.1817]	N/A	−0.0584 [−0.8951, 2.4926]
	h	0.6632 [0.3213, 1.704]	N/A	0.5089 [0.3913, 8.449]
Mexiletine	pIC_{50}	N/A	5.0478 [4.9484, 5.1128]	N/A
	h	N/A	1.409 [1.041, 1.846]	N/A
Quinidine	pIC_{50}	5.4575 [5.3999, 5.511]	5.0261 [4.9062, 5.1077]	4.909 [4.6683, 5.0426]
	h	1.282 [1.049, 1.585]	1.337 [1.034, 1.7]	1.494 [1.004, 2.236]
Ondansetron	pIC_{50}	2.9901 [−0.8308, 4.4636]	4.7172 [4.6073, 4.8]	4.2391 [3.5217, 4.6469]
	h	0.9891 [0.4407, 9.691]	1.035 [0.8001, 1.399]	1.02 [0.5024, 8.671]
Diltiazem	pIC_{50}	−0.4506 [−0.922, 2.6212]	4.6602 [4.5116, 4.7776]	3.9551 [3.2876, 4.8315]
	h	0.1696 [0.1551, 0.364]	0.6779 [0.5485, 0.9082]	0.7022 [0.4484, 9.337]
Chlorpromazine	pIC_{50}	1.754 [−0.6914, 4.776]	5.341 [5.2543, 5.4232]	5.3433 [5.221, 5.4298]
	h	0.3654 [0.2318, 8.56]	0.9379 [0.7797, 1.148]	1.995 [1.628, 3.064]

The optimal fitted values are shown with 95% CIs obtained using Markov-chain Monte Carlo simulation. IC_{50}-values are log-transformed as $pIC_{50} = -log_{10}(IC_{50}/c_0)$, where $c_0 = 10^9$ nM. Not applicable (N/A) indicates that IC_{50}-values were not defined in Li et al. (2017), so the amount of block was assumed to always be 0%.

particular drug were assumed to be independent and were combined in AP simulations to assess the uncertainty in qNet (see section Simulation Protocol for TdP Risk Evaluation). One sample from each distribution was selected in sequential order (e.g., the first sample from each distribution) to form a set of parameters that defined a single sample from the drug-effect probability distribution. This was repeated until all parameter samples were exhausted, generating a sampling distribution of 2,000 drug-effect samples per drug (referred to as uncertainty inputs), which. Each input was simulated with the CiPAORdv1.0 model to assess variability in AP model outputs (qNet, see section Simulation Protocol for TdP Risk Evaluation). Variability in qNet was quantified with 95% CIs. Sampling distributions of qNet were visualized with violin plots.

Cross Validation

Leave-one-out cross validation (LOOCV) (Hastie et al., 2009) was used to assess the accuracy of TdP risk stratification at each simulated concentration relative to C_{max}. The CiPA Low, Intermediate, and High TdP risk levels (**Table 1**) were given numerical category values of 0, 1, and 2, respectively. At each concentration ($1-25\times$ C_{max}), a classifier was trained on all samples from the qNet distributions of all but one of the training drugs. The classifier was based on proportional odds logistic regression using the lrm function from version 4.5-0 of the rms package (Harrell, 2016). The numerical tolerance was set to 10^{-10} and the maximum number of iterations was set to 10^6 for fitting. Each sample of the remaining, "left out" drug was then assigned to the category with the highest probability based on logistic regression results. The predicted probability of each category [P(x), where x is 0, 1, or 2] for the "left out" drug was computed as the fraction of samples assigned to that category, and the prediction error for that drug was computed as the mean absolute difference between the assigned and actual TdP category over all samples. This procedure was repeated for all 12 training drugs, and the mean and standard deviation of prediction errors at each concentration were computed to evaluate overall TdP risk stratification performance.

Software and Data

The software and data used in this study are available at https://github.com/FDA/CiPA.

RESULTS

Uncertainty in Drug-hERG Binding Kinetics

Bootstrapping was performed with voltage clamp data from Li et al. (2017) in order to estimate the joint probability distribution of fitted drug-hERG dynamic binding parameters. The 95% CIs of hERG binding parameters for the 12 CiPA training drugs (**Table 1**) are listed in **Table 2**. Parameter fitting results for bepridil are illustrated in **Figure 1A**. The rate of bepridil unbinding (K_u) had a relatively narrow 95% CI [$10^{-3.8713}$, $10^{-3.671}$ ms^{-1}], indicating that this parameter was well-constrained by the experimental data and uncertainty in its value was low. In contrast, the pairwise scatter plot of $\log_{10}(K_{max})$ and $\log_{10}(EC_{50}{}^n)$ revealed a strong correlation between the two parameters, and their fitted ranges spanned several orders of magnitude. The pairwise scatter plots for other training drugs displayed similar correlations between $\log_{10}(K_{max})$ and $\log_{10}(EC_{50}{}^n)$ (panel A in Figures S1–S11).

The large uncertainty in K_{max} and $EC_{50}{}^n$ did not produce a similar degree of variability in the kinetics of hERG block, however. In **Figure 1B** and panel B of Figures S1–S11, shaded areas indicate the 95% CI of the block predicted by parameters in **Figure 1A** and panel A of Figures S1–S11. The variability in hERG block was much more limited than the variability in K_{max} or $EC_{50}{}^n$, which was not surprising because Li et al. (2017) showed that for most of the 12 training drugs, there was a near-linear relationship between drug concentration and binding rate, occurring when the fitted EC_{50}-value was much greater than the maximum drug concentration tested. For example, the optimal EC_{50}-value of bepridil was $10^{8.7}$ nM, and the bootstrap-estimated 95% CI was [$10^{7.0}$, $10^{9.7}$], but the maximum bepridil concentration tested was 300 nM, or roughly $10^{2.5}$ nM. In such cases, the E_{max} equation defining the sigmoidal dose-response relationship of drug binding [$E_{max} = K_{max}{}^*(D^n/(D^n{+}EC_{50}{}^n))$] was linearly approximated by $E_{max}{\approx}(K_{max}/EC_{50}{}^n){}^*D^n$, and the ratio $K_{max}/EC_{50}{}^n$ effectively becomes a single identifiable parameter. Thus, the 95% CIs for $\log_{10}(K_{max}/EC_{50}{}^n)$ were much narrower than the 95% CIs for $\log_{10}(K_{max})$ and $\log_{10}(EC_{50}{}^n)$ (**Table 2**). The E_{max} equation was chosen to model drug binding because of its flexibility in accommodating both linear and sigmoidal dose-response relationships. As a result, for those compounds whose drug binding mode is actually linear, the ratio but not the individual values of the two correlated parameters were identifiable (Li et al., 2017).

In addition, multimodality (the presence of multiple peaks in the sampling distribution) was frequently observed in other hERG kinetics parameters (Figures S1–S11), in particular with $V_{halftrap}$. In the hERG binding model, $V_{halftrap}$ is a drug trapping parameter that determines the steady-state fraction of open-bound (untrapped) to close-bound (trapped) channels. Li et al. (2017) demonstrated that the High- and Low-risk CiPA training drugs could be separated by this single parameter ($V_{halftrap} > -65$ mV for High-risk drugs, while $V_{halftrap} < -85$ mV for Low-risk drugs). The multimodality identified in $V_{halftrap}$ sampling distributions raised the question of whether this trend still holds under uncertainty analysis. As shown in **Figure 2**, the 95% CIs of $V_{halftrap}$ were quite wide for most drugs, but much of this variability covered ranges where the ratio of open- to close-bound channels (O_{bound}/C_{bound}) at -80 mV was relatively flat, near 1 for Low-risk drugs (green bars) or near 0 for High-risk drugs (red bars). In the steepest region of the O_{bound}/C_{bound} curve, $V_{halftrap}$ distributions of High- vs. Low-risk drugs were well-separated (upper credible bounds < -77 mV for Low-risk drugs, lower credible bounds > -75 mV for High-risk drugs). Thus, UQ identified consistently low or high levels of trapping for Low- vs. High-risk drugs, respectively, providing increased confidence in the $V_{halftrap}$ trend identified by Li et al. (2017). Note that with or without UQ, the $V_{halftrap}$-values of Intermediate-risk drugs (blue bars and points) other than chlorpromazine were generally indistinguishable from Low-risk drugs, and chlorpromazine was indistinguishable from High-risk drugs, indicating that the

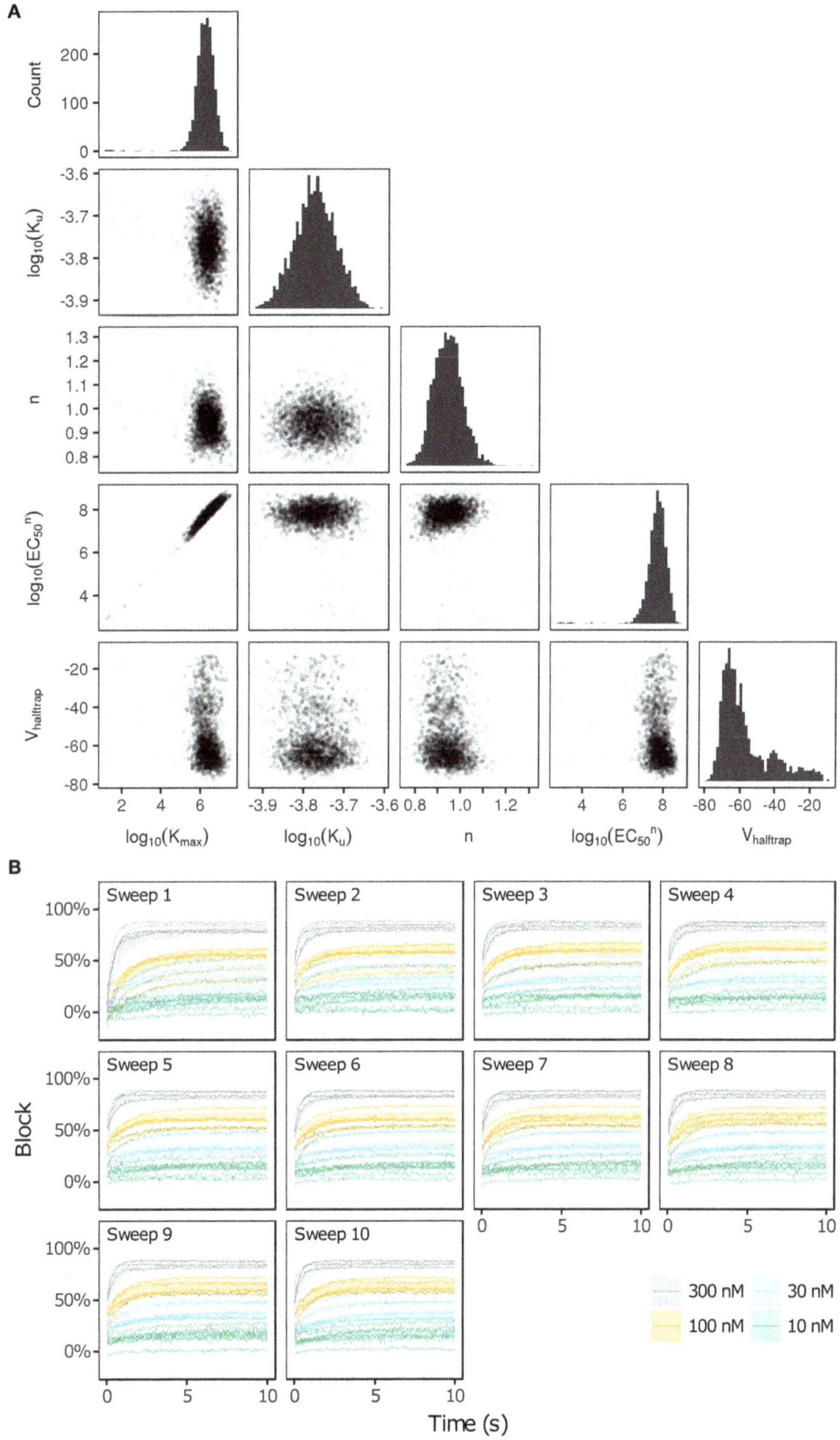

FIGURE 1 | Uncertainty in bepridil-hERG binding kinetics. **(A)** The joint probability distribution of K_{max} (maximum drug effect at saturating concentrations), K_u (rate of drug unbinding), *n* (Hill coefficient of drug binding), EC_{50}^n (nth power of the half-maximal drug concentration), and $V_{halftrap}$ (drug trapping potential) was estimated by bootstrapping. Plots on the diagonal show the marginal histograms of each parameter (log-transformed in some cases). Plots below the diagonal show pairwise scatter plots of the fitted parameters for 2,000 bootstrap samples. **(B)** Kinetics of hERG block during 10 sweeps of a modified Milnes voltage-clamp protocol (Milnes et al., 2010; Li et al., 2017). Shaded areas show the range of block produced by the parameters from **(A)**. Lines show the experimental results used to fit the data (down-sampled 5× for clarity).

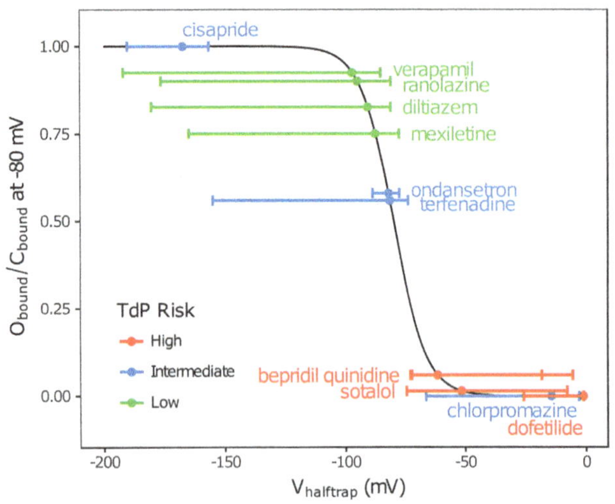

FIGURE 2 | Uncertainty in drug trapping for the 12 CiPA training drugs. Fitted $V_{halftrap}$-values (points) are plotted along the curve defining the resulting steady-state fraction of open-bound to close-bound channels (O_{bound}/C_{bound}) at $V_m = -80$ mV. The 95% CIs (horizontal error bars) were estimated with bootstrapping. High TdP-risk drugs are in red, Intermediate-risk drugs are in blue, and Low-risk drugs are in green. Intermediate-risk drugs were indistinguishable from Low- and High-risk drugs.

degree of drug trapping is not sufficient to stratify compounds into the three CiPA risk levels.

Uncertainty in Dose-Response Curves

Bayesian inference was used to estimate the joint probability distribution of Hill equation parameters characterizing steady-state I_{Na}, I_{CaL}, I_{NaL}, I_{to}, I_{Ks}, and I_{K1} block by each of the 12 CiPA training drugs. MCMC simulation was not performed for drug-current combinations that did not have defined IC_{50}-values in Li et al. (2017), which were assumed to have 0% block. Parameter fitting results are summarized in **Table 3**. Some MCMC simulations produced joint sampling distributions with a single well-defined peak, such as, that of ranolazine-I_{NaL} (**Figure 3A**). The mean parameter values of this distribution ($pIC_{50} = 5.0958$, $h = 0.9594$) were close to the optimal fitted values ($pIC_{50} = 5.1033$, $h = 0.945$), and the 95% CIs [pIC_{50} (4.9859, 5.2079), h (0.7247, 1.256)] were relatively narrow, indicating that uncertainty in these parameters was low. Consequently, the variability in dose-response curves defined by these parameters was also low. At any given concentration, uncertainty in ranolazine-I_{NaL} block (i.e., the width of its 95% CI) was <16% (**Figure 3B**, shaded area), reflecting the variability observed in experiments (circles). Note that uncertainty in ranolazine- I_{NaL} block did not increase at concentrations beyond the highest tested (23 μM) because the well-constrained dose-response curve allowed for extrapolation beyond experimentally tested concentrations.

For other MCMC simulations such as, dofetilide-I_{NaL}, an inverse relationship of possible IC_{50}- and h-values was observed, without a defined peak (**Figure 3C**). Furthermore, many MCMC samples reached near the bounds imposed on IC_{50} and h during fitting [95% CIs for pIC_{50} (−0.754, 7.8227] and h [0.1543, 9.49)]. This was symptomatic of having insufficient experimental data to constrain IC_{50}-values, as the maximum measured I_{NaL} block was 12.1% at 3× C_{max}, the highest concentration tested (**Figure 3D**, circles). Although an optimal fit could be defined using least squares (solid line), confidence in the fitted parameters was low, and uncertainty in predicted block increased abruptly above 3× C_{max}. At 10× and 25× C_{max}, the 95% CIs of predicted block were [0, 82.8%] and [0, 99.8%], respectively, reaching close to the maximum possible range (shaded area). Thus, under circumstances where insufficient current block was achieved in experiments, uncertainty in the dose-response relationship became very high when extrapolating beyond the tested concentrations. Similar findings were obtained with other drug-current combinations (**Table 3** and Figures S12–S62).

The amount of uncertainty in predicted block (measured as the width of the 95% CI) was examined as a function of the mean block achieved at the highest tested concentration (C_{high}). **Table 4** lists the mean block measured in experiments at 1× C_{high} for the 12 CiPA training drugs (some drugs had a different C_{high} for different channels). The resulting uncertainty in the amount of drug block at concentrations above C_{high} is depicted in **Figure 4**. At 1× C_{high}, uncertainty was <25% for all drug-current combinations, indicating that variability in the experimental observations was low. When uncertainty was quantified at extrapolated concentrations (2×, 3×, and 10× C_{high}), differences were observed between experiments with low and high amounts of block at 1× C_{high}. When <30% mean block was measured at 1× C_{high}, uncertainty was >25% for most dose-response curves and reached close to 100% in several cases. But when >60% mean block was measured at 1× C_{high}, uncertainty at the extrapolated concentrations was <16%. Thus, UQ results for this dataset suggest that >60% block should be achieved experimentally if dose-response curves are to predict drug effects beyond the tested concentrations. Although >60% block was achieved in hERG experiments with the 12 CiPA training drugs, none of the training drugs were tested at concentrations producing >60% block for all six non-hERG ionic currents (which would be unlikely other than for quinidine, given the selectivity of these compounds). This analysis therefore suggested that drug effects could only be reliably predicted at the highest experimentally tested concentration for which data on all six non-hERG ionic currents were available (**Table 4**).

Propagation of Uncertainty to AP Simulations

Uncertainty in drug-hERG kinetics and dose-response curves was propagated to AP simulations to explore its impact on TdP risk stratification for the 12 CiPA training drugs. For each drug, the optimal drug-hERG parameters and Hill equation parameters (referred to as fixed inputs) were used to simulate APs, as in previous studies (Dutta et al., 2017; Li et al., 2017). In addition, a total of 2,000 drug-effect uncertainty samples per drug (referred to as uncertainty inputs) were simulated in order to estimate the distribution of drug effects derived from uncertainty characterization (see section Uncertainty in

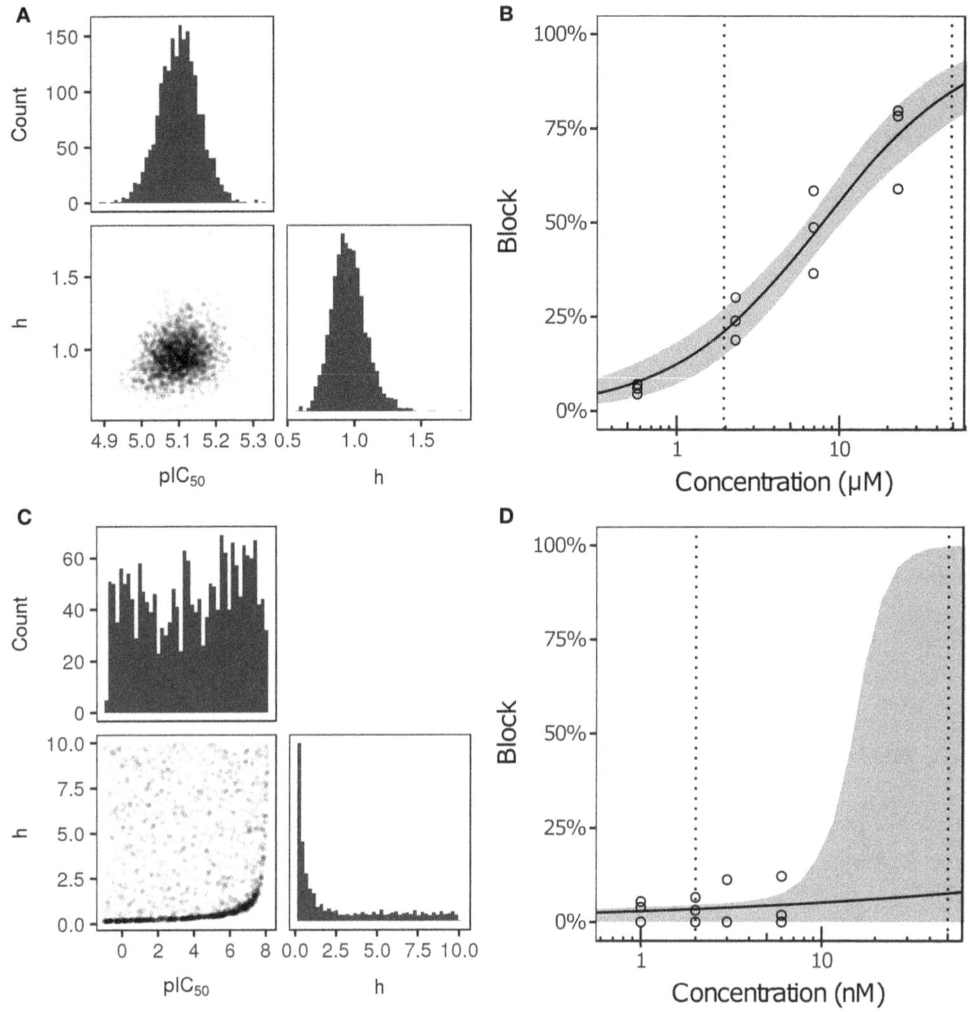

FIGURE 3 | Uncertainty in the dose-response relationship of late sodium current (I_{NaL}) block by ranolazine **(A,B)** and dofetilide **(C,D)**. **(A,C)** show the joint distribution of pIC_{50} and Hill coefficient (h)-values, estimated with a Bayesian inference approach. Marginal histograms are displayed on the diagonal plots, and pairwise scatter plots are below the diagonal (2,000 samples per drug). IC_{50}-values are in nM. **(B,D)** show the dose-response relationships for the two drugs. Solid lines show the Hill equation defined by IC_{50}- and h-values from Li et al. (2017). Shaded areas denote the 95% CI of the percentage block at each concentration, as determined by the parameters in **(A,C)**. Circles are the experimental values used to fit the dose-response curves. Vertical dotted lines indicate the limits of the concentration range used in AP simulations (1–25× C_{max}).

Drug-hERG Binding Kinetics–Uncertainty in Dose-Response Curves). Individual beats were classified as having normal APs, EADs, or depolarization failure (**Figure 5A**), and each simulation was classified as having EADs, complete depolarization failure, or normal otherwise (see section Simulation Protocol for TdP Risk Evaluation). As drug concentration increased from 1 to 25× C_{max} in uncertainty-input simulations, repolarization and depolarization abnormalities became more frequent for some training drugs. EADs occurred in quinidine, dofetilide, and ranolazine simulations (**Figure 5B**), and depolarization failure occurred in quinidine, dofetilide, ranolazine, and verapamil simulations (**Figure 5C**). However, the frequency of these events was generally low except in quinidine simulations, which had EADs in >90% of simulations at 3–10× C_{max} and depolarization failure in >50% of simulations at ≥20× C_{max}. While EADs are mechanistically linked to TdP, depolarization failure constitutes a different type of rhythm disturbance; therefore, simulations with depolarization failure were removed from further analysis. The remaining simulations represented the conditional distribution of drug effects, given that depolarization failure did not occur at a particular concentration.

Impact of Uncertainty on TdP Risk Stratification

Although EADs are a mechanistic marker for TdP risk, stratification based on EADs was not possible because they occurred very rarely in simulations, and not at all for many High Risk compounds at free C_{max}. Instead, Dutta et al. (2017) proposed to use the *in silico* metric qNet (the net charge carried by major AP currents during one paced beat at steady state) as

TABLE 4 | Mean current block at the highest drug concentrations tested in experiments (C_{high}).

Drug	C_{high}	× C_{max}	I_{CaL} (%)	I_{K1} (%)	I_{Ks} (%)	I_{Na} (%)	I_{NaL} (%)	I_{to} (%)
Dofetilide	6 nM	3	1.2	3.4	0.2	2.5	4.6	27.0
Bepridil	3 uM	90.9	50.7	0.5	16.2	51.7	67.0	2.4
Sotalol	2100 uM	143.0	26.0	38.6	30.6	3.9	11.0	11.4
Quinidine	5.4 uM	1.7	20.2	5.6	55.5	22.3	31.8	64.2
Cisapride	125 nM	48.1	0.7	5.3	1.8	2.4	0.0	13.2
Terfenadine	800 nM	200	52.0	0.0	3.3	14.0	12.7	20.6
Ondansetron	20 uM	143.9	47.4	3.0	9.9	25.5	51.6	2.0
Chlorpromazine	10.5 uM	276.3	55.4	51.1	5.2	84.2	69.2	6.0
Verapamil	1 uM	12.3	85.7	3.9	–	0.5	12.0	9.9
	500 nM	6.2	–	–	2.4	–	–	–
Ranolazine	23 uM	11.8	2.5	0.3	2.1	17.4	72.3	–
	69 uM	35.4	–	–	–	–	–	26.5
Mexiletine	10 uM	2.4	19.5	0.6	0.0	6.1	51.9	1.0
Diltiazem	12.5 uM	102.5	97.0	4.6	0.0	17.7	40.6	11.0

Concentrations are also expressed as multiples of the maximum therapeutic concentration (× C_{max}). Because some ionic current experiments used different test concentrations, verapamil and ranolazine both have two entries in the table.

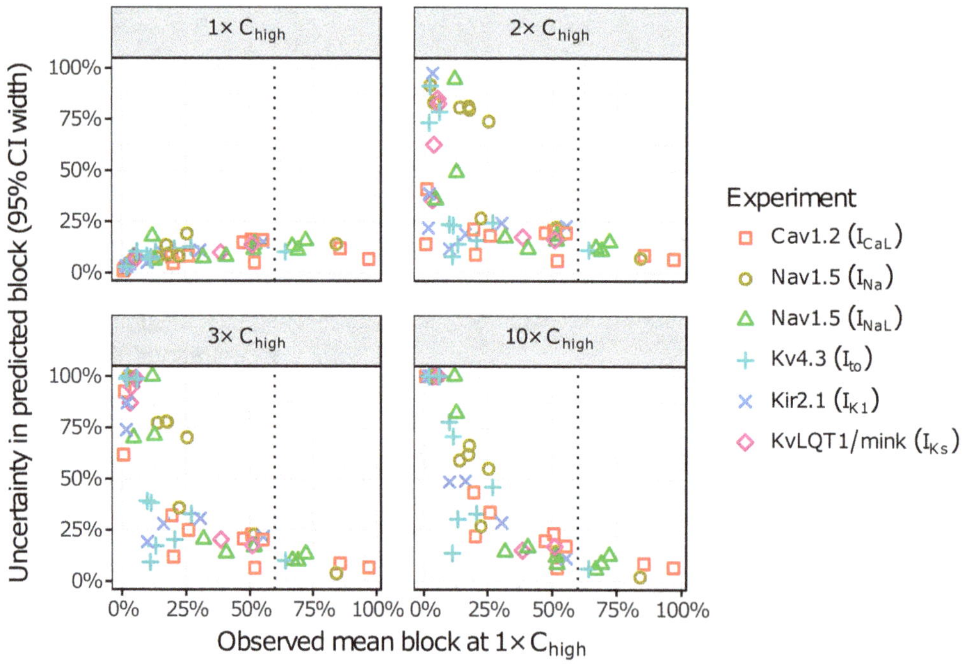

FIGURE 4 | Uncertainty in dose-response curves at extrapolated drug concentrations. Current block experiments were performed for six ionic currents (see legend) with the 12 CiPA training drugs (72 drug-current combinations total with 19 excluded, see **Table 3**). Dose-response curves were fitted for each experiment and extrapolated above the highest experimentally tested drug concentration (C_{high}). Uncertainty in dose-response curves was quantified at 1×, 2×, 3×, and 10× C_{high} as the width of the 95% CI for the predicted percentage block, plotted as a function of the mean experimentally observed block at 1× C_{high}. Vertical dotted line is drawn at 60% observed mean block, denoting an approximate lower limit on the mean block that was observed at 1× C_{high} in experiments for which uncertainty remained low (<16%) at higher concentrations.

an indicator of how far a cell is at a particular drug concentration from producing an EAD. The qNet metric was used in the present study as a marker of TdP risk because it successfully stratified the 12 CiPA training drugs at a range of concentrations in the previous study by Dutta et al. (2017). The calculation of qNet was updated to include simulations in which EADs occurred (see section Simulation Protocol for TdP Risk Evaluation) so that the sampling distributions of qNet would accurately reflect the uncertainty in drug parameters (excluding those that produced depolarization failure). As expected, the values of qNet obtained

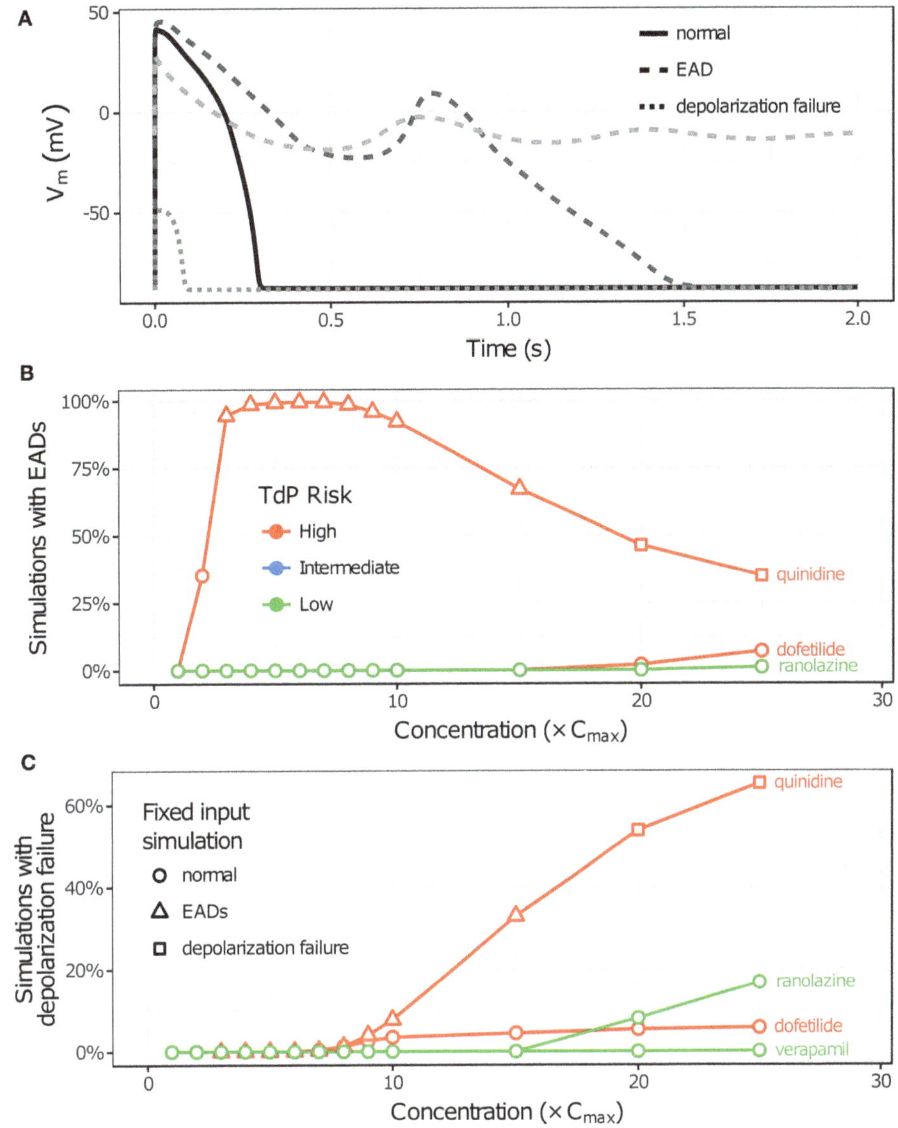

FIGURE 5 | Repolarization and depolarization abnormalities in AP simulations. **(A)** Traces showing representative examples of beats with normal APs (solid), EADs (dashed), or depolarization failure (dotted). **(B,C)** The percentage of uncertainty-input simulations (2,000 total) in which EADs occurred **(B)** or which had complete depolarization failure **(C)** is shown as a function of drug concentration in **(B,C)**, respectively. Only results for drugs that had these events at the simulated concentrations (1–25× C_{max}) are plotted. (Note that ranolazine had 19 simulations with EADs at 25× C_{max}; verapamil only had one instance of depolarization failure occurring at 25× C_{max}.) Markers indicate whether simulations with fixed inputs produced normal Aps (circles), EADs (triangles), or depolarization failure (squares).

with uncertainty-input simulations trended according to TdP risk (**Figures 6A,B**). At a given concentration, median qNet-values decreased between the Low, Intermediate, and High TdP-risk drugs, indicating that outward currents were diminished and inward currents became increasingly dominant at higher risk levels. Note also that extreme negative values of qNet occurred when EADs were present (**Figure 6B**), reflecting the higher TdP risk evident in these simulations.

Variability in qNet increased as uncertainty in drug effects increased. At 1× C_{max}, the distribution of qNet-values for each drug was relatively narrow, and as a result, only a small amount of overlap was observed between adjacent TdP risk levels (**Figure 6A**). At 10× C_{max}, however, the distribution of qNet-values for dofetilide (a High-risk drug) contained several outliers, which encompassed the values for all other drugs except the most negative quinidine values (**Figure 6B**). These outliers resulted from the high degree of uncertainty in dose-response curves for dofetilide above the highest concentration tested (3× C_{max}), particularly with inward currents. As discussed in section Uncertainty in Dose-Response Curves, uncertainty in I_{NaL} block by dofetilide increased dramatically above 3× C_{max} (**Figure 3D**, shaded area). A similar pattern occurred for I_{CaL} block by dofetilide (Figure S12), with high uncertainty in predicted block at 10× C_{max} [95% CI (0%, 97.6%)]. Because qNet reflects the

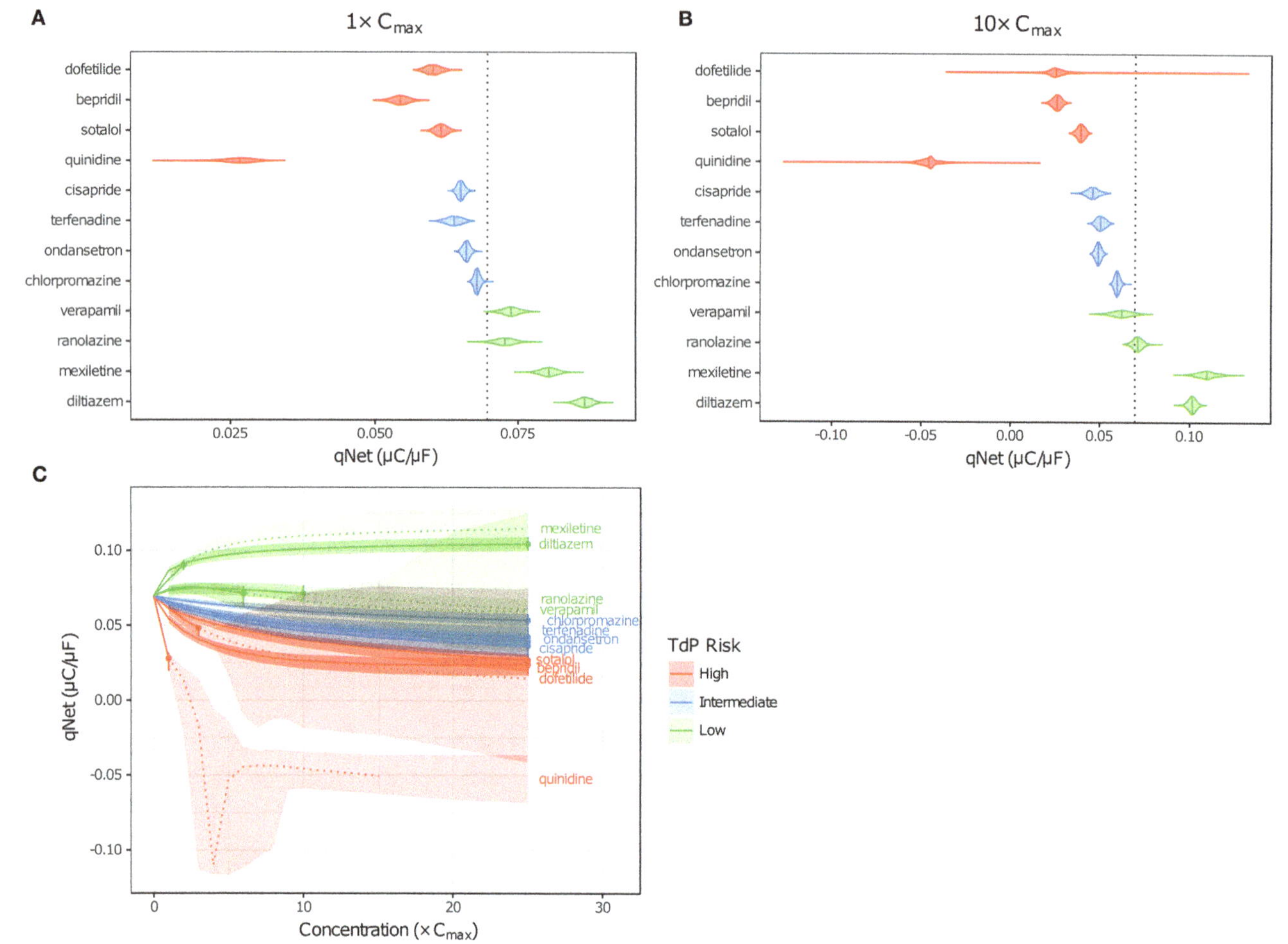

FIGURE 6 | Uncertainty in qNet for the 12 CiPA training drugs. Violin plots are shown for qNet distributions at 1× **(A)** and 10× **(B)** C_{max}, based on uncertainty-input simulations. Dotted line indicates the control (no drug) value of qNet. **(C)** qNet at 1–10× C_{max} (1× increments) and 15–25× C_{max} (5× increments). Shaded areas indicate the 95% CIs of qNet obtained from uncertainty-input simulations. Points indicate the highest simulated concentration for which complete experimental data on six non-hERG currents were available. Fixed-input results are shown below (solid lines) or above (dotted lines) this concentration. Likewise, uncertainty-input results are indicated below (dark shaded areas) or above (light shaded areas) this concentration. Simulations with depolarization failure (**Figure 5B**) were excluded from the results. For all panels, High TdP-risk drugs are in red, Intermediate-risk drugs are in blue, and Low-risk drugs are in green.

balance of inward currents (I_{NaL} and I_{CaL}) and outward currents (mainly I_{Kr}), the effects of I_{Kr} block by dofetilide were offset in simulations with significant block of I_{NaL} or I_{CaL}, resulting in the "safe" outliers for dofetilide at 10× C_{max} with very high qNet-values. On the other hand, simulations with very little I_{NaL} or I_{CaL} block led to "dangerous" outliers with very low or negative qNet-values.

Poor separation of qNet between TdP risk levels was apparent at higher drug concentrations, due primarily to the increased uncertainty in drug effects. Dutta et al. (2017) showed that with fixed model simulations, perfect separation in qNet occurred for the 12 CiPA training drugs at 1–25× C_{max}. However, our analysis of dose-response uncertainty in section Uncertainty in Dose-Response Curves suggests that qNet may be highly variable above experimentally tested concentrations. In **Figure 6C**, fixed-input simulation results are shown for concentrations up to (solid lines) and including (point) the maximum simulated concentrations for which complete drug block data on all six non-hERG ionic currents was available; above these concentrations, fixed-input results are plotted as dotted lines. At 1× C_{max}, data were available for all 12 CiPA training drugs. Above 1× C_{max}, however, some data were unavailable for quinidine (>1.7× C_{max}), mexiletine (>2.4× C_{max}), dofetilide (>3× C_{max}), verapamil (>6.2× C_{max}), and ranolazine (>11.8× C_{max}; see **Table 4**). Nevertheless, near 1× C_{max}, the 95% CIs of qNet remained largely separated between TdP risk levels, indicating that uncertainty at these concentrations was low enough to stratify the training drugs (shaded areas). At >4× C_{max}, however, overlap between different risk levels increased due to the higher variability in qNet sampling distributions, particularly for verapamil and dofetilide. However, increased uncertainty in qNet was not the sole factor affecting TdP risk separation. The qNet-values for verapamil and ranolazine (Low-risk drugs) also drifted closer to those of chlorpromazine (Intermediate-risk) at >4× C_{max}, further increasing the overlap between these risk levels, though qNet-values for fixed-input results remained separate.

The accuracy of TdP risk stratification as a function of concentration was assessed using LOOCV. At each concentration relative to C_{max}, a classifier was trained on qNet uncertainty samples for 11 of the 12 training drugs and then used to predict the probabilities of each TdP risk level for the remaining drug (see section Cross Validation). At 1× C_{max}, the maximum probability always occurred at the correct TdP risk level, but several drugs had non-zero probabilities for the incorrect TdP risk level (**Table 5**). In contrast, when LOOCV was performed at 1× C_{max} in Dutta et al. (2017), two drugs (terfenadine and chlorpromazine) were misclassified on the basis of fixed-input results (equivalent to a predicted 100% probability of the drug being in the wrong category). As a result, although LOOCV prediction errors were non-zero for more drugs when uncertainty was considered, the overall mean prediction error was lower as compared to fixed-input results (0.09 vs. 0.17). At 10× C_{max}, however, mean prediction error was higher when the classifier was trained on uncertainty-input results rather than fixed-input results (0.23 vs. 0.08) because of increased prediction errors for dofetilide, sotalol, cisapride, and verapamil. This was due to the low level of block achieved experimentally for many non-hERG currents, which led to high uncertainty in qNet when drug effects were extrapolated above the tested concentrations. Thus, uncertainty analysis produced more robust TdP risk predictions near concentrations with experimental data for all currents but less robust predictions at concentrations for which extrapolation of drug effects was unreliable due to insufficient levels of block (<60%) measured experimentally.

LOOCV results for the 12 training drugs at 1–25× C_{max} are summarized in **Figure 7A**. As concentration increased, prediction errors improved for some drugs and worsened for others. Terfenadine's prediction error was the highest of all drugs at 1× C_{max} (0.4545) but decreased to <0.01 at 4× C_{max} (blue diamonds). On the other hand, prediction errors for chlorpromazine (blue circles), sotalol (red triangles), verapamil (green triangles), cisapride (blue × s), and dofetilide (red squares) all generally increased from 1 to 10× C_{max}. Above 10× C_{max}, prediction errors for dofetilide and ranolazine (green crosses) increased, while prediction errors for sotalol decreased. As a result of these trends, both the mean and the standard deviation of prediction errors were lowest at 1–4× C_{max} (**Figure 7A**, black points and error bars), near the concentrations for which experimental data on all currents were available for the 12 training drugs.

TABLE 5 | Leave-one-out cross validation for TdP risk prediction at 1× C_{max}.

	Left-out drug	Category	P(0)	P(1)	P(2)	Prediction error
1× C_{max}	Dofetilide	2	0	0.033 (0)	0.967 (1)	0.033 (0)
	Bepridil	2	0	0	1	0
	Sotalol	2	0	0.3475 (0)	0.6525 (1)	0.3475 (0)
	Quinidine	2	0	0	1	0
	Cisapride	1	0	1	0	0
	Terfenadine	1	0	0.5455 (0)	0.4545 (1)	0.4545 (1)
	Ondansetron	1	0	1	0	0
	Chlorpromazine	1	0.1575 (1)	0.8425 (0)	0	0.1575 (1)
	Verapamil	0	0.9995 (1)	0.0005 (0)	0	0.0005 (0)
	Ranolazine	0	0.9215 (1)	0.0785 (0)	0	0.0785 (0)
	Mexiletine	0	1	0	0	0
	Diltiazem	0	1	0	0	0
10× C_{max}	Dofetilide	2	0.0373 (0)	0.0580 (0)	0.9047 (1)	0.1326 (0)
	Bepridil	2	0	0	1	0
	Sotalol	2	0	0.712 (0)	0.288 (1)	0.712 (0)
	Quinidine	2	0	0	1	0
	Cisapride	1	0	0.728 (1)	0.272 (0)	0.272 (0)
	Terfenadine	1	0	1	0	0
	Ondansetron	1	0	1	0	0
	Chlorpromazine	1	0.9945 (1)	0.0055 (0)	0	0.9945 (1)
	Verapamil	0	0.3075 (1)	0.6925 (0)	0	0.6925 (0)
	Ranolazine	0	1	0	0	0
	Mexiletine	0	1	0	0	0
	Diltiazem	0	1	0	0	0

The TdP risk levels were assigned category values of 2 (High), 1 (Intermediate), and 0 (Low). A classifier was trained on 11 of 12 drugs and then used to predict the category probabilities [P(x), where x is the category value] and to obtain an overall prediction error for the remaining drug (see section Cross Validation). Uncertainty model simulations were used for training and prediction. For comparison, probabilities, and prediction errors from Dutta et al. (2017) are shown in parentheses when they differed from uncertainty results.

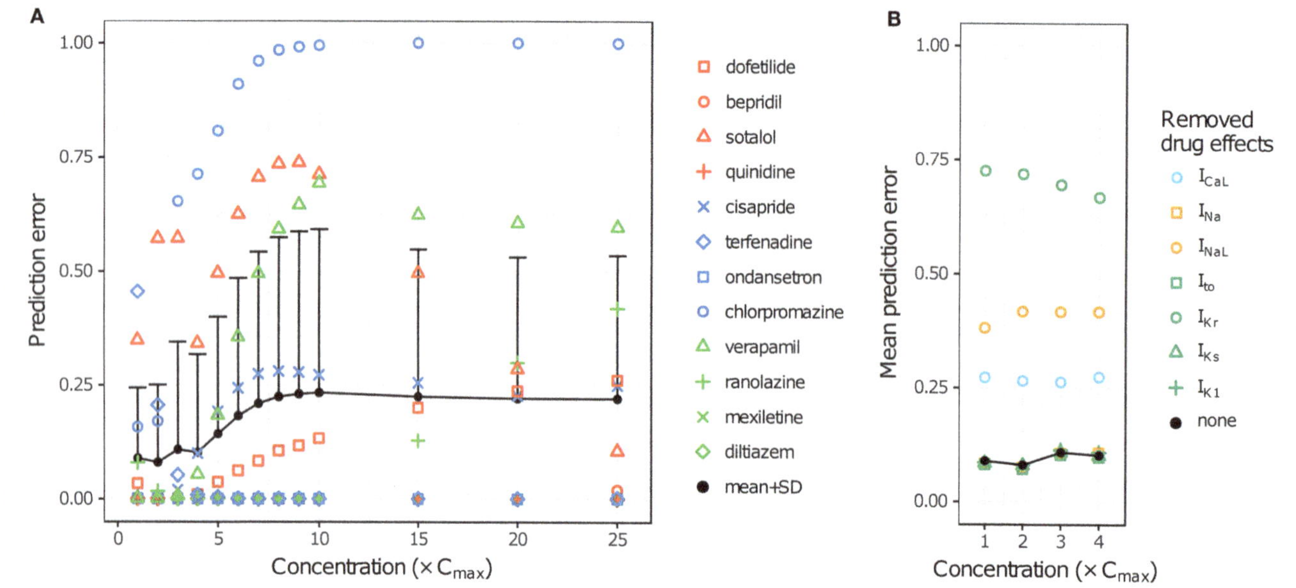

FIGURE 7 | Cross validation of TdP risk stratification with uncertainty quantification. LOOCV was performed at each concentration to assess TdP risk stratification performance. Prediction error for each drug was obtained by training on qNet distribution samples from all other drugs and calculating the mean classification error of the test drug's samples. **(A)** LOOCV at 1–25× C_{max}. Markers show the prediction errors for each drug when it was "left out," as indicated in the legend. Black points and error bars are the mean + standard deviation (SD) of prediction errors at each concentration. High TdP-risk drugs are in red, Intermediate-risk drugs are in blue, and Low-risk drugs are in green. **(B)** LOOCV at 1–4× C_{max} was repeated with the drug effects for a particular ionic current removed. Black points are the mean prediction errors from **(A)**. Markers show the mean prediction errors that resulted when drug effects on the ionic current indicated in the legend were omitted from simulations.

To explore the impact of different ionic currents on TdP risk stratification, LOOCV was repeated for a set of simulations in which drug effects on a particular ion channel were removed. This analysis was limited to 1–4× C_{max} in order to avoid concentrations at which uncertainty was due primarily to the lack of experimental data. When drug effects on I_{Na}, I_{to}, I_{Ks}, or I_{K1} were removed, prediction errors were virtually unchanged (**Figure 7B**). However, when drug effects on I_{CaL}, I_{NaL}, or I_{Kr} were removed, prediction errors increased dramatically, indicating that TdP risk stratification of the 12 CiPA training compounds depended primarily on the drug effects for these three currents. Because most of the training compounds (other than quinidine) did not block I_{Na}, I_{to}, I_{Ks}, or I_{K1} substantially at 1–4× C_{max}, their resulting impact on TdP risk stratification was expected to be minimal.

DISCUSSION

Although many potential sources of uncertainty exist within the CiPA paradigm, the primary concern for the *in silico* component is uncertainty related to *in vitro* measurements of pharmacological effects on ionic currents. This study presents methods for conducting UQ within the framework of the CiPA *in silico* assay. Previously, Dutta et al. (2017) showed that the metric qNet, derived from fixed-input AP simulations incorporating multiple ion channel pharmacology, could be used to stratify the CiPA training set of 12 compounds by relative TdP risk. This study examined the impact of uncertainty in drug effects on simulation predictions. Bootstrapping and Bayesian inference were used to estimate the joint probability distributions of drug parameters in order to quantify the variability in mean drug effects. This variability was then propagated to a set of uncertainty-input AP simulations to assess the robustness of risk stratification with qNet. UQ revealed that some drug effects were insufficiently constrained at higher concentrations to be able to stratify TdP risk with high confidence. Near therapeutic concentrations, however, TdP risk stratification was robust to the uncertainty in drug effects. This study illustrates the benefits of applying UQ under the CiPA paradigm, both during model validation and when model-based predictions are used in regulatory decision making.

UQ helped to identify challenges concerning model calibration and parameter identification that will inform future model development. Such issues are frequently encountered in models of cardiac electrophysiology but are not often addressed during model development (Fink and Noble, 2009; Shotwell and Gray, 2016). In the Li et al. (2017) I_{Kr} Markov model, drug-hERG binding kinetics was characterized by six parameters, but one parameter (drug trapping rate, K_t) was fixed at a value of 3.5×10^{-5} ms^{-1}. UQ revealed that three of the remaining five parameters (K_{max}, $EC_{50}{}^{n}$, and $V_{halftrap}$) could not be precisely estimated based on the available data. Although the current model structure was designed to allow for both linear and sigmoidal drug binding as well as drug trapping, this flexibility comes at the expense of parameter identifiability and presents difficulties for UQ. To address these issues, model recalibration and/or simplification may be warranted, as was done for a model of I_{Na} inactivation in Pathmanathan et al. (2015).

On the other hand, for some drugs, the observed hERG block kinetics could not be accurately captured by the I_{Kr} Markov model. For instance, at 10 nM cisapride, hERG block developed more slowly in the experimental traces than in fitted model, even when uncertainty was considered (Figure S4B). This suggests that alternative (and possibly more complex) model structures might be needed to characterize certain drugs. Thus, the challenge for CiPA is to define a one-size-fits-all model that is simple enough to be estimable but still accurate enough to predict TdP risk. The current approach attempts to strike an appropriate balance between the two concerns, combining the flexible dynamic representation of I_{Kr} block with a simplified pore-block approach for other currents. The final assessment of the model will depend on its validation with an additional 16 compounds, which will determine its suitability for CiPA (Colatsky et al., 2016).

Many IC_{50}-values could not be reliably estimated from the current data, an issue raised previously by Johnstone et al. (2016a). This occurred when fitted IC_{50}-values were well above the tested concentrations, resulting in high levels of uncertainty in the upper concentration ranges simulated by Li et al. (2017) and Dutta et al. (2017). The impact of this uncertainty is illustrated in results for the High-risk drug dofetilide, which is known to be a selective hERG blocker. Because its hERG selectivity could not be confirmed above 3× C_{max} with the current dataset (see **Figure 3D** and Figures S12–S15), uncertainty-input simulations of dofetilide above 10× C_{max} resulted in highly variable qNet-values, including very "safe" values similar to Low-risk drugs (**Figure 6B**). Although the impact of dofetilide on non-hERG currents is likely small, such assumptions cannot be made for new compounds, particularly if such currents and higher concentration ranges are deemed relevant for TdP risk prediction. To avoid these assumptions, *in silico* model predictions should be limited to concentrations less than or equal to the highest tested experimentally, unless the amount of drug block can be reliably extrapolated from data at lower concentrations (generally, if >60% block is achieved experimentally, see **Figure 4**). Thus, UQ highlights the importance of obtaining the appropriate data for generating reliable model predictions within the CiPA paradigm. For the current training set, TdP risk prediction appeared to depend solely on I_{CaL}, I_{NaL}, and I_{Kr} data (**Figure 7B**), so this "60% rule" may potentially only need apply to these three currents. However, the importance of I_{Na}, I_{to}, I_{Ks}, and I_{K1} cannot be discounted entirely because most of the training compounds did not substantially affect these currents. Further sensitivity analysis of qNet and testing with additional compounds may provide insight into the importance of these currents for TdP risk prediction.

Hierarchical UQ approaches may account for some of the discrepancies between observed experimental variability and the estimated variability of model outputs in the present study. For example, at the highest bepridil concentration (300 nM), the kinetics of I_{Kr} block in a few cells was noticeably faster than that of other cells and the fitted bootstrap traces. Although it is unlikely that any single method could capture all observed variability, hierarchical approaches to quantify inter-individual variability may provide a more accurate representation of the true physiological variability than do population-averaged approaches (Pathmanathan et al., 2015). Recently, Johnstone et al. (2016a) used a hierarchical statistical model to assess the inter-experiment variability of drug block data from Crumb et al. (2016). Such an approach could be explored in the future if complete dose-response data for all ionic currents become available. In the present study, however, the IC_{50} of most currents could not be reliably estimated, so a further hierarchical analysis was not warranted. For the Li et al. (2017) I_{Kr} Markov model, hierarchical methods would be more experimentally and computationally challenging. Experimentally, this would require obtaining hERG block data for each cell at multiple concentrations in order to estimate individual dose-dependent kinetics. However, due to stability and time limitations associated with the current experimental protocol, cells were only recorded at a single concentration. The computational demands of estimating hierarchical model parameters for dynamic models would also be very high because of the need to integrate differential equations. Addressing these difficulties may be unnecessary for CiPA, however, if a population-averaged approach to UQ is shown to provide sufficient information for robust TdP risk prediction.

The UQ results presented in this study illustrate the need to evaluate model predictions in the context of uncertainty. Previously, Dutta et al. (2017) demonstrated that qNet could separate the CiPA training drugs by TdP risk better than metrics based on AP or Ca^{2+} transient morphology. In addition, the mean LOOCV prediction error of qNet was lower when drugs were simulated at 10× and 20× C_{max} than at 1× C_{max}, suggesting that higher concentrations could provide better risk separation. However, this assessment was based only on fixed-input simulations. When uncertainty inputs were used to classify drugs, mean LOOCV prediction error was lowest at 1–4× C_{max} and worsened as concentration increased above 4× C_{max} (**Figure 7A**). In part, the differences in LOOCV results for fixed vs. uncertainty inputs were due to the high uncertainty in qNet for drugs such as, dofetilide and verapamil above 4× C_{max} (**Figure 6C**). However, these differences also arose because when uncertainty was low, classification with qNet probability distributions was more robust than with fixed qNet-values, which improved the mean LOOCV prediction error at 1× C_{max} (**Table 5**). UQ also provided an indication of the degree to which drugs could be separated, so LOOCV was more sensitive to subtle changes in qNet. Risk stratification of the training drugs at >4× C_{max} may be improved if additional *in vitro* data are obtained at higher concentrations and incorporated into the model. However, it is important to keep in mind that the CiPA-assigned TdP risk levels for the 12 training and 16 validation compounds are not absolute; these relative risks are mainly based on years of clinical evidence and expert opinion rather than a quantitative measure of real-world data. Effort is ongoing within the CiPA framework to develop more objective and quantitative TdP risk categorization systems based on postmarket data, which will help to refine the model and metric for more accurate TdP risk assessment.

This study did not address the issue of model uncertainty related to physiological variability because the focus of CiPA is on drug screening and obtaining an estimate of proarrhythmic risk that can be used to assess overall drug safety, not on predicting risk in specific individuals or subpopulations. However, this is an important topic for many safety pharmacology applications involving mathematical modeling. In pharmacokinetics, non-linear mixed effects (NLME) models have routinely been applied to quantify intersubject variability (Fitzmaurice et al., 2008). However, methods for quantifying physiological variability in more complex cardiac electrophysiology models are not well-established. One approach has been to use a "population" of *in silico* cardiac cell models, generated by randomly varying model parameters, to explore mechanisms underlying physiological variability and to predict the resulting variability in drug responses, such as, hERG block-induced changes in APD (Sarkar and Sobie, 2011; Britton et al., 2013). The aim of UQ is to estimate model parameters within a statistical framework and then to give probabilistic predictions. Pathmanathan et al. (2015) used data from 10 to 16 cells and NLME modeling to perform a thorough UQ analysis of a single model parameter, steady-state I_{Na} inactivation. But applying similar approaches to whole cell models, which typically have dozens of parameters, would require large amounts of data and, most likely, simpler models, as discussed by Pathmanathan et al. (2015). Nevertheless, such studies on physiological variability can be considered in complement with the results in this study concerning UQ of drug effects, providing insight into how multiple sources of uncertainty may impact variability in drug responses.

One additional issue that was not explored in this study was the effect of the number of experimental repeats on parameter uncertainty. For the manual patch clamp data used in this study, 4–10 repeats were obtained per drug concentration for the hERG experiments, and 3–4 repeats were obtained for non-hERG experiments. Thus, based on the current dataset, 3–4 experimental repeats appeared sufficient to constrain the model parameters for TdP risk prediction. However, data obtained from multiple labs or using automated, high-throughput systems can be much more variable, and more experimental repeats may be needed to accurately estimate the mean drug effect with these types of data (Elkins et al., 2013). These issues may be addressed in the future CiPA *in silico* validation phase.

In summary, risk stratification of the CiPA training drugs with the currently available data was most reliable near the maximum clinical concentration. This was because most of the *in vitro* experiments were designed around known therapeutic concentrations that often did not block the major ionic currents, and measurements at significantly higher concentrations were not consistently obtained for all drugs. The lack of experimental data produced a large degree of uncertainty in drug effects, which negatively impacted the ability to distinguish between drugs of different TdP risk at higher concentrations. Hence, our findings suggest that for new compounds, the CiPA *in silico* assay will require *in vitro* measurements at much higher drug concentrations that can achieve significant ionic current block if the model is expected to provide TdP risk predictions with high confidence. Whether this will be necessary for all seven ion channels that have been suggested as part of CiPA, however, remains to be determined.

AUTHOR CONTRIBUTIONS

KC designed and carried out the study and wrote the manuscript. SD, GM, KB, and ZL contributed to the study design and analysis. ZL supervised the project. ZL, DS, SD, GM, KB, and TC revised the manuscript. JS, PT, MW, and WW collected the data and provided guidance on interpretation of the data.

FUNDING

This project was supported by an appointment to the Research Participation Program at CDER, administered by the Oak Ridge Institute for Science and Education (ORISE) through an interagency agreement between the US Department of Energy and the FDA. The perspectives presented in this work are those of the authors and do not represent the views of the FDA or its employees. GM gratefully acknowledges personal support from a Sir Henry Dale Fellowship jointly funded by the Wellcome Trust and The Royal Society (Grant Number 101222/Z/13/Z).

ACKNOWLEDGMENTS

The authors would like to thank Dr. Norman Stockbridge for his helpful discussions and feedback on the manuscript.

REFERENCES

Antzelevitch, C., Belardinelli, L., Zygmunt, A. C., Burashnikov, A., Di Diego, J. M., Fish, J. M., et al. (2004). Electrophysiological effects of ranolazine, a novel antianginal agent with antiarrhythmic properties. *Circulation* 110, 904–910. doi: 10.1161/01.CIR.0000139333.83620.5D

Britton, O. J., Bueno-Orovio, A., Van Ammel, K., Lu, H. R., Towart, R., Gallacher, D. J., et al. (2013). Experimentally calibrated population of models predicts and explains intersubject variability in cardiac cellular electrophysiology. *Proc. Natl. Acad. Sci. U.S.A.* 110, E2098–E2105. doi: 10.1073/pnas.1304382110

Canty, A., and Ripley, B. D. (2016). *boot: Bootstrap R (S-Plus) Functions*. R package version 1.3–18.

Chézalviel-Guilbert, F., Davy, J.-M., Poirier, J.-M., and Weissenburger, J. (1995). Mexiletine antagonizes effects of sotalol on QT interval duration and its proarrhythmic effects in a canine model of Torsade de Pointes. *J. Am. Coll. Cardiol.* 26, 787–792. doi: 10.1016/0735-1097(95)00234-U

Colatsky, T., Fermini, B., Gintant, G., Pierson, J. B., Sager, P., Sekino, Y., et al. (2016). The comprehensive *in vitro* proarrhythmia assay (CiPA) initiative - update on progress. *J. Pharmacol. Toxicol. Methods* 81, 15–20. doi: 10.1016/j.vascn.2016.06.002

Crumb, W. J. Jr., Vicente, J., Johannesen, L., and Strauss, D. G. (2016). An evaluation of 30 clinical drugs against the comprehensive *in vitro* proarrhythmia assay (CiPA) proposed ion channel panel. *J. Pharmacol. Toxicol. Methods* 81, 251–262. doi: 10.1016/j.vascn.2016.03.009

Davison, A. C., and Hinkley, D. V. (1997). *Bootstrap Methods and Their Applications*. (Cambridge: Cambridge University Press).

Duff, H. J., Mitchell, L. B., Manyari, D., and Wyse, D. G. (1987). Mexiletine-quinidine combination: electrophysiologic correlates of a favorable antiarrhythmic interaction in humans. *J. Am. Coll. Cardiol.* 10, 1149–1156. doi: 10.1016/S0735-1097(87)80360-1

Dutta, S., Chang, K. C., Beattie, K. A., Sheng, J., Tran, P. N., Wu, W. W., et al. (2017). Optimization of an *in silico* cardiac cell model for proarrhythmia risk assessment. *Front. Physiol.* 8:616. doi: 10.3389/fphys.2017.00616

Efron, B., and Tibshirani, R. (1986). Bootstrap methods for standard errors, confidence intervals, and other measures of statistical accuracy. *Stat. Sci.* 1, 54–75. doi: 10.1214/ss/1177013815

Elkins, R. C., Davies, M. R., Brough, S. J., Gavaghan, D. J., Cui, Y., Abi-Gerges, N., et al. (2013). Variability in high-throughput ion-channel screening data and consequences for cardiac safety assessment. *J. Pharmacol. Toxicol. Methods* 68, 112–122. doi: 10.1016/j.vascn.2013.04.007

Fermini, B., Hancox, J. C., Abi-Gerges, N., Bridgland-Taylor, M., Chaudhary, K. W., Colatsky, T., et al. (2016). A new perspective in the field of cardiac safety testing through the comprehensive *in vitro* proarrhythmia assay paradigm. *J. Biomol. Screen.* 21, 1–11. doi: 10.1177/1087057115594589

Fink, M., and Noble, D. (2009). Markov models for ion channels: versatility versus identifiability and speed. *Philos. Trans. A Math. Phys. Eng. Sci.* 367, 2161–2179. doi: 10.1098/rsta.2008.0301

Fitzmaurice, G., Davidian, M., Verbeke, G., and Molenberghs, G. (2008). *Longitudinal Data Analysis*. New York, NY: CRC Press.

Gintant, G., Sager, P. T., and Stockbridge, N. (2016). Evolution of strategies to improve preclinical cardiac safety testing. *Nat. Rev. Drug Discov.* 15, 457–471. doi: 10.1038/nrd.2015.34

Guo, D., Zhao, X., Wu, Y., Liu, T., Kowey, P. R., and Yan, G.-X. (2007). L-type calcium current reactivation contributes to arrhythmogenesis associated with action potential triangulation. *J. Cardiovasc. Electrophysiol.* 18, 196–203. doi: 10.1111/j.1540-8167.2006.00698.x

Hansen, N. (2006). "The CMA evolution strategy: a comparing review," in *Towards a New Evolutionary Computation: Advances in the Estimation of Distribution Algorithms*, eds J. A. Lozano, P. Larra-aga, I. Inza, and E. Bengoetxea (Berlin; Heidelberg: Springer Berlin Heidelberg), 75–102.

Harrell, F. E. Jr. (2016). *Rms: Regression Modeling Strategies*. R package version 4.5–0.

Hastie, T., Tibshirani, R., and Friedman, J. H. (2009). *The Elements of Statistical Learning: Data Mining, Inference, and Prediction*. New York, NY: Springer.

January, C. T., and Moscucci, A. (1992). Cellular mechanisms of early afterdepolarizationsa. *Ann. N. Y. Acad. Sci.* 644, 23–32. doi: 10.1111/j.1749-6632.1992.tb30999.x

January, C. T., and Riddle, J. M. (1989). Early afterdepolarizations: mechanism of induction and block. A role for L-type Ca^{2+} current. *Circ. Res.* 64, 977–990. doi: 10.1161/01.RES.64.5.977

Johnstone, R. H., Bardenet, R., Gavaghan, D. J., and Mirams, G. R. (2016a). Hierarchical bayesian inference for ion channel screening dose-response data. *Wellcome Open Res.* 1, 6. doi: 10.12688/wellcomeopenres.9945.1

Johnstone, R. H., Chang, E. T. Y., Bardenet, R., de Boer, T. P., Gavaghan, D. J., Pathmanathan, P., et al. (2016b). Uncertainty and variability in models of the cardiac action potential: can we build trustworthy models? *J. Mol. Cell. Cardiol.* 96, 49–62. doi: 10.1016/j.yjmcc.2015.11.018

Li, Z., Dutta, S., Sheng, J., Tran, P. N., Wu, W., Chang, K., et al. (2017). Improving the *in silico* assessment of proarrhythmia risk by combining hERG (Human ether-à-go-go-related gene) channel–drug binding kinetics and multichannel pharmacology. *Circ. Arrhythm. Electrophysiol.* 10:e004628. doi: 10.1161/CIRCEP.116.004628

Li, Z., Dutta, S., Sheng, J., Tran, P. N., Wu, W., and Colatsky, T. (2016). A temperature-dependent *in silico* model of the human ether-a-go-go-related (hERG) gene channel. *J. Pharmacol. Toxicol. Methods* 81, 233–239. doi: 10.1016/j.vascn.2016.05.005

Milnes, J. T., Witchel, H. J., Leaney, J. L., Leishman, D. J., and Hancox, J. C. (2010). Investigating dynamic protocol-dependence of hERG potassium channel inhibition at 37 degrees C: cisapride versus dofetilide. *J. Pharmacol. Toxicol. Methods* 61, 178–191. doi: 10.1016/j.vascn.2010.02.007

Mirams, G. R., Pathmanathan, P., Gray, R. A., Challenor, P., and Clayton, R. H. (2016). White paper: uncertainty and variability in computational and mathematical models of cardiac physiology. *J. Physiol.* 594, 6833–6847. doi: 10.1113/JP271671

O'Hara, T., Virág, L., Varró, A., and Rudy, Y. (2011). Simulation of the undiseased human cardiac ventricular action potential: model formulation and experimental validation. *PLoS Comput. Biol.* 7:e1002061. doi: 10.1371/journal.pcbi.1002061

Pathmanathan, P., and Gray, R. A. (2013). Ensuring reliability of safety-critical clinical applications of computational cardiac models. *Front. Physiol.* 4:358. doi: 10.3389/fphys.2013.00358

Pathmanathan, P., Shotwell, M. S., Gavaghan, D. J., Cordeiro, J. M., and Gray, R. A. (2015). Uncertainty quantification of fast sodium current steady-state inactivation for multi-scale models of cardiac electrophysiology. *Prog. Biophys. Mol. Biol.* 117, 4–18. doi: 10.1016/j.pbiomolbio.2015.01.008

R Core Team (2016). *R: A Language and Environment for Statistical Computing*. R version 3.3.

Sarkar, A. X., and Sobie, E. A. (2011). Quantification of repolarization reserve to understand interpatient variability in the response to proarrhythmic drugs: a computational analysis. *Heart Rhythm.* 8, 1749–1755. doi: 10.1016/j.hrthm.2011.05.023

Shotwell, M. S., and Gray, R. A. (2016). Estimability analysis and optimal design in dynamic multi-scale models of cardiac electrophysiology. *J. Agric. Biol. Environ. Stat.* 21, 261–276. doi: 10.1007/s13253-016-0244-7

Soetaert, K., and Petzoldt, T. (2010). Inverse modelling, sensitivity and monte carlo analysis in R using package FME. *J. Stat. Softw.* 33, 1–28. doi: 10.18637/jss.v033.i03

Soetaert, K., Petzoldt, T., and Setzer, R. W. (2010). Solving differential equations in r: package desolve. *J. Stat. Softw.* 33, 1–25. doi: 10.18637/jss.v033.i09

Trautmann, H., Mersmann, O., and Arnu, D. (2011). *cmaes: Covariance Matrix Adapting Evolutionary Strategy*. R package version 1.0–11.

Wickham, H. (2009). *ggplot2: Elegant Graphics for Data Analysis*. New York, NY: Springer-Verlag New York.

Yan, G.-X., Wu, Y., Liu, T., Wang, J., Marinchak, R. A., and Kowey, P. R. (2001). Phase 2 early afterdepolarization as a trigger of polymorphic ventricular tachycardia in acquired long-QT syndrome. Direct evidence from intracellular recordings in the intact left ventricular wall. *Circulation* 103, 2851–2856. doi: 10.1161/01.cir.103.23.2851

3

The Clinical Pharmacokinetics and Pharmacodynamics of Warfarin when Combined with Compound Danshen: A Case Study for Combined Treatment of Coronary Heart Diseases with Atrial Fibrillation

*Chunxiao Lv[1], Changxiao Liu[2], Zhuhua Yao[3], Xiumei Gao[4], Lanjun Sun[5], Jia Liu[1], Haibo Song[6], Ziqiang Li[1], Xi Du[1], Jinxia Sun[1], Yanfen Li[1], Kui Ye[7], Ruihua Wang[1] and Yuhong Huang[1]**

[1] Department of Clinical Pharmacology, Second Affiliated Hospital of Tianjin University of Traditional Chinese Medicine, Tianjin, China, [2] State Key Laboratory of Drug Delivery Technology and Pharmacokinetics, Tianjin Institute of Pharmaceutical Research, Tianjin, China, [3] Department of Cardiology, People's Hospital of Tianjin, Tianjin, China, [4] Engineering Research Center of Modern Chinese Medicine Discovery and Preparation Technique, Tianjin University of Traditional Chinese Medicine, Tianjin, China, [5] Department of Cardiology, Second Affiliated Hospital of Tianjin University of Traditional Chinese Medicine, Tianjin, China, [6] National Center for ADR Monitoring of China, Center for Drug Reevaluation of CFDA, Beijing, China, [7] Department of Vascular Surgery, Tianjin 4th Center Hospital, Tianjin, China

***Correspondence:**
Yuhong Huang
hyh101@126.com

Warfarin is used as anticoagulant and Compound Danshen prescription (CDP) is able to promote blood circulation. The combination might produce a synergic effect for patients of coronary heart diseases (CHDs) with atrial fibrillation (AF). Whether the combination increases the bleeding risk of warfarin is unclear, so the effects of Compound Danshen dripping pill (CDDP) on the pharmacokinetics (PK) and pharmacodynamics (PD) profiles of warfarin was investigated in patients. The dose and blood concentrations of warfarin, the four indicators of blood coagulation, prothrombin time, activated partial thromboplatin time, thrombin time, fibrinogen, and international normalized ratio value were compared when with and without CDDP treatment. The population PK (PPK) and PPK-PD models were established to assess patient demographics, genetic polymorphisms and CDDP as covariates. And the Seattle Angina Questionnaire was used to evaluate clinical efficacy, and the bleeding risk of combination was analyzed. The results indicated that CDDP had little influence on PK and PD profiles of warfarin in most patients and the combination of CCDP and warfarin would be a promising alternative regime for CHD with AF patients. The study was registered on China Clinical Trial Registry with number ChiCTR-ONRC-13003523.

Keywords: warfarin, compound Danshen dripping pill, pharmacokinetics, pharmacodynamics, patients, coronary heart diseases, atrial fibrillation

INTRODUCTION

It was reported that about 10%~15% patients in coronary heart diseases (CHDs) would be associated with atrial fibrillation (AF). Moreover, about 30% patients in AF would be associated with CHD (Jason et al., 2014). The main hazard of AF is thromboembolic complications. Anticoagulants may reduce the risk of death rate in AF patients by 38% (Alpesh, 2013), so about 70–80% patients with AF are suitable for long-term use of warfarin, which was initially used in humans in the early 1950s as vitamin K antagonist (Liu et al., 2014; Darcy et al., 2017).

It is more than 100 years history in China that Compound Danshen prescription (CDP) has being applied to treat CHD, which consists of *Radix salvia miltiorrhizae*, *Radix notoginseng*, and *Borneolum* (Xin et al., 2013). In order to get market approval in the United States, the Compound Danshen dripping pill (CDDP), one Chinese patent drug of CDP, had recently completed a multinational phase III clinical trial. Pre-clinical and clinical studies have suggested that CDDP may increase coronary flow-rate and superoxide dismutase activity, expand blood vessel, promote blood circulation, relieve blood stasis, improve microcirculation, and improve hemorheological property, as well as decrease myocardial oxygen consumption (Pei et al., 2004; Zheng et al., 2007).

Concurrent use of CDDP with warfarin may be a desirable combination that may produce a synergistic effect, to relieve the symptoms of CHD with AF by CDDP part and meanwhile to decrease the incidence of thromboembolic complication by warfarin. Warfarin treatment is difficult to handle due to its narrow therapeutic window with a large inter-individual variability in the dose-response relationship (Zeng et al., 2016). Both pharmacodynamic (PD) and pharmacokinetic (PK) factors may contribute to more than 10–20 fold inter-individual variability in dose requirement (Hamberg et al., 2007; Steven et al., 2011; Zeng et al., 2016). Whether the CDDP could have impact on the PK and/or PD characteristics of warfarin increasing the bleeding risk as a result, is not clear. It is necessary, therefore, to get the information about the interactions between CDDP and warfarin. Only one literature report has been retrieved to address the interactions between CDDP and warfarin in rats (Chu et al., 2011), but any information on such interactions in humans has not been reported.

We conducted the study to explore the potential effects of CDDP on the PK and PD of warfarin in patients. During two periods on and off CDDP, we collected the dose and blood concentration of warfarin, the four indicators of blood coagulation, international normalized ratio (INR) value, and to establish appropriate population pharmacokinetics (PPK) and population pharmacodynamics (PPD) models to assess patient demographics, genetic polymorphisms and CDDP as covariates to evaluate the interaction effects of CDDP on warfarin. The seattle angina questionnaire (SAQ) was used to evaluate the effect of warfarin combined with CDDP on CHD with AF patients. In addition, 2 years follow-up was done after the two periods to learn about the drug compliance, the incidence of bleeding and other important outcomes, such as myocardial infarction, severe arrhythmia, revascularization, death and so on. We hope the study could provide useful clinical information for patients of CHD with AF.

MATERIALS AND METHODS

Patients

The study was conducted in four hospitals in Tianjin from November 2013 to January 2016. Participants, suffered from CHD with AF, had been administrated warfarin with a long time. The study included two periods, in the first period patients took warfarin (Orion Corporation, Finland) at dose titration manner guided by INR values on the daily determined basis to guarantee the INR value maintained in the range of 2–3. When the INR value reached stable and maintained for successive 2 weeks on the fixed dose of warfarin, then the participants switched to the second period, in which, 10 dripping pills of CDDP (Tianjin Tasly Group Co., Ltd, China) were added orally to patients three times per day for at least 4 weeks. The dose of warfarin was re-adjusted according to the changed INR value, until the INR value was stable again and the dose of warfarin was retained for 2 weeks. Four blood samples (4*3 ml) were collected at the end of each period for warfarin concentration assay. The sampling time points were arranged at trough (before the administration of warfarin), at peak, two random times on elimination phase (before the next dose of warfarin). All the time points of blood sampling and warfarin dosing were recorded accurately.

This study was carried out in accordance with the recommendations of Ethics committees of the Second Affiliated Hospital of Tianjin University of TCM with written informed consent from (ICF) all subjects. All subjects gave written informed consent in accordance with the Declaration of Helsinki. The protocol was approved by the Ethics committees of the Second Affiliated Hospital of Tianjin University of TCM in August 2013.

Genotyping

The information of genes which affect the metabolism of warfarin was obtained by literatures (Lin G.G. et al., 2015; Zeng et al., 2016). In this study, genotyping of *VKORC1*, *CYP2C9*3*, *CYP4F2*, *EPHX1*, and *PROC* were detected. Genomic DNA was isolated from peripheral blood leukocytes using a Genomic DNA Purification kit. Individual single-nucleotide polymorphism (SNP) loci were amplified using the polymerase chain reaction, which provided a template for allele-specific primer extension. All genotyping were performed using the gene sequencing methods (Kumar et al., 2008; Jorgensen et al., 2009; Steven et al., 2011; Lin G.G. et al., 2015). The *VKORC1* was classified by detection of 1173 C > T variant (rs9923231), the *CYP2C9*3* was classified by detection of 1075 A > C variant (rs1057910), the *CYP4F2* was classified by detection of C > T variant (rs2108622), the *EPHX1* was classified by detection of G > A variant (rs2292566), the *PROC* was classified by detection of G > T variant (rs5936).

Bioanalysis

Plasma warfarin concentrations were determined using a high-performance liquid chromatography tandem mass spectrometry method. Good chromatographic separation was achieved on an Astec CHIROBIOTIC V column (250 mm × 4.6 mm i.d., particle size 5 μm) with acetonitrile-5 mm ammonium acetate with 0.1% acetic acid in water (30:70, v/v) as the mobile phase at a flow rate of 0.50 mL/min (Jin et al., 2012). The column effluent was analyzed using a mass spectrometer in multiple reactions monitoring (MRM) mode by AB Triple Quad 5500 system in positive mode. S-warfarin, R-warfarin, and Tolglybutamide (Internal standard, IS) were extracted from plasma samples by protein precipitation with acetonitrile. Calibration curves were linear with 50.00–2000 ng/ml for S-warfarin and R-warfarin. Both intra-day and inter-day precision and accuracy of S-warfarin and R-warfarin were well within acceptance criteria (15%). The mean absolute extraction recoveries of S-warfarin, R-warfarin, and IS from human plasma were all more than 60.00%. The validated method has been successfully applied to determine of S-warfarin and R-warfarin in human plasma. Then total warfarin was the sum of S-warfarin and R-warfarin.

Software

The population PK and PK-PD models were developed using a nonlinear mixed-effect modeling approached with the NONMEM^{TM} (nonlinear mixed-effect modeling, version VII, level 2.0, ICON Development Solutions, Ellicott City, MD, United States). Goodness-of-fit diagnostic plots were prepared with R software (3.2.1, R-project. org). All models were run using the first-order conditional estimation method with interaction (FOCEI).

PK Model Development

Structural Model

After inspection of the PK profiles, a one-compartment model with first-order absorption was adopted as the optimal base model for warfarin, R-warfarin, and S-warfarin. Structural PK model was fit to plasma concentrations, and typical values of absorption rate constant (Ka), apparent volume of distribution (V/F), and oral clearance (CL/F) were calculated (where F denotes bioavailability). In this study, each individual parameter was expressed approximately as a coefficient of variation to be a log-normal distribution with the mean of population parameters according to results of previous researches (Maria et al., 2003; Eunice et al., 2010; Mark et al., 2010; Juno et al., 2013).

$$P_{ij} = P_{TV\,j} \cdot Exp(\eta_{ij}) \tag{1}$$

Where P_{ij} was the PK Parameters j for ith individual, P_{TVj} was mean of predicted population of PK Parameters j, η_{ij} was a between-subject random variable distributed normally. PK Parameters j was just about Ka, V/F, or CL/F.

The residual error model was assumed to be a mixed error model as following:

$$C_{Obs} = C_{Pred} \cdot (1 + \varepsilon_1) + \varepsilon_2 \tag{2}$$

Where C_{Obs} was the observed plasma concentration, C_{Pred} was the model prediction concentration. Both of multiplicative residual error (ε_1) and additive residual error (ε_2) were assumed as a normal distribution.

Covariate Models

These covariates were first explored graphically and each potential covariate individually added to the base model if graphical trends were shown. For the covariate models, stepwise of a forward inclusion step and a backward elimination step method was used. When a variable was considered for entering in the final model, it must reduce the objective function value (OFV) by more than 3.84 if $p < 0.05$ (5% significance level assuming a one degree of freedom, $\Delta OFV > 3.84$, df = 1; $\Delta OFV > 5.99$, df = 2; $\Delta OFV > 7.81$, df = 3). The variable that had the biggest impact on the OFV could enter first and subsequent variables added according to their impact on the OFV. The forward process described above was repeated again until no further covariates were incorporated into the model. Then, the backward elimination step was implementing. The variables were retained in the model if its removal caused an increase in OFV at least 6.63 if $p < 0.05$($\Delta OFV > 6.63$, df = 1). The relative contribution of each covariate to the goodness of fit was evaluated by deleting it from the full model. With these restrictive criteria, only covariates showing statistically significant and clinically relevant contributions were kept in the population PK (PPK) model.

In our research, the covariate of weight was described by allometric scaling equation:

$$P_{i,j} = P_{TV} \cdot (\frac{WT}{\overline{WT}})^{\theta_2} \cdot Exp(\eta_{i,j}) \tag{3}$$

Where $P_{i,j}$ was the PPK parameters, P_{TV} was a reference value of PPK parameters, WT was weight, $\overline{WT}$ was median of WT,θ_2 was effect value of WT to PPK parameter.

Other covariates (except weight) were divided into categorical covariates (gender, genotyping, administrated CDDP) and continuous covariates (age, BMI, ALT, AST, BUN, CRE, CRCL).

For the categorical covariates, the following equation was adopted:

$$If(COV = l)\ P_{i,j} = (P_{TV} + \theta_l) \cdot Exp(\eta_{i,j})\, l = 2, ...m \tag{4}$$

Where COV was a categorical covariate which had m levels, θ_l was adjusted value for P_{TV} to $P_{i,j}$.

For categorical covariates, the linear models were employed:

$$P_{i,j} = P_{TV} \cdot (1 + (COV - \overline{COV}) \cdot \theta_3) \cdot Exp(\eta_{i,j}) \tag{5}$$

Where COV was continuous covariates, $\overline{COV}$ was median of continuous covariate, θ_3 was a coefficient for the effect of covariate to parameter.

PK–PD Model Development

The PK–PD model was developed only for S-warfarin, because S-warfarin is the main active ingredient, which is 3–5 times more potent than R-warfarin. According to the plot of relationship between INR and concentration of S-warfarin, the Emax model was selected as the PD model. For the covariate models, stepwise of forward and backward method was used as mentioned in PK model.

Model Evaluation

Model Diagnostics

The PK models for warfarin, R-warfarin, S-warfarin, and PK-PD model for S-warfarin was evaluated by the goodness of fit of these models using visual inspection of diagnostic scatter plots of the observed plasma concentrations (DV) versus mean population predicted plasma concentrations (PRED), DV versus individual predicted plasma concentrations (IPRED), conditional weighted residuals (CWRES) versus time, individual weighted residuals (IWRES) versus population predictions (PRED).

TABLE 1 | The demographic profile summary for subjects.

Characteristics	Values (Range)
Number of patients	59
Number of plasma concentration points	404
Number of international normalized ratio (INR)	600
Dose of warfarin (mg)	3.41 (0.75 – 7.50)
Concentration of S-warfarin (mg/L)	0.43 (0.10 – 1.74)
Concentration of R-warfarin (mg/L)	0.89 (0.19 – 3.11)
Concentration of Total-warfarin (mg/L)	1.32 (0.29 – 4.85)
INR	2.17 (0.89 – 4.83)
Gender (male/female)	38/21
Age (year)	63 (49 – 79)
Weight (WT, Kg)	73 (50 – 99)
BMI (kg/m^2)	25.70 (16.03 – 34.48)
VKORC1 (%)	
T/T	54 (91.53%)
C/T	5 (8.47%)
*CYP2C9*3* (%)	
A/A	51 (86.44%)
A/C	8 (13.56%)
CYP4F2 (%)	
C/C	35 (59.32%)
C/T	19 (32.20%)
T/T	5 (8.47%)
EPHX1 (%)	
A/A	2 (3.39%)
A/G	33 (55.93%)
G/G	24 (40.68%)
PROC (%)	
G/G	11 (18.64%)
T/T	13 (22.03%)
T/G	35 (59.32%)
Alanine aminotransferase, ALT (U/L)	28.7 (10 – 137)
Aspartate aminotransferase, AST (U/L)	22.9 (8 – 80)
Blood urea nitrogen, BUN (mmol/L)	5.45 (2.30 – 13.70)
Creatinine, CRE (mmol/L)	81.64 (48 – 278)
Creatinine clearance rate, CRCL (ml/min)	85.39 (19.15 – 158.7)
Systolic blood pressure, SBP (mmhg)	126.73 (93 – 180)
Diastolic blood pressure, DBP (mmhg)	78.09 (60 – 105)
Long use (LU) of warfarin	32 (54.24%)

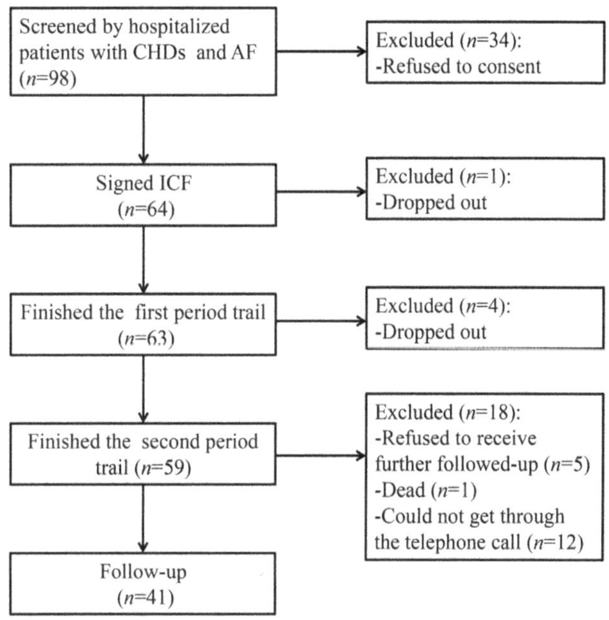

FIGURE 1 | The participant flow chart.

Model Validation

Visual predictive check (VPC)

A visual predictive check (VPC) was performed to evaluate the prediction of PK models for warfarin, R-warfarin, S-warfarin, and PK-PD model for S-warfarin. The VPC were conducted by comparing 1000 datasets simulated from the final parameters with the observed plasma concentrations. The 95% predicted intervals (PIs) obtained from the simulation were superimposed and compared with the observations.

Bootstrap

A nonparametric bootstrap analysis was used to assess the stability of the parameter estimates and to confirm the robustness of the models. The 1000 bootstrap sample datasets were re-sampled from random sampling with replacement from the original data using individual as sampling unit. Next, population parameters of final PK and PK-PD models for each dataset were estimated. Then, the median and 95% confidence intervals (CI) were constructed by obtaining the 2.5th and 97.5th smallest values out of 1000 parameters estimated from bootstrap sample datasets. Comparing with the mean and 95% CI, each estimated parameter derived from the mean and its standard error of the final parameters.

SAQ and Follow-Up

The SAQ was applied to evaluate clinical symptoms of patients. The score of SAQ was collected after each period of clinical trial, and compared by paired *t*-test. In order to learn about more information about warfarin and CDDP administration, the follow-ups were done every 6 months and lasted for 2 years. The contents of follow-up included the length of taking the combination of warfarin and CDDP and some important and

TABLE 2 | The fixed dose and blood concentrations for patients in the first and second period.

	Mean	SD	P
Fixed doe of warfarin (mg)			
First period	3.39	1.04	0.691
Second period	3.36	0.92	
Blood concentrations of warfarin (mg/L)			
First period (warfarin)	1.2225	0.5329	0.587
Second period (warfarin)	1.1849	0.4949	
First period (R-warfarin)	0.8337	0.3597	0.650
Second period (R-warfarin)	0.8128	0.3132	
First period (S-warfarin)	0.3887	0.2253	0.535
Second period (S-warfarin)	0.3721	0.2301	

main outcomes, such as bleeding, myocardial infarction, severe arrhythmia, revascularization, ACS, TIA, stroke, heart failure, death, and other conditions causing hospitalization.

RESULTS

Patients

Sixty-four patients were enrolled from four hospitals in Tianjin from November 2013 to January 2016. Fifty-nine patients completed the trial, among which 21 patients were female, and the mean age was 63 years (49–79 years). The demographic information of the patients was presented in **Table 1**. There were 404 samples and 600 INR values available for analysis from the 59 patients. About 41 patients completed the follow-up. The participant flow chart was shown in **Figure 1**.

Fixed Dose and Concentration of Warfarin

In the two periods, the fixed doses of warfarin were 3.39 ± 1.04 mg and 3.36 ± 0.92 mg ($P = 0.691$), respectively. The steady-state concentration in the two periods was 1.2225 ± 0.5329 mg kg^{-1} and 1.1849 ± 0.4949 mg kg^{-1} ($P = 0.587$) for warfarin, 0.8337 ± 0.3597 mg kg^{-1} and 0.8128 ± 0.3132 mg kg^{-1} ($P = 0.650$) for R- warfarin, 0.3887 ± 0.2253 mg kg^{-1} and 0.3721 ± 0.2301 mg kg^{-1} ($P = 0.535$) for S-warfarin. So, the fixed dose and the steady-state concentration of warfarin were no statistically different between warfarin alone and warfarin plus CDDP. The results were shown in **Table 2**.

Four Indicators of Blood Coagulation and INR Value

The results were shown in **Table 3**. The four indicators of blood coagulation, prothrombin time (PT), activated partial thromboplatin time (APTT), thrombin time (TT), fibrinogen (FIB), and INR value between the two periods at the fixed warfarin dose had no statistical differences which was compared by paired *t*-test.

TABLE 3 | The INR value, four indicators of blood coagulation, and seattle angina questionnaire (SAQ) for patients in the first and second period.

Mean ± SD	INR value	PT (s)	APTT (s)	TT (s)	FIB (g/L)	SAQ (Score)
First period	2.42 ± 0.29	25.92 ± 2.43	47.74 ± 10.48	16.95 ± 1.64	3.47 ± 0.55	19.71 ± 5.05
Second period	2.40 ± 0.61	25.64 ± 5.01	49.24 ± 9.03	17.49 ± 1.60	3.49 ± 0.80	21.02 ± 5.07
P	0.893	0.803	0.514	0.120	0.874	0.002

TABLE 4 | The covariates of pharmacokinetics (PK) models for Warfarin, R-warfarin, and S-warfarin.

Warfarin			R-warfarin			S-warfarin		
Description	**Estimate**	**RSE (%)**	**Description**	**Estimate**	**RSE (%)**	**Description**	**Estimate**	**RSE (%)**
Ka	0.999	43.7	Ka	0.586	129.4	Ka	1.69	74.6
CL/F	0.117	8	CL/F	0.158	3.7	CL/F	0.357	4.6
V/F	11.3	16	V/F	17.8	17.9	V/F	25.5	15.1
PROC on Ka(G/G)	1		*PROC* on Ka(G/G)	1		*PROC* on Ka(G/G)	1	
PROC on Ka(T/T)	0.0355	45.6	*PROC* on Ka(T/T)	0.055	120.9	*PROC* on Ka(T/T)	0.21	98.1
PROC on Ka(T/G)	4.29	60.1	*PROC* on Ka(T/G)	4.52	121.2	*PROC* on Ka(T/G)	15.7	67.5
PROC on CL(G/G)	1					CDDP* on Ka	−0.796	13.9
PROC on CL(T/T)	0.764	9.4				*CYP2C9*3* on CL(A/A)	1	
PROC on CL(T/G)	0.941	9.1				*CYP2C9*3* on CL(A/C)	0.686	14.2
IIVKa/F	0(FIX)		IIVKa/F	0.206	115.3	IIVKa/F	2.29	39.1
IIV CL/F	0.0552	8.8	IIV CL/F	0.072	9.4	IIV CL/F	0.105	7
IIV V/F	0.501	17	IIV V/F	0.588	18.9	IIV V/F	0.438	20
Prop.RE (sd)	0.172	8.8	Prop.RE (sd)	0.182	10.9	Prop.RE (sd)	0.18	7.3
Add.RE (sd)	0(FIX)		Add.RE (sd)	0(FIX)		Add.RE (sd)	0(FIX)	

When CDDP was 0 represented the first period that patients was not administrated CDDP, and CDDP was 1 represented the second period that patients was administrated CDDP.

Structural Model for PK Models

The PK profile of warfarin was in accordance with one-compartment model (Eunice et al., 2010; Steven et al., 2011) or two-compartment model (Jiang et al., 2006; Hamberg et al., 2007) based on literatures, including warfarin, S-warfarin, and R-warfarin. One-compartment and two-compartment models were both investigated for warfarin, S-warfarin and R-warfarin in this study. By comparing OFVs, goodness of fit to the models, as well as rational of parameters, one-compartment was chosen as the optimal ones for initial structure models for warfarin, S-warfarin, and R-warfarin.

Covariate Models for PK Models

Once the base structural models were established, potentially significant covariates were evaluated as described. The OFVs of structure models for warfarin, R-warfarin, and S-warfarin were -622.414, -897.240, and −1448.94. When the covariate of weight was on CL, OFV were -623.958, -898.783, and -1449.40 for warfarin, R-warfarin, and S-warfarin, respectively. When the covariate of weight was on V, OFV were -622.423, -897.335, and -1448.94 for warfarin, R-warfarin and S-warfarin, respectively. Comparing with structural models, these OFVs were not more than 3.84, so weight was not the significantly covariates for warfarin, R-warfarin, and S-warfarin.

For warfarin models, in the forward models, three covariates were brought in, *PROC* on CL, LU on CL, *PROC* on Ka, but in the backward models, LU on CL was eliminated. At last, the covariates of *PROC* on Cl and *PROC* on Ka were in the model. For R-warfarin models, *PROC* on Ka and *PROC* on CL were in the models, then *PROC* on CL was removed, so *PROC* on Ka was the significantly covariate. For S-warfarin model, the covariates *PROC* on Ka, CDDP on KA, *CYP2C9*3* on CL, *EPHX1* on V and *VKORC1* on CL were in the forward models, then two covariates were rejected, *PROC* on Ka, CDDP on KA and *CYP2C9*3* on CL were in the models as the significantly covariates. The detail information about the covariates for warfarin, R-warfarin, and S-warfarin were shown in **Table 4**.

PK–PD Model

On the basis of the final PK model, individual estimates of S-warfarin concentrations were predicted and used in the development of PD model. Graphical analyses of the INR observations versus time for S-warfarin demonstrated the Emax model may be more suitable for PD model. So direct Emax models, as well as BIOPH Emax models were investigated in our research. The parameters of the two models were all within a reasonable range, but OFV of BIOPH Emax model decreased 16.35 compared with direct Emax model. Moreover, there was a considerable time delay between INR response and drug concentration. Therefore, BIOPH Emax model was at last considered as the PD model of S-warfarin.

Once the basic structural model was established, potentially significant covariates were evaluated. From the consequence of forward and backward method and the reasonable parameters, AST was finally brought on KE0 of PD model for S-warfarin. The detail information about covariates of PK-PD model for S-warfarin was shown in **Table 5**.

Model Evaluation

Model Diagnostics

The model diagnostic plots were shown in **Figure 2**. **Figures 2A,B** demonstrated that all the data points distributed uniformly in both sides of line $y = x$. **Figures 2C,D** demonstrated that CWRES and IWRES distributed uniformly in both sides of line $y = 0$, and the absolute value were less than 4. So, these models adequately described the plasma concentrations, suggesting good fitness of the PK models for warfarin, R-warfarin, S-warfarin, and PK-PD model for S-warfarin.

Visual Predictive Check

The VPC plots were shown in **Figure 3**. Most of the observations were in the 95% PIs, so the fit of the models were acceptable in terms of visual or statistical biases for the prediction.

Bootstrap

The estimated parameters and 95% values from all bootstrap runs for the PK models of warfarin, R-warfarin, and PK-PD model of S-warfarin were given in **Table 6**. The data indicated that the parameter estimated in PK models and PK-PD model had little bias and the models were fairly robust.

The Results of SAQ and Follow-Up

The results of SAQ were shown in **Table 3**. The score of SAQ during trail were 19.71 ± 5.05 for the first period and

TABLE 5 | The covariates of pharmacokinetics–pharmacodynamics (PK–PD) models for S-warfarin.

Description	Estimate	RSE (%)
KA	1.44	44.2
CL/F	0.356	4.7
V/F	26.1	14.3
PROC on Ka(T/T)	0.272	64
PROC on Ka(T/G)	12.2	65.1
CDDP* on Ka	− 0.728	20.1
*CYP2C9*3* on CL(A/C)	0.69	14.5
KE0	0.0365	48.2
E0	1.21	4.9
EMAX	3.54	81.1
EC50	0.889	113.6
AST ON KE0	0.0006	0.7
IIV KA	2.14	58.9
IIV CL/F	0.0984	14.5
IIV V/F	0.503	41.6
IIVE0	0.0196	54.6
IIVEC50	0.198	31.6
Residual errors		
PK Prop.RE (*SD*)	0.014	7.7
PK Add.RE (*SD*)	0 (FIX)	
PD Prop.RE (*SD*)	0.0112	5.3
PD Add.RE (*SD*)	0 (FIX)	

**When CDDP was 0 represented the first period that patients was not administrated CDDP, and CDDP was 1 represented the second period that patients was administrated CDDP.*

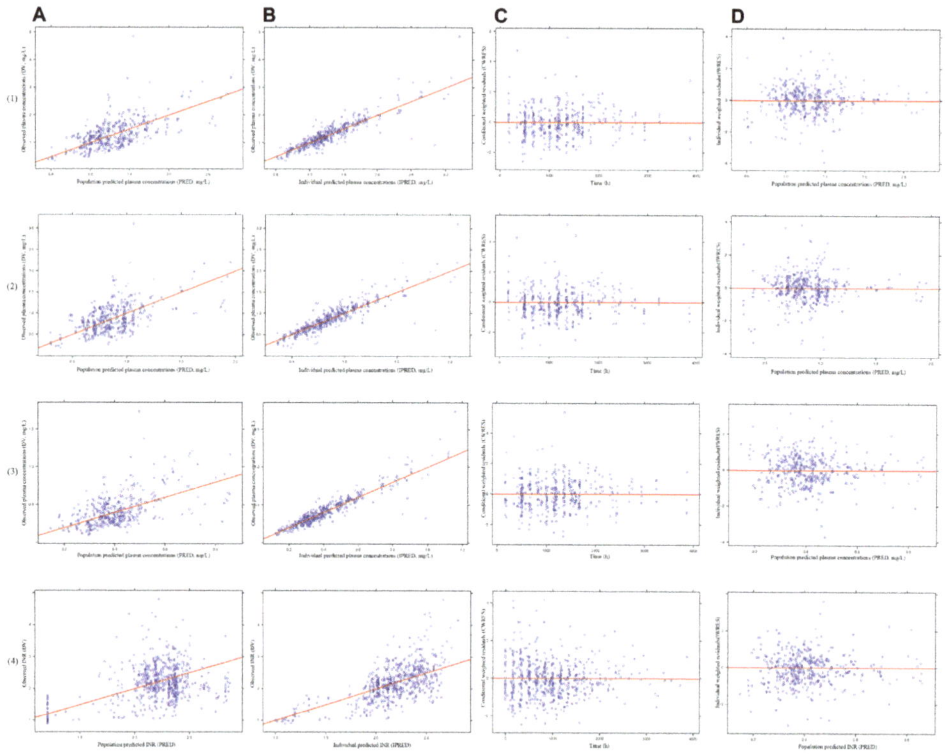

FIGURE 2 | The model diagnostics plots of pharmacokinetics (PK) models for warfarin (1), R-warfarin (2) and S-warfarin (3) and pharmacokinetics–pharmacodynamics (PK–PD) model for S-warfarin (4). **(A)** The observed plasma concentrations (DV) versus mean population predicted plasma concentrations (PRED), **(B)** The DV versus individual predicted plasma concentrations (IPRED), **(C)** The conditional weighted residuals (CWRES) versus time, **(D)** The individual weighted residuals (IWRES) versus population predictions (PRED).

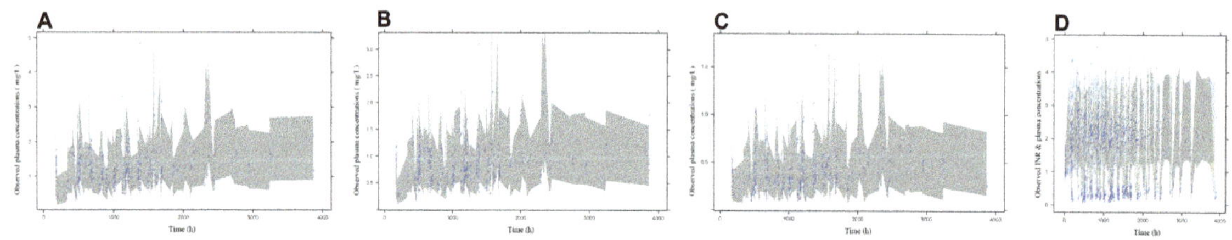

FIGURE 3 | The VPC plots of PK models for warfarin **(A)**, R-warfarin **(B)**, and S-warfarin **(C)** and PK-PD model for S-warfarin **(D)**. The Shadows were the 95th PIs.

21.02 ± 5.07 for the second period. There was significant difference between two periods ($P = 0.002$). During 2 years of follow-up, the mean length of taking CDDP is 0.96 ± 0.80 years and 1.70 ± 0.83 years for warfarin. Severe arrhythmia occurred in one patient, revascularization in two patients, death in one patient, and 16 patients were hospitalized due to other conditions. The incidence of severe arrhythmia, revascularization, death, and hospitalization were 2.44% (1/41), 4.88% (2/41), 2.44% (1/41), and 39.02% (16/41).

DISCUSSION

In this study a total of 404 blood samples, instead of 472 as required by protocol (eight for each patient), were collected for warfarin assay. There were 600 INR values obtained in the study. Being serious in nature of the heart disease, the compliance of the enrolled patients in the study was relatively low. With the limited number of patients enrolled in this study, we use the principle of PPK algorithm with more detail information collected from the participants, as described in the Guidance for Industry PPK published by FDA which states "Since patients are studied in more detail in this design, the design requires fewer subjects, and the relationship of trough levels to patient characteristics can be evaluated with more precision". Similarly, in some other PPK-PPD studies (Hamberg et al., 2007; Parker et al., 2015; Agarwal et al., 2016; Pier et al., 2017), these numbers of subjects enrolled were comparable to our study.

These CHD patients with AF had been taking warfarin for a long period of time to decrease the risk of thromboembolic

TABLE 6 | The bootstrap results of PK models for warfarin, R-warfarin and PK-PD model for S-warfarin.

Warfarin					R-Warfarin					S-Warfarin				
Description	Model	Bootstrap (95%CI)			Description	Model	Bootstrap (95%CI)			Description	Model	Bootstrap (95%CI)		
	Median	Median	2.5%	97.5%		Median	Median	2.5%	97.5%		Median	Median	2.5%	97.5%
Ka	0.999	0.839	0.114	3.42	Ka	0.586	0.258	0.0695	0.965	KA	1.44	1.82	0.613	11.9
CL/F	0.117	0.116	0.094	0.145	CL/F	0.158	0.158	0.151	0.169	CL/F	0.356	0.359	0.333	0.381
V/F	11.3	10.6	7.36	14.7	V/F	17.8	15.3	10.5	23.7	V/F	26.1	24.4	18.3	33.1
PROC on Ka(T/T)	0.0355	0.0478	0.0102	1.12	*PROC* on Ka(T/T)	0.055	0.108	0.0224	0.400	*PROC* on Ka(T/T)	0.272	0.171	0.00849	2.93
PROC on Ka(T/G)	4.29	4.42	0.689	45.6	*PROC* on Ka(T/G)	4.52	8.11	1.68	59.6	*PROC* on Ka(T/G)	12.2	7.69	1.25	58.74
PROC on CL(T/T)	0.764	0.772	0.608	0.957						CDDP* on Ka	-0.728	-0.756	-0.866	0.095
PROC on CL(T/G)	0.941	0.922	0.691	1.13						*CYP2C9*3* on CL(A/C)	0.69	0.65	0.52	0.95
										KE0	0.0365	0.0331	0.0254	0.0367
										E0	1.21	1.30	1.16	1.48
										EMAX	3.54	3.63	3.23	3.79
										EC50	0.889	0.921	0.723	1.31
										AST ON KE0	0.0006	0.0004	0.0001	0.0011
IIVKa/F	0(FIX)	0	0	0	IIVKa/F	0.206	0.275	0.00280	0.974	IIV KA	2.14	2.35	0.52	5.08
IIV CL/F	0.0552	0.0514	0.0307	0.0772	IIV CL/F	0.072	0.063	0.046	0.089	IIV CL/F	0.0984	0.0936	0.0724	0.118
IIV V/F	0.501	0.538	0.193	1.162	IIV V/F	0.588	0.483	0.284	0.791	IIV V/F	0.503	0.396	0.145	0.917
										IIVE0	0.0196	0.015	0.009	0.024
										IIVEC50	0.198	0.141	0.124	0.297
Prop.RE (sd)	0.172	0.168	0.134	0.201	Prop.RE (sd)	0.182	0.196	0.153	0.230	PK Prop.RE(sd)	0.014	0.017	0.015	0.020
Add.RE (sd)	0(FIX)	0	0	0	Add.RE (sd)	0(FIX)	0	0	0	PK Add.RE (sd)	0(FIX)	0	0	0
										PD Prop.RE (sd)	0.0112	0.013	0.0089	0.018
										PD Add.RE (sd)	0(FIX)	0	0	0

complications. The underlying conditions included hypertension (28.8%), diabetes (18.7%), and cerebral ischemic stroke (16.9%) in the study. Various medications were concomitantly used in the patients due to its complicated property of the disease. More frequently used drugs included β-blockers (39.0%), nitric esters (33.9%), statins (22.0%), diuretics (22.0%), cardiac glycosides (18.7%), calcium channel blockers (15.3%), and antidiabetic drugs (15.3%). Identification of the effect of CDDP on profiles of PK and PD of warfarin were established on a self-control design, maintaining all concomitant medications except warfarin from beginning to end of trial. The INR value, fixed warfarin doses and trough concentration of plasma warfarin had not significantly difference ($P > 0.05$) with or without CDDP. That suggested there is no drug-drug interaction between CDDP and warfarin in human, and CDDP did not affect anticoagulant mechanism of warfarin because CDDP did not interfere metabolic process of warfarin in human.

The PPK models for warfarin, S-warfarin and R-warfarin and PPD model for S-warfarin were developed with assessing patient demographics, genetic polymorphisms and CDDP as covariates. The PK behavior of warfarin, S-warfarin and R-warfarin was in accordance with one-compartment model or two-compartment model based on literatures (Jiang et al., 2006; Hamberg et al., 2007; Eunice et al., 2010; Steven et al., 2011). The One-compartment models were more optimal and reasonable for warfarin, either S-warfarin or R-warfarin in our study. The consequence of *CYP2C9*3* on CL of S-warfarin was identical to other researches (Chanan et al., 2016; Darcy et al., 2017), but the age, gender, weight had no significant effects on S-warfarin or R-warfarin which were inconsistent with some research (Hamberg et al., 2007; John et al., 2012; Lin R.F. et al., 2015). The gene of *CYP4F2*, *PROC*, *VKOR*, *CYP2C9*3*, and *EPHX1* were investigated in this research. There was no precise conclusion about the effects of gene subtypes on PK and PD characteristics of warfarin due to limited distribution rate of each individual subtype, which was consistent with other literatures (Özer et al., 2011; Radka et al., 2015). The change of the fixed dose of warfarin in EPHXI gene subtype A/A is higher than the other gene types. Because only two patients with *EPHX1* gene subtype A/A were enrolled, it is difficult to make the conclusion that CDDP affect the PK and PD characteristics of warfarin on this kind of patient.

The study result also suggested by PPK model and PPD model that there may be no influence of CDDP on PK and PD of warfarin in patients, although CDDP was as a covariate on Ka of S-warfarin. There had a great variation of Ka with a higher RSE (43.7%, 129.4%, 74.6% for PK models of warfarin, R- warfarin, and S- warfarin) meaning an incredible consequence about absorption. The bioavailability of warfarin is more than 95% (Mark et al., 2010; Juno et al., 2013), some reports had applied 100% bioavailability when developing models (Maria et al., 2003; Hamberg et al., 2007; Steven et al., 2011). Moreover, there were few reports to evaluate the absorption of warfarin due to its high bioavailability.

The SAQ was applied to evaluate efficacy effect of the co-treatment of warfarin and CDDP in the patients of CHD with AF. It's showed that there was significant difference in the SAQ score with or without CDDP. It may indicate that CDDP can improve the life quality of CHD with AF patients when both INR and dose of warfarin are stable. During 2 years follow-up, many patients still took the combination for a long time, and there were no report about bleeding. So, the combination of CDDP with warfarin might relieve clinical symptoms and provide benefits for patients with CHD and AF. However, this was not a randomized clinical trial, some researches would be needed to further demonstrate the clinical efficacy.

CONCLUSION

In summary, robust and stable PK-PD models have been successfully developed for evaluating the effect of CDDP on the PK and PD of warfarin. The results indicated that CDDP did not influence the INR stability and PK characteristic of warfarin when warfarin was administrated simultaneously with CDDP in most CHDs patients. Moreover, The SAQ and follow-up results showed the CDDP combined with warfarin might provide benefit in clinical practice for patients. This study would provide some useful information of the combined regimen of CDDP and warfarin for the treatment of CHDs with AF, but the result in Chinese genetic subtypes of *EPHX1* and the clinical efficacy study need to be confirmed further.

AUTHOR CONTRIBUTIONS

CLv and YH wrote the manuscript. CLiu, YH, XG, and HS designed the research. ZY, LS, XD, JS, YL, and KY performed research. CLv, JL, ZL, and RW analyzed data.

ACKNOWLEDGMENTS

This study was supported by the Chinese National Natural Science Foundation (No. 81273936). We wish to thank all those who volunteered to participate in this study.

REFERENCES

Agarwal, N., McPherson, J. P., Bailey, H., Gupta, S., Werner, T. L., Reddy, G., et al. (2016). A phase I clinical trial of the effect of belinostat on the pharmacokinetics and pharmacodynamics of warfarin. *Cancer Chemother. Pharmacol.* 77, 299–308. doi: 10.1007/s00280-015-2934-1

Alpesh, A. (2013). Oral anticoagulation to reduce risk of stroke in patients with atrial fibrillation: current and future therapies. *Clin. Interv. Aging* 8, 75–84. doi: 10.2147/CIA.S37818

Chanan, S., Simcha, B., Mordechai, M., Meir, B., and Yoseph, C. (2016). Quantitative assessment of *CYP2C9* genetic polymorphisms effect on the oral clearance of S-Warfarin in healthy subjects. *Mol. Diagn. Ther.* 21, 75–83. doi: 10.1007/s40291-016-0247-7

Chu, Y., Zhang, L., Wang, X. Y., Guo, J. H., Guo, Z. X., and Ma, X. H. (2011). The effect of compound Danshen dripping pills, a Chinese herb medicine, on the pharmacokinetics and pharmacodynamics of warfarin in rats. *J. Ethnopharmacol.* 137, 1457–1461. doi: 10.1016/j.jep.2011.08.035

Darcy, R. F., Allan, E. R., Richard, C. B., and Timothy, S. T. (2017). CYP2C9 genotype-dependent warfarin pharmacokinetics: impact of CYP2C9 genotype on R- and S-warfarin and their oxidative metabolites. *J. Clin. Pharmacol.* 57, 382–393. doi: 10.1002/jcph.813

Eunice, Y., Ivelina, G., Stephen, W., Danny, S., and Leon, A. (2010). Ethnic differences in the population pharmacokinetics and pharmacodynamics of warfarin. *J. Pharmacokinet. Pharcodyn.* 37, 3–24. doi: 10.1007/s10928-009-9138-4

Hamberg, A. K., Dahl, M. L., Barban, M., Scordo, M. G., Wadelius, M., Pengo, V., et al. (2007). A PK-PD model for predicting impact of age, *CYP2C9* and *VKORC1* genotype on individualization of Warfarin therapy. *Clin. Pharmacol. Ther.* 81, 529–538. doi: 10.1038/sj.clpt.6100084

Jason, A., Paul, K., Dobromir, D., and Stanley, N. (2014). The clinical profile and pathophysiology of atrial fibrillation relationships among clinical features, epidemiology, and mechanisms. *Circ. Res.* 114, 1453–1467. doi: 10.1161/CIRCRESAHA.114.303211

Jiang, X. M., Elaine, Y. L. B., and Andrew, J. M. (2006). Investigation of the effects of herbal medicines on warfarin response in healthy subjects: a population pharmacokinetic-pharmacodynamic modeling approach. *J. Clin. Pharmacol.* 46, 1370–1378. doi: 10.1177/0091270006292124

Jin, S., Zhang, Y. F., Chen, X. Y., Liu, K., and Zhong, D. F. (2012). Enantioselective determinination of R-warfarin/S-warfarin in human plasma using liquid chromatography-tandem mass spectrometry and its application in a drug-drug interaction study. *Acta Pharm. Sin.* 47, 105–109.

John, M., Andrew, A. S., Berit, P. J., Heather, M. J., Melanie, G., and Paul, E. R. (2012). The pharmacokinetics and pharmacodynamics of single dose (R)- and (S)-warfarin administered separately and together: relationship to *VKORC1* genotype. *Br. J. Clin. Pharmacol.* 75, 208–216. doi: 10.1111/j.1365-2125.2012.04335.x

Jorgensen, A., Al-Zubiedi, S., Zhang, E., Keniry, A., Hanson, A., Hughes, D., et al. (2009). Genetic and environmental factors determining clinical outcomes and cost of warfarin therapy: a prospective study, accepted. *Pharmacogenet. Genomics* 19, 800–812. doi: 10.1097/FPC.0b013e3283317ab5

Juno, Y., Rengarajan, B., and Yoo, B. K. (2013). Self-nanoemulsifying drug delivery system of lutein: physicochemical properties and effect bioavailability of warfarin. *Biomol. Ther.* 21, 173–179. doi: 10.4062/biomolther.2013.011

Kumar, V., Brundage, R. C., Oetting, W. S., Leppik, I. E., and Tracy, T. S. (2008). Differential genotype dependent inhibition of Cyp2c9 in humans. *Drug Metab. Dispos.* 36, 1242–1248. doi: 10.1124/dmd.108.020396

Lin, G. G., Yi, L., Zhang, K., Sun, Y., Wang, L. N., Zhang, R., et al. (2015). Improvements in CYP2C9 genotyping accuracy are needed: a report of the first proficiency testing for warfarin-related CYP2C9 and VKORC1 genotyping in China. *J. Cardiovasc. Pharmacol.* 66, 129–134. doi: 10.1097/FJC.0000000000000254

Lin, R. F., Lin, W. W., Wang, C. L., Huang, P. F., and Fang, S. J. (2015). Population pharmacokinetic/pharmacodynamic modeling of warfarin by nonlinear mixed effects model. *Acta Pharm. Sin.* 50, 1280–1284.

Liu, X. B., Huang, H. M., Yu, J. H., Gao, G. L., Feng, L. L., Xu, Q., et al. (2014). Warfarin compared with aspirin for older Chinese patients with stable coronary heart diseases and atrial fibrillation complications. *Int. J. Clin. Pharm. Ther.* 52, 454–459. doi: 10.5414/CP201996

Maria, P., Eva, M. P., Leon, A., and Malcolm, R. (2003). A Bayesian method based on clotting factor activity for the prediction of maintenance warfarin dosage regimens. *Ther. Drug Monit.* 25, 36–40. doi: 10.1097/00007691-200302000-00005

Mark, K., Dennis, G., and Veronica, M. (2010). Warfarin bioavailability with feeding tubes and enteral formula. *JPEN J. Parenter Enteral Nutr.* 34, 300–304. doi: 10.1177/0148607109337257

Özer, M., Demirci, Y., Sarikaya, S., Karalti, L., Kaspar, C., Hizel, C., et al. (2011). The effect of polymorphisms in CYP2C9, CYP4F2, EPHX1 and VKORC1 on warfarin dose in Turkish patients. *Curr. Opin. Biotechnol.* 22, S125–S125. doi: 10.1016/j.copbio.2011.05.408

Parker, S. L., Frantzeskakic, F., Wallisa, S. C., Diakakic, C., Giamarelloue, H., Koulentia, D., et al. (2015). Population pharmacokinetics of fosfomycin in critically Ill patients. *Antimicrob. Agents Chemother.* 59, 6471–6476. doi: 10.1128/AAC.01321-15

Pei, W. J., Zhao, X. F., Zhu, Z. M., Lin, C. Z., Zhao, W. M., and Zheng, X. H. (2004). Study of the determination and pharmacokinetics of compound Danshen dripping pills in human serum by column switching liquid chromatography electrospray ion trap mass spectrometry. *J. Chromatogr. B* 809, 237–242. doi: 10.1016/S1570-0232(04)00512-4

Pier, G. C., Anna, C., Virginia, R. M., Davide, L., Maria, E. Z., Renato, F., et al. (2017). Population pharmacokinetics and dosing considerations for the use of daptomycin in adult patients with haematological malignancies. *J. Antimicrob. Chemother.* 72, 2342–2350. doi: 10.1093/jac/dkx140

Radka, V., David, J. H., and Pavel, S. (2015). Microsomal epoxide hydrolase 1 (EPHX1): gene, structure, function, and role in human disease. *Gene* 571, 1–8. doi: 10.1016/j.gene.2015.07.071

Steven, L., Sameh, A. Z., Ellen, H., Ivan, M., Andrea, L. J., Panos, D., et al. (2011). The population pharmacokinetics of *R*- and *S*-warfarin: effect of genetic and clinical factors. *Br. J. Clin. Pharmacol.* 73, 66–76. doi: 10.1111/j.1365-2125.2011.04051.x

Xin, X., Zou, H. M., Zheng, N. M., Xu, X. C., Liu, Y. M., Wang, X. X., et al. (2013). Metabonomic strategy to the evaluation of Chinese medicine compound Danshen dripping pills interfering myocardial ischemia in rats. *Evid. Based Complement. Alternat. Med.* 2013:718305. doi: 10.1155/2013/718305

Zeng, W. T., Xu, Q., Li, C. H., Chen, W. Y., Sun, X. T., Wang, X., et al. (2016). Influence of genetic polymorphisms in cytochrome P450 oxidoreductase on the variability in stable warfarin maintenance dose in Han Chinese. *Eur. J. Clin. Pharmacol.* 72, 1327–1334. doi: 10.1007/s00228-016-2098-x

Zheng, X. H., Zhao, X. F., Zhao, X., Wang, S. X., Wei, Y. M., and Zheng, J. B. (2007). Determination of the main bioactive metabolites of *Radix Salvia miltiorrhizae* in compound Danshen dripping pills and the tissue distribution of Danshensu in rabbit by SPE-HPLC-MSn. *J. Sep. Sci.* 30, 851–857. doi: 10.1002/jssc.200600287

4

Determinants of Isoform-Specific Gating Kinetics of hERG1 Channel: Combined Experimental and Simulation Study

Laura L. Perissinotti[1†], Pablo M. De Biase[1†], Jiqing Guo[2†], Pei-Chi Yang[3†], Miranda C. Lee[1], Colleen E. Clancy[3*], Henry J. Duff[2*] and Sergei Y. Noskov[1*]*

[1] Centre for Molecular Simulations, Department of Biological Sciences, Faculty of Science, University of Calgary, Calgary, AB, Canada, [2] Libin Cardiovascular Institute of Alberta, Faculty of Medicine, University of Calgary, Calgary, AB, Canada, [3] Department of Physiology and Membrane Biology, University of California, Davis, Davis, CA, United States

***Correspondence:**
Laura L. Perissinotti
laura.perissinotti@ucalgary.ca
Colleen E. Clancy
ceclancy@ucdavis.edu
Henry J. Duff
hduff@ucalgary.ca
Sergei Y. Noskov
snoskov@ucalgary.ca

† These authors have contributed equally to this work.

I_{Kr} is the rapidly activating component of the delayed rectifier potassium current, the ion current largely responsible for the repolarization of the cardiac action potential. Inherited forms of long QT syndrome (LQTS) (Lees-Miller et al., 1997) in humans are linked to functional modifications in the Kv11.1 (hERG) ion channel and potentially life threatening arrhythmias. There is little doubt now that hERG-related component of I_{Kr} in the heart depends on the tetrameric (homo- or hetero-) channels formed by two alternatively processed isoforms of hERG, termed hERG1a and hERG1b. Isoform composition (hERG1a- vs. the b-isoform) has recently been reported to alter pharmacologic responses to some hERG blockers and was proposed to be an essential factor pre-disposing patients for drug-induced QT prolongation. Very little is known about the gating and pharmacological properties of two isoforms in heart membranes. For example, how gating mechanisms of the hERG1a channels differ from that of hERG1b is still unknown. The mechanisms by which hERG 1a/1b hetero-tetramers contribute to function in the heart, or what role hERG1b might play in disease are all questions to be answered. Structurally, the two isoforms differ only in the N-terminal region located in the cytoplasm: hERG1b is 340 residues shorter than hERG1a and the initial 36 residues of hERG1b are unique to this isoform. In this study, we combined electrophysiological measurements for HEK cells, kinetics and structural modeling to tease out the individual contributions of each isoform to Action Potential formation and then make predictions about the effects of having various mixture ratios of the two isoforms. By coupling electrophysiological data with computational kinetic modeling, two proposed mechanisms of hERG gating in two homo-tetramers were examined. Sets of data from various experimental stimulation protocols (HEK cells) were analyzed simultaneously and fitted to Markov-chain models (M-models). The minimization procedure presented here, allowed assessment of suitability of different Markov model topologies and the corresponding parameters that describe the channel kinetics. The kinetics modeling pointed to key differences in the gating kinetics that were linked to the full channel structure. Interactions between soluble domains and the transmembrane part of the channel appeared to be critical determinants of the gating kinetics. The structures of the full channel in the open and closed states were compared for the first time using the recent Cryo-EM resolved structure for full open hERG channel and an homology model for the closed state, based on the highly homolog EAG1 channel. Key potential interactions which emphasize the importance of electrostatic interactions between N-PAS cap, S4-S5, and C-linker are suggested based on the structural analysis. The derived kinetic parameters were later used in higher order models of cells and tissue to track down the effect of varying the ratios of hERG1a and hERG1b on cardiac action potentials and computed electrocardiograms. Simulations suggest that the recovery from inactivation of hERG1b may contribute to its physiologic role of this isoform in the action potential. Finally, the results presented here contribute to the growing body of evidence that hERG1b significantly affects the generation of the cardiac I_{Kr} and plays an important role in cardiac electrophysiology. We highlight the importance of carefully revisiting the Markov models previously proposed in order to properly account for the relative abundance of the hERG1 a- and b- isoforms.

Keywords: long-QT, hERG Isoforms, gating kinetics, arrhythmias, computational models, Markov process

INTRODUCTION

The I_{Kr} current is a primary contributor to the repolarization of the human cardiac muscle, a delayed rectifier potassium current conducted by the Kv11.1 ion channel (more commonly referred to as human ether-a-go-go-related gene, or hERG1) (Sanguinetti et al., 1995; Li et al., 1996). The Kv11.1 channel is homologous in structure to other voltage-gated potassium channels (**Figure 1**) and is assembled as a tetramer to become a fully functioning ion channel, but has very different kinetics compared to other potassium channels. Inactivation is much faster than activation, and consequently, current is suppressed at positive potentials but rebounds on repolarization as channels quickly recover from inactivation and slowly close. During an action potential, this gating behavior produces a resurgent current that peaks during the repolarization phase. Mutations, channels block by drugs and/or impaired trafficking of Kv11.1 channels to the cell membrane lead to prolongation of the QT interval on the surface electrocardiogram (LQTS), leading to a potentially life threatening ventricular arrhythmia (Behere et al., 2014). Since the physiological role of I_{Kr} is to repolarize the late phase of cardiac action potentials, hERG1 has a clear link to these arrhythmias (Robertson et al., 2008; Gustina and Trudeau, 2009; Robertson, 2012; Vandenberg et al., 2012). That is, if I_{Kr} is reduced, due to loss-of-function mutations or action of small molecules (drugs), patients are more likely to develop severe arrhythmias initiated by premature beats.

Up to date, our understanding of how I_{Kr} contributes to the ventricular repolarization is based primarily on studies utilizing heterologous expression of the originally identified hERG1 a-isoform (Sanguinetti et al., 1995; Trudeau et al., 1995; Smith et al., 1996; Wang et al., 1997). More recent studies showed that native I_{Kr} result from hetero-tetramers formed by the co-assembly of two hERG isoforms termed hERG1a and hERG1b. Two splice variants—hERG1a and hERG1b are co-expressed not only in cardiac tissue, but also in neurons and smooth muscles (Chiesa et al., 1997; Ohya et al., 2002). Importantly, isoforms display very different gating kinetics (Lees-Miller et al., 2003). The hERG gating is modulated by the cytoplasmic domains (N-terminal or PAS domain, CNBD and C-linker) in a way that still remains largely unknown but of a critical importance for unraveling structural mechanisms responsible for QT prolongation. In particular, a mutation in the N-terminal of hERG1b was discovered in a patient with long QT Syndrome (LQTS), highlighting the importance of this isoform in cardiac repolarization (Robertson et al., 2008; Robertson, 2012).

Many drugs are known to block ion current across Kv11.1 channels, resulting in an acquired form of LQTS (Larsen et al., 2010). Many blockers exhibit state-dependent activity and hence their propensity to later hERG currents is related to the channel's gating kinetics. It has recently been shown that EA4031, a selective blocker of hERG1 currents, differs in effectiveness on homo-tetrameric vs. hetero-tetrameric channels formed of different isoforms (Sale et al., 2008). Similar findings were also reported for hERG1 activators. Larsen et al. (2010) showed that activators such as NS1643 display differential effects on the homo-tetrameric channels formed by two hERG1 isoforms (Holzem et al., 2016). Due to the therapeutic risks hidden in hERG1 blockers and potential of hERG1 activators, establishing differences in gating mechanisms of two isoforms is critically important. Structurally, the two isoforms differ only in the N-terminal region located in the cytoplasm: hERG1b is 340 residues shorter than hERG1a and the initial 36 residues of hERG1b are unique to this isoform (Lees-Miller et al., 1997; Splawski et al., 1998) (**Figure 1**). As mentioned above, the channel gating is modulated by the cytoplasmic domains (PAS, CNBD, and C-linker) in a way that still remains unknown (Trudeau et al., 2011; Ng et al., 2014; Morais-Cabral and Robertson, 2015; Perry et al., 2015). Consequently, as hERG1b is lacking the entire PAS/Pas-cap domains, it has a different gating behavior compared to hERG1a.

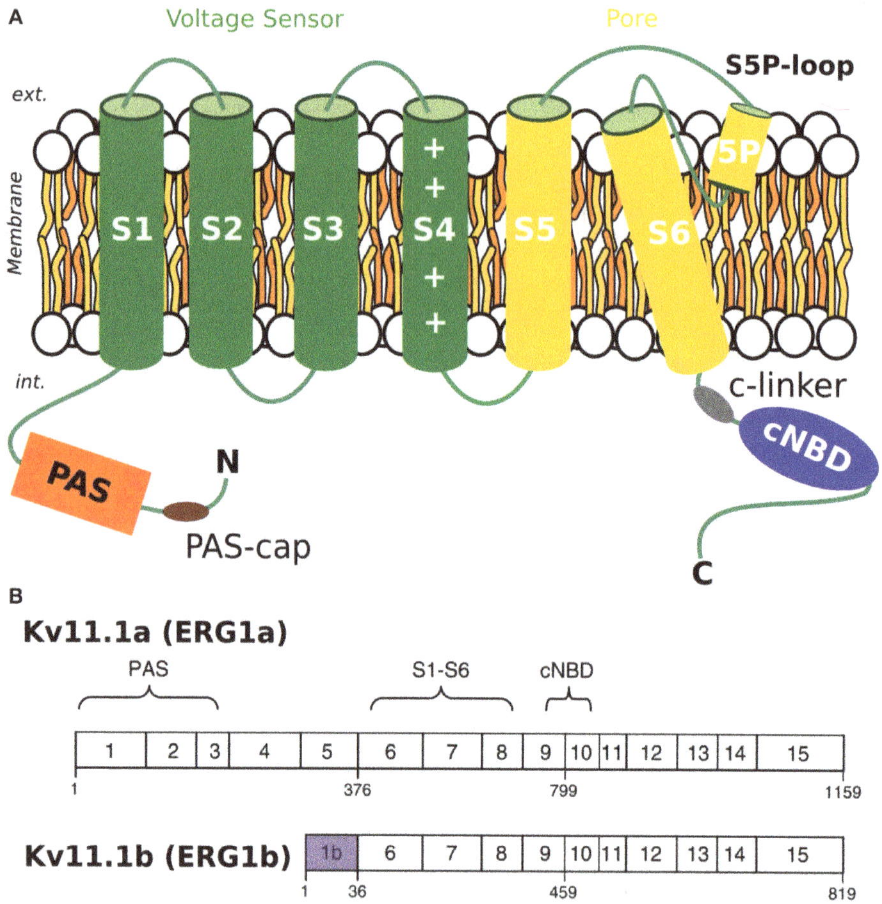

FIGURE 1 | (A) Topology of Kv11.1 or hERG channel. **(B)** Comparison of a-isoform and b-isoform. Exons of each of the two splice variants, with a-isoform on the top and b-isoform on the bottom.

The isoform originally discovered was hERG1a which is considered the full length transcript of the associated gene, and is often referred to simply as hERG1 when not being compared to other isoforms. Additionally, these isoforms are present in relatively fixed ratios, which depend on the cellular environment (Larsen et al., 2007, 2008). Deviations from these ratios, leading to abnormal abundance of a particular Kv11.1 isoform, may result in heart beat anomalies (Larsen et al., 2008; Kannankeril et al., 2010; Robertson, 2012).

Recently, hERG1b was found to be critical for human cardiac repolarization and a 1b-specific mutation associated with intrauterine fetal death was discovered (Jones et al., 2014, 2015, 2016). Additionally, the relative levels of expression appear to be greater in the young compared with the adult heart (Wang et al., 2008; Crotti et al., 2013). Evidence supports that when hERG1a and hERG1b are present in heterologous expression systems, they co-assemble to form hetero-tetrameric channels, although it is unknown if there is a preferred stoichiometry of these channels (London et al., 1997).

As previously mentioned, the two isoforms gating properties differ substantially. The hERG1 b- isoform is characterized by faster kinetics of activation, recovery from inactivation, and most prominently, deactivation (Larsen et al., 2008, 2010). These differences in gating kinetics are due mainly to the differences in the N-terminal regions of the two isoforms. More specifically, steady state activation is affected by the absence of the proximal N-terminal region in hERG1b, and the activation rate is suggested to be dependent on a short sequence of residues in the proximal portion of the hERG1a N-terminus (Saenen et al., 2006; Trudeau et al., 2011). Consequently, activation rates are much faster in hERG1b channels where these residues are missing (Larsen et al., 2008). Regarding deactivation, it has been suggested that the slow deactivation of hERG1a channels might be facilitated by the first 16 residues of the N-terminus, among other factors (Wang et al., 2008). According to that, faster deactivation rates in hERG1b can be explained by the presence of a unique N-terminal. The inactivation rate was shown to be similar between the two isoforms (Larsen et al., 2008). This finding is expected, as the mechanism by which fast inactivation occurs has been proposed to rely mainly on voltage induced changes in the structure of the outer mouth of the pore (Schönherr and Heinemann, 1996; Perry et al., 2013a,b; Thomson et al., 2014) and the sequence spanning this region is identical in both isoforms. Lastly, recovery from inactivation is significantly faster in hERG1b compared

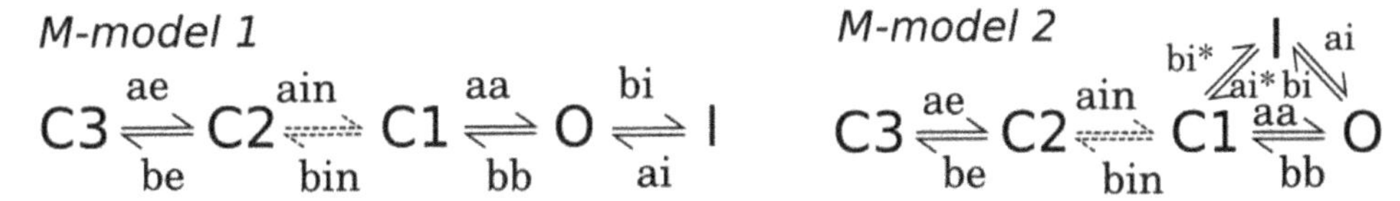

FIGURE 2 | Proposed kinetic mechanisms using Markov models (M-models) for WT hERG (Perissinotti et al., 2015; Romero et al., 2015) showing the transition rates with the corresponding labels.

to hERG1a, potentially implying that by some means, the N-terminus contributes to this process with already proposed stabilizing interactions (Saenen et al., 2006; Gustina and Trudeau, 2011).

Despite the evidence that heterometric hERG 1a/1b channels underlie cardiac I_{kr}, little is known about the gating and pharmacological properties of these channels, how hERG1a channels differ from hERG1b homomers, 1a/1b heteromers, or which role hERG1b might play in disease. Two broadly accepted gating mechanisms were established on the basis of kinetic modeling driven by the experimental data from electrophysiology studies of Kv11.1a channel. The first gating mechanism that successfully describes gating kinetics was proposed by Rasmusson, and later refined by Fink et al. and Romero et al. (termed M-model 1, **Figure 2**) (Wang et al., 1997; Fink et al., 2008; Romero et al., 2015). The modified M-model 1 (Fink et al., 2008) for hERG1 channel has been combined with the cardiac cell model (Ten-Tusscher Model; Ten Tusscher and Panfilov, 2006) in order to reproduce, and explain in terms of kinetics, measurements in oocytes, and HEK cells and showed overall good performance. The second hERG1 current scheme with different connectivity between gating states was developed by both Clancy et al. (Clancy and Rudy, 2001; Clancy et al., 2007) and Mazhari et al. (2001) (termed M-model2, **Figure 2**) on the basis of M-model originally proposed by Kiehn et al. (1999).

There are only a limited number of studies that employ kinetic modeling to understanding of gating kinetics in hERG1 isoforms. Sale et al. (2008) previously attempted to study the hetero channels formed by hERG1a/1b in HEK cells in presence and absence of E-4031 blocker. The M-model 2 was used to describe gating process in a-isoform and a-,b- heteromer. To explain apparent challenges in fitting experimental currents, Sale et al. proposed that the presence of the extended N termini in all 4 subunits in hERG 1a may alter gating process; hence an alternative gating mode ("N-mode") was considered. Another previous work modified the M-model 1 parameters proposed by Fink et al. (2008) and implemented them in the cardiac cell model (Ten Tusscher and Panfilov, 2006) in order to reproduce, and explain measurements in oocytes and HEK cells. However, none of the previous works (Robertson et al., 2008; Sale et al., 2008; Larsen et al., 2010; Holzem et al., 2016) tested the quality of the proposed kinetic models in fitting the hERG1b homo-tetramer experimental data, nor attempted to derive the set of model parameters for this isoform or suggest structural mechanisms explaining differences in isoform gating kinetics (Wacker et al., 2017).

The rapid progress in the structural biology finally resulted in the Cryo-EM high-resolution structure of hERG1 channel. The structure of the full hERG1 channel in its open state together with other highly homologous channels EAG1 and other closely-related channels from CNG and HCN families were published in 2016-2017 (Whicher and Mackinnon, 2016; Lee and Mackinnon, 2017; Li et al., 2017; Wang and Mackinnon, 2017). The availability of this new structural data provides a unique opportunity to connect well-established kinetic models of hERG1 channel to its structural determinant.

This work is striving to achieve several goals. First goal is the methodological one, where we developed and compared optimal gating schemes for hERG a- and b- isoforms. The second goal is to provide a perspective view on the potential structural mechanisms responsible for apparent kinetic differences between two isoforms and then to explore and discuss its implications at the tissue level. To achieve our methodological goal we systematically compared two gating schemes using available and novel electrophysiological recordings performed in HEK cell lines. The kinetic schemes illuminated profound differences in deactivation kinetics between two isoforms. To understand underlying reasons for different deactivation process, we employed structural modeling of hERG1 channel in open and closed-states using recently published structures of EAG1 and hERG1 channels from Cryo-EM (Whicher and Mackinnon, 2016; Wang and Mackinnon, 2017). We found that the available structures allowed identification of potential mutants with altered kinetics in good agreement with developed kinetic models. Finally, to provide a perspective on the potential role of isoforms in cellular dynamics, we undertook the cardiac cell simulations to reveal the conditions (i.e., isoform composition of hERG channels) leading to QT alterations. To provide initial glimpses into cellular roles of different isoform expression, a selected kinetic model, together with the optimized parameters, was incorporated into a higher dimensional model of the cardiac cell (O'hara et al., 2011) to simulate cellular and tissue dynamics effects as function of hERG isoform ratio.

MATERIALS AND METHODS

Expression of hERG1a and hERG1b in HEK Cells

Lees-Miller et al. first reported the electrophysiology of the hERG1 b-isoform (Lees-Miller et al., 1997). The hERG1 b-isoform was cloned from human atrium. hERG1 isoforms were cloned into the pIRES-hr green fluorescent protein-1a vector (Agilent Technologies, Santa Clara, CA) for co-expression

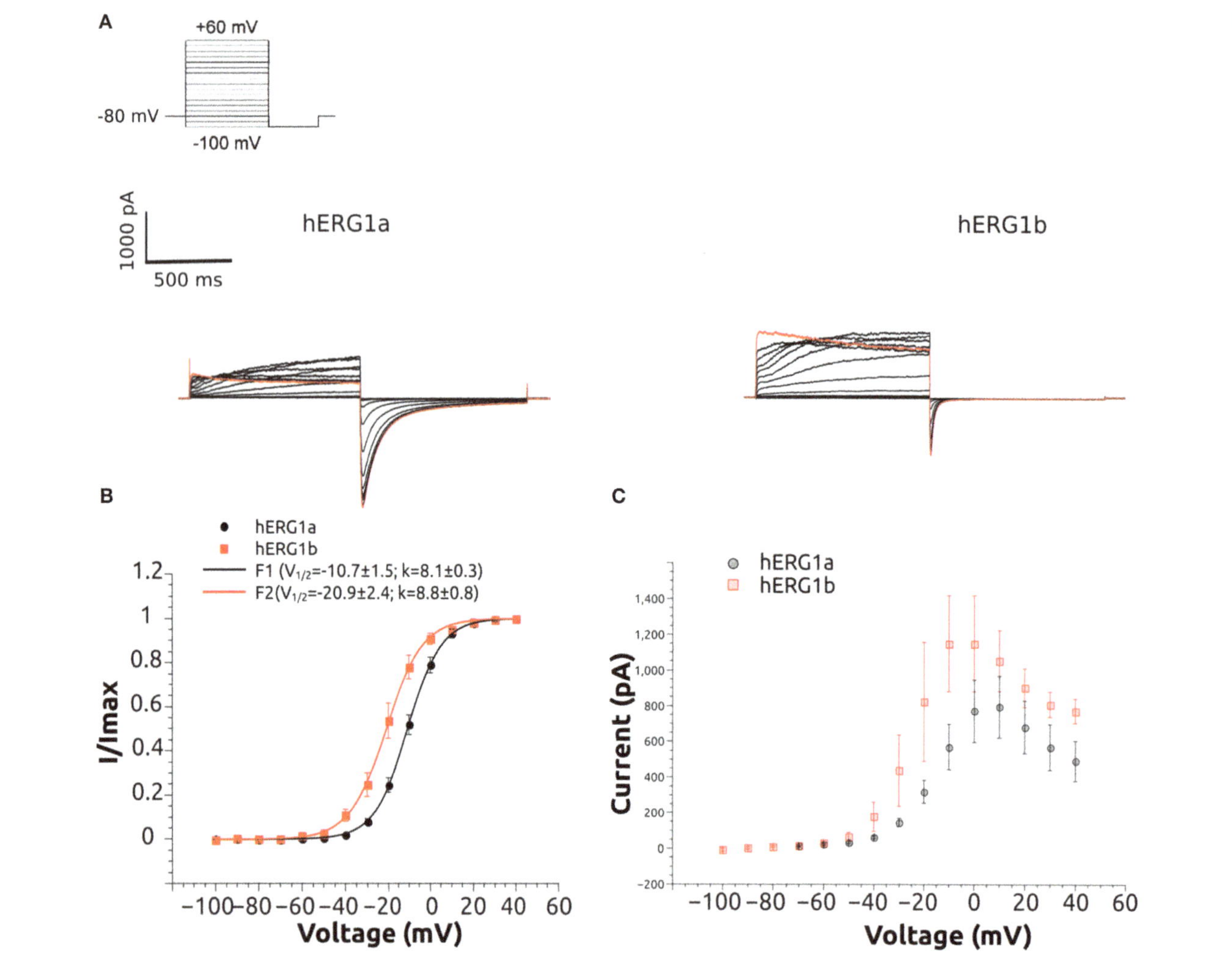

FIGURE 3 | Representative current traces of hERG1a and hERG1b channels and their current-voltage relationship at room temperature. **(A)** Selected current traces recorded from HEK cells and elicited by the voltage protocol shown in the top. **(B)** Normalized tail currents against voltage. The solid lines correspond to the fitted Boltzmann functions and symbols correspond to data. All data are listed as mean ± SEM. hERG1a ($n = 10$), hERG1b ($n = 10$). **(C)** Currents measured at the end of each step were used to construct the current-voltage (I-V) relationship. All data are shown as mean ± SEM. hERG1a ($n = 10$), hERG1b ($n = 10$).

with humanized Renilla reniformis GPF. Human embryonic kidney (HEK) 293 cells were transfected by using calcium phosphate and cultured in Dulbecco's modified Eagle's medium supplemented with 10% horse serum (Invitrogen, Carlsbad, CA). Transfection was monitored by green fluorescence. HEK cells were chosen because their background potassium currents are small. More importantly, no dofetilide-sensitive tail current has been observed by using the voltage-clamp protocol in untransfected HEK cells.

General Setup for Electrophysiological Recordings

Transfected HEK cells on glass coverslips were placed in a chamber mounted on a modified stage of an inverted microscope. The chamber was superfused at a rate of 2 ml/min with a normal external solution. Micropipettes were pulled from borosilicate glass capillary tubes on a programmable horizontal puller (Sutter Instrument Company, Novato, CA). Standard patch-clamp methods were used to measure the whole-cell currents of hERG1 mutants expressed in HEK 293 cells by using the Axopatch 200B amplifier (Molecular Devices, Sunnyvale, CA) (Lees-Miller et al., 2009). The pipette solution contained the following: 10 mM KCl, 110 mM K-aspartate, 5 mM $MgCl_2$, 5 mM Na_2ATP, 10 mM ethylene glycol-bis(β-aminoethyl ether)-N,N,N′,N′tetraacetic acid, 5 mM HEPES, and 1 mM $CaCl_2$. The solution was adjusted to pH 7.2 with KOH. The EC solution contained the following: 140 mM NaCl, 5.4 mM KCl, 1 mM $CaCl_2$, 1 mM $MgCl_2$, 5 mM HEPES, and 5.5 mM glucose. The solution was adjusted to pH 7.4 with NaOH. In patch clamp experiments, serious resistance and capacitance during the whole cell patch clamp recording were compensated to 90% through Axopatch 200B patch clamp amplifier. Whole cell patch clamp experiments were performed when access resistance was <10 MOme. No leak subtraction was performed. The junction potential of −10 mV was adjusted on all the membrane potentials recorded. All experiments were conducted at room temperature.

Voltage Protocols

Voltage-dependence of activation

From a holding potential of −80 mV cells were depolarized for 1 s to a range of voltages from −100 to +40 mV followed by a step to −100 mV (1 s) to record the tail currents (**Figure 3**). The isochronal tail current-voltage plots were fit to a single Boltzmann function (1):

$$\frac{I}{I_{max}} = \frac{1}{(1 + exp[\frac{(V_{\frac{1}{2}} - V_m)}{k}])} \quad (1)$$

Where I / I_{max} is the normalized current, $V_{1/2}$ is voltage of the half-maximal activation, k is the slope factor and V_m is the membrane potential.

Envelope of tails

The activation of hERG1a and hERG1b channels was examined at +40 mV in HEK cells. The protocol is shown in **Figure 4**. The measurements were carried out by activating the channels at +40 mV for various durations of time (from 5 to 500 ms) and then measuring the tail current at −100 mV (3 s). The peak amplitude of the tail current was used as a measure of the relative amount of activated channels at a given time point. The peak amplitudes were normalized to the maximum amplitude and plotted as a function of the duration of the activating step.

Deactivation

Deactivation of hERG1a/1b tail current was measured by activating channels al +40, followed with a short (5 ms) repolarization step to −120 mV and deactivating step at −120, −100, −60, −40 mV. Currents at different voltages were normalized and averaged (n = 10) time course data was plotted for each isoform at the different voltages (**Figure 5**).

Statistical analysis

Statsview (Abacus Concepts, Berkeley, CA) or QTIplot (Vasilef, 2013), Grace (http://plasma-gate.weizmann.ac.il/Grace/) were used to analyze the data. Data are presented as mean ± SEM.

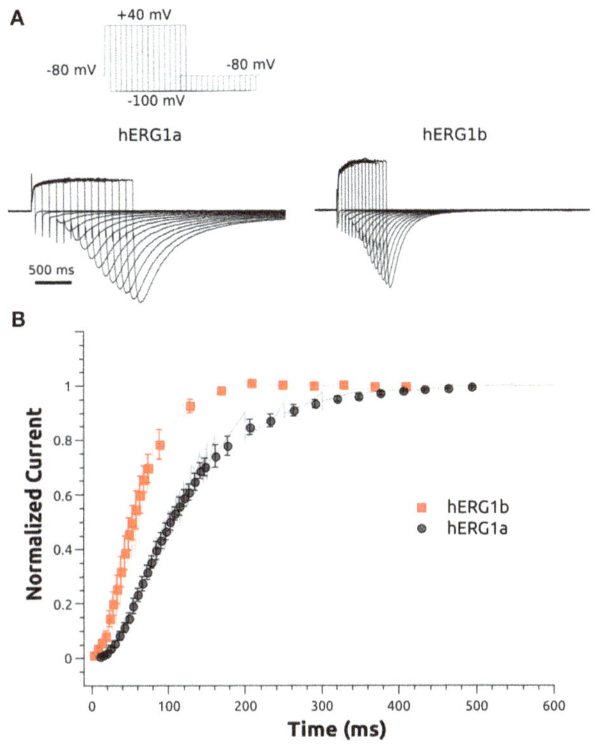

FIGURE 4 | Activation kinetics of hERG1a and hERG1b channels expressed in HEK cells. An envelope of tails protocol was used to measure the activation properties at +40 mV. **(A)** Representative current traces elicited by the protocol shown at the top corresponding to 5–500 ms of activation are shown. **(B)**The data were normalized to the maximum amplitude of the tail current and plotted against time. hERG1a (n = 10); hERG1b (n = 10). All data are shown as mean ± SEM.

Computational Methods

Kinetic Modeling: Vgckimo Program Package[1]

The dominant paradigm for ion transport over the past 60 years has been based on the seminal experiments of Hodgkin and Huxley (Hodgkin and Huxley, 1952; Hodgkin et al., 1952). However, a much more detailed picture of the mechanisms underlying membrane excitation can be described in terms of Markov models (M-models) (Rudy and Silva, 2006; Moreno et al., 2011), where the conducting and non-conducting states are interconnected by rate constants dependent on the membrane potential. The essence of M-models is that, for any single step in the gating mechanism, the transition probability (i.e., the microscopic equivalent of the rate constant) is time independent. In an M-model of ion channels, transition rates define the interstate dynamics. These rates may depend on environmental variables such us membrane potential or ligand concentration.

The state probabilities in the model are calculated by solving the following differential equation (Equation. 2):

$$\frac{d\vec{p}}{dt} = Q\vec{p} \quad (2)$$

where $\vec{p}$ is the vector of state probabilities and Q is the system matrix of the transition rate constants. Each transition rate constant is assumed to have the following expression:

$$k_i = \alpha_i e^{\beta_i V} \quad (3)$$

where $\alpha_i = \frac{k_B T}{h} \bullet e^{\frac{\Delta S_i}{R} - \frac{\Delta H_i}{RT}}$ (ms^{-1}), $\beta_i = \frac{z_i F}{RT}$ (mV^{-1}); V is the external electric potential in mV; z_i is the effective valence of moving charges; T(K) is the temperature; ΔH_i (J/M) the change in enthalpy; ΔS_i(J/M/K) the change in entropy. k_B =

[1]Voltage-Gated Ion Channels Kinetic Modeling from whole-cell voltage-clamp data (VGC-KiMo) is a standalone tool written in C++ language, working on Linux machines and parallelized with OpenMP (see the Supporting Material for the scalability benchmarks). VGC-KiMo code is distributed under GNU General Public License thus freely available for download from https://github.com/vgckimo/vgckimo, together with documentation and tutorial files. See Supporting Material for a complete description of the code.

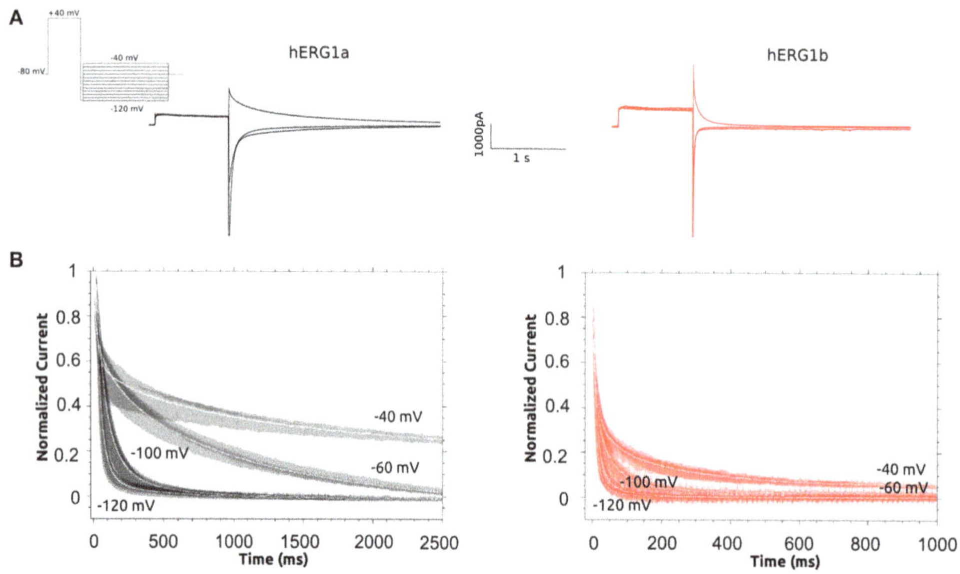

FIGURE 5 | Deactivation Kinetics of hERG1a and hERG1b channels measured in HEK cells. **(A)** Representative current traces elicited by the voltage protocol shown in the top for both isoforms. **(B)** Superimposed raw deactivation time courses for voltages −40, −60, −100, and −120 mV for hERG1a (n = 10) and hERG1b (n = 10). Average time course is shown with a solid white line.

1.381 10^{-23} J K^{-1} (Boltzmann constant); h = 6.626 10^{-34} J s^{-1} (Planck constant); R = 8.315 $Jmol^{-1}$ K^{-1} (ideal gas constant); F = 96785 C M^{-1} (Faraday constant).

Once Equation (2) is solved, the probability of being in the open state (pO: conducting state) is found and the current is calculated using the following equations:

$$I_{Kr} = g_{Kr} p_O (V - E_k) \tag{4}$$

$$g_{Kr} = g^0_{Kr} (aT + b) \left(\frac{[K+]_O}{5.4\,mM} \right)^{\frac{1}{2}} \tag{5}$$

Where g^0_{Kr} =0.024 pA/pF/mV, a = 1/35, and b = −55/7, O is the open probability (see SM and (Fink et al., 2008) for more details).

Through the Global-Fitting procedure described in Balser et al. (1990) and implemented in VGC-KiMo[1], the rate constants of a given M-model can be estimated from macroscopic ion channel currents in voltage-clamped membranes. The use of comprehensive and extensive data sets of experimental information from a broad range of ion current responses to multiple voltage stimulations conditions (voltage protocols, membrane potentials, temperature, etc.), shrinks the universe of possible solutions to the model system mechanism ensuring the robustness of the parameter set. Although several methods exist for analyzing voltage dependent currents (Wang et al., 1997; Mazhari et al., 2001; Fink et al., 2008; Bett et al., 2011; Moreno et al., 2011; Ben-Shalom et al., 2012) most of them are published only as a set of equations without the simulation tools. Others, from the neurophysiology field, are designed to use the full current traces, data that are neither commonly available nor easy to extract from published literature (Gurkiewicz and Korngreen, 2007; Ben-Shalom et al., 2012).

In the current form, VGC-KiMo[1] source code includes two Markov formulations for the Kv11.1, best known as the hERG K^+ channel. Any other channel can be added to the source code in addition to the current one, as well as different Markov models and other voltage protocols. The experimental data chosen for the model validation was not used for the development of the model's parameters and belongs to a different cell line than the one used to originally derive the parameters for the M-model (HEK cells), see SM (Section 2: Validation). The performance of the original parameters is fairly good but corrections were needed to reproduce the data from CHO cell line, suggesting that the published set of parameters is robust and reliable. A preliminary version of VGC-KiMo has also been used recently to simulate WT hERG and a variant using experimental data from HEK cell line (Guo et al., 2015; Perissinotti et al., 2015).

Cell Simulations

An I_{Kr} Markov model (Romero et al., 2015) was incorporated into the O'Hara-Rudy human ventricular action potential model(O'hara et al., 2011) and its maximum conductance (gKr = 0.0422) was scaled to elicit a close value of the peak Ikr as the original O'Hara model at 1 Hz. Physiological action potential simulations were subsequently performed at 37°C. b-Isoform and a-Isoform transition rate constants together with the corresponding temperature correction are shown in Table S12.

Simulated action potentials (APs) were recorded in endocardial cells at the 1000th paced beat (BCL = 1000 ms). The numerical method used for updating the voltage was forward Euler. All the Simulations were encoded in C/C++ and run on Mac Pro 3.06 GHz 12-Core computers. The time step was set to 0.00005 ms during AP upstroke, otherwise the time step was 0.005 ms. Numerical results were visualized using MATLAB R2014a by The Math Works, Inc.

Transmural fiber simulations

We simulated a transmural fiber composed of 165 ventricular cells ($\Delta x = \Delta y = 100\,\mu m$) connected by resistances to simulate gap junctions (Faber and Rudy, 2000). The fiber contains an endocardial (cells 1 to 60), M-cell (cells 61 to 105), and epicardial (cells 106 to 165) regions, as described by O'Hara et al. The fiber was paced at BCL = 1,000 ms for 2,000 beats. The stimulus was applied to the first cell. Current flow is described by the following equation:

$$\frac{\partial V(x,t)}{\partial t} = D\frac{\partial^2 V(x,t)}{\partial x^2} - \frac{I_{ion}\_I_{stim}}{C_m} \tag{6}$$

Where V is the membrane potential, t is time, D is the tissue diffusion coefficient [0.00092 cm^2/ms, calculated from Shaw and Rudy (Shaw and Rudy, 1997)], I_{ion} is the sum of transmembrane ionic currents, I_{stim} is the stimulus current (300 $\mu A/cm^2$ for 0.5 ms), and C_m is the membrane capacitance (1 $\mu F/cm^2$).

ECG computation

Extracellular unipolar potentials (Φ_e) generated by the fiber in an extensive medium of conductivity σ_e, were computed from the transmembrane potential V_m using the integral expression as in Gima and Rudy (Gima and Rudy, 2002):

$$\Phi_e(x',y',z') = \frac{a^2\sigma_i}{4\sigma_e}\int(-\nabla V_m)\bullet\left[\nabla\frac{1}{r}\right]dx \tag{7}$$

$$r = \left[(x-x')^2 + (y-y')^2 + (z-z')^2\right]^{1/2} \tag{8}$$

where ∇V is the spatial gradient of V_m, a is the radius of the fiber, σ_i is the intracellular conductivity, σ_e is the extracellular conductivity, and r is the distance from a source point (x, y, z) to a field point (x', y', z'). Φ_e was computed at an "electrode" site 2.0 cm away from the distal end along the fiber axis.

Structural Modeling

Recently published full hERG ($hERG_T$) open channel solved by Cryo-EM at 3.8 angstrom resolution (PDB ID 5VA2) was used for the structural analysis. The construct used for structural studies has functional properties very similar to WT but is lacking residues between 141 and 350, that correspond to the structure between PAS and S1; and 871-1005 (C-terminal). The structure was cut right after CNBD ends and missing residues at the outer pore mouth were added and modeled as extracellular loops that were minimized using NAMD2.10 (Phillips et al., 2005). The 3D structure of the closed-state hERG channel used in this study is based on the homology modeling to EAG1 Cryo-EM structure (PDB ID 5K7L) determined at 3.78 angstrom resolution (Yang et al., 2017). This structure represents the closed pore while the voltage sensing domain (VSD) displays an open conformation (Whicher and Mackinnon, 2016). The SWISS-MODEL homology modeling program (Arnold et al., 2006) was used for the development of the hERG closed model from the available EAG1 channel structure as described previously (Yang et al., 2017). Sequence alignment was performed using the CLUSTALW algorithm (Larkin et al., 2007; Goujon et al., 2010). Protein models were generated from the alignment in a stepwise manner. The generated model was later minimized using NAMD2.10 (Phillips et al., 2005).

TABLE 1 | Experimental data for HEK cells at room temperature.

	hERG1a	hERG1b
ACTIVATION PARAMETERS		
$V_{1/2}$ (mV);	−10.7 ± 1.5 (*n* = 10)	−20.9 ± 2.4 (*n* = 10)
slope (mV)	8.1 ± 0.3	8.8 ± 0.8
RECOVERY FROM INACTIVATION, τ (ms)		
−100 mV	3.6 ± 0.2 (*n* = 7)	1.1 ± 0.1 (*n* = 6)
−50 mV	11.0 ± 0.8 (*n* = 4)	2.1 ± 0.5 (*n* = 3)

Each value is an average of n experiments. Equation (1) was used to obtain $V_{1/2}$ and k, data are presented as mean ± SEM.

RESULTS AND DISCUSSIONS

Experimental Measurements

The whole-cell patch clamp configuration at room temperature was used to study the voltage-dependent activation by applying a standard step protocol described in the methodology. The normalized tail currents measured at −100 mV were plotted against the membrane potential of the previous step and fitted to a Boltzmann function. The $V_{1/2}$ of activation is shifted around 10 mV in the negative direction for hERG1b compared to hERG1a (**Figure 3**, **Table 1**). The mean current levels measured at the end of the 1-s depolarizing pulse to +40 mV were used to construct the current-voltage (I-V) relationship (**Figure 3C**). Similar to what is observed for hERG1a, the b-isoform shows a strong inward rectification, resulting in the characteristic bell-shaped curve. Kinetics of activation was studied by applying an envelope of tails protocol, as described in the methodology section. The b-isoform shows a similar sigmoid shape of activation, but a much faster rate compared to the a-isoform (**Figure 4**).

Deactivation kinetics was characterized by recording tail currents at potentials ranging from −40 to −120 mV after an activating step to +40 mV (see methods). Current traces for selected voltages are shown in **Figure 5**. The deactivating currents were best fitted to a double exponential function and time constants corresponding to the fast and slow deactivation processes are shown in Table S13. Both deactivating components are significantly reduced for hERG1b. The observed reduction depends on the voltage, at −60 mV, the slow and fast components are around 10 to 14 times faster for hERG1b while the difference is around 4 to 7 times for −40 and −100 mV, respectively. As it was found before for CHO cells by Larsen et al. (2008), the relative contribution of the fast component of deactivation depends on the voltage and is much more pronounced for hERG1b compared to hERG1a, in fact at −120 mV there is no slow component according to the experimental fit. Regarding

TABLE 2 | M-model 1 rate constants for transitions within hERG gating for a-isoform and b-isoform.

Transition	Parameter name		Rates		ratio b/a
			b-Isoform	a-Isoform	
C3→ C2	ae	α	4.71 E-2	3.39 E-2	**1.39**
		β	9.36 E-3	1.04 E-2	0.90
C2→ C3	be	α	7.43 E-2	4.82 E-2	**1.54**
		β	−5.05 E-2	−6.91 E-2	0.73
C2→ C1	ain	α	5.01 E-2	2.20 E-2	**2.28**
C1→ C2	bin	α	2.95 E-2	1.36 E-2	**2.17**
I→ O	**ai**	α	2.80 E-2	6.63 E-3	**4.23**
		β	−3.06 E-2	−3.89 E-2	0.79
O→ I	bi	α	7.41 E-2	7.41 E-2	1.00
		β	1.88 E-2	2.80 E-2	0.67
C1→ O	**aa**	α	1.71 E-2	4.94 E-3	**3.46**
		β	3.05 E-2	4.31 E-2	0.71
O→ C1	**bb**	α	1.61 E-3	2.06 E-4	**7.83**
		β	−3.44 E-2	−3.76 E-2	0.91

*α (1/ms) indicates voltage independent rate, and β (1/mV) indicates voltage dependent rate as follows: k = α*exp(β*V) The transitions between O and I states are also dependent on extracellular potassium concentration $[K^+]^0$ That dependence is accounted for in the model by modifying the transition rate for inactivation (O → I, bi) as: $k_{bi}([K^+]^0)=k'_{bi}(5.4mM/[K^+]^0)^{0.4}$. Bold values indicate moderate change of the corresponding transitions calculated as a ratio. Transitions that are strongly affected are shown in bold red. Transitions that are affected the most are shown as underlined red bold values. For details of the optimizations, original model parameters and optimization from CHO data see Tables S1–S4.*

TABLE 3 | M-model 2 rate constants for transitions within hERG gating for a-isoform and b-isoform.

Transition	Parameter name		Rates		ratio b/a
			b-Isoform	a-Isoform	
C3→ C2	ae	α	1.19 E-2	3.77 E-3	**3.17**
		β	2.17 E-2	3.29 E-2	0.66
C2→ C3	be	α	1.82 E-2	2.44 E-2	0.74
		β	−3.79 E-2	−6.77 E-2	0.56
C2→ C1	ain	α	9.29 E-2	3.59 E-2	**2.59**
C1→ C2	bin	α	1.09 E-1	1.65 E-2	**6.62**
I→ O	**ai**	α	5.11 E-2	1.74 E-2	**2.93**
		β	2.09 E-2	2.87 E-2	0.73
O→ I	bi	α	1.79 E-2	9.26469 E-3	1.94
		β	−2.15 E-2	−2.347 E-2	0.92
C1→ O	**aa**	α	1.55 E-1	8.80 E-2	**1.76**
		β	9.60 E-3	1.02 E-2	0.94
O→ C1	**bb**	α	7.82 E-2	5.11 E-3	**15.28**
		β	−3.54 E-2	−4.44 E-2	0.80
C1→ I	**bi***	α	9.32E-07	1.02E-09	**910.41**
		β	1.621E-05	7.99E-06	2.03

*α (1/ms) indicates voltage independent rate, and β (1/mV) indicates voltage dependent rate as follows: k= α*exp(β*V). *Constraint by microscopic reversibility. Bold values indicate moderate change of the corresponding transitions calculated as a ratio. Transitions that are strongly affected are shown in bold red. Transitions that are affected the most are shown as underlined red bold values. For additional details on the optimizations and original model parameters see Tables S1–S4.*

the inactivation process, there was not significant difference and was not further investigated here (Larsen et al., 2008) (data not shown). Time constants for recovery from inactivation for a-isoform and b-isoform display a significant difference and are collected in **Table 1**.

Markov Kinetic Models to Describe hERG a- and b-Isoforms

The most pronounced difference evident from the experimental raw current traces is the markedly faster deactivation rate and the faster activation rate of hERG1b compared to hERG1a. This is in agreement to what was also found for CHO cells (Larsen et al., 2008). The experimental measurements in the HEK cell line focus in these events and the M-models were fitted to the data presented in the above section. All transition rates were defined using Equation (3). The previously derived values for α_i and β_i were used for initial guess (see Table S1 in Supplemental Materials). For M-model 1, the initial guess values were derived using the comprehensive experimental data-set from Berecki et al. at room temperature and 37°C respectively (Berecki et al., 2005). Two correction terms, *a* and *b* were introduced to α and β parameters for quality monitoring during optimization routine (Equation 9). α and β were set to the constant values, while ***a*** and ***b*** parameters were introduced as free variables for optimization routine.

$$k_i = \boldsymbol{a}_i \alpha_i e^{\boldsymbol{b}_i \beta_i V} \tag{9}$$

Correction to individual parameters ($\mathbf{a}_i$, $\mathbf{b}_i$: Equation 5) from Fink et al. and Mazhari et al. has been done to reproduce available data from HEK-cell measurements at room temperature (23). All fitted parameters for the kinetic mechanism considered, can be found in **Tables 2**, **3** and Tables S4, S5. Note that ***β*** was set to zero for transitions a_{in} and b_{in} (**Figure 2**) and thus, these transitions are modeled as voltage independent. Maximum single channel conductance was assumed to be the same for hERG1a and hERG1b, so all differences are attributed to channel kinetics.

Three and/or four different voltage protocols were included simultaneously in the optimization protocol (see Supplementary Materials for a complete description of the voltage protocols). Different optimization routines were performed and the correction factors were defined for each of the parameters. All parameters required corrections to the initial guesses. The best fits are shown in **Tables 2**, **3** for two isoforms and each model, respectively. Further improvement of the optimizations was achieved by using the random initial guess generator around the already fitted values and assigning different weight to the partial cost function. In all the cases, the stability analysis showed that all values were well-converged. The simulated voltage protocols and computed currents are in reasonable agreement with the measured ones, meaning that voltage dependence and curve shapes are qualitatively well-reproduced. Overall, both gating mechanisms from the literature were able to reproduce the gating kinetics for both isoforms. However, the optimized parameters showed some interesting differences and limitations in quantitatively reproducing the time course of the deactivation kinetics at different voltages.

Performance of M-Model 1

The M-model 1 implies linear connectivity between different gating states. The channel has to go through the open state to fully inactivate. The experimental basis for this scheme was extensively discussed in the literature (Bett et al., 2011). Assuming that both isoforms follow same kinetic scheme (Sale et al., 2008), the key differences between the a-isoform and b-isoform kinetics lie essentially in the highlighted steps shown in **Table 2**. According to the results collected in **Table 2**, the best fit within M-model 1 indicates that the main difference between two hERG isoforms is in the late deactivation step. The late deactivation is about eight times faster for the b-isoform. These parameters also show an increase in the activation rate steps, together with an increase in the recovery from inactivation rate in agreement with the experimental data (**Table 1**). Simulated data from CHO cell line (SM) also display a good agreement with the optimal fit (Tables S3, S4, S9). **Figure 6** shows the simulated data together with the experiments. An excellent agreement is obtained for the activation and Steady State Activation curves for both isoforms (**Figure 9**). However, the main challenges are in the modeling of the deactivation kinetics for different voltage protocols (−40, −60, −100, −120 mV). For b-isoform in particular, the quality of the optimization is limited, although it qualitatively reproduces the behavior at the different voltages.

Performance of M-Model 2

This model, in contrast to the M-model 1, is not linear, but instead, includes a direct transition to the inactivated state from the closed state immediately preceding the open state. In one of the previous formulations (Mazhari et al., 2001), this transition is negligible compared to the transition to the open state and so, numerically, this model is almost linear. In our work, M-model 2 was tested assuming a range of different values for this transition and in all the cases a very small rate was obtained for both isoforms. Although the obtained value was small and almost negligible, it is almost 1000 times faster for the b-isoform. The M-model 2 shows a similar performance compared to the M-model 1 although the fit quality is consistently lower than that of M-model 1. The differences between a-isoform and b-isoform are distributed over the activation steps but mainly in the late deactivation and the new extra step considered in this scheme (**Table 3**). Simulated current traces elicited by the voltage protocols and the activation curves are well-reproduced by this model (**Figure 7**). Similar to what was observed for M-model 1, the quality of the optimization is poor, although it qualitatively reproduces the behavior at the different voltages.

Taking together the results from M-model 1 and 2, we conclude that both models capture the main kinetic difference between the isoforms. The pivotal feature of isoform kinetics is a considerable increase in the late deactivation step. Both models point to a moderate increase in the activation and recovery from inactivation steps, the changes and their magnitudes depend on the model. The current traces simulated by each model and elicited by the SSA voltage protocol are shown in **Figure 8**. It can be seen that they qualitatively reproduce the experimental behavior shown in **Figure 3**. The b-isoform displays larger currents, an increased activation rate, faster recovery from inactivation and clearly shows a much faster deactivation rate under the repolarizing pulse. The simulated I-V relationships show the typical curve shape and qualitatively reproduce the experimental differences characteristic of each isoform, although they show significant deviations for voltages above 10 mV. At these voltages background currents are relatively high, while hERG current is relatively small. The combination of these two factors presents a natural challenge and led to the discussed discrepancy between simulated and experimental data.

The best optimization for M-model 1 which also shows fair agreement with the fit to CHO data (Table S9), suggests that although the main difference is in the late deactivation step, being eight times faster for the b-isoform when compared to a-isoform, early and late activation are also increased by a factor of ~2 and 4, respectively. According to this fit, the voltage independent rates are increased in forward and backward directions by a factor of 2 and the recovery from inactivation rate by a factor of 4. M-model 2 suggests similar changes and fair agreement with CHO data (Table S10); late deactivation is 15 times faster for the b- compared to the a-isoform, but also early and late activation, being 3 and 2 times faster respectively. It also shows a three-fold increase for the recovery from inactivation and an increase for both voltage insensitive rates, being 2.5 times faster in the deactivating direction.

Limitations of the Kinetic Modeling

It is important to mention that the time course of deactivation was not well-fitted by the M-models used in this work for both HEK and CHO cell lines. We observed that the quality of the fit is different for different voltages. To improve modeling of the deactivation kinetics, a number of different conditions were tested for both models, i.e., randomization of initial values, constraints, boundaries, etc., but no further improvement was achieved. The reason could be related to the amount of data used in the fitting procedure, experimental limitations in the data acquisition (temperature, cell-line variability, resolution of electrophysiological recordings), or indicate that the M-models should be revisited. It is important to mention that some inconsistencies between the deactivation experimental data and these models were previously discussed by other authors (Fink et al., 2008). Another example can be found in a recently developed Markov model that reproduces biophysical

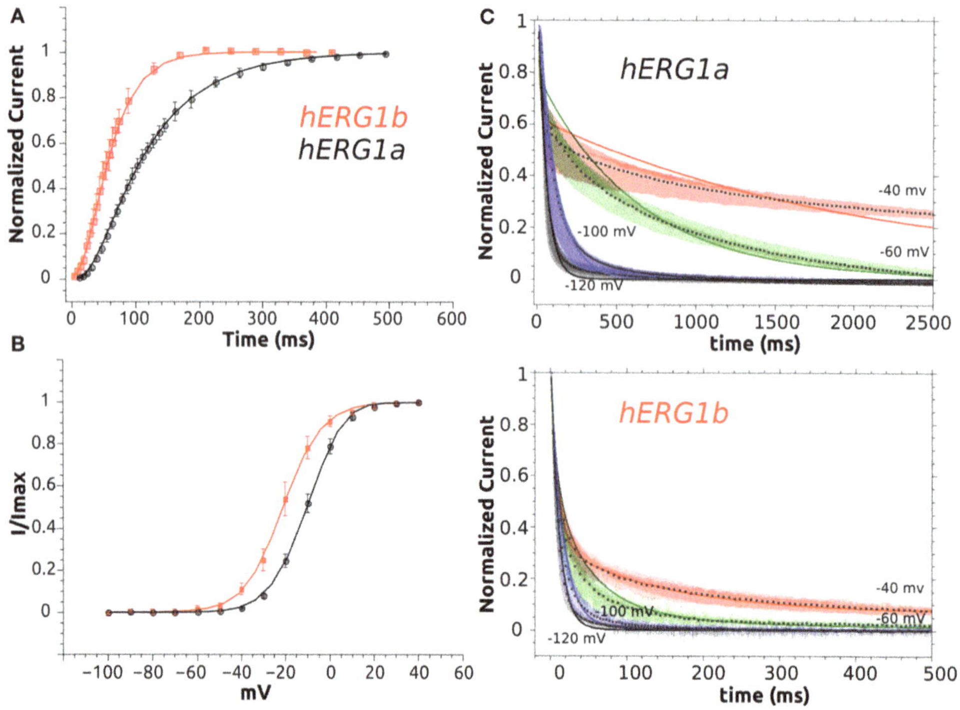

FIGURE 6 | M-model 1 optimization to experimental data. **(A)** Activation curve of a-isoform and b-isoform. **(B)** Steady State Activation curve for both isoforms. **(C)** Simulated deactivation curves at −120, −100, −60, and −40 mV. Simulated data is shown as solid lines and symbols are used for experimental time course data (average, $n = 10$). Superimposed raw time course data ($n = 10$) is shown in the background for deactivation at each voltage.

experimental data at room temperature with CHO cell line includes two closed (C1, C2), one open (O) and corresponding inactivated states (IC1, IC2, IO) (Di Veroli et al., 2013). This model also faces difficulties in fitting deactivation at different voltages. Interestingly, the 6-states model with closed loops can be reduced to a 4-states cyclic model (C1, O, IC, IO) at 37°C, as different closed states could not be resolved. However, unless explicitly introducing temperature-dependent parameters, all of the available models cannot account for temperature-dependent hERG channel activity changes. A modification of the Di Veroli model was done recently by Li et al. (Li et al., 2016), and can recapitulate macroscopic hERG channel gating behavior for a temperature range from 20 to 37°C. Providing the better performance for the temperature range, different states and connectivity, it would be interesting to test the performance of this new model in reproducing the experimental data for both isoforms. It is important to emphasize that having a complete and more reliable M-model is of key importance for modeling and predicting differential and temperature dependent effects of drugs on the delayed rectifier potassium "I_{kr}" current.

Structural Underpinnings of Isoform Function

The kinetic modeling discussed above isolates principal differences in gating kinetics of hERG a- and hERG b-isoforms. The recent Cryo-EM structures allowed the structural modeling for open- and closed states of hERG1 channel enabling molecular-level description of the determinants of this apparent isoform-specific differences. Homology models (Wacker et al., 2017) and chimera constructs were very useful in the past (Dhillon et al., 2014) for understanding structure-function relationships in K+ channels. However, most of the models were focusing on the trans-membrane section of hERG1 channel only (Wacker et al., 2017). The recently-solved hERG structure shows an open pore, while the EAG1 channel solved by Cryo-EM is captured with the pore closed due to the presence of Ca2+ and calmodulin, which lock the pore closed while the VSD is supposed to be in its depolarized state (Wang and Mackinnon, 2017). The hERG closed model presented here was built using EAG1 structure as a representative template for hERG's closed pore. Given the fact that conformational differences between these two states of VSD are relatively small compared to structures and models of open- and closed states found in K^+ channels from Shaker family (Li et al., 2014); then the question is, if this is a good representation of hERG closed state, what kind of VSD movement could result in that same conformational change in the pore?. As Wang et al. (Wang and Mackinnon, 2017) pointed out, there are key structural differences in the arrangement of the VSD (non-domain swapped) in hERG and EAG1. It seems that an S4 inward movement toward the cytoplasm and centric displacement toward the pore axis driven by the membrane electric field could produce a similar pore closure. In that scenario, there is almost not translation of S4

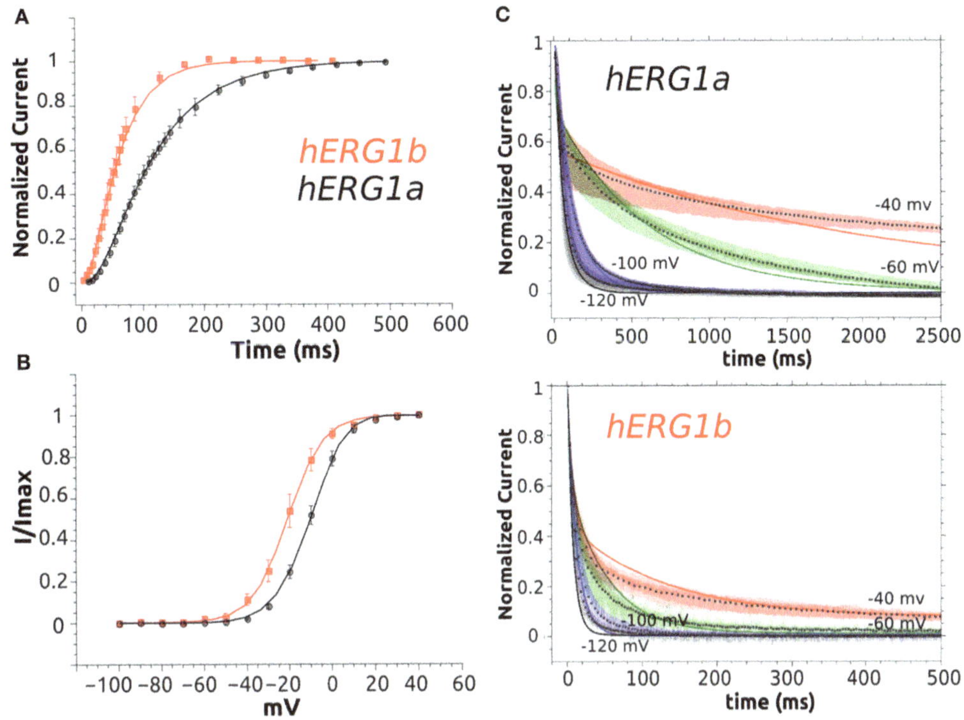

FIGURE 7 | M-model 2 fit to experimental data. **(A)** Activation curve of a-isoform and b-isoform. **(B)** Steady State Activation curve for both isoforms. **(C)** Simulated deactivation curves at −120, −100, −60, and −40 mV. Simulated data is shown as solid lines and symbols are used for experimental time course data (average, $n = 10$). Superimposed raw time course data ($n = 10$) is shown in the background for deactivation at each voltage.

across the membrane, S5 maintains an extensive antiparallel contact with S6 and the VSD would transmit force through the S5-S6 interface as the movement of S4 would compress the S5 helices and close the S6 gate. This proposed mechanism is different than the lever mechanism proposed for Shaker-like Kv channels and the cytoplasmic domains may play a crucial role in it. It is important to mention that functional measurements also point to substantial differences in the total gating charge, being much less for hERG, which implies that the VSD conformational changes are smaller in hERG channel (Zhang et al., 2004; Li et al., 2014). These rapid developments in hERG structural biology emphasized important roles of PAS and CNBD domains in gating kinetics. As it was shown previously for Kv1.2-Kv2.1 (Morais-Cabral and Robertson, 2015), PAS-CNBD complex published for mEAG1 (Haitin et al., 2013), and all the recent structures; the PAS (**Figure 9**, in orange) domain is far away from the VSD. In stark contrast, hERG structures show (Whicher and Mackinnon, 2016; Wang and Mackinnon, 2017), that the N-terminus of the PAS domain (absent in b-isoform) is directed toward the VSD and S4-S5 linker (**Figure 9B**) and most likely interacts with the gating machinery. NMR studies previously suggested that the N-terminal cap shows a high degree of structural variability and is long enough to reach the voltage sensor, the S4-S5 linker or the C-linker (Muskett et al., 2011; Ng et al., 2011, 2014) (**Figure 9B**). As it was mentioned before, the new structures present new topology of VSD-pore domain packing, which is different from the domain-swapped architecture and might suggest a new paradigm for voltage dependent gating. It was recently proposed for EAG1, a mechanism in which the VSD interacts with the cytoplasmic domains to gate the channel. Combined with the data from isoform kinetic modeling described above, models of hERG in open and closed state may provide better understanding of stabilizing interactions present or missing in a particular isoform.

The arrangement of cytoplasmic domains in the open state and closed state models are shown in **Figure 9**. The PAS domain is interacting with CNBD in a similar way it was found previously for homologous channels (Lee and Mackinnon, 2017; Li et al., 2017; Wang and Mackinnon, 2017). Similar to the previously solved structures for CNBD domains (Ng et al., 2011; Adaixo et al., 2013; Brelidze et al., 2013; Haitin et al., 2013), a portion of the hERG sequence occupies the cyclic nucleotide binding site, which prevents the cyclic nucleotide binding. In addition to that, the N-terminus of PAS Domain (N-cap), which influences the rate of voltage dependent channel opening and closing, is directed toward the VSD (Wang and Mackinnon, 2017) (**Figures 9B, 10B**). When the channel is in its open state, the C-linker region is packed against the transmembrane domain (**Figure 10A**) interacting with the S4-S5 linker and VSD. A novel interaction pinpointed by the structural analysis is the salt-bridge formed between Glu544 and Arg681 (**Figures 10C,D**). This salt-bridge is missing in the closed state model of the channel as the C-linker is slightly rotated with respect to the S4-S5 linker. Hence, we hypothesize that it might be one of the open-state

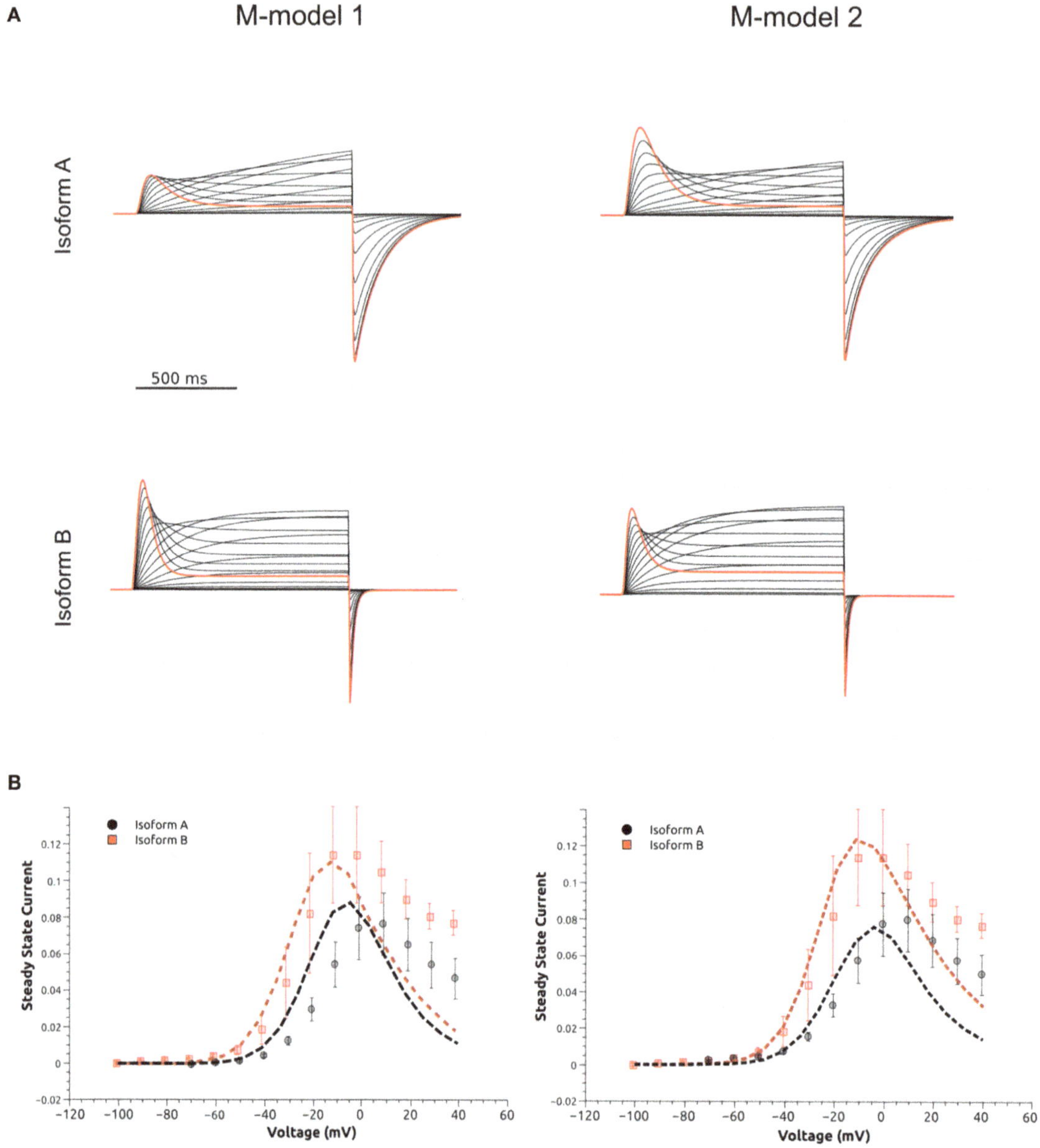

FIGURE 8 | Simulated currents M-model 1 and M-model 2. **(A)** Simulated currents elicited by the SSA voltage protocol **(Figure 3)** for both M-models and Isoforms. **(B)** Simulated I-V steady state current (x10^4 pA) relationship for M-model 1 and 2. a-Isoform is shown as black dashed line and b-isoform as red dashed line. Experimental data is shown in the background as symbols with the corresponding error bar **(Figure 3)**.

stabilizing interactions that it is affected in the absence or the PAS domain (b-isoform), note that N-cap (Val 3) is close to E544 and might indirectly affect the E544-R681 interaction. Unfortunately, solved structures are missing significant part of the PAS domain sequence and further refinement of hERG1 PAS domain is essential future goal for structural modeling. Nevertheless, the previously studied E544L mutant (Durdagi et al., 2012) shows an increase in the deactivation rate. Even though is not as much as for the b-isoform (**Figure 10E**), it highlights a potential key role of this residue. When transitioning from closed to open state, the transmembrane and cytoplasmic domains slightly rotate with respect to each other (**Figures 9**, **10B**), we suggest that the interplay between PAS, VSD: S4-S5, and C-linker during such rotation might be of key importance in modulation the gating.

While more work is still required to decipher gating kinetics of hERG1, the structural models already show enhanced interactions between the cytoplasmic and the transmembrane (TM) domain for the open state of the channel. Analysis of structural differences between open and closed states suggests that a slight rotational movement changing packing of the cytoplasmic domains against the TM part of the channel is required as part of activation/deactivation process. This is in

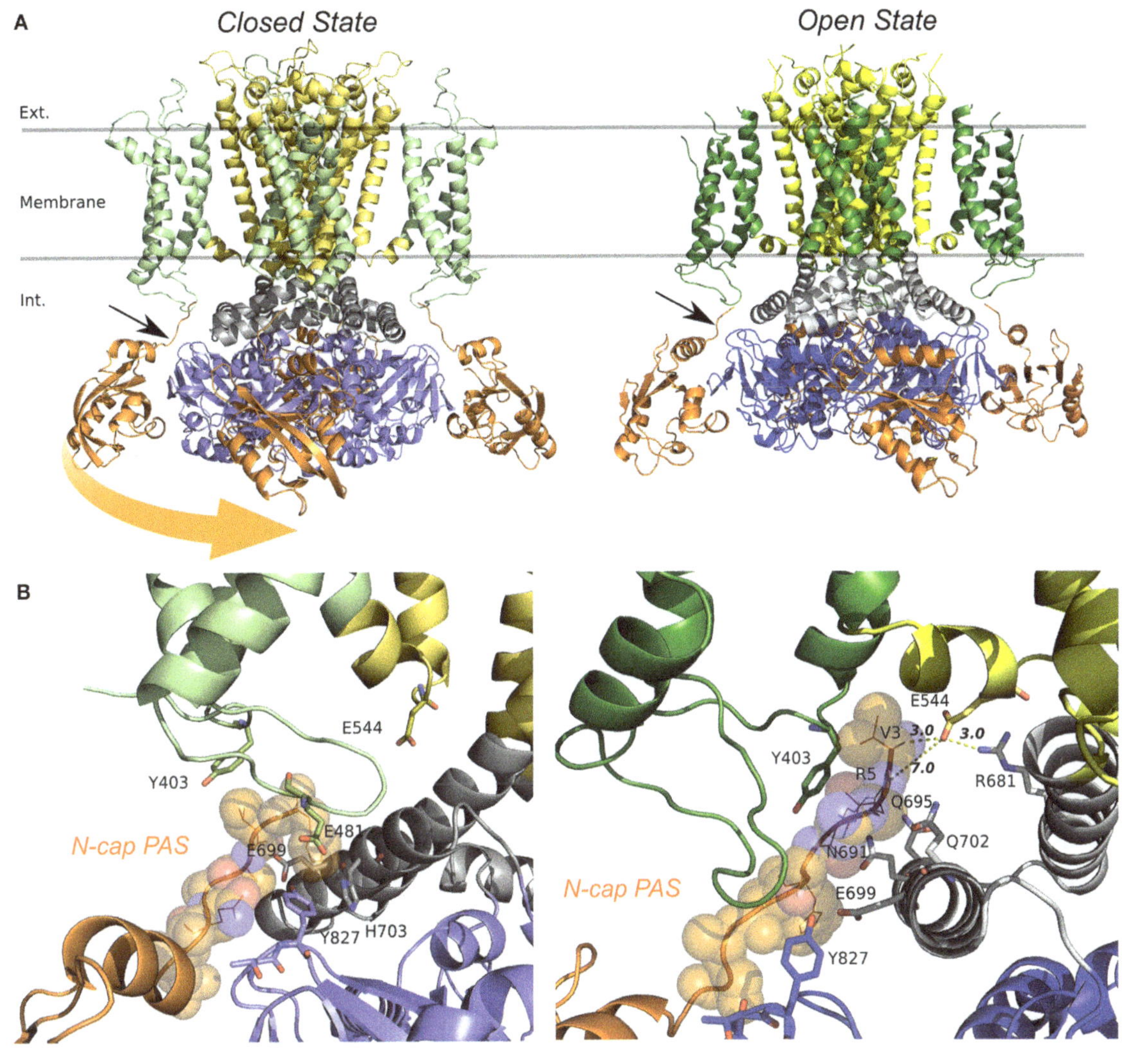

FIGURE 9 | Models of the quaternary structure of homomeric hERG tetramers. Side view **(A)** of closed state model in the left panel and open state hERG Cryo-EM structure, right panel. In both structures N-cap PAS can be seen interacting with VSD (black arrow). When the TM domain is aligned, cytoplasmic domains are slightly rotated respects each other. Orange arrow show the rotation direction when transitioning from closed to open states. **(B)** N-cap PAS interaction with VS (S1 & potentially S4-S5), CNBD, and C-linker for closed in the left panel and open states, right panel.

line with the finding that the conformational change that VSD is undergoing during gating cycle might be small compared to other potassium channels. This would allow the CNBD to close the channel independent of the VSD conformation (as it was observed for EAG1) and provide an added level of regulation through the interaction of intracellular domains with the voltage dependent gating machinery (Whicher and Mackinnon, 2016). These structural insights, although preliminary, lead us to the hypothetic gating mechanism summarized in **Figure 11**. The similar mechanism of gating modulated by soluble domains has been proposed for MolK1, a prokaryotic potassium channel lacking the C-linker and PAS domain (Kowal et al., 2014).

These structural models also raise another point. In other channels, PAS and CNBD domains serve a regulatory function in which the binding of small molecules or signaling proteins is transduced into conformational changes. It is not known whether or not this could be happening for hERG. These new models align to what was suggested previously (Morais-Cabral and Robertson, 2015), and that points to the possibility that the C-linker-CNBD-PAS serves as an anchor to correctly position the N-pas terminal cap during the gating process. Can we explain observed differences in the deactivation kinetics between hERG a- and b-isoforms observed with kinetic modeling? Any of the functional alterations due to mutations or truncations in the N-terminal cap or the entire PAS Domain (b-isoform) would ultimately lead to a loss of N-terminal cap position and severely-altered gating kinetics. The lack of stabilizing interactions between soluble and trans-membrane domains is expected to impact the opening probability and stability of the open state. It may explain observed rapid transitions between open and closed states present in the b-isoform.

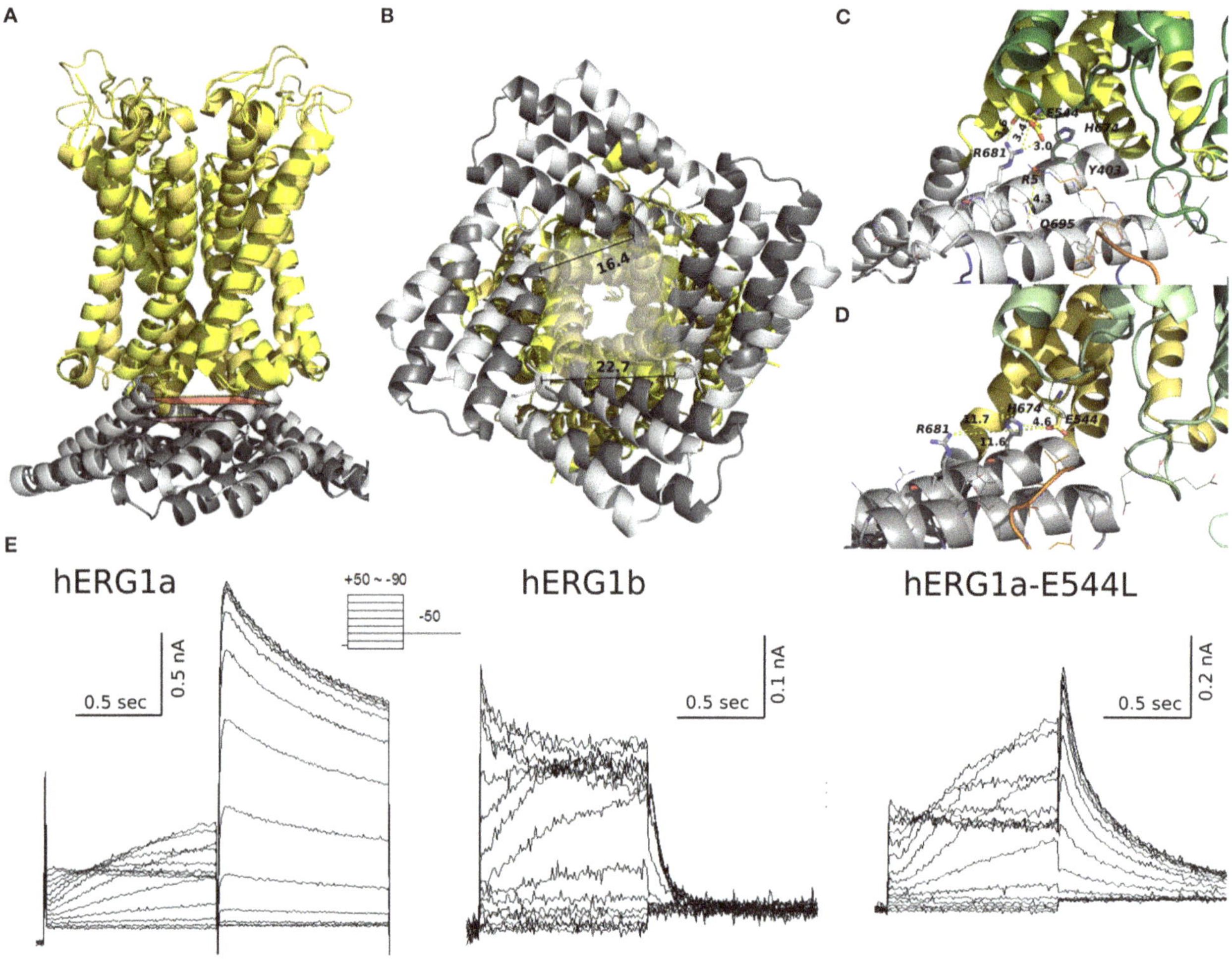

FIGURE 10 | Structural alignment of closed (light colors) and open (dark colors) models of hERG. TM and C-linker side view shows that the C-linker/TM are closer to each other in the open state compared to the closed **(A)**. Distances between residues Gly669 show that a closer C-linker is a consequence of a more open pore in the open state **(B)**. Key salt bridge interactions between Glu544 and Arg681 can only be found in the open state **(C)** but not in the closed state **(D)**. **(E)** Current traces from experiments previously published by Durdagi et al. for hERG1a, hERG1b, and hERG1a-E544L elicited by the voltage protocol at the top. E544L mutant displays a faster deactivation rates than WT but not as much as hERG1b.

Cardiac Cell Models: Functional Implications of Different Isoform Ratios in the Heart

The improved kinetic models allowed us to directly address physiological questions like whether or not hERG isoform composition in ventricular myocytes has a potential to alter QT duration and, hence, to pre-dispose a patient for drug-induced QT prolongation. To specifically address the functional implication of having homomeric hERG1a or hERG1b in the heart we conducted simulations including our M-model 1 parameters in the cardiac cell (O'Hara-Rudy human cardiac ventricular myocyte Model) (O'hara et al., 2011; Romero et al., 2015). The final parameters from the fittings were then used as input values in the cardiac cell and tissue model (O'hara et al., 2011) in order to simulate the shape of the action potential and ECG signal for both isoforms (**Figure 12**). The M-model 1 and its parameters from the optimization were introduced in the cardiac cell model in order to test the way in which they affect the shape and duration of action potential. As it was found previously (Larsen and Olesen, 2010), the results of the ventricular cardiomyocyte simulations showed that kinetic changes in I_{kr} corresponding to homomeric hERG1b resulted in much shorter action potential duration (APD). **Figure 12B** shows the action potential (Dhillon et al.) shape and duration considering the extreme situation of I_{kr} corresponding only to hERG1 a- or b- isoforms. Intermediate cases, where weighed contributions from both isoforms were considered, are shown in **Figure 12A**. I_{kr} currents are also shown in **Figure 12A** and, as it can be seen, the currents became larger and peak earlier when transitioning from pure a- to b- isoforms.

Mechanistic inspection of the changes in the channel state occupancy revealed several differences. Figures S9, S11 show the proportion of channels in the different states. The

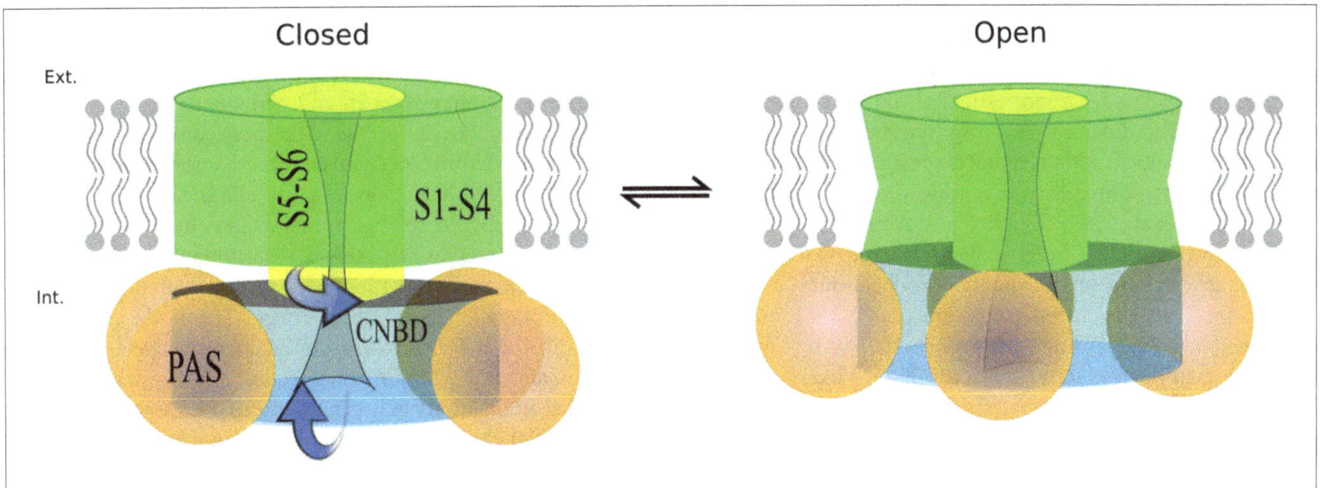

FIGURE 11 | Proposed mechanism based on the structures modeled. When the channel opens the cytoplasmic domains rotate toward the membrane as the S6 end twists in the same direction.

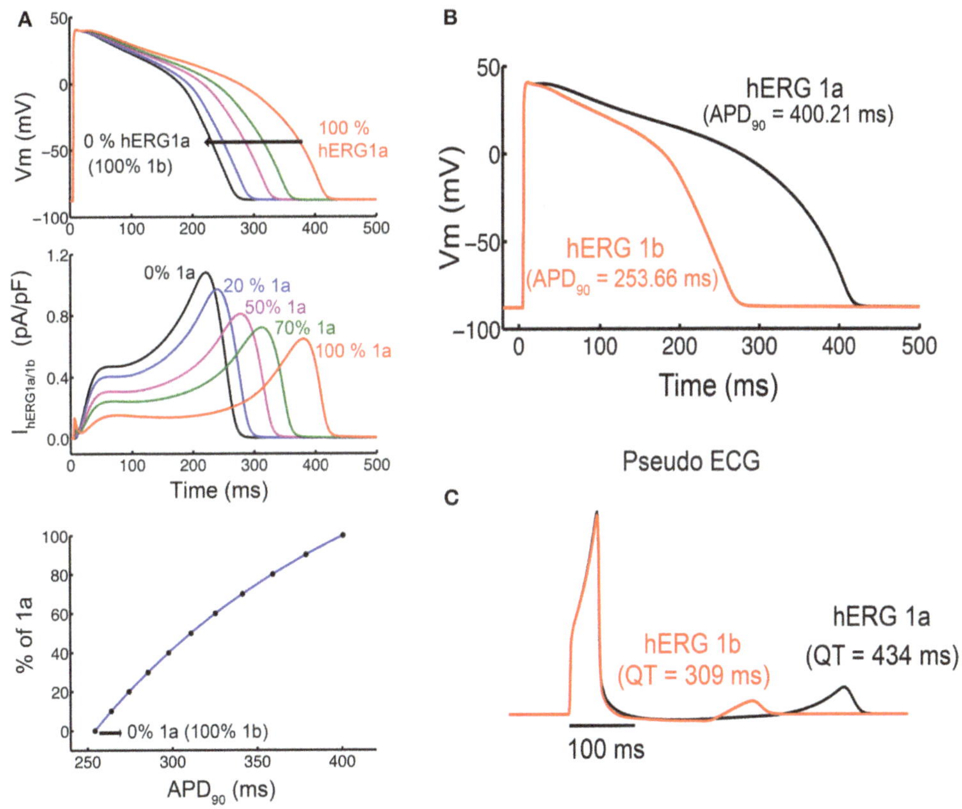

FIGURE 12 | Simulated action potential duration (APD) in cells and virtual pseudo-ECGs in a transmural 1-D tissue model. **(A)** Single cells simulations show concentration response for different ratios of a- and b-isoforms. **(B)** APD for the 1,000th paced beat at 1 Hz in single endocardial cells. hERG 1a shows a longer APD compared to hERG 1b. **(C)** The Pseudo ECGs of hERG 1b (red) indicates shorter QT intervals than hERG 1a.

most prominent difference lies in the occupancy of open and inactivated states when comparing a-isoform to b-isoform. The AP shortening is mainly due to an increase in the open state occupancy and a reduction in the inactivated states occupancy for hERG1b compared to hERG1a. Finally, the M-model 1 was also introduced in the tissue model (cable) and the ECG signal was simulated for both homomers (**Figure 12C**). As expected, virtual hERG1b expression resulted in a reduction in the QT interval on the computed pseudo-ECG.

Experimental investigations have revealed many sources of heterogeneity and associated regulation in the heart. Distinct regions with associated cell types that are distinguishable by morphology and action potential duration have been documented. The different cell types have been shown to arise from heterogeneities in ion channel expression, which have been modeled and used in cell-type specific predictive simulations (Viswanathan et al., 1999) (Shimizu and Antzelevitch, 1999). In the left ventricle of the heart, cellular heterogeneity from the endocardium to mid-myocardium to endocardium exists and arises from heterogeneity in potassium currents (Shimizu and Antzelevitch, 1999) (Liu and Antzelevitch, 1995). The differences in stoichiometry between hERG1a and hERG1b likely constitute a novel source of cardiac heterogeneity that may vary in terms of distribution and be subject to regulation by as yet unknown mechanisms.

The kinetic modeling in section Markov Kinetic Models to Describe hERG a- and b-Isoforms shows a profound difference in hERG1a and hERG1b deactivation rates, where the quantitatively fitted parameters to the data suggested that the hERG1b late deactivation rate is between 8 and 15 times faster than hERG1a. One of the most interesting and counterintuitive findings in the results shown above is that this difference did not result in effects on the action potential duration that would expected from the observed changes alone. The dominant presence of the hERG1 b-isoform results in faster deactivation, which by itself would result in fewer channels in the open state as the channels close more quickly. The anticipated effect on the action potential duration would be less repolarizing current and consequently, shorter APD. In fact, the opposite was observed both in our modeling predictions with M-model 1 and in a previous experimental study (Larsen and Olesen, 2010). The reason is that the hERG1 b-isoform has both faster activation kinetic and faster recovery from inactivation kinetics that results in a net increase current compared to the hERG1 a-isoform.

CONCLUSIONS

We investigated structural and biophysical properties of hERG1a and 1b homo-tetramers in the context of previously proposed Markov models and new data measured in the HEK cell line. Two M-models were tested and fitted to the experimental data. For the first time a set of parameters were provided for both isoforms. The models' parameters were then used to investigate effects of various homo-tetramers ratios formed by two isoforms in cardiac cells and tissue to track isoform-specific effects on emergent behaviors that occur in higher dimensions. The minimization procedure presented here, allowed assessment of suitability of different Markov model topologies and the corresponding parameters that describe the channel kinetics. In terms of the gating kinetics, we found that both M-models were able to qualitatively capture the kinetics of two isoforms. The kinetic modeling showed a profound difference in hERG1a and hERG1b deactivation rates, where the quantitatively fitted parameters to the data suggested that the hERG1b late deactivation rate is between 8 and 15 times faster than hERG1a.

In order to gain insight and link the observed isoforms' differences to the structure, full channel structural models were developed and analyzed for open and closed states. From the structural point of view, open and closed structural models for the full channel were for the first time compared providing hypothetical structural mechanism for transitions between closed to open states of hERG channel. In line with the kinetic modeling, interactions between soluble domains and the TM part of the channel appeared to be critical determinants of the gating kinetics allowing explanation of apparent differences in the deactivation rates between two isoforms. The model emphasized importance of the electrostatic interactions between N-cap of PAS domain and TM domain. To test the proposed role of stabilizing interactions between N-cap of PAS domain and the gating machinery in TM, we examined gating kinetics of E544L. Introduction of charge neutralizing resulted in significantly enhanced deactivation rates, reminiscent of isoform-specific differences. We attribute it to interactions between E544 and R681 missing in E544L mutant. Importantly, this interaction is present in both hERG1 a-isoform and hERG1 b-isoform, however b-isoform is missing the of PAS domain who might contribute to stabilize that interaction. While this work was under review, another publication by de la Peña et al. (2018) showed that hERG gating profiles can be reconsiled from non-covalently linked VSD and Pore Domain. Their findings, in line to what is presented in this work, challenge the classical view of the S4–S5 linker acting as lever to open the gate, supporting the hypothesis that the S4–S5 linker might integrate signals coming from the cytoplasmic domains (c-linker/PAS). Importantly, those split-channels disconnected at the S4–S5 linker show a destabilization of the closed state, in particular one of the split shown to be near E544 position discussed in our submission. Our structural modeling is providing a first structural glimpse of the structural underpinnings of the peculiar isoforms' gating and suggesting potential key interactions between S4–S5 linker, C-linker and PAS. Equally important question discussed in our study is the potential impact on the Action Potential from different ratios of isoform expression in the myocytes. The AP simulations performed in our study suggest that recovery from inactivation of hERG1 B may contribute to its physiologic role of b-isoform in the action potentials. Both structural and functional models were exploratory in nature aiming to provide a perspective for future multi-scale modeling studies.

In conclusion, the results and in-depth review of modeling, structural and functional data presented here contribute to the growing body of evidence that hERG1b significantly affects the generation of the cardiac I_{kr} and plays an important role in cardiac electrophysiology.

AUTHOR CONTRIBUTIONS

JG: Performed all of the electrophysiological recordings and mutagenesis experiments, analyze results and wrote the manuscripts. LP and PD: Wrote the software; LP, ML, and P-CY: Performed simulations and analyzed the data; CC, SN, and HD:

Supervised the research; LP, HD, CC, and SN: Designed the research. All authors wrote the article.

ACKNOWLEDGMENTS

This work was supported by the Canadian Institutes of Health Research (to SN); and the Discovery grant from Natural Scientific and Engineering Research Council of Canada (to HD). CC was supported by the National Institutes of Health Grants R01HL128170, U01HL126273 and R01HL128537 (together with SN). The computational support for this work was provided by West-Grid and Compute Canada through a resource allocation award and NSERC-RTI award to SN.

REFERENCES

Adaixo, R., Harley, C. A., Castro-Rodrigues, A. F., and Morais-Cabral, J. H. (2013). Structural properties of pas domains from the KCNH potassium channels. *PLoS ONE* 8:e59265. doi: 10.1371/journal.pone.0059265

Arnold, K., Bordoli, L., Kopp, J., and Schwede, T. (2006). The Swiss-Model workspace: a web-based environment for protein structure homology modelling. *Bioinformatics* 22, 195–201. doi: 10.1093/bioinformatics/bti770

Balser, J. R., Roden, D. M., and Bennett, P. B. (1990). Global parameter optimization for cardiac potassium channel gating models. *Biophys. J.* 57, 433–444. doi: 10.1016/S0006-3495(90)82560-1

Behere, S. P., Shubkin, C. D., and Weindling, S. N. (2014). Recent advances in the understanding and management of long QT syndrome. *Curr. Opin. Pediatr.* 26, 727–733. doi: 10.1097/MOP.0000000000000161

Ben-Shalom, R., Aviv, A., Razon, B., and Korngreen, A. (2012). Optimizing ion channel models using a parallel genetic algorithm on graphical processors. *J. Neurosci. Methods* 206, 183–194. doi: 10.1016/j.jneumeth.2012.02.024

Berecki, G., Zegers, J. G., Verkerk, A. O., Bhuiyan, Z. A., De Jonge, B., Veldkamp, M. W., et al. (2005). HERG channel (dys)function revealed by dynamic action potential clamp technique. *Biophys. J.* 88, 566–578. doi: 10.1529/biophysj.104.047290

Bett, G. C. L., Zhou, Q., and Rasmusson, R. L. (2011). Models of HERG gating. *Biophys. J.* 101, 631–642. doi: 10.1016/j.bpj.2011.06.050

Brelidze, T. I., Gianulis, E. C., Dimaio, F., Trudeau, M. C., and Zagotta, W. N. (2013). Structure of the C-terminal region of an ERG channel and functional implications. *Proc. Natl. Acad. Sci. U.S.A.* 110, 11648–11653. doi: 10.1073/pnas.1306887110

Chiesa, N., Rosati, B., Arcangeli, A., Olivotto, M., and Wanke, E. (1997). A novel role for HERG K+ channels: spike-frequency adaptation. *J. Physiol.* 501, 313–318. doi: 10.1111/j.1469-7793.1997.313bn.x

Clancy, C. E., and Rudy, Y. (2001). Cellular consequences of HERG mutations in the long QT syndrome: precursors to sudden cardiac death. *Cardiovasc. Res.* 50, 301–313. doi: 10.1016/S0008-6363(00)00293-5

Clancy, C. E., Zhu, Z. I., and Rudy, Y. (2007). Pharmacogenetics and anti-arrhythmic drug therapy: a theoretical investigation. *Am. J. Physiol. Heart Circul. Physiol.* 292, H66–H75. doi: 10.1152/ajpheart.00312.2006

Crotti, L., Tester, D. J., White, W. M., Bartos, D. C., Insolia, R., Besana, A., et al. (2013). Long QT syndrome-associated mutations in intrauterine fetal death. *JAMA* 309, 1473–1482. doi: 10.1001/jama.2013.3219

de la Peña, P., Domínguez, P. and Barros, F. (2018). Gating mechanism of Kv11.1 (hERG) K+ channels without covalent connection between voltage sensor and pore domains. *Pflugers Arch. Eur. J. Physiol.* 470:517. doi: 10.1007/s00424-017-2093-9

Dhillon, M. S., Cockcroft, C. J., Munsey, T., Smith, K. J., Powell, A. J., Carter, P., et al. (2014). A functional Kv1.2-hERG chimaeric channel expressed in *Pichia pastoris*. *Sci. Rep.* 4:4201. doi: 10.1038/srep04201

Di Veroli, G. Y., Davies, M. R., Zhang, H. G., Abi-Gerges, N., and Boyett, M. R. (2013). High-throughput screening of drug-binding dynamics to HERG improves early drug safety assessment. *Am. J. Physiol.* 304, H104–H117. doi: 10.1152/ajpheart.00511.2012

Durdagi, S., Guo, J. Q., Lees-Miller, J. P., Noskov, S. Y., and Duff, H. J. (2012). Structure-guided topographic mapping and mutagenesis to elucidate binding sites for the human ether-a-go-go-related gene 1 potassium channel (KCNH2) activator NS1643. *J. Pharmacol. Exp. Therapeut.* 342, 441–452. doi: 10.1124/jpet.111.189159

Faber, G. M., and Rudy, Y. (2000). Action potential and contractility changes in Na+ (i) overloaded cardiac myocytes: a simulation study. *Biophys. J.* 78, 2392–2404. doi: 10.1016/S0006-3495(00)76783-X

Fink, M., Noble, D., Virag, L., Varro, A., and Giles, W. R. (2008). Contributions of HERG K+ current to repolarization of the human ventricular action potential. *Prog. Biophys. Mol. Biol.* 96, 357–376. doi: 10.1016/j.pbiomolbio.2007.07.011

Gima, K., and Rudy, Y. (2002). Ionic current basis of electrocardiographic waveforms: a model study. *Circ. Res.* 90, 889–896. doi: 10.1161/01.RES.0000016960.61087.86

Goujon, M., Mc william, H., Li, W., Valentin, F., Squizzato, S., Paern, J., et al. (2010). A new bioinformatics analysis tools framework at EMBL-EBI. *Nucleic Acids Res.* 38, W695–W699. doi: 10.1093/nar/gkq313

Guo, J., Cheng, Y. M., Lees-Miller, J. P., Perissinotti, L. L., Claydon, T. W., Hull, C. M., et al. (2015). NS1643 interacts around L529 of hERG to alter voltage sensor movement on the path to activation. *Biophys. J.* 108, 1400–1413. doi: 10.1016/j.bpj.2014.12.055

Gurkiewicz, M., and Korngreen, A. (2007). A numerical approach to ion channel modelling using whole-cell voltage-clamp recordings and a genetic algorithm. *PLoS Comput. Biol.* 3, 1633–1647. doi: 10.1371/journal.pcbi.0030169

Gustina, A. S., and Trudeau, M. C. (2009). A recombinant N-terminal domain fully restores deactivation gating in N-truncated and long QT syndrome mutant hERG potassium channels. *Proc. Natl. Acad. Sci. U.S.A.* 106, 13082–13087. doi: 10.1073/pnas.0900180106

Gustina, A. S., and Trudeau, M. C. (2011). hERG potassium channel gating is mediated by N- and C-terminal region interactions. *J. Gen. Physiol.* 137, 315–325. doi: 10.1085/jgp.201010582

Haitin, Y., Carlson, A. E., and Zagotta, W. N. (2013). The structural mechanism of KCNH-channel regulation by the eag domain. *Nature* 501, 444–448. doi: 10.1038/nature12487

Hodgkin, A. L., and Huxley, A. F. (1952). A quantitative description of membrane current and its application to conduction and excitation in nerve. *J. Physiol.* 117, 500–544. doi: 10.1113/jphysiol.1952.sp004764

Hodgkin, A. L., Huxley, A. F., and Katz, B. (1952). Measurement of current-voltage relations in the membrane of the giant axon. *J. Physiol.* 116, 424–448.

Holzem, K. M., Gomez, J. F., Glukhov, A. V., Madden, E. J., Koppel, A. C., Ewald, G. A., et al. (2016). Reduced response to IKr blockade and altered hERG1a/1b stoichiometry in human heart failure. *J. Mol. Cell. Cardiol.* 96, 82–92. doi: 10.1016/j.yjmcc.2015.06.008

Jones, D. K., Liu, F., Dombrowski, N., Joshi, S., and Robertson, G. A. (2016). Dominant negative consequences of a HERG 1B mutation associated with intrauterine fetal death. *Prog. Biophys. Mol. Biol.* 120, 67–76. doi: 10.1016/j.pbiomolbio.2016.01.002

Jones, D. K., Joshi, S., Liu, F., and Robertson, G. A. (2015). Dominant negative consequences of a HERG 1B mutation associated with intrauterine fetal death. *Biophys. J.* 108, 196A. doi: 10.1016/j.bpj.2014.11.1083

Jones, D. K., Liu, F., Vaidyanathan, R., Eckhardt, L. L., Trudeau, M. C., and Robertson, G. A. (2014). hERG 1b is critical for human cardiac repolarization. *Proc. Natl. Acad. Sci. U.S.A.* 111, 18073–18077. doi: 10.1073/pnas.1414945111

Kannankeril, P., Roden, D. M., and Darbar, D. (2010). Drug-induced long QT syndrome. *Pharmacol. Rev.* 62, 760–781. doi: 10.1124/pr.110.003723

Kiehn, J., Lacerda, A. E., and Brown, A. M. (1999). Pathways of HERG inactivation. *Am. J. Physiol. Heart Circul. Physiol.* 277, H199–H210. doi: 10.1152/ajpheart.1999.277.1.H199

Kowal, J., Chami, M., Baumgartner, P., Arheit, M., Chiu, P.-L., Rangl, M., et al. (2014). Ligand-induced structural changes in the cyclic nucleotide-modulated potassium channel MloK1. *Nat. Commun.* 5:3106. doi: 10.1038/ncomms4106

Larkin, M. A., Blackshields, G., Brown, N. P., Chenna, R., Mc gettigan, P. A., Mc william, H., et al. (2007). Clustal W and clustal X version 2.0. *Bioinformatics* 23, 2947–2948. doi: 10.1093/bioinformatics/btm404

Larsen, A. P., Bentzen, B. H., and Grunnet, M. (2010). Differential effects of K(v)11.1 activators on K(v)11.1a, K(v)11.1b and K(v)11.1a/K(v)11.1b channels. *Br. J. Pharmacol.* 161, 614–628. doi: 10.1111/j.1476-5381.2010.00897.x

Larsen, A. P., Jespersen, T., Grunnet, M., and Olesen, S. P. (2007). Electrophysiological characterization of hERG1a and hERG1b Homo- and heteromeric channels. *J. Mol. Cell. Cardiol.* 42, S17–S18. doi: 10.1016/j.yjmcc.2007.03.050

Larsen, A. P., and Olesen, S.-P. (2010). Differential expression of hERG1 channel isoforms reproduces properties of native I-Kr and modulates cardiac action potential characteristics. *PLoS ONE* 5:e9021. doi: 10.1371/journal.pone.0009021

Larsen, A. P., Olesen, S.-P., Grunnet, M., and Jespersen, T. (2008). Characterization of hERG1a and hERG1b potassium channels - a possible role for hERG1b in the I(Kr) current. *Pflugers Arch. Eur. J. Physiol.* 456, 1137–1148. doi: 10.1007/s00424-008-0476-7

Lee, C. H., and Mackinnon, R. (2017). Structures of the human HCN1 hyperpolarization-activated channel. *Cell* 168, 111.e1–120.e1. doi: 10.1016/j.cell.2016.12.023

Lees-Miller, J. P., Guo, J. Q., Somers, J. R., Roach, D. E., Sheldon, R. S., Rancourt, D. E., et al. (2003). Selective knockout of mouse ERG1 B potassium channel eliminates I-Kr in adult ventricular myocytes and elicits episodes of abrupt sinus bradycardia. *Mol. Cell. Biol.* 23, 1856–1862. doi: 10.1128/MCB.23.6.1856-1862.2003

Lees-Miller, J. P., Kondo, C., Wang, L., and Duff, H. J. (1997). Electrophysiological characterization of an alternatively processed ERG K+ channel in mouse and human hearts. *Circ. Res.* 81, 719–726. doi: 10.1161/01.RES.81.5.719

Lees-Miller, J. P., Subbotina, J. O., Guo, J., Yarov-Yarovoy, V., Noskov, S. Y., and Duff, H. J. (2009). Interactions of H562 in the S5 helix with T618 and S621 in the pore helix are important determinants of hERG1 potassium channel structure and function. *Biophys. J.* 96, 3600–3610. doi: 10.1016/j.bpj.2009.01.028

Li, G. R., Feng, J. L., Yue, L. X., Carrier, M., and Nattel, S. (1996). Evidence for two components of delayed rectifier K+ current in human ventricular myocytes. *Circ. Res.* 78, 689–696. doi: 10.1161/01.RES.78.4.689

Li, M., Zhou, X., Wang, S., Michailidis, I., Gong, Y., Su, D., et al. (2017). Structure of a eukaryotic cyclic-nucleotide-gated channel. *Nature* 542, 60–65. doi: 10.1038/nature20819

Li, Q. F., Wanderling, S., Paduch, M., Medovoy, D., Singharoy, A., Mcgreevy, R., et al. (2014). Structural mechanism of voltage-dependent gating in an isolated voltage-sensing domain. *Nat. Struct. Mol. Biol.* 21, 244–252. doi: 10.1038/nsmb.2768

Li, Z. H., Dutta, S., Sheng, J. S., Tran, P. N., Wu, W., and Colatsky, T. (2016). A temperature-dependent *in silico* model of the human ether-a-go-go-related (hERG) gene channel. *J. Pharmacol. Toxicol. Methods* 81, 233–239. doi: 10.1016/j.vascn.2016.05.005

Liu, D. W., and Antzelevitch, C. (1995). Characteristics of the delayed rectifier current (IKr and IKs) in canine ventricular epicardial, midmyocardial, and endocardial myocytes. A weaker IKs contributes to the longer action potential of the M cell. *Circ. Res.* 76, 351–365. doi: 10.1161/01.RES.76.3.351

London, B., Trudeau, M. C., Newton, K. P., Beyer, A. K., Copeland, N. G., Gilbert, D. J., et al. (1997). Two isoforms of the mouse ether-a-go-go-related gene coassemble to form channels with properties similar to the rapidly activating component of the cardiac delayed rectifier K+ current. *Circ. Res.* 81, 870–878. doi: 10.1161/01.RES.81.5.870

Mazhari, R., Greenstein, J. L., Winslow, R. L., Marbán, E., and Nuss, H. B. (2001). Molecular interactions between two long-QT syndrome gene products, HERG and KCNE2, rationalized by *in vitro* and *in silico* analysis. *Circ. Res.* 89, 33–38. doi: 10.1161/hh1301.093633

Morais-Cabral, J. H., and Robertson, G. A. (2015). The enigmatic cytoplasmic regions of KCNH channels. *J. Mol. Biol.* 427, 67–76. doi: 10.1016/j.jmb.2014.08.008

Moreno, J. D., Zhu, Z. I., Yang, P.-C., Bankston, J. R., Jeng, M.-T., Kang, C., et al. (2011). A computational model to predict the effects of class I anti-arrhythmic drugs on ventricular rhythms. *Sci. Transl. Med.* 3:98ra83. doi: 10.1126/scitranslmed.3002588

Muskett, F. W., Thouta, S., Thomson, S. J., Bowen, A., Stansfeld, P. J., and Mitcheson, J. S. (2011). Mechanistic insight into human ether-a-go-go-related gene (hERG) K+ channel deactivation gating from the solution structure of the EAG domain. *J. Biol. Chem.* 286, 6184–6191. doi: 10.1074/jbc.M110.199364

Ng, C. A., Hunter, M. J., Perry, M. D., Mobli, M., Ke, Y., Kuchel, P. W., et al. (2011). The N-Terminal tail of hERG contains an amphipathic alpha-helix that regulates channel deactivation. *PLoS ONE* 6:e16191. doi: 10.1371/journal.pone.0016191

Ng, C. A., Phan, K., Hill, A. P., Vandenberg, J. I., and Perry, M. D. (2014). Multiple interactions between cytoplasmic domains regulate slow deactivation of Kv11.1 channels. *J. Biol. Chem.* 289, 25822–25832. doi: 10.1074/jbc.M114.558379

O'hara, T., Virág, L., Varró, A., and Rudy, Y. (2011). Simulation of the undiseased human cardiac ventricular action potential: model formulation and experimental validation. *PLoS Comput. Biol.* 7:e1002061. doi: 10.1371/journal.pcbi.1002061

Ohya, S., Horowitz, B., and Greenwood, I. A. (2002). Functional and molecular identification of ERG channels in murine portal vein myocytes. *Am. J. Physiol. Cell Physiol.* 283, C866–C877. doi: 10.1152/ajpcell.00099.2002

Perissinotti, L. L., Guo, J., De Biase, P. M., Clancy, C. E., Duff, H. J., and Noskov, S. Y. (2015). Kinetic model for NS1643 drug activation of WT and L529I variants of Kv11.1 (hERG1) potassium channel. *Biophys. J.* 108, 1414–1424. doi: 10.1016/j.bpj.2014.12.056

Perry, M. D., Ng, C.-A., Mann, S. A., Sadrieh, A., Imtiaz, M., Hill, A. P., et al. (2015). Getting to the heart of hERG K+ channel gating. *J. Physiol.* 593, 2575–2585. doi: 10.1113/JP270095

Perry, M. D., Ng, C. A., and Vandenberg, J. I. (2013a). Pore helices play a dynamic role as integrators of domain motion during Kv11.1 channel inactivation gating. *J. Biol. Chem.* 288, 11482–11491. doi: 10.1074/jbc.M113.461442

Perry, M. D., Wong, S., Ng, C. A., and Vandenberg, J. I. (2013b). Hydrophobic interactions between the voltage sensor and pore mediate inactivation in Kv11.1 channels. *J. Gen. Physiol.* 142, 275–288. doi: 10.1085/jgp.201310975

Phillips, J. C., Braun, R., Wang, W., Gumbart, J., Tajkhorshid, E., Villa, E., et al. (2005). Scalable molecular dynamics with NAMD. *J. Comput. Chem.* 26, 1781–1802. doi: 10.1002/jcc.20289

Robertson, G. A. (2012). hERG subunit-specific contributions to gating and disease. *Biophys. J.* 102, 212A. doi: 10.1016/j.bpj.2011.11.1157

Robertson, G. A., Sale, H., Tester, D., O'hara, T. J., Phartiyal, P., Wang, J., et al. (2008). hERG 1b as a potential target for inherited and acquired long QT syndrome. *Circulation* 118:S525.

Romero, L., Trenor, B., Yang, P.-C., Saiz, J., and Clancy, C. E. (2015). *In silico* screening of the impact of hERG channel kinetic abnormalities on channel block and susceptibility to acquired long QT syndrome. *J. Mol. Cell. Cardiol.* 87, 271–282. doi: 10.1016/j.yjmcc.2015.08.015

Rudy, Y., and Silva, J. R. (2006). Computational biology in the study of cardiac ion channels and cell electrophysiology. *Q. Rev. Biophys.* 39, 57–116. doi: 10.1017/S0033583506004227

Saenen, J. B., Labro, A. J., Raes, A., and Snyders, D. J. (2006). Modulation of HERG gating by a charge cluster in the N-terminal proximal domain. *Biophys. J.* 91, 4381–4391. doi: 10.1529/biophysj.106.087247

Sale, H., Wang, J., O'hara, T. J., Tester, D. J., Phartiyal, P., He, J.-Q., et al. (2008). Physiological properties of hERG 1a/1b heteromeric currents and a hERG 1b-specific mutation associated with long-QT syndrome. *Circ. Res.* 103, E81–E95. doi: 10.1161/CIRCRESAHA.108.185249

Sanguinetti, M. C., Jiang, C. G., Curran, M. E., and Keating, M. T. (1995). A mechanistic link between an inherited and an acquired cardiac arrhythmia: HERG encodes the IKr potassium channel. *Cell* 81, 299–307. doi: 10.1016/0092-8674(95)90340-2

Schönherr, R., and Heinemann, S. H. (1996). Molecular determinants for activation and inactivation of HERG, a human inward rectifier potassium channel. *J. Physiol.* 493, 635–642. doi: 10.1113/jphysiol.1996.sp021410

Shaw, R. M., and Rudy, Y. (1997). Electrophysiologic effects of acute myocardial ischemia. A mechanistic investigation of action potential conduction and conduction failure. *Circ. Res.* 80, 124–138. doi: 10.1161/01.RES.80.1.124

Shimizu, W., and Antzelevitch, C. (1999). Cellular basis for long QT, transmural dispersion of repolarization, and torsade de pointes in the long QT syndrome. *J. Electrocardiol.* 32, 177–184. doi: 10.1016/S0022-0736(99)90077-8

Smith, P. L., Baukrowitz, T., and Yellen, G. (1996). The inward rectification mechanism of the HERG cardiac potassium channel. *Nature* 379, 833–836. doi: 10.1038/379833a0

Splawski, I., Shen, J. X., Timothy, K. W., Vincent, G. M., Lehmann, M. H., and Keating, M. T. (1998). Genomic structure of three long QT syndrome genes: KVLQT1, HERG, and KCNE1. *Genomics* 51, 86–97. doi: 10.1006/geno.1998.5361

Ten Tusscher, K. H. W. J., and Panfilov, A. V. (2006). Cell model for efficient simulation of wave propagation in human ventricular tissue under normal and pathological conditions. *Phys. Med. Biol.* 51, 6141–6156. doi: 10.1088/0031-9155/51/23/014

Thomson, S. J., Hansen, A., and Sanguinetti, M. C. (2014). Concerted All-or-none subunit interactions mediate slow deactivation of human ether-a-go-go-related gene K+ channels. *J. Biol. Chem.* 289, 23428–23436. doi: 10.1074/jbc.M114.582437

Trudeau, M. C., Leung, L. M., Roti, E. R., and Robertson, G. A. (2011). hERG1a N-terminal eag domain-containing polypeptides regulate homomeric hERG1b and heteromeric hERG1a/hERG1b channels: a possible mechanism for long QT syndrome. *J. Gen. Physiol.* 138, 581–592. doi: 10.1085/jgp.201110683

Trudeau, M. C., Warmke, J. W., Ganetzky, B., and Robertson, G. A. (1995). hERG, a human inward rectifier in the voltage-gated potassium channel family. *Science* 269, 92–95. doi: 10.1126/science.7604285

Vandenberg, J. I., Perry, M. D., Perrin, M. J., Mann, S. A., Ke, Y., and Hill, A. P. (2012). hERG K+ channels: structure, function, and clinical significance. *Physiol. Rev.* 92, 1393–1478. doi: 10.1152/physrev.00036.2011

Vasilef, I. (2013). *Data Analysis and Scientific Visualization.* Utrecht: Universiteit Utrecht.

Viswanathan, P. C., Shaw, R. M., and Rudy, Y. (1999). Effecs of IKr and IKs heterogeneity on action potential duration and its rate dependence. *Circulation* 99, 2466–2474. doi: 10.1161/01.CIR.99.18.2466

Wacker, S., Noskov, S. Y., and Perissinotti, L. L. (2017). Computational models for understanding of structure, function and pharmacology of the cardiac potassium channel Kv11.1 (hERG). *Curr. Top Med. Chem.* 17, 2681–2702. doi: 10.2174/1568026617666170414143430

Wang, S. M., Liu, S. G., Morales, M. J., Strauss, H. C., and Rasmusson, R. L. (1997). A quantitative analysis of the activation and inactivation kinetics of HERG expressed in *Xenopus oocytes. J. Physiol.* 502, 45-60. doi: 10.1111/j.1469-7793.1997.045bl.x

Wang, W. W., and Mackinnon, R. (2017). Cryo-EM structure of the open human ether-a-go-go-related K+ channel hERG. *Cell* 169, 422.e10–430.e10. doi: 10.1016/j.cell.2017.03.048

Wang, X., Xu, R., Abernathey, G., Taylor, J., Alzghoul, M. B., Hannon, K., et al. (2008). Kv11.1 channel subunit composition includes MinK and varies developmentally in mouse cardiac muscle. *Dev. Dyn.* 237, 2430–2437. doi: 10.1002/dvdy.21671

Whicher, J. R., and Mackinnon, R. (2016). Structure of the voltage-gated K+ channel Eag1 reveals an alternative voltage sensing mechanism. *Science* 353, 664–669. doi: 10.1126/science.aaf8070

Yang, P. C., Perissinotti, L. L., López-Redondo, F., Wang, Y., Demarco, K. R., Jeng, M. T., et al. (2017). A multiscale computational modelling approach predicts mechanisms of female sex risk in the setting of arousal-induced arrhythmias. *J. Physiol.* 595, 4695–4723. doi: 10.1113/JP273142

Zhang, M., Liu, J., and Tseng, G. N. (2004). Gating charges in the activation and inactivation processes of the hERG channel. *J. Gen. Physiol.* 124, 703–718. doi: 10.1085/jgp.200409119

5

Synergistic Anti-Arrhythmic Effects in Human Atria with Combined Use of Sodium Blockers and Acacetin

*Haibo Ni[1, 2, 3], Dominic G. Whittaker[1], Wei Wang[1], Wayne R. Giles[4], Sanjiv M. Narayan[5] and Henggui Zhang[1, 2, 3, 6]**

[1] Biological Physics Group, University of Manchester, Manchester, United Kingdom, [2] Space Institute of Southern China, Shenzhen, China, [3] Key Laboratory of Medical Electrophysiology, Ministry of Education, Collaborative Innovation Center for Prevention and Treatment of Cardiovascular Disease/Institute of Cardiovascular Research, Southwest Medical University, Luzhou, China, [4] Faculties of Kinesiology and Medicine, University of Calgary, Calgary, AB, Canada, [5] Department of Medicine, Stanford University School of Medicine, Stanford, CA, United States, [6] School of Computer Science and Technology, Harbin Institute of Technology, Harbin, China

***Correspondence:**
Henggui Zhang
henggui.zhang@manchester.ac.uk

Atrial fibrillation (AF) is the most common cardiac arrhythmia. Developing effective and safe anti-AF drugs remains an unmet challenge. Simultaneous block of both atrial-specific ultra-rapid delayed rectifier potassium (K^+) current (I_{Kur}) and the Na^+ current (I_{Na}) has been hypothesized to be anti-AF, without inducing significant QT prolongation and ventricular side effects. However, the antiarrhythmic advantage of simultaneously blocking these two channels vs. individual block in the setting of AF-induced electrical remodeling remains to be documented. Furthermore, many I_{Kur} blockers such as acacetin and AVE0118, partially inhibit other K^+ currents in the atria. Whether this multi-K^+-block produces greater anti-AF effects compared with selective I_{Kur}-block has not been fully understood. The aim of this study was to use computer models to (i) assess the impact of multi-K^+-block as exhibited by many I_{Kur} blokers, and (ii) evaluate the antiarrhythmic effect of blocking I_{Kur} and I_{Na}, either alone or in combination, on atrial and ventricular electrical excitation and recovery in the setting of AF-induced electrical-remodeling. Contemporary mathematical models of human atrial and ventricular cells were modified to incorporate dose-dependent actions of acacetin (a multichannel blocker primarily inhibiting I_{Kur} while less potently blocking I_{to}, I_{Kr}, and I_{Ks}). Rate- and atrial-selective inhibition of I_{Na} was also incorporated into the models. These single myocyte models were then incorporated into multicellular two-dimensional (2D) and three-dimensional (3D) anatomical models of the human atria. As expected, application of I_{Kur} blocker produced pronounced action potential duration (APD) prolongation in atrial myocytes. Furthermore, combined multiple K^+-channel block that mimicked the effects of acacetin exhibited synergistic APD prolongations. Synergistically anti-AF effects following inhibition of I_{Na} and combined I_{Kur}/K^+-channels were also observed. The attainable maximal AF-selectivity of I_{Na} inhibition was greatly augmented by blocking I_{Kur} or multiple K^+-currents in the atrial myocytes. This enhanced anti-arrhythmic effects of combined block of Na^+- and K^+-channels were also seen in 2D and 3D simulations; specially, there was an enhanced efficacy in terminating re-entrant excitation waves, exerting improved antiarrhythmic effects in the human atria as compared to a single-channel block. However, in the human ventricular myocytes and tissue, cellular repolarization and computed QT intervals were modestly affected in the presence of actions of acacetin and I_{Na} blockers (either alone or in combination). In conclusion, this study demonstrates synergistic antiarrhythmic benefits of combined block of I_{Kur} and I_{Na}, as well as those of I_{Na} and combined multi K^+-current block of acacetin, without significant alterations of ventricular repolarization and QT intervals. This approach may be a valuable strategy for the treatment of AF.

Keywords: atrial-selective block, atrial fibrillation, sodium and potassium current block, multiscale simulation, synergistic antiarrhythmic effect

INTRODUCTION

Despite recent advances in the management of Atrial fibrillation (AF), the world's most common cardiac arrhythmia (Dobrev et al., 2012; Nattel and Dobrev, 2017), developing effective and safe antiarrhythmic drugs for treatment of AF remains challenging (Aguilar-Shardonofsky et al., 2012; Aguilar et al., 2015). Frequently these antiarrhythmic agents promote ventricular arrhythmias (Dobrev et al., 2012; Woods and Olgin, 2014; Voigt and Dobrev, 2016) by prolonging cellular action potential durations (APDs). The associated QT-interval prolongation can lead to life-threatening consequences. Developing atrial-selective drugs is acknowledged to be a current strategy for the treatment of AF (Burashnikov et al., 2007).

Atrial and ventricular tissues show intrinsic regional differences in their cellular ion channel properties, thus suggesting a basis for developing atrial-selective drugs. For example, the atrial and ventricular fast sodium (Na^+) channel currents (I_{Na}) exhibit different voltage-dependent inactivation properties, opening the opportunity for atrial-selective Na^+ channel blockade (Burashnikov et al., 2007; Antzelevitch and Burashnikov, 2009; Zygmunt et al., 2011). Previous simulation studies have demonstrated that by optimizing state-dependent Na^+-channel blocking dynamics (i.e., drug-channel interaction parameters), atrial-selective block of I_{Na} could be achieved and that could maximize pharmaceutical effects on the atria while minimizing their proarrhythmic actions in the ventricles (Aguilar-Shardonofsky et al., 2012; Aguilar et al., 2015).

Another tissue-specific difference between the atria and ventricles is that the ultra-rapid delayed rectifier potassium current (I_{Kur}, carried by the $K_V1.5$ channel) contributes to repolarization in the atria but plays little role in the ventricles (Tamargo et al., 2009; Ravens and Wettwer, 2011). Recent studies suggest that atrial-selective blockade of I_{Kur} may be an effective pharmacological treatment of AF (Li et al., 2008; Pavri et al., 2012; Loose et al., 2014; Ford et al., 2016). Although the efficacy of I_{Kur} block in the treatment of AF remains controversial (Burashnikov and Antzelevitch, 2008), multiple I_{Kur} blockers have been developed (Tamargo et al., 2009; Loose et al., 2014; Wettwer and Terlau, 2014; Ford et al., 2016). Interestingly, these I_{Kur} blockers actually target multiple channels, and are known to inhibit other K^+ currents including I_{to} and $I_{K,ACh}$ in the atria (Burashnikov and Antzelevitch, 2008). Examples of such blockers include AVE0118 (Gögelein et al., 2004), AVE1231 (Wirth et al., 2007), AZD7009 (Persson et al., 2005), and acacetin (Li et al., 2008). Among these channel blockers, acacetin, a natural flavone initially isolated from a traditional Chinese medicine *Xuelianhua*, potently blocks I_{Kur}, I_{to}, and $I_{K,ACh}$, and has a smaller potency in inhibiting I_{Kr} and I_{Ks} (Li et al., 2008), similar to AVE0118 (Gögelein et al., 2004; Haan et al., 2006). Acacetin is regarded as a promising atrial-selective agent for the treatment of AF (Li et al., 2008). However, the actions of acacetin on atrial electrophysiology, especially its effects following AF-induced electrical remodeling of atrial electrophysiological properties (Dobrev et al., 2012), remain to be elucidated. Furthermore, since most I_{Kur} blockers inhibit other K^+ channels, the question whether the "additional" inhibitive actions produce favorable antiarrhythmic effects has not been addressed thoroughly. A better understanding of these effects of modulating multiple ion channels on atrial excitation and recovery/repolarization may provide insights into evaluating and developing antiarrhythmic drugs.

Interestingly, simultaneous multiple-channel blocking of both depolarization and repolarization currents is attracting more attention since empirical observations suggest that such multi-channel blockers generally mediate more effective antiarrhythmic effects (Kirchhoff et al., 2015; Reiffel et al., 2015; Hartmann et al., 2016). A recent numerical and experimental study on the canine heart (Aguilar et al., 2015) suggested that blocking K^+ currents enhanced the anti-arrhythmic effects and AF-selectivity of I_{Na} blockade. In their study, I_{Kur} block was modeled using a simple pore block scheme by reducing the conductance of the channel. As the kinetics of drug action plays an important role in the effects of I_{Kur} blockers (Scholz et al., 2013; Ellinwood et al., 2017), in simulating I_{Kur} block a state-dependent block model reproducing a realistic blocker is more favorable. Once again, the effects of combined I_{Na} and I_{Kur} block on the human atria, especially in the setting of AF-induced electrical remodeling which reduced I_{Kur}, remain to be elucidated. It is also unclear how multiple-channel blockade may affect QT interval.

In the present study, it was hypothesized that combined block of I_{Na} and K^+-currents (predominantly I_{Kur}) could produce antiarrhythmic benefits compared with the application of either blocker alone in the setting of AF-induced electrical remodeling. We have tested the hypothesis with the following three aims: (i) to identify and illustrate the effects of the realistic I_{Kur}

blocker, acacetin, on atrial electrophysiology following AF-related remodeling; (ii) to assess whether combined I_{Na} and I_{Kur} block produce synergistic antiarrhythmic effects; and (iii) to investigate the action of such drug combinations on ventricular electrophysiology.

METHODS

Modeling Electrophysiology of the Human Heart

To simulate human atrial electrophysiology, an updated Colman et al. model for atrial electrophysiology (Colman et al., 2013, 2017) was used. For *in silico* study of effects of chronic AF-(cAF) induced electrophysiological remodeling on the atria, we incorporated the cAF model parameters from our previous study (Colman et al., 2013) into the updated atrial single cell model (for details please see Online Supplement Material 1.1).

To assess the effects of the anti-AF drugs on the human ventricles, simulations were performed to investigate the actions of the anti-AF drugs on the ventricular AP, I_{Na} and QT intervals in the electrograms. In these simulations, the mathematical model developed by O'Hara et al. (2011) was used to represent the ventricular electrophysiology. Additionally, the I_{Na} formulation in the model was replaced by the one in the Luo–Rudy model (Luo and Rudy, 1994), which enabled electrical excitation to propagate in the tissue model.

More detailed descriptions of the electrophysiological models of human atrial and ventricular cells are given in Online Supplementary Material 1.1.

Modeling State-Dependent I_{Na} Block

As in previous studies (Aguilar-Shardonofsky et al., 2012; Aguilar et al., 2015), I_{Na} block was simulated using a guarded receptor model with dynamical drug-channel interactions. This approach allows for investigations of the role of the specified parameters for selected I_{Na} blockers, and effects of combined I_{Kur} block on the atrial selectivity of Na^+-channel block. The guarded receptor model considers the binding and unbinding kinetics of the drug to I_{Na} channels in a drug concentration-dependent manner. They can be described by first-order transition equations (Aguilar-Shardonofsky et al., 2012; Aguilar et al., 2015). It was also assumed that the drug predominantly binds to the activated and/or inactivated states of I_{Na}. The blockade of I_{Na} is given by Aguilar-Shardonofsky et al. (2012) and Aguilar et al. (2015):

$$I_{Na} = g_{Na}\,(1 - B_A - B_I)\, m^3 hj\,(V_m - E_{Na}) \quad (1)$$

$$\frac{dB_A}{dt} = K_A\,[D_{Na^+}]\, m^3 hj\,(1 - B_A - B_I) - L_A B_A \quad (2)$$

$$\frac{dB_I}{dt} = K_I\,[D_{Na^+}]\,(1 - h)\,(1 - B_A - B_I) - L_I B_I \quad (3)$$

where g_{Na} is the maximum conductance of I_{Na}; B_A and B_I are the fractional blockade of activation and inactivation channels; m is the activation gate state variable, h and j are the inactivation gate state variables; V_m the transmembrane potential; E_{Na} the reversal potential of Na^+; K_A, K_I the binding constants and L_A, L_I the unbinding constants; $[D_{Na^+}]$ is the concentration of a Na^+-blocker. As in previous studies (Aguilar-Shardonofsky et al., 2012; Aguilar et al., 2015), a concentration of 60 μM was utilized unless otherwise stated; this concentration was chosen based on previous experimental and modeling studies (Zhu et al., 2006; Moreno et al., 2011; Aguilar-Shardonofsky et al., 2012; Aguilar et al., 2015); a parameter set ($K_A = 100\ ms^{-1}\cdot M^{-1}$, $K_I = 100\ ms^{-1}\cdot M^{-1}$, $L_A = 1\ ms^{-1}$, $L_I = 0.01\ ms^{-1}$) was first used to represent the kinetics of an I_{Na}-selective blocker.

In our investigations of the AF-selectivity of I_{Na} block following AF-remodeling, the binding and unbinding constants of the I_{Na} blockers were varied to evaluate the dependence of I_{Na} block on these parameters, and whether an atrial-selective anti-AF action could be achieved in cAF-remodeled myoctes. The AF-selectivity of Na^+-channel blockade was defined as the product of atrial-selectivity, rate-selectivity and block efficacy. With fractional block (B_f) by Na^+-channel blockers being measured as the relative reduction in the peak of I_{Na}, the rate-selectivity was defined as the ratio of B_f measured in an atrial myocyte paced at 6 Hz to that paced at 1 Hz (Aguilar-Shardonofsky et al., 2012; Aguilar et al., 2015). Atrial-selectivity was used to determine the extent of atrial-ventricular difference in response to each drug. This was represented by the ratio of B_f observed from an atrial myocyte to that of a ventricular cell both paced at 1 Hz. In this study, we defined block efficacy (E) as:

$$E = \frac{1.0}{1.0 + \left(\frac{0.5}{B_{f,6Hz}}\right)^4} \quad (4)$$

where $B_{f,6Hz}$ is the fractional block of I_{Na} measured in an atrial cell paced at 6 Hz. Different from Aguilar et al. (2015), we introduced block efficacy to constrain the measure of AF-selectivity when the fractional block observed in a ventricular cell paced was minimal (and could result in a great atrial-selectivity), which otherwise could give a great value in AF-selectivity regardless of a small $B_{f,6Hz}$.

To assess the dependence of the AF-selectivity of I_{Na} block on the drug action kinetics, the unbinding constants L_A and L_I were first varied over a parameter space from 10^{-5} to $10^0\ ms^{-1}$, while K_A and K_I were fixed (see Figure S6 of online Supplementary Materials for more details). The resultant unbinding constants were used in subsequent optimizations varying K_A and K_I. The parameter space was {1, 10, 100, 500, 2,500, 10,000} for K_A and {1, 10, 100, 200, 500, 2,500} for K_I. The parameter space fell into a likely range of I_{Na} blockers as summarized in Aguilar-Shardonofsky et al. (2012).

Modeling Effects of Acacetin on Atrial and Ventricular Electrophysiology

Acacetin was the chosen I_{Kur} blocker in the present study. To reveal the functional effects of (i) pure I_{Kur} block vs. (ii) the effects of combined K^+ currents block by acacetin on human atrial electrophysiology, the actions of acacetin were modeled by considering its effects on (a) I_{Kur} only, and (b) all the respective K^+ currents as detailed in **Table 1**. This approach allows for modeling the effects of the selective I_{Kur} block as well as uncovering the role of "additional" inhibitory effects of acacetin on other K^+ currents.

TABLE 1 | Concentration-dependent block of K^+-currents by acacetin (Li et al., 2008; Wu et al., 2011).

	I_{Kur}	I_{to}	I_{Kr}	I_{Ks}
IC_{50} (μM)	3–3.2	9.3	32.4	81.4
Hill coefficient	0.8	0.9	0.9	0.8
Fractional inhibition at 3.2 μM	50%	28%	11%	7%

Modeling Effect of Acacetin on I_{Kur}

Previous modeling studies have demonstrated the important role of the kinetic properties of drug actions in I_{Kur} block (Tsujimae et al., 2008; Almquist et al., 2010; Scholz et al., 2013). In addition, the pharmaceutical effects of acacetin on I_{Kur} are characterized by use- and rate-dependencies (Wu et al., 2011), which have also been observed in other I_{Kur} blockers (Pavri et al., 2012; Ford et al., 2016). Therefore, it was necessary to adopt a state-dependent block model (Brennan et al., 2009) for simulating the blockade of I_{Kur} by acacetin. Similar to our approach for modeling I_{Na} block, the binding and unbinding kinetics of a drug was described by a first-order transition equation, in contrast to simulating I_{Kur} block by reducing its conductance in Aguilar et al. (2015). Experimental studies revealed that acacetin binds to both the open and closed gates of $K_V1.5$ (Wu et al., 2011). Therefore, following the guarded receptor formulas given in Equations (1–3), the formulation of inactivation-state binding and unbinding kinetics in I_{Na} block was modified to simulate the closed-state block of I_{Kur} by acacetin. The guarded receptor model of I_{Kur} block by acacetin is given by:

$$I_{Kur} = g_{Kur}\left(1 - B_O - B_C\right) ai \left(V_m - E_K\right) \tag{5}$$

$$\frac{dB_O}{dt} = K_O \exp\left(Z_{KO}\frac{V_mF}{RT}\right)\left[D_{K^+}\right] ai \left(1 - B_O - B_c\right) - L_O \exp\left(-Z_{LO}\frac{V_mF}{RT}\right) B_O \tag{6}$$

$$\frac{dB_c}{dt} = K_c \exp\left(Z_{Kc}\frac{V_mF}{RT}\right)\left[D_{K^+}\right]\left(1 - a\right) i \left(1 - B_O - B_c\right) - L_c \exp\left(-Z_{Lc}\frac{V_mF}{RT}\right) B_c \tag{7}$$

where g_{Kur} is the conductance of I_{Kur}; B_o and B_C are the fractional block on open and closed state variables, respectively; a and i are the activation and inactivation gate variables; E_K is the reversal potential of potassium; F, R, and T are the Faraday's constant, universal gas constant and temperature respectively. K_O and K_c are the binding constants; L_O and L_c are the unbinding constants; Z_{KO}, Z_{LO}, Z_{Kc} and Z_{Lc} are the drug charge parameters for the corresponding binding or unbinding processes; $[D_{K^+}]$ is the concentration of acacetin applied. The binding and unbinding parameters were obtained by fitting the model to the experimental data on the rate-dependent blockade of I_{Kur} by acacetin (Wu et al., 2011), as detailed in Online Supplementary Material 1.1.

Figure 1 shows a simulated frequency-dependent block of I_{Kur} by acacetin, and this is compared to the experimental data (**Figures 1A,B**). As shown, repeating the voltage command (**Figure 1B**, insert) at 0.5 Hz resulted in an approximately 50% blockade in this current after application of 3 μM acacetin. Increasing the voltage command rate to 4 Hz significantly increased the relative fractional block to approximately 63% (**Figure 1C**).

Modeling Effect of Acacetin on I_{to}, I_{Kr}, and I_{Ks}

In addition to inhibiting I_{Kur} in the atria, acacetin potently blocks both I_{to} and $I_{K,ACh}$, and also modulates I_{Kr} and I_{Ks}, exhibiting multiple K^+-current block. The parameters of Hill equations describing use-dependent inhibitions of these channels by acacetin are shown in **Table 1**. In the simulations, the effects of acacetin on these channels were modeled using a simple pore block model (Yuan et al., 2015). In the present study, we did not simulate the effects of acacetin on $I_{K,ACh}$ inhibitions as the role of autonomic regulation on AF is beyond the scope of the study.

Simulations of the Effects of Acacetin on Human Ventricle

The effects of acacetin on human ventricular APs are unknown, although experimental data demonstrated that acacetin at 30 μM did not affect the heart rate and QT interval in isolated rabbit hearts (Li et al., 2008). In the present study, it was assumed that similar effects on the K^+ currents (I_{to}, I_{Kr}, I_{Ks}) in atrial myocytes could be extrapolated to the ventricular myocytes. We acknowledge that I_{Kur} is negligible in ventricles (Ravens and Wettwer, 2011), therefore in simulations of blocking I_{Kur} alone, the ventricular electrophysiology was not affected.

Tissue Models

The effects of acacetin and I_{Na} blockers on atrial and ventricular electrophysiology were further evaluated using tissue models. The monodomain equation (Clayton et al., 2011) was employed to simulate the excitation wave propagation in the myocardium. 1D models of human atrial strands were used to quantify the effects of channel blockers on atrial conduction velocity and APD restitution properties. Changes in ventricular depolarization and repolarization in response to these drugs were evaluated using a 1D model representing a transmural strand of ventricular tissue. In order to evaluate the antiarrhythmic effects of the channel blockers on re-entrant excitations in atria in the setting of cAF-induced remodeling, both idealized 2D models representing an isotropic slab of atrial tissue and an anatomically accurate 3D model of the human atria (Aslanidi et al., 2011; Colman et al., 2013, 2017; Whittaker et al., 2017) were employed to simulate the behavior of re-entrant excitations in atrial tissue. Pseudo-ECGs (pECGs) (Gima and Rudy, 2002; Baher et al., 2006) were computed as a measure of the excitation rates of in-tissue with sprial excitation waves. Detailed descriptions of these tissue models and pECGs are given in Online Supplementary Material 1.2, 1.3.

RESULTS

The updated Colman et al. human atrial model was first used to simulate effects cAF-induced remodeling on the

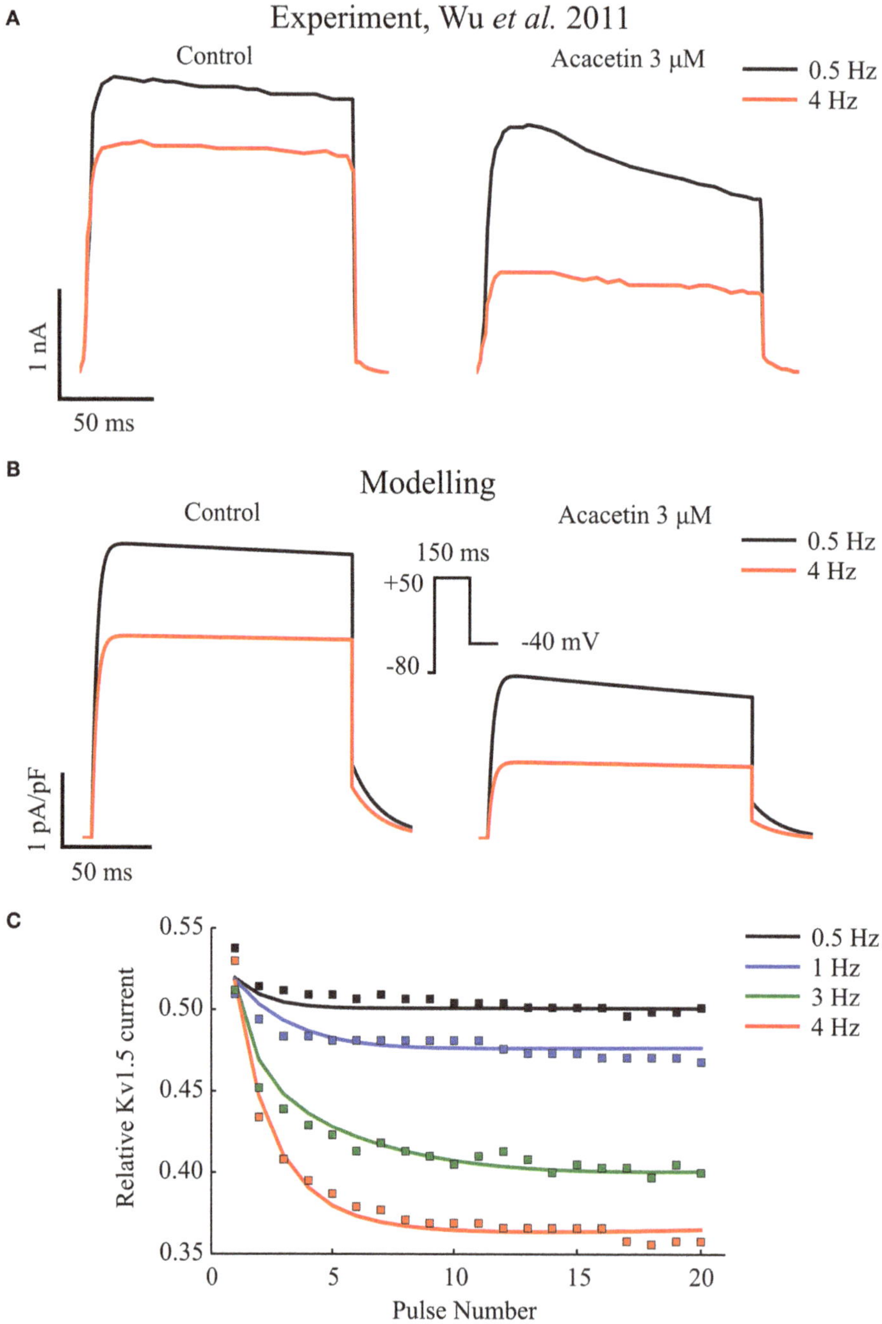

FIGURE 1 | Frequency-dependent inhibition of I_{Kur} by acacetin. **(A)** Experimental and **(B)** simulated traces of $K_V1.5$ channel current elicited from the 20th voltage step repeating at 0.5 and 4 Hz in control (left) and after exposure to 3 μM of acacetin (right). **(C)** Relative remaining I_{Kur} following application of acacetin at various frequencies plotted against the pulse number of the voltage step. The simulated data (lines) were compared with experimental values (squares). The relative fraction was obtained by normalizing the end-step current measured from each pulse following application of acacetin to that of control. Experimental data were digitalized from Wu et al. (2011).

action potential (AP) and calcium transient (CaT). Details are presented in Online Supplementary Material 2.1. The resultant changes in APD, APD restitution and CaT following cAF-induced remodeling as compared to those under the normal condition showed good agreement with previous experimental (Bosch et al., 1999; Osaka et al., 2000; Workman et al., 2001; Dobrev and Ravens, 2003; Voigt et al., 2012) and simulation studies (Zhang et al., 2005; Grandi et al., 2011; Colman et al., 2013, 2017; Wilhelms et al., 2013).

Effects of Application of Acacetin on Human Atrial Cells

To reveal the roles of inhibition of individual channels by acacetin in modulating cellular AP by acacetin, both the individual and combined block of I_{to}, I_{Kr}, I_{Kur}, and I_{Ks} by acacetin (3.2 μM) in simulated SR at cycle length 1,000 ms without (normal) or with cAF-related electrical remodeling were simulated. **Figures 2A,B** illustrates the effects of individual and combined K^+-channel block by acacetin on AP waveform. The alterations to APD relative to the control are summarized in **Figures 2C,D**.

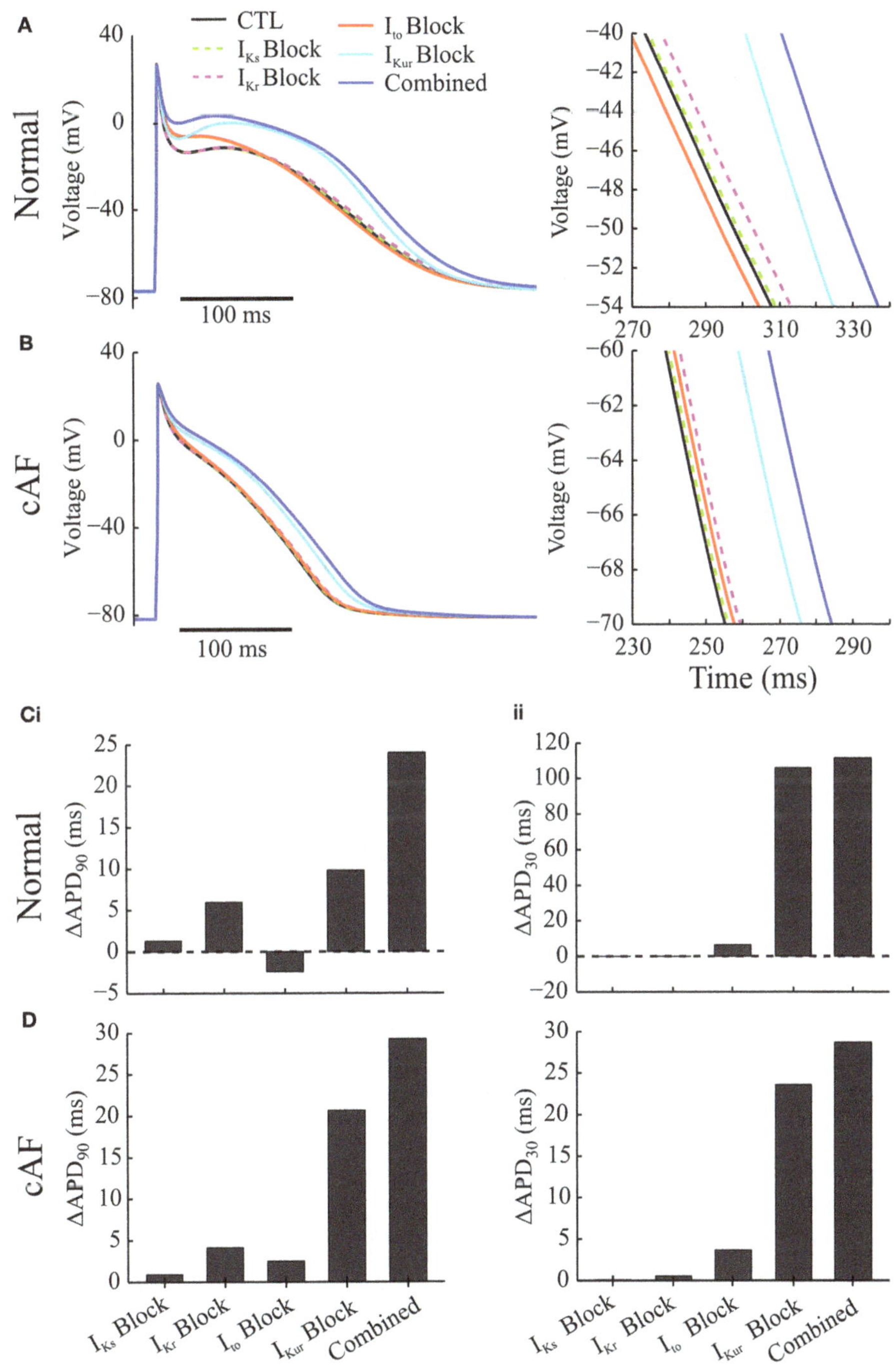

FIGURE 2 | Effects of individual vs. combined block of K^+-currents by acacetin (3.2 μM) on the human atrial AP in normal and cAF-remodeled myocytes paced at 1 Hz. **(A,B)** Effects on the atrial AP in **(A)** normal and **(B)** cAF-remodeled myocytes; a zoomed-in view for the traces of AP during phase-3 is plotted to the right. **(C,D)** Alterations in the **(i)** APD_{90} and **(ii)** APD_{30} by the simulated block obtained from atrial cells in **(C)** normal and **(D)** cAF-remodeled myocytes.

In the absence of electrical remodeling, in normal myocytes at a cycle length of 1,000 ms, simulated I_{Ks} or I_{Kr} block by acacetin (3.2 μM) presented no significant alterations to the atrial AP: although the atrial repolarization was delayed by 1.3 and 5.9 ms, respectively, the plateau phase was not affected, which is consistent with the minimal potency of acacetin on these channels (**Table 1**). Similar effects were also obtained from our simulated I_{Kr} and I_{Ks} block by the compound in the cAF-remodeled atrial cells.

Selective block of I_{to} (alone) by acacetin elevated the atrial plateau potential in both normal and cAF-remodeled myocytes paced at 1 Hz, and this led to modest prolongations in APD_{30} (by 6.4 and 3.6 ms for normal and AF-remodeling myocytes, respectively). The changes in APD_{90} due to I_{to} block varied between the two conditions: under normal conditions the atrial APD_{90} was shortened by 2.4 ms, whereas it was prolonged by 3.7 ms following cAF-remodeling at a stimulus rate of 1 Hz.

In contrast, blocking I_{Kur} alone by acacetin resulted in a pronounced alteration to the shape and duration of the AP in both normal and cAF-remodeled myocytes. The inhibition in I_{Kur} significantly elevated the plateau potential of atrial AP (by 7.1 and 5.7 mV in normal and cAF-remodeled myocytes, respectively), and this was accompanied by marked prolongations in APD_{30} (by 105.9 and 23.6 ms in normal and cAF-remodeled myocytes, respectively). The prolongation in APD_{90} induced by the I_{Kur} block was 9.8 ms for normal atrial cells, and was more pronounced (23.6 ms) in cAF-remodeled myocytes, despite that I_{Kur} was down-regulated by cAF-remodeling.

We note that combined effects of acacetin (3.2 μM) on multiple K^+-currents produced greater alterations to the AP than those of any individual blocking effect. We have quantified effects produced by the combined block and compared it with the sum of the changes seen in each individual block. Synergistic effects were observed in the changes in APD_{90}, represented by a further prolongation of 9.3 and 1.1 ms in APD_{90} in normal and cAF-remodeled myocytes, respectively. Additionally, the effects of I_{Kur} block dominated the AP-modulation by the compound, which is consistent with the high potency of acacetin on the channel (**Table 1**).

Effects of Sodium Blocker and Acacetin on cAF-Remodeled Atrial Myocytes and Ventricular Cells

Effects on Single Myocyte AP and I_{Na}

Individual and combined effects of Na^+-block (indicated by Bl·I_{Na}) and K^+-block by acacetin (3.2 μM) on human atrial electrophysiology after cAF-remodeling were simulated to assess any anti-AF benefits. Effects of acacetin (representing K^+-block) were simulated in different settings: (i) I_{Kur} block alone (denoted by Bl·I_{Kur}) and (ii) combined block of all K^+-currents in **Table 1** (denoted by Comb·Bl·I_X). In addition, the effects of Na^+- and K^+- block on human ventricular myocytes were also studied to assess the atrial-selectivity of the block. The results are shown in **Figures 3A–C** and quantitative measurements are shown in **Figures 4A–C**.

For atrial myocytes paced at 1 Hz, Bl·I_{Kur}, and Comb·Bl·I_X prolonged atrial APD (**Figure 4Ai** and as presented in Effects of Application of Acacetin on Human Atrial Cells) whilst their effects on peak I_{Na} were minimal (reducing peak I_{Na} by less than 0.3%). Bl·I_{Na} alone slightly reduced the peak I_{Na} by 1.63% without affecting the APD. The fractional inhibition in I_{Na} by I_{Na}-block was slightly increased by the addition of Bl·I_{Kur} or Comb·Bl·I_X (**Figure 4Aii**). In the ventricles, the simulated application of acacetin induced a prolongation of 19.5 ms in APD_{90} compared with that in control (drug-free) condition (**Figures 3B, 4Ci**). Bl·I_{Na} alone showed a negligible inhibitory effect on the ventricular I_{Na} (by 0.42%), which was also not affected by combining Bl·I_{Na} and Comb·Bl·I_X (**Figure 4Cii**).

In atrial myocytes paced at 6 Hz, AP alternans were observed under the drug-free condition (**Figure 3Ci**): the APD varied between 100.1 and 88.1 ms. In the presence of AP alternans, the changes in APD by the Na^+- and K^+- blockers were quantified by comparing the corresponding big APs at baseline and after drug actions. These values were selected based on the characteristics of AP (APD prolongations seen in the long AP, and reduced I_{Na} for the short AP) that may be anti-arrhythmic. The fractional reductions in peak I_{Na} were calculated from the I_{Na} associated with the shorter APs. The results showed that applying Bl·I_{Kur} or Comb·Bl·I_X alone both abolished the AP alternans while prolonging the APD to 116.3 and 126.3 ms and reducing the peak I_{Na} by 5.9 and 20.1%, respectively. The application of Bl·I_{Na} alone produced a minor APD prolongation (3.5 ms) and a reduction of 16.2% in peak I_{Na}. Combining block of I_{Na} with Bl·I_{Kur} or Comb·Bl·I_X promoted the genesis of AP alternans, resulting in substantial prolongations in the APD of the big APs (by 35.4 ms for Bl·I_{Kur} + Bl·I_{Na}, and 55.6 ms for Comb·Bl·I_X + Bl·I_{Na}) and dramatic decreases in the peak I_{Na} (by 57.5% for Bl·I_{Kur} + Bl·I_{Na} and 88.2% for Comb·Bl·I_X + Bl·I_{Na}) in the corresponding small APs. These results suggest that the combined block of Bl·I_{Na} and Comb·Bl·I_X/Bl·I_{Kur} exhibited synergistic antiarrhythmic effects manifested by prolongation in APD and reduction in peak I_{Na}. However, an increased susceptibility to AP alternans was observed at a fast pacing rate of 6 Hz, which may be potentially proarrhythmic at fast heart rates.

Effects on Steady-State Restitutions of APD and Conduction Velocity

Steady-state APD restitutions of cAF-remodeled human atria were simulated at both the cellular and tissue levels. In single myocyte simulations (Figure S5 in Online Supplementary Material 2.2), APD was prolonged over the entire range of simulated basic cycle lengths (BCL) for Bl·I_{Kur} and Comb·Bl·I_X as compared to the control (drug-free) conditions. The reduction in peak I_{Na} in Bl·I_{Na} was rate-dependent and significantly greater at fast pacing rates. K^+-block alone (Bl·I_{Kur} or Comb·Bl·I_X) slightly shifted the rate-dependence of peak I_{Na} to larger BCLs. In comparison to the effects of individual current block scenarios, synergistic reductions in peak I_{Na} were observed following combined blocks of Bl·I_{Na} with Bl·I_{Kur} or Comb·Bl·I_X over a wide range of BCLs. As compared to the drug-free conditions, AP alternans were observed at greater BCLs after K^+-block, and this was further increased by combined Na^+- and K^+-block (Figure S5 in Online Supplementary Material 2.2).

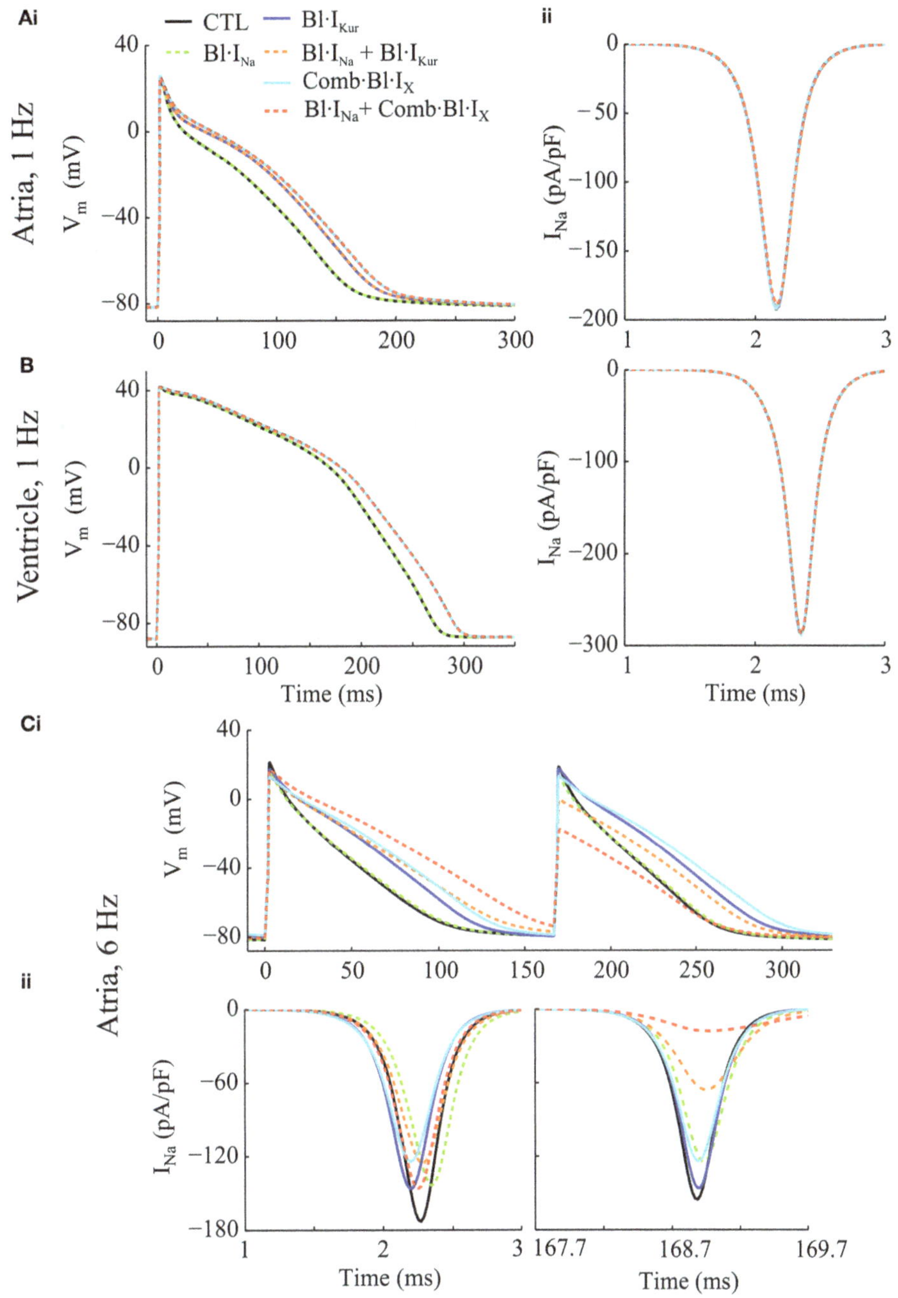

FIGURE 3 | Simulated AP and I_{Na} traces of cAF-remodeled atrial myocytes and ventricular cells in response to Na^+- and K^+- block regimens. **(Ai)** APs from cAF-remodeled atrial myocytes paced at 1 Hz; **(Aii)** Time courses of corresponding I_{Na} during the upstroke phase. **(B)** Simulated time courses of AP and I_{Na} of a ventricular cell paced at 1 Hz. **(C)** Illustration of **(i)** APs and **(ii)** the corresponding time courses of I_{Na} of a cAF-remodeled myocyte paced at 6 Hz. In these simulations, rate constants for I_{Na} blocker were: $K_A = 100\ \text{ms}^{-1} \cdot \text{M}^{-1}$, $K_I = 100\ \text{ms}^{-1} \cdot \text{M}^{-1}$, $l_A = 1\ \text{ms}^{-1}$, $l_I = 0.01\ \text{ms}^{-1}$.

Using a 1D model of atrial strands, the atrial APD and conduction velocity (CV) restitutions, as well as the rate-adaptation of in-tissue upstroke velocity (V_{max}), were evaluated (**Figure 5**). The atrial activation-recovery interval (ARI) was not affected by Bl·I_{Na} alone, whereas it was substantially lengthened by K^+-block as compared to control (**Figure 5A**). Applying K^+-block alone also shifted the CV and V_{max} restitution curves rightwards (i.e., to higher BCLs) (**Figures 5B,C**). These rate-adaptations of V_{max} and CV were progressively enhanced by Bl·I_{Na} and the combined block over a wide range of BCLs. Synergistically enhanced rate-dependent reductions in V_{max} and CV were observed in response to the combined blocks. Furthermore, K^+-block increased the critical BCLs for conduction block as compared to the drug-free condition (**Figure 5C**).

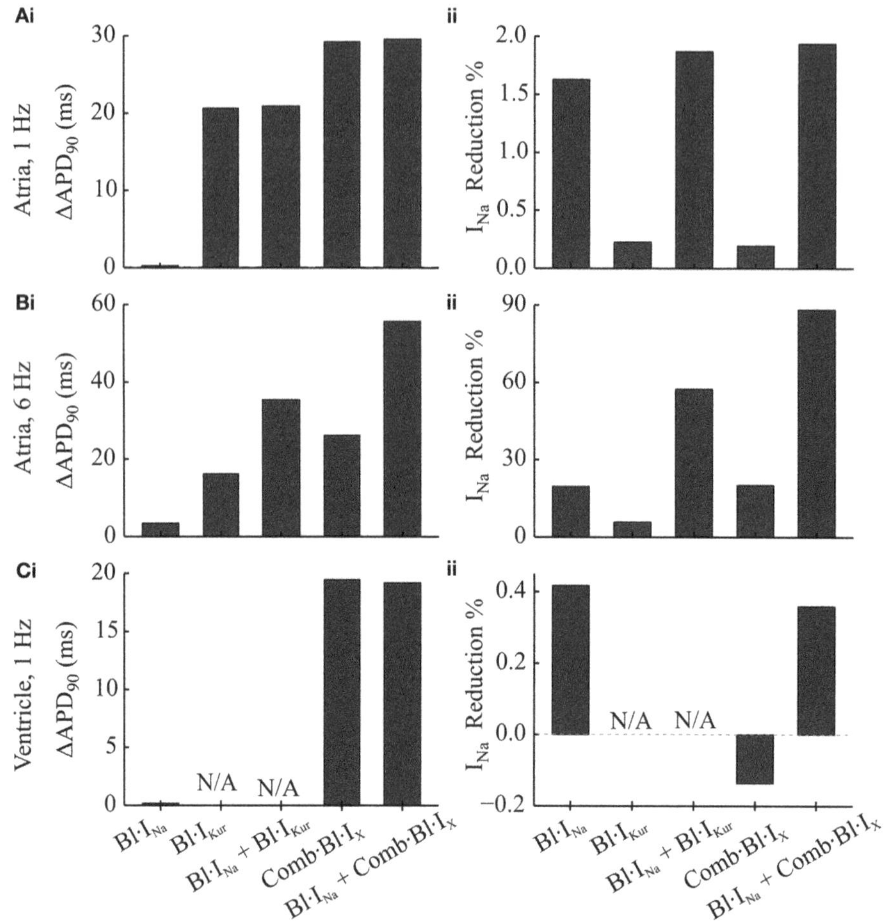

FIGURE 4 | Simulated changes in the APD and peak I_{Na} following the applications of Na^+- and K^+- block in comparison to the drug-free condition in cAF-remodeled atrial myocytes or ventricular cells. **(A,B)** Changes in **(i)** APD and **(ii)** peak I_{Na} measured from a cAF-remodeled atrial myocyte paced at **(A)** 1 Hz and **(B)** 6 Hz. In the presence of alternans, the changes in APD were quantified by comparing the corresponding longer APs. The fractional reductions in peak I_{Na} were calculated from the I_{Na} of the corresponding shorter APs. **(C)** Changes in **(i)** APD and **(ii)** peak I_{Na} measured from an *in silico* ventricular myocyte paced at 1 Hz.

Effects of Combined Na^+- and K^+- Block on the AF-Selectivity of I_{Na} block

AF-selectivity of Na^+ blockers in cAF-remodeled hearts was examined by varying the drug binding and unbinding constants over wide parameters spaces to provide information concerning drug-Na^+-channel interactions for various drug candidates. This was done by independently changing L_A and L_I for fixed $\{K_A, K_I\}$ (Online Supplementary Material 2.3); and then varying K_A and K_I for fixed $\{L_A, L_I\}$. In this way we obtained the maximum AF-selectivity over the parameter space of drug binding and unbinding kinetics. Simulations with varied K_A and K_I were repeated for Bl·I_{Na} + Bl·I_{Kur} and Bl·I_{Na} + Comb·Bl·I_X.

Figures 6A–D illustrates the block efficacy (defined in Equation 4), rate-selectivity, atrial-selectivity and the resultant AF-selectivity for Bl·I_{Na} alone and the combined block as a function of K_A and K_I. For Bl·I_{Na} alone, the block efficacy increased with increase of K_I, whereas the rate-selectivity was reduced by increasing K_A or K_I. The AF-selectivity reached a maximum value of 9 at $K_A = 1$ and $K_I = 500\ ms^{-1} \cdot M^{-1}$. The combined blocks achieved significantly greater AF-selectivity than Bl·I_{Na} alone: the maximum attainable AF-selectivity was increased by nearly 6-fold for Bl·I_{Kur} + Bl·I_{Na} and more than 14-fold for Comb·Bl·I_X + Bl·I_{Na} as compared to Bl·I_{Na} alone (**Figure 6C**). These dramatic increases were attributed to the significantly greater values in all metrics contributing to the AF-selectivity. The maximal block efficacy achieved by Bl·I_{Na} alone was 0.77, and was increased to 0.81 and 0.94 for Bl·I_{Kur} + Bl·I_{Na} and Comb·Bl·I_X + Bl·I_{Na}, respectively. A more appreciable increase in the maximal rate-selectivity was observed by the combined blocks as compared to Bl·I_{Na} alone (8-fold for Bl·I_{Kur} + Bl·I_{Na} and nearly 10-fold for Comb·Bl·I_X + Bl·I_{Na}). Additionally, the atrial-selectivity was also increased by the combined block, although to a lesser extent. Bl·I_{Kur} + Bl·I_{Na} exhibited a greater atrial-selectivity than that of Comb·Bl·I_X + Bl·I_{Na} since Bl·I_{Kur} was assumed to have no effect on the ventricles.

Furthermore, these simulations revealed that the block efficacy, rate-selectivity and atrial-selectivity were strongly

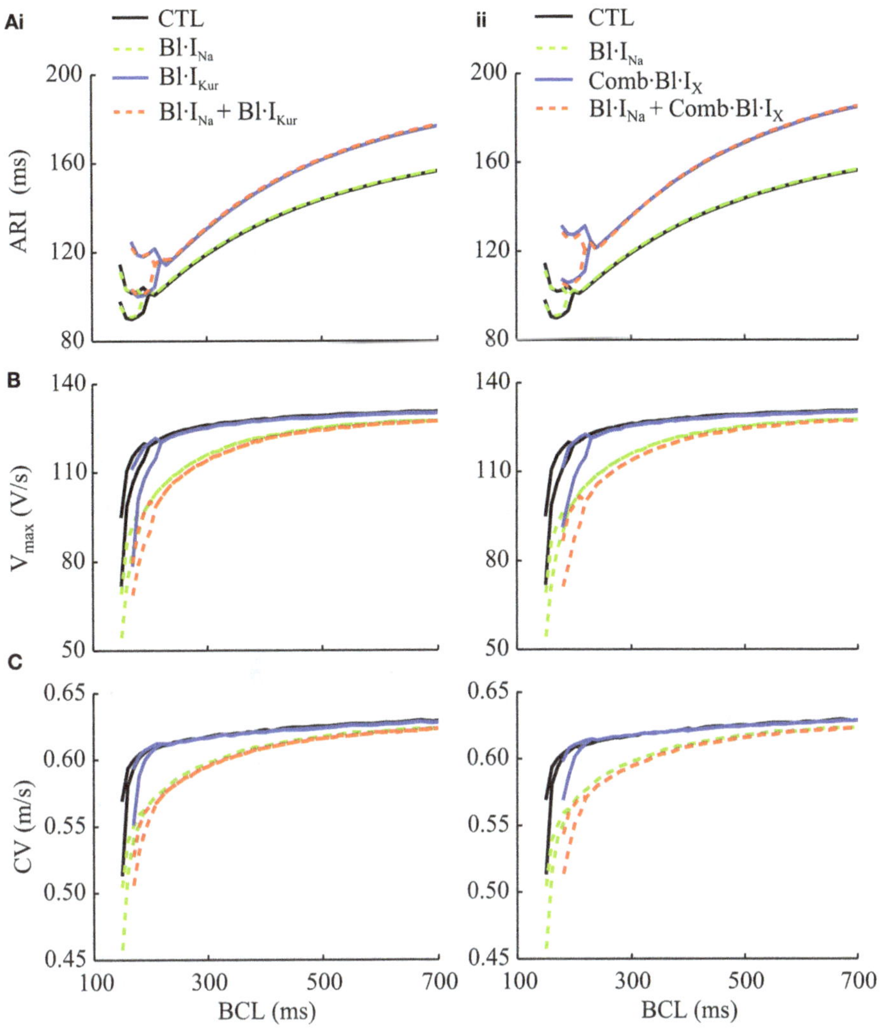

FIGURE 5 | Simulated activation-recovery intervals (ARI) **(A)**, V_{max} **(B)**, and CV (conduction velocity) **(C)** measured in 1D cAF-remodeled atrial strand models as a function of BCL for control (drug-free), individual and combined Na^+- and **(i)** I_{Kur} block and **(ii)** action of acacetin. ARI values were measured as the interval between the time at which the AP depolarizes to −20 mV and the time it reaches a 90% repolarization.

dependent on the inactivation state binding rate K_I. These measures were also dependent on the open-state binding kinetics K_A, but to a much lesser extent. The block efficacy was mainly determined by K_I: an increase in K_I led to a significant increase in the block efficacy. In combined block, the maximal rate- and atrial-selectivity were observed for $K_A = K_I = 1\ ms^{-1} \cdot M^{-1}$ and increases in K_I resulted in substantial reductions in the rate- and atrial-selectivity. In Bl·I_{Na} alone, the parameter set $K_A = 1\ ms^{-1} \cdot M^{-1}$, $K_I = 200\ ms^{-1} \cdot M^{-1}$ produced a maximal value in atrial-selectivity. Collectively, the optimal K_I that maximized AF-selectivity was $200\ ms^{-1} \cdot M^{-1}$ for Bl·I_{Na} and Bl·I_{Kur} + Bl·I_{Na}, and smaller ($100\ ms^{-1} \cdot M^{-1}$) for Comb·Bl·$I_X$ + Bl·I_{Na}. The optimal $K_A = 1\ ms^{-1} \cdot M^{-1}$ was seen for all conditions. Increasing K_A consistently resulted in a smaller rate- and atrial-selectivity and therefore reduced AF-selectivity. These results suggest that the inactivation-state binding rate might be a more favorable targeting parameter than the open-state binding kinetics in optimizing AF-selectivity of Na^+-blockers.

Effects of I_{Na} and I_{Kur} Block on Spiral Excitation Events in cAF-Remodeled Atria

Two-Dimensional Simulations

Using the cross-shock protocol, spiral waves were initiated in a 2D model representing a tissue slab of cAF-remodeled human atria. For each condition, a 10-s episode of electrical activity was simulated. Representative snapshots of the re-entrant waves in control (drug-free) and following application of drugs are presented in **Figure 7A**. The trajectories of the tips of re-entrant rotors under these conditions were traced and are shown in **Figure 7B**. The number of rotors during the time course of wave evolution was also measured (**Figure 7C**). The simulated pseudo-ECGs, membrane potential traces extracted from a representative

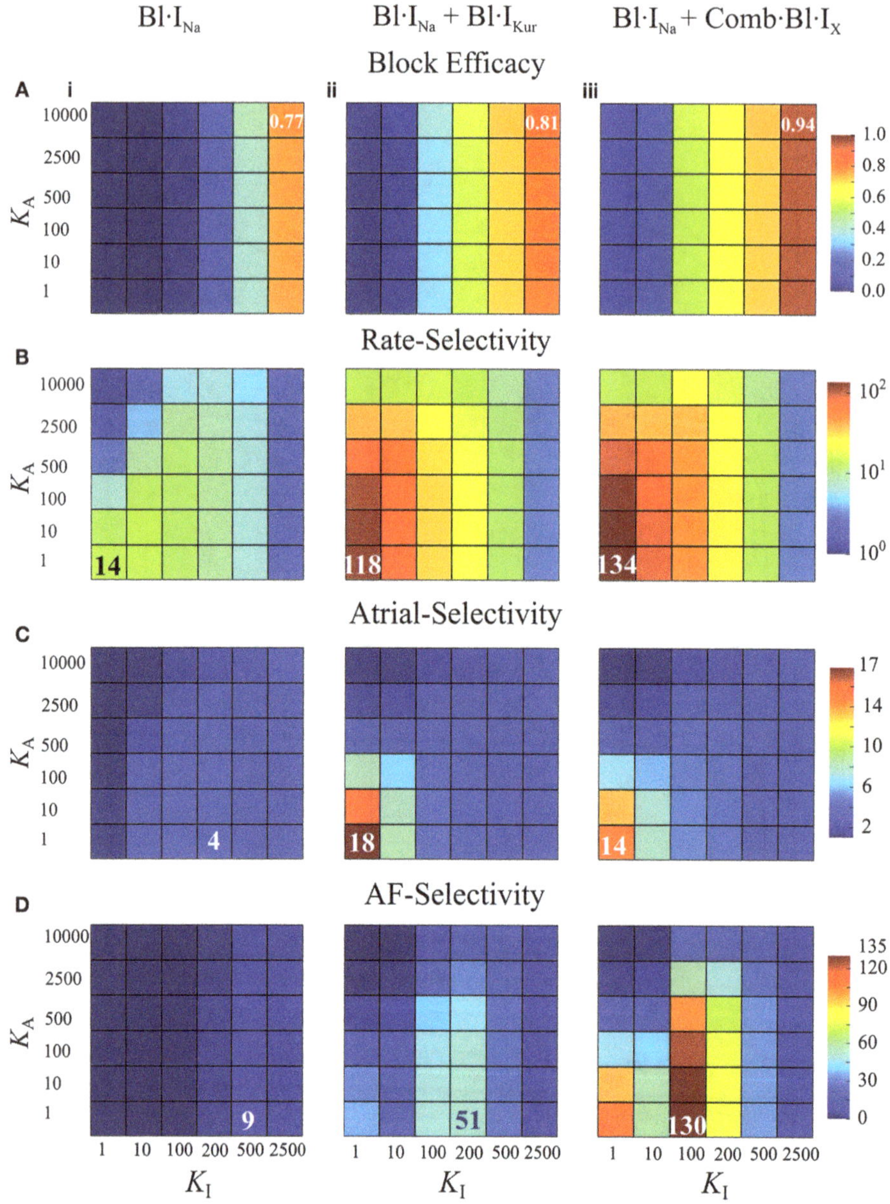

FIGURE 6 | Block efficacy, and the rate-, atrial-, and AF-selectivity as a function of the open- and inactivated- state binding rates (K_A, K_I) for Na^+-block or combined Na^+- and K^+-block computed from cAF-remodeled atrial myocytes or ventricular myocytes. **(A)** Block efficacy; **(B)** rate-selectivity; **(C)** atrial-selectivity, and **(D)** AF-selectivity. In each column shown are data from Bl·INa **(i)**, combined Bl·INa and Bl·IKur **(ii)**, and combined Bl·INa and Comb·Bl·IX **(iii)**. $L_A = 1\ ms^{-1}, L_I = 0.01\ ms^{-1}$. Unit of K_A, K_I: $ms^{-1} \cdot M^{-1}$.

myocyte and the corresponding fractional block of I_{Na} and I_{Kur} are detailed in Online Supplementary Material 2.4.

Under the control (drug-free) condition, a single rotor was formed at approximately $t = 630$ ms; this broke into two spiral waves at $t = 830$ ms. These two rotors were stably anchored with star-shaped tip trajectories at the bottom half of the slab and persisted throughout the rest of the simulated 10-s episode (**Figures 7Ai,Bi,C**). In simulating drug actions, each drug was applied at $t = 2{,}500$ ms. For Bl·I_{Na} the dual rotors progressively became unstable, and the tips of the spiral waves meandered out of the tissue at approximately $t = 6{,}000$ ms, leading to self-termination of the re-entrant waves (**Figures 7Aii,Bii,C**). The dual rotors persisted throughout the period of the simulation after applying Bl·I_{Kur} alone (**Figures 7Aiii,Biii,C**). For Bl·I_{Na} + Bl·I_{Kur}, the rotor at the bottom left corner of the slab became unstable and meandered out of the tissue at approximately $t = 3{,}800$ ms, whereas the trajectory of the second rotor was confined to a small tissue area until $t = 7{,}000$ ms and then gradually became chaotic, forming up to 3 transient rotors that self-terminated at $t = 8{,}334$ ms (**Figures 7Aiv,Biv,C**). A

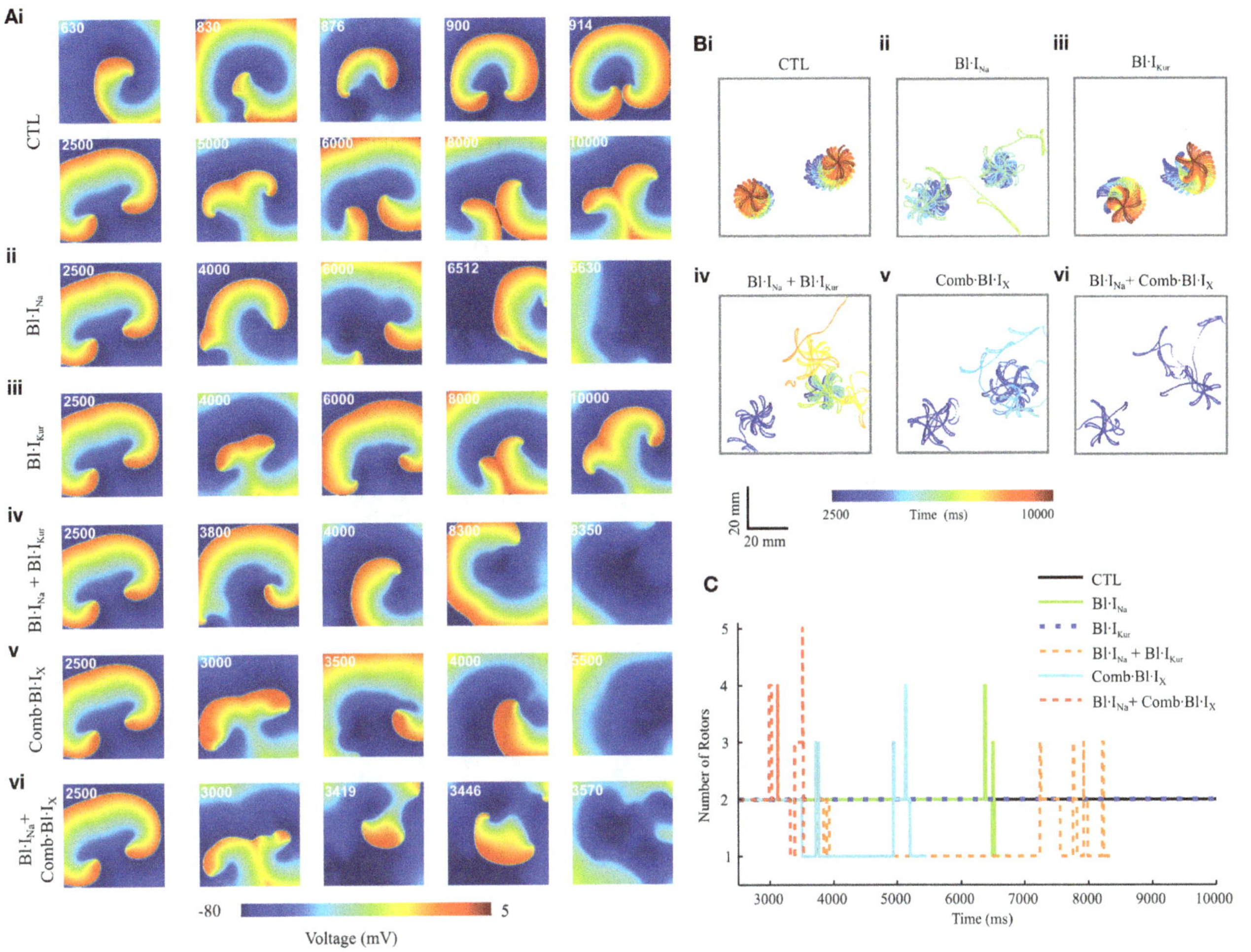

FIGURE 7 | Snapshots of simulated re-entrant excitation events, tip trajectories of re-entrant waves and the number of rotor in a 2D model of cAF-remodeled atrial tissue slab in drug-free condition or after applying the drugs. **(A)** Snapshots of simulated re-entrant excitation events; The time sequence (ms) is indicated at the top left corner of each screenshot. **(B)** Tip trajectories of re-entrant waves. **(C)** Temporal evolution of total number of rotors represented by the number of spiral wave tips in tissue. In both **(A,B)**, **(i)** Drug-free (CTL) condition, **(ii)** $Bl{\cdot}I_{Na}$ alone, **(iii)** $Bl{\cdot}I_{Kur}$ alone, **(iv)** Combined $Bl{\cdot}I_{Na}$ and $Bl{\cdot}I_{Kur}$, **(v)** Applying $Comb{\cdot}Bl{\cdot}I_X$ alone, and **(vi)** Combined $Bl{\cdot}I_{Na}$ and $Comb{\cdot}Bl{\cdot}I_X$. Rate constants for I_{Na} block: $K_A = 1\ ms^{-1} \cdot M^{-1}, K_I = 100\ ms^{-1} \cdot M^{-1}, L_A = 1\ ms^{-1},\ L_I = 0.01\ ms^{-1}$.

similar but more marked effect was seen in the simulations that addressed the aggregate effects of acacetin: the bottom left rotor quickly meandered out of the tissue at $t = 3{,}510$ ms whilst the tip trajectory of the other rotor became chaotic and terminated at $t = 5{,}439$ ms (**Figures 7Av,Bv,C**). We note that the combined $Bl{\cdot}I_{Na}$ and $Comb{\cdot}Bl{\cdot}I_X$ exerted the strongest potency in terminating re-entrant excitations in these simulations: the two rotors transiently turned unstable and chaotic and self-terminated at $t = 3{,}555$ ms, with up to 5 rotors during the excitation in the slab (**Figures 7Avi,Bvi,C**).

The anti-arrhythmic benefits of combined Na^+- and K^+-block were clearly revealed by additional simulations assuming the use of a different Na^+-blocker ($K_A = 1\ ms^{-1} \cdot M^{-1}, K_I = 200\ ms^{-1} \cdot M^{-1}, L_A = 1\ ms^{-1}, L_I = 0.01\ ms^{-1}$) and at a reduced dose (75%) of both Na^+-blocker and acacetin. The life span of re-entrant excitations was measured and shown in **Figure 8A**. Also, the pECG was computed and the segment from $t = 3{,}000$ ms to 500 ms before the termination of re-entries (or the end of the simulation if the rotor sustained) was analyzed using the Fast Fourier Transform to obtain the dominant frequency (DF) of the re-entrant excitations, which is illustrated in **Figure 8B**.

At the simulated doses of acacetin, applying $Bl{\cdot}I_{Kur}$ alone did not lead to termination of re-entrant waves within the duration of the simulation (7,500 ms after T_{Drug}), whereas the rotors were terminated in the simulations for $Comb{\cdot}Bl{\cdot}I_X$ at both doses (**Figure 8Ai–iv**), thus demonstrating enhanced anti-AF benefits of combined K^+-channel block. For the simulated $Bl{\cdot}I_{Na}$ alone, the Na^+-blocker with $K_I = 100\ ms^{-1} \cdot M^{-1}$ led to termination of AF at the control dose (lifespan of 4,102 ms) but not at the reduced dose; increasing K_I of the Na^+-blocker to $200\ ms^{-1} \cdot M^{-1}$ resulted in a reduced lifespan (1,305 and 1,459 ms for $[D_{Na^+}] =$ 60 and 45 μM, respectively). The lifespan for the combined $Bl{\cdot}I_{Na} + Comb{\cdot}Bl{\cdot}I_X$ was consistently shorter than that of any individual applications of $Bl{\cdot}I_{Na}$ or $Comb{\cdot}Bl{\cdot}I_X$ alone in all cases.

A similar augmented anti-arrhythmic effect (shown as shortened lifespan of re-entry) was also observed for the combined Bl·I_{Na} + Bl·I_{Kur} for $[D_{Na^+}] = 45$ μM and $K_I = 200$ $ms^{-1} \cdot M^{-1}$ (**Figure 8Aiv**) but not for the rest of the cases.

A consistent decrease in the DF was observed in the drug-modulated re-entrant excitations as compared to those in the drug-free condition (**Figure 8Bi–iv**). In the drug-free condition, the DF extracted from the pECG was 8.63 Hz, which is within the range of similar clinical data (Jarman et al., 2012). Applying Na^+- or K^+- block individually resulted in slowing of the rate of the rotors, and this was dependent on the concentrations and parameters of the blockers. For Bl·I_{Kur} the DF was 8.25 Hz

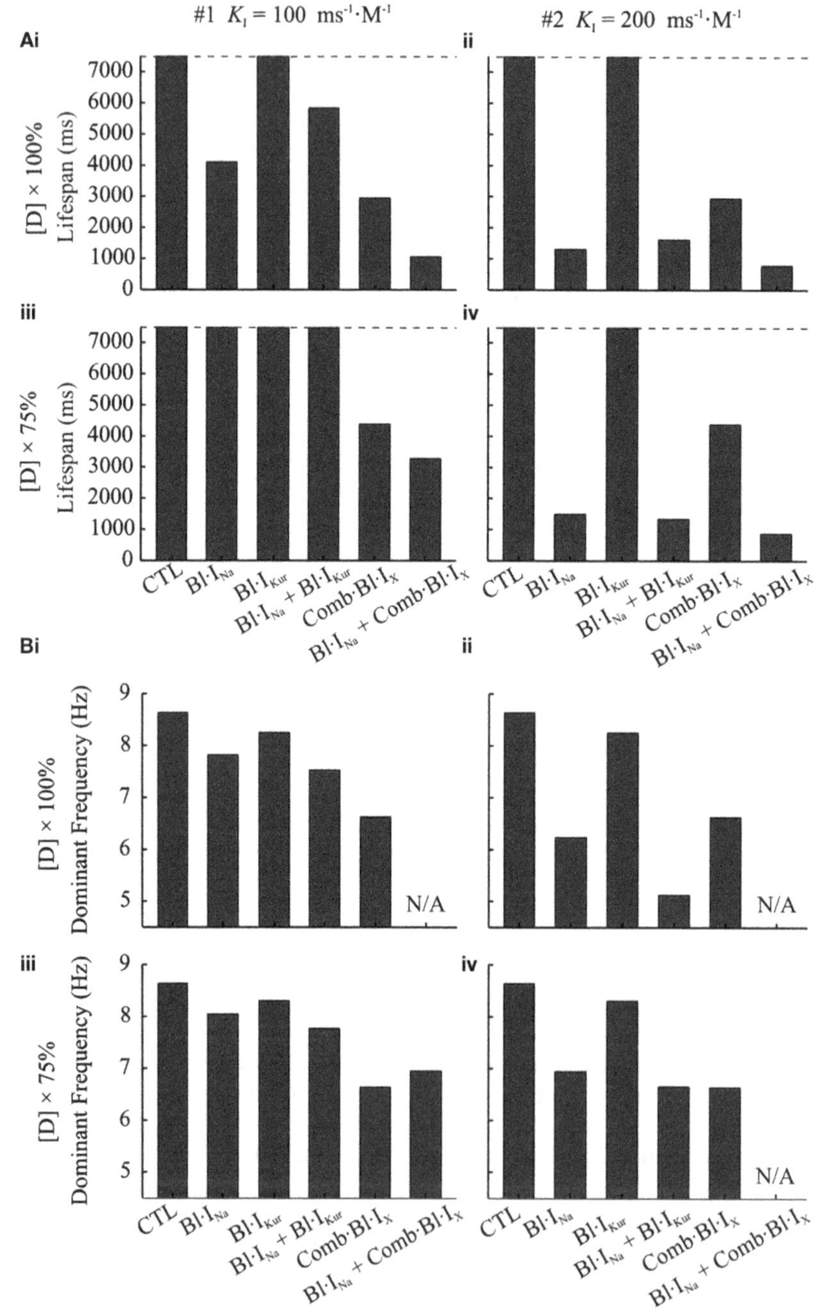

FIGURE 8 | Dominant frequency and lifespan of re-entrant waves in 2D simulations using the cAF-remodeled atrial tissue model in the drug-free condition or after applying drugs. **(A)** Lifespan of the spiral waves. **(B)** DF of spiral waves. The results of K^+-block alone are shown in both left and right panels for the purpose of comparison. In the left column **(i,iii)** of **(A,B)**, Bl·I_{Na} was simulated with $K_I = 100$ $ms^{-1} \cdot M^{-1}$; in the right column **(ii,iv)**, $K_I = 200$ $ms^{-1} \cdot M^{-1}$. In the top panels **(i,ii)** of **(A,B)**, $[D_{K^+}] = 3.2$ μM, $[D_{Na^+}] = 60$ μM; in the bottom panels **(iii,iv)**, $[D_{K^+}] = 2.4$ μM, $[D_{Na^+}] = 45$ μM. In all panels, $K_A = 1$ $ms^{-1} \cdot M^{-1}$, $L_A = 1$ ms^{-1}, $L_I = 0.01$ ms^{-1}.

with the control dose and 8.30 Hz for the reduced dose. In the simulations with Comb·Bl·I_X, the DF was 6.63 Hz and was not affected by the 25% reduction in the dose of the compound. For Bl·I_{Na} alone the DF was 7.81 Hz and substantially smaller (6.24 Hz) for Na^+-blockers of $K_I = 100\ ms^{-1} \cdot M^{-1}$ and $K_I = 200\ ms^{-1} \cdot M^{-1}$, respectively. An enhanced deceleration of the rotors was observed for Bl·I_{Na} + Bl·I_{Kur} in all cases. The DF for simulations with Comb·Bl·I_X + Bl·I_{Na} was not computed due to the short lifespan in these events.

3D Simulations

The antiarrhythmic effects of acacetin and Na^+-block on the re-entrant waves in the cAF-remodeled atria were also evaluated using our 3D anatomical model of the human atria (Colman et al., 2013, 2017). A 10-s episode of sustained re-entrant excitation was first initiated in the cAF-remodeled atria in the drug-free condition; this produced the initial conditions of the 3D model for additional 10-s episode simulations. Next, the behavior of electrical waves of another 10-s episode simulation in the drug-free condition and after applying the selected blockers was analyzed and compared. **Figure 9A** shows snapshots of excitation wave evolution following the 10-s episode of re-entrant excitation events. pECGs computed from the excitation waves are shown in **Figure 9Bi–iv**. **Figures 9C,D** illustrates power spectrum analyses of the pECGs and a comparison of the lifespan of the electrical waves in the drug-free condition and after applying the drugs/blockers. In the drug-free condition, stable re-entrant waves around the pulmonary veins and left atrium were observed; the power spectrum density (PSD) manifests a single-focused peak around 8.16 Hz. Following applying Bl·I_{Na}, the re-entrant waves became less organized and also decelerated. This was characterized by a smaller dominant frequency (6.58 Hz) and less focused PSD distribution; the excitation was not terminated. Following the application of Comb·Bl·I_X, the re-entrant wave soon became unstable and eventually disappeared after $t =$ 3,279 ms. Note that the peak PSD amplitude was much smaller and its distribution was much broader as compared to the drug-free condition. The combined drugs further destabilized the re-entrant waves and reduced the lifespan to approximately 1,120 ms.

Simulated Effects of Acacetin and Na^+-Current Blocker on the QT Interval

Further simulations were performed using a 1D ventricular transmural strand model to evaluate the changes in the waveform of electrograms in consequence of applying the drugs. A comparison of the computed electrogram waveforms are illustrated in **Figures 10A,B**, and the QT intervals are quantified in **Figure 10C**. Blocking small fractions of I_{Kr}, I_{Ks} and I_{to} in the human ventricles by acacetin slightly increased the QT interval by 21 ms. The electrograms were not noticeably affected by applications of the Na^+-blocker with the simulated parameters. Results from both cases did not show dramatic QT prolongation, indicating no dramatic effects affecting ventricular repolarization process which might promote ventricular arrhythmias.

DISCUSSION

Even decades after goal-directed work, successful development of effective and safe antiarrhythmic drugs for treating AF has not been accomplished and remains a major unmet clinical need. In a recent study on the canine heart, enhanced anti-arrhythmic effects and AF-selectivity of I_{Na} blockade by additional I_{Kur} block was demonstrated (Aguilar et al., 2015). Whether similar effects could be obtained in the human atria, especially following cAF-induced electrical remodeling which reduces I_{Kur}, remained unclear. How the combined Na^+ and K^+-block modulates the QT interval also remained incompletely understood. In this study, the effects of I_{Kur} (combined with a modest block in I_{to}, I_{Kr}, and I_{Ks} as presented by acacetin, a compound shown to be effective in anti-AF treatment) and I_{Na} block (two potentially effective atrial-selective block on human atrial electrophysiology) were investigated *in silico* using multiscale models of the human atria and state-dependent block scheme. The simulation results demonstrate that both Na^+-block and K^+-block exhibited anti-arrhythmic effects in the atria following cAF-remodeling, despite reduced I_{Kur} by the remodeling. The present study highlighted that in addition to combined Na^+- and K^+-block, combined multi-K^+-channels also exerted beneficial synergistic antiarrhythmic effects when compared with single channel block whilst having modest impact on ventricular repolarization (QT interval). This study suggests that multi-channel block (either combined Na^+-K^+-block, or combined multi-K^+-block) may be a favorable strategy for the development of novel pharmaceutical therapies for AF.

Effects of I_{Na} block

An atrial-ventricular difference in the properties of I_{Na}, especially in the voltage dependence of steady-state inactivation, has been reported (Li et al., 2002; Burashnikov et al., 2007; Chen et al., 2016; Fan et al., 2016; Caves et al., 2017). In these studies, the voltage dependent steady-state inactivation curves for I_{Na} were found to be negatively shifted (by 5–16 mV) in atrium as compared to the ventricular parameters. This difference gave rise to an on-going interest in developing an atrial-selective blocker of I_{Na} as a strategy in terminating AF (Burashnikov et al., 2007; Antzelevitch and Burashnikov, 2009; Zygmunt et al., 2011; Morotti et al., 2016; Caves et al., 2017). As was done in previous studies (Aguilar-Shardonofsky et al., 2012; Aguilar et al., 2015), in this study, the kinetic parameters in drug actions of Na^+-blockers were varied over wide parameter spaces to reveal AF-selectivity of Na^+-blockers in the ventricles and fibrillating atria. Our results demonstrated that in the presence of AF-remodeling, an atrial-selective block of I_{Na} could produce different effects between atrial and ventricular cells (**Figures 3**, **4**) and that the AF-selectivity could be maximized by optimizing the binding and unbinding rates of the Na^+-blocker (**Figure 6**). Note also that, the fractional inhibition of I_{Na} by the Na^+-blocker exhibited a substantial dependence on the rate of pacing (**Figures 3**, **4** and Online Supplementary Material 2.2), which was quantified using the rate-selectivity (**Figure 6**).

At the cellular level, Na^+-block resulted in a significant inhibition in I_{Na} at fast pacing rates, but minor effects within

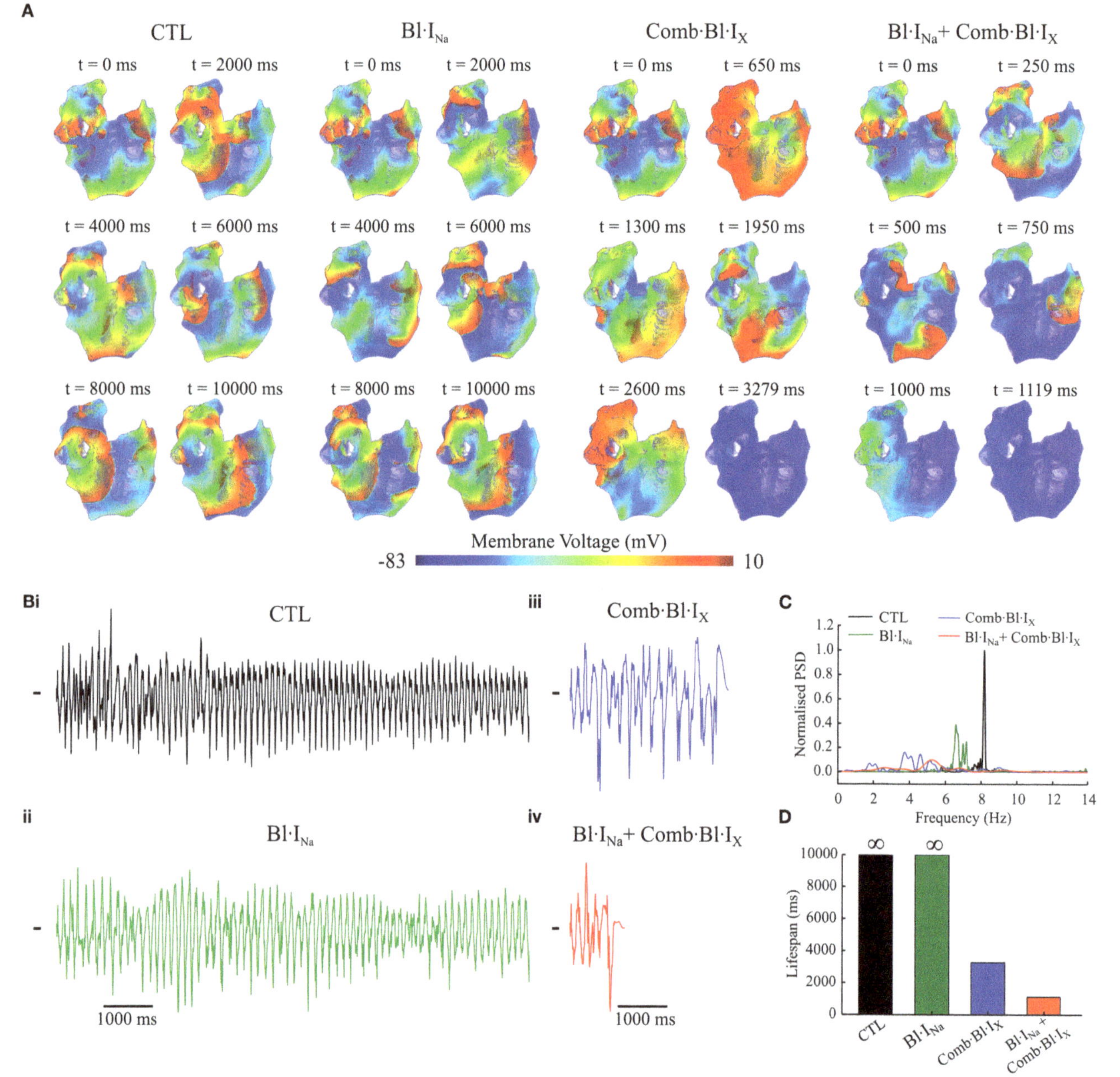

FIGURE 9 | Simulated re-entrant excitations computed using the 3D anatomical model of the cAF-remodeled human atria in response to application of channel blockers as compared to that of the drug-free (CTL) condition. **(A)** Snapshots of electrical excitation waves. Drugs were applied at $t = 0$ ms. **(B)** Simulated pECGs. **(C)** Power spectrum density (PSD) obtained from the pECGs. PSDs were normalized to the maximum value of that in control. **(D)** Lifespan of re-entrant excitations in these simulated atria for various conditions. The symbol ∞ indicates the spiral waves were sustained throughout the 10-s episode of simulation. $K_A = 1\ \text{ms}^{-1} \cdot \text{M}^{-1}$, $K_I = 100\ \text{ms}^{-1} \cdot \text{M}^{-1}$, $L_A = 1\text{ms}^{-1}$, $L_I = 0.01\ \text{ms}^{-1}$; $[D_{K+}] = 3.2\mu\text{M}$, $[D_{Na+}] = 60\mu\text{M}$.

the range of normal heart rates in the atria (**Figures 5**, **6**). The antiarrhythmic effects of these changes were demonstrated in simulations of multicellular atrial tissue. In a 1D atrial strand model, applying Na^+-block progressively enhanced the rate-adaptations of V_{max} and CV over a larger range of BCLs, whereas the atrial APD was not affected. At fast pacing rates, V_{max} and CV were decreased significantly, suggesting reduced excitabilities of atrial myocytes (**Figure 5**). These results are in concordance with the recent study (Aguilar et al., 2015) where similar effects of Na^+-block on the canine atria were demonstrated *in silico* and experimentally in coronary-perfused hearts.

In 2D tissue simulations, this Na^+-block shortened the lifespan and caused slowing in the excitation rate of the spiral waves (**Figures 7**, **8**). In the 3D anatomical model, applying Na^+-block alone produced antiarrhythmic effects by slowing the re-entrant excitations (**Figure 9**). Furthermore,

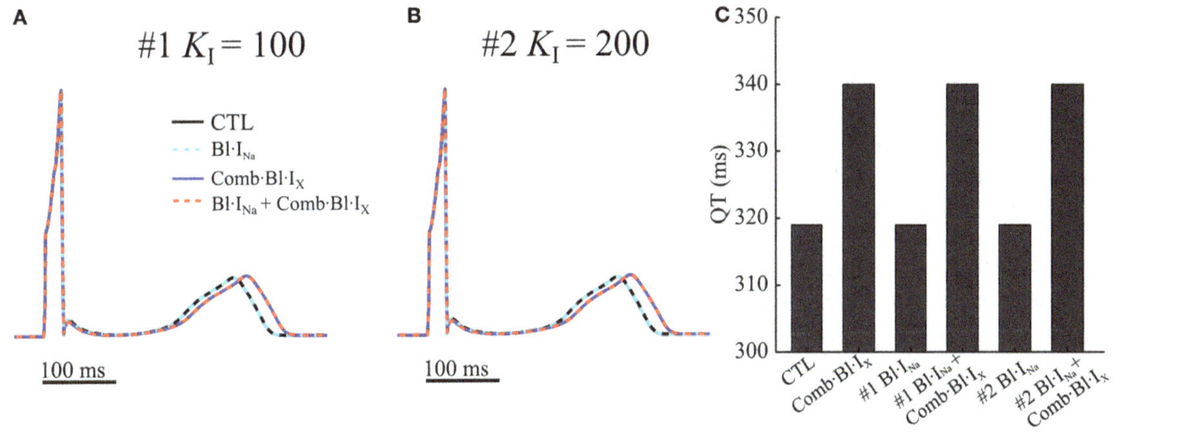

FIGURE 10 | Computed pECGs from a 1D strand model for human ventricular transmural strands in drug-free (CTL) condition and in response to anti-arrhythmic drugs. In **(A,B)** two sets of parameters (#1 $K_I = 100\ ms^{-1}\cdot M^{-1}$, #2 $K_I = 200\ ms^{-1}\cdot M^{-1}$) for I_{Na} block were simulated. **(C)** QT intervals measured from the pECGs.

in our 1D model of transmural ventricular strand, the simulations suggested that the Na^+-block had minimal impact on ventricular repolarization, as judged by modest QT interval prolongation. These results demonstrated that Na^+-block could be beneficial in suppressing re-entrant activities in the cAF-remodeled atria, with modest impact on ventricular repolarization.

Effects of K^+-Current Block

K^+-current blockers delay the repolarization phase of the AP and thus prolong atrial APD and refractory period. This can cause disruptions and eventually termination of the re-entrant circuits (Hancox et al., 2016). However, K^+-channel blockers such as dofetilide and sotalol (which potently inhibit I_{Kr}) have a substantial risk of prolonging QT interval and promoting *Torsades de pointes* arrhythmias (Hondeghem and Snyders, 1990; Yap and Camm, 2003). In principle, blocking atrial-specific K^+-channels may exert antiarrhythmic effects in the atria while minimizing potential risks of adverse effects in the ventricles. I_{Kur} is believed to be such an atrial-selective substrate for drug interventions, and effects of I_{Kur} block have been extensively studied (Burashnikov and Antzelevitch, 2008; Li et al., 2008; Tsujimae et al., 2008; Almquist et al., 2010; Pavri et al., 2012; Scholz et al., 2013; Loose et al., 2014; Ford et al., 2016). Interestingly, many existing I_{Kur} blockers potently block other K^+-channels including I_{to} and $I_{K,ACh}$ (Gögelein et al., 2004; Wirth et al., 2007; Burashnikov and Antzelevitch, 2008; Li et al., 2008). The additional blockades of these channels may contribute to the antiarrhythmic effects of those drugs, which warrant further investigations.

In this study, acacetin, a compound initially isolated from the traditional Chinese medicine *Xuelianhua*, was selected as a representative I_{Kur} blocker. The effects of acacetin on atrial electrophysiology were evaluated in two ways: (a) the effects of acacetin blocking I_{Kur} only; and (b) the full actions of acacetin on the targeting channels (I_{to}, I_{Kur}, I_{Kr}, and I_{Ks}) (Li et al., 2008). This approach allowed for investigations into the effects of I_{Kur} block alone as well as the potential benefits of additional-but-modest inhibition of other K^+-currents in the human atria.

Selective I_{Kur} Block

Blocking I_{Kur} with 3.2 μM acacetin exerted APD prolongation (9.8 ms) under the baseline/normal conditions (**Figure 2**). Experimental data show that dependent on the baseline AP waveform the effect of I_{Kur} block on human atrial APD_{70-90} under normal (SR) conditions can manifest as prolongation or shortening in the APD, (Workman et al., 2001; Wettwer et al., 2004; Schotten et al., 2007; Burashnikov and Antzelevitch, 2008; Loose et al., 2014). Additionally, the prolongation in APD by I_{Kur} block observed in the present study is similar to our previous paper (Colman et al., 2017) concerning the effects of genetically down-regulated I_{Kur}. Moreover, inhibiting I_{Kur} under normal conditions elevated the AP plateau potential and prolonged APD_{30} (**Figure 2**). Both effects matched well with experimental studies (Workman et al., 2001; Wettwer et al., 2004; Schotten et al., 2007; Burashnikov and Antzelevitch, 2008; Loose et al., 2014) and our simulation study (Colman et al., 2017).

We note that in the cAF-remodeling cells, a more pronounced prolongation in APD (by 23.6 ms for 1 Hz and 16.2 ms at 6 Hz, **Figure 4**) was observed in the presence of 3.2 μM acacetin, despite that this current was down-regulated by cAF-remodeling (Wagoner et al., 1997; Brandt et al., 2000; Christ et al., 2008). These results are in accordance with previous experimental results of blocking I_{Kur} with MK-0448 (Pavri et al., 2012; Loose et al., 2014). In addition, I_{Kur} block exhibited enhanced rate-dependent adaptations in APD both at the cellular (Online Supplementary Material 2.2) and 1D strand models (**Figure 5**). Importantly, the CV restitution curve shifted toward higher BCLs, indicating that this tissue is less capable of conduction of atrial excitation waves at high rate while maintaining conduction of slow waves (**Figure 5**). In 2D tissue simulations, applying I_{Kur} block alone (3.2 μM acacetin) destabilized the cores of rotors (i.e., potential organizing centers for AF), and slightly slowed their excitation rates, but failed to terminate them (**Figure 7**), suggesting a limited efficacy of terminating AF by I_{Kur} block alone. Similarly, a recent modeling study by Aguilar et al. (2017) suggested that the antiarrhythmic efficacy of I_{Kur} block was substantially decreased in the presence of AF-induced electrical remodeling. Also, the experimental study (Burashnikov and Antzelevitch, 2008) showed that block of I_{Kur} by 4-AP of small doses had limited efficacy in suppressing AF in canine atria. This may represent the fact that I_{Kur} is reduced at high frequencies (as discussed/suggested in Feng et al., 1998a; Burashnikov and Antzelevitch, 2008; Wu et al., 2011) and shown in **Figure 1**) as well as by cAF-induced remodeling (Wagoner et al., 1997; Brandt et al., 2000; Christ et al., 2008). In addition, I_{Kur} is primarily active during phase 2 of AP, and hence pure I_{Kur} block exerted a relatively greater prolongation in APD_{30} than APD_{90} (**Figure 3**), in contrast to other K^+-block including dofetilide which mediates anti-AF effects by prolonging the terminal phase of the AP (Roukoz and Saliba, 2007).

In this study, I_{Kur} block was simulated using a state-dependent block model, which successfully reproduced the use- and rate-dependent inhibition of acacetin (**Figure 1**). The rate-dependent block of I_{Kur} exerted a higher fractional inhibition in the current at faster pacing rates, which likely produces greater anti-AF effects in the presence of high-frequency excitations as seen during AF. Along with the previous modeling studies on investigating effects of I_{Kur} block (Almquist et al., 2010; Scholz et al., 2013; Ellinwood et al., 2017), this study demonstrated the importance of explicitly considering the kinetic properties of the block in computational efforts of understanding the consequences and underlying mechanisms of I_{Kur} block.

Effects of Combined K^+-Current Block

The combined K^+-block (as exhibited by acacetin and many other I_{Kur} blockers) resulted in synergistic APD prolongation as well as an increased efficacy in terminating re-entry in tissue as compared to the pure I_{Kur} block.

Note that at the single myocyte level, the combined actions of acacetin produced greater prolongation in atrial APD than the sum of changes due to drug-induced block of individual channel in normal and cAF-remodeled myocytes (**Figure 2**). Additionally, the combined K^+-block increased the rate-additivity of APD as compared to the pure I_{Kur} block (Online Supplementary Material 2.2). This was also consistently observed in the 1D simulation (**Figure 5**). In the setting of pure I_{Kur} block, the elevated and prolonged plateau phase of the AP could promote the activation of I_{Kr}/I_{Ks}, which in return may accelerate the repolarization of AP-phase 3 (Colman et al., 2017). Therefore, additional inhibition in I_{Kr} by an identical fraction is expected to result in a greater APD prolongation than a pure I_{Kur} or I_{Kr}/I_{Ks} block.

In 2D simulations, the combined K^+-block produced an enhanced efficacy in suppressing AF compared with the pure I_{Kur} block: promoting meandering of rotor tips (**Figure 7B**), shortening the lifespan of re-entries (**Figure 8A**) and slowing of spiral wave excitations (**Figure 8B**). Rotor meandering is one mechanism by which spiral waves may meet non-conducting boundaries to extinguish re-entry (Narayan et al., 2013; Pandit and Jalife, 2013; Rappel et al., 2015).

The effects of acacetin (3.2 μM) on the ventricular AP and QT interval was assessed in a single cell model and 1D transmural strand model by assuming similar blockade effects of the compound on the human ventricles and atria. It was shown that following applying acacetin, the ventricular repolarization and QT interval was both preserved with slight prolongations around 21 ms (**Figure 10**). Our results are close to the previous experimental study (Li et al., 2008) showing that QT intervals were not prolonged by acacetin in isolated rabbit hearts and anesthetised dogs.

The synergistic effects demonstrated by the combined K^+-blocks have implications on developing novel pharmaceutical anti-AF therapies. Given that I_{to}, I_{Kr} and I_{Ks} contribute to the repolarizations of ventricular APs, inhibitions in these channels may promote risks of side effects in the ventricles. In this regard, combined block of atrial-specific K^+ channels may be favorable. Recently, another two families of K^+-channels that are dominantly expressed in the atria have been acknowledged: the small-conductance Ca^{2+}-activated K^+ (SK) channels (I_{SK}) (Qi et al., 2014), and the two-pore K^+ (K2P3.1) channel (I_{TASK-1}) (Schmidt et al., 2015), further to the well-known constitutively active acetylcholine-activated K^+ current ($I_{K,ACh}$). Combined block of these atrial-specific channels may exert greater and safer antiarrhythmic effects in the atria, warranting future investigations.

Synergistic Effects of Combined Na^+- and K^+- Block

The present study reveals novel and significant synergistic effects of combined block of Na^+- and K^+-currents (I_{Na} and pure-I_{Kur}/multi-K^+-block) and demonstrates the additional synergistic anti-arrhythmic effects derived from the multi-K^+ channel block in cAF-remodeled atria.

In cAF-remodeled atria, combined Na^+- and K^+-block significantly increased the fractional I_{Na} inhibition and APD prolongation (**Figures 3, 4**) and promoted pronounced AP alternans at 6 Hz, with complex effects in human AF (Narayan et al., 2011). In the simulations varying the blockade kinetics of I_{Na} block, the combined block dramatically augmented the attainable maximal AF-selectivity in consequence of enhanced atrial-selectivity and rate-selectivity as compared to the pure Na^+-block (**Figure 6**).

In the 1D model of an atrial strand, combined Na^+ and K^+-block produced synergistic reductions in V_{max} and CV; the threshold of BCL allowing a 1:1 conduction was increased as compared to the control conditions (**Figure 5**). In simulated re-entrant waves in 2D and 3D atria, the combined Bl·I_{Na} + Comb·Bl·I_X exhibited a greater efficacy in suppressing AF, with a decreased lifespan of rotors as compared to that by either individual block (**Figures 7–9**). Although the combined Bl·I_{Na} + Bl·I_{Kur} did not further reduce the lifespan of spiral waves as compared to the Bl·I_{Na} alone, the combination did lead to the extinction of one of the two rotors (**Figures 7Aiv,Biv**) and deceleration of re-entrant activations (**Figure 8B**). Follow-up simulations showed that consistent synergistic antiarrhythmic effects could be obtained with reduced doses of Na^+- and K^+-blockers.

The non-specific multi-channel blockade is increasingly recognized as a strategy for pharmaceutical therapy of AF both experimentally (Sicouri et al., 2010; Aguilar et al., 2015;

Kirchhoff et al., 2015; Hartmann et al., 2016) and clinically (Koskinas et al., 2014; Reiffel et al., 2015). In a previous study (Aguilar et al., 2015), synergistic anti-arrhythmic effects were demonstrated both *in silico* and experimentally in healthy canine hearts. Additionally, the favorable synergistic antiarrhythmic effects have also been reported in combined block of I_{SK} and I_{Na} in an experimental atrial-fibrillated guinea pig model (Kirchhoff et al., 2015). Also, the recent HARMONY trial (Reiffel et al., 2015) revealed synergistic AF-suppressing effects for combined use of ranolazine and dronedarone. While revealing the synergistic effects of combined Na^+- and K^+- block in cAF-remodeled human atria, this study supports and adds insights into the on-going efforts in developing multi-channel block as a strategy for the treatment of AF.

Limitations and Future Work

In the absence of the required detailed experimental data, when simulating effects of acacetin on I_{to}, I_{Ks} and I_{Kr}, the dose-dependence block of acacetin was assumed to be identical in both human atrial and ventricular cells. This assumption may warrant further investigations. In addition, the parameters of atrial I_{to} have been reported to be different from those of ventricular I_{to} in human (Amos et al., 1996). Previous studies reported that the IC_{50} of 4-AP block of atrial I_{to} was one-third of that of ventricular I_{to} (Amos et al., 1996; Nattel et al., 2000). If a similar atrial-vs.-ventricular difference in the IC_{50} of I_{to} and/or I_{Kr}/I_{Ks} could exist for acacetin, the effects of acacetin on the ventricular electrophysiology would be less significant than our simulations, which might result in to a smaller change in ventricular I_{Na} and APD for the combined block of Bl·I_{Na} and Comb·Bl·I_X, and thus enhance the computed atrial-selectivity and AF-selectivity of the combined block. Given that applying acacetin *in vivo* did not prolong QT intervals in isolated rabbit hearts and anesthetised dogs (Li et al., 2008), any significant prolongation of the ventricular APD and QT interval is unlikely (**Figures 3B**, **4C**, **10**). Therefore, our assumption of no atrial-ventricular difference in the potency of acacetin on K^+-currents may not affect our conclusions concerning the atrial-selectivity of combined Na^+- and K^+-block.

Additionally, in the absence of detailed experimental data for state-dependent block of I_{to}, I_{Kr}, and I_{Ks} by acacetin, the block of these channels was modeled using a single pore block model. The IC50 values (**Table 1**) were determined by fitting the concentration-response relation of the step current at 40 mV in previous experimental studies (Li et al., 2008; Wu et al., 2011). A recent study suggests that the IC50 values may be dependent on the voltage protocols applied, and this cannot be reflected by single pore models. In future studies, the pore block model for I_{to}, I_{Kr}, and I_{Ks} can be replaced by a state-dependent block model when such experimental data become available. Also, the present work did not attempt to model the effects of acacetin on $I_{K,ACh}$, although the study shows the current is potently blocked by the compound. The 2D and 3D simulations of atrial tissue, while validated, may not fully capture the complexity of fibrosis-tissue interfaces which are seen in structurally remodeled atria and were not simulated in these monodomain experiments.

Thirdly, our simulation results showed a moderate QT prolongation of around 20 ms following applying both I_{Na} blocker and acacetin. While a QT prolongation of less than 5 ms does not raise a regulatory concern (Committee for Medicinal Products for Human Use, 2012), implications of QT prolongations between 5 and 20 ms remain inconclusive (Committee for Medicinal Products for Human Use, 2005). In the present study, though the extent of QT prolongation of 20 ms is far less than the threshold of discontinuation criteria of 60 ms as indicated in Committee for Medicinal Products for Human Use (2005), it would indeed raise a positive flag in thorough QT tests and necessitate extended safety assessment and intensive patient monitoring during late stages of trials (Committee for Medicinal Products for Human Use, 2012). On the other hand, the approach we used in accounting for the effects of acacetin on ventricular myocytes may result in upper bound of QT prolongation, since the potency of acacetin was assumed to be identical in atria and ventricles.

Fourthly, the threshold in BCL inducing AP alternans was increased by K^+-block (**Figure 5**, Figure S5). However, AP alternans seen at slower pacing rates has been linked with occurrence of AF (Narayan et al., 2002, 2011). Therefore, the increased threshold in BCL developing AF by K^+-block can be potentially proarrhythmic. The safety of K^+-block and its proarrhythmic potential in the atria should be addressed in future studies.

Fifthly, there are limitations in the approaches used in simulating the I_{Na} blockers in single myocytes and tissue. Similar to previous studies (Aguilar-Shardonofsky et al., 2012; Aguilar et al., 2015), in our simulations, the drug action on I_{Na} was modeled through a state-dependent block assuming drugs binding to both activated and inactivated states of I_{Na}, and the gating variables of I_{Na} were modeled using an Hodgkin-Huxley scheme. The limitations in this approach outlined in Aguilar-Shardonofsky et al. (2012) therefore apply in the present study. The results of the use-dependent block may be affected by the models used (Aguilar-Shardonofsky et al., 2012). However, the previous study (Aguilar-Shardonofsky et al., 2012) compared this modeling scheme with simulations using a Markov model, showing qualitative agreement in major findings. Therefore, the major conclusions drawn from this study may not be affected by the selected modeling approach for I_{Na} and drug interactions. Furthermore, in optimizing the AF-selectivity of the I_{Na} and K^+-current blockers, the concentrations of Na^+ and K^+ blockers were fixed at 60 uM. This may potentially impose limitations in discomposing the role of the binding parameters in the modulatory effects of the blockers because of the very slow kinetics of the drug binding to its targeted channel at this high concentration. It warrants further studies by varying the concentration of blockers to simulate the optimized effects of the AF-selectivity of I_{Na} blocker. In tissue simulations, effects of drugs were modeled by increasing their doses homogeneously, simultaneously and instantaneously. The realistic actions of I_{Na} blockers in tissue, however, may be different. Also, in tissue simulations a homogenous cell model was used. As previous study (Feng et al., 1998b) showed atria are electrically heterogeneous, future work is needed to assess how tissue heterogeneities affect the efficacy of atrial-selective pharmaceutical interventions. Furthermore, the current simulations did not take the cardiac autonomic regulation into account in order to take into considerations of acacetin on I_{KACh}. Future studies on interactions of atrial-selective anti-arrhythmic drug actions and autonomic systems may also render valuable findings.

It is important to acknowledge that administration of class Ic agents for Na^+-block can cause cardiac arrhythmia and increased mortality (Echt et al., 1991). Further investigations are therefore warranted to assess the safety of the simulated Na^+-block in the heart, especially in the ventricles.

CONCLUSIONS

By using state-dependent drug block models and our mathematical models of the human atria, the antiarrhythmic effects of atrial selective Na^+- and K^+-blockers on the cAF-remodeled atria were evaluated. The combined block of multiple K^+-currents as well as simultaneous block of Na^+- and K^+-currents produced synergistic antiarrhythmic effects. Our results suggest that developing multi-channel (multiple K^+ currents and/or combined Na^+- and K^+-current) block is a potentially valuable strategy for the treatment of AF.

AUTHOR CONTRIBUTIONS

HZ and HN conceived the study. HN designed experiments, developed and validated computational models, and performed numerical experiments. HN, DW, and WW analyzed data. HN, DW, WW, WG, SN, and HZ interpreted data and wrote the manuscript.

FUNDING

This work was supported by grants from the British Heart Foundation FS/14/5/30533, EPSRC (UK) (EP/J00958X/1; EP/I029826/1), MC-IRSES CORDIS3D (317766), NSFC (61179009), Shenzhen Science and Technology Innovation Committee (JCYJ20151029173639477; JSGG20160229125049615). SN is supported by grants from the National Institutes of Health (R01 Hl83359).

REFERENCES

Aguilar, M., Feng, J., Vigmond, E., Comtois, P., and Nattel, S. (2017). Rate-dependent role of IKur in human atrial repolarization and atrial fibrillation maintenance. *Biophys. J.* 112, 1997–2010. doi: 10.1016/j.bpj.2017.03.022

Aguilar, M., Xiong, F., Qi, X. Y., Comtois, P., and Nattel, S. (2015). Potassium channel blockade enhances atrial fibrillation-selective antiarrhythmic effects of optimized state-dependent sodium channel blockade. *Circulation* 132, 2203–2211. doi: 10.1161/CIRCULATIONAHA.115.018016

Aguilar-Shardonofsky, M., Vigmond, E. J., Nattel, S., and Comtois, P. (2012). *In silico* optimization of atrial fibrillation-selective sodium channel blocker pharmacodynamics. *Biophys. J.* 102, 951–960. doi: 10.1016/j.bpj.2012.01.032

Almquist, J., Wallman, M., Jacobson, I., and Jirstrand, M. (2010). Modeling the effect of Kv1.5 block on the canine action potential. *Biophys. J.* 99, 2726–2736. doi: 10.1016/j.bpj.2010.08.062

Amos, G. J., Wettwer, E., Metzger, F., Li, Q., Himmel, H. M., and Ravens, U. (1996). Differences between outward currents of human atrial and subepicardial ventricular myocytes. *J. Physiol.* 491, 31–50. doi: 10.1113/jphysiol.1996.sp021194

Antzelevitch, C., and Burashnikov, A. (2009). Atrial-selective sodium channel block as a novel strategy for the management of atrial fibrillation. *J. Electrocardiol.* 42, 543–548. doi: 10.1016/j.jelectrocard.2009.07.007

Aslanidi, O. V., Colman, M. A., Stott, J., Dobrzynski, H., Boyett, M. R., Holden, A. V., et al. (2011). 3D virtual human atria: a computational platform for studying clinical atrial fibrillation. *Prog. Biophys. Mol. Biol.* 107, 156–168. doi: 10.1016/j.pbiomolbio.2011.06.011

Baher, A., Qu, Z., Hayatdavoudi, A., Lamp, S. T., Yang, M.-J., Xie, F., et al. (2006). Short-term cardiac memory and mother rotor fibrillation. *Am. J. Physiol. Heart Circ. Physiol.* 292, H180–H189. doi: 10.1152/ajpheart.00944.2005

Bosch, R. F., Zeng, X., Grammer, J. B., Popovic, K., Mewis, C., and Kühlkamp, V. (1999). Ionic mechanisms of electrical remodeling in human atrial fibrillation. *Cardiovasc. Res.* 44, 121–131. doi: 10.1016/S0008-6363(99)00178-9

Brandt, M. C., Priebe, L., Böhle, T., Südkamp, M., and Beuckelmann, D. J. (2000). The ultrarapid and the transient outward K^+ current in human atrial fibrillation: their possible role in postoperative atrial fibrillation. *J. Mol. Cell. Cardiol.* 32, 1885–1896. doi: 10.1006/jmcc.2000.1221

Brennan, T., Fink, M., and Rodriguez, B. (2009). Multiscale modelling of drug-induced effects on cardiac electrophysiological activity. *Eur. J. Pharm. Sci.* 36, 62–77. doi: 10.1016/j.ejps.2008.09.013

Burashnikov, A., and Antzelevitch, C. (2008). Can inhibition of IKur promote atrial fibrillation? *Heart Rhythm* 5, 1304–1309. doi: 10.1016/j.hrthm.2008.05.020

Burashnikov, A., Diego, J. M. D., Zygmunt, A. C., Belardinelli, L., and Antzelevitch, C. (2007). Atrium-selective sodium channel block as a strategy for suppression of atrial fibrillation differences in sodium channel inactivation between atria and ventricles and the role of ranolazine. *Circulation* 116, 1449–1457. doi: 10.1161/CIRCULATIONAHA.107.704890

Caves, R. E., Cheng, H., Choisy, S. C., Gadeberg, H. C., Bryant, S. M., Hancox, J. C., et al. (2017). Atrial-ventricular differences in rabbit cardiac voltage-gated Na^+ currents: basis for atrial-selective block by ranolazine. *Heart Rhythm.* 14, 1657–1664. doi: 10.1016/j.hrthm.2017.06.012

Chen, K.-H., Xu, X.-H., Sun, H.-Y., Du, X.-L., Liu, H., Yang, L., et al. (2016). Distinctive property and pharmacology of voltage-gated sodium current in rat atrial versus ventricular myocytes. *Heart Rhythm.* 13, 762–770. doi: 10.1016/j.hrthm.2015.11.022

Christ, T., Wettwer, E., Voigt, N., Hála, O., Radicke, S., Matschke, K., et al. (2008). Pathology-specific effects of the IKur/Ito/IK,ACh blocker AVE0118 on ion channels in human chronic atrial fibrillation. *Br. J. Pharmacol.* 154, 1619–1630. doi: 10.1038/bjp.2008.209

Clayton, R. H., Bernus, O., Cherry, E. M., Dierckx, H., Fenton, F. H., Mirabella, L., et al. (2011). Models of cardiac tissue electrophysiology: progress, challenges and open questions. *Prog. Biophys. Mol. Biol.* 104, 22–48. doi: 10.1016/j.pbiomolbio.2010.05.008

Colman, M. A., Aslanidi, O. V., Kharche, S., Boyett, M. R., Garratt, C., Hancox, J. C., et al. (2013). Pro-arrhythmogenic effects of atrial fibrillation-induced electrical remodelling: insights from the three-dimensional virtual human atria. *J. Physiol.* 591, 4249–4272. doi: 10.1113/jphysiol.2013.254987

Colman, M. A., Ni, H., Liang, B., Schmitt, N., and Zhang, H. (2017). *In silico* assessment of genetic variation in KCNA5 reveals multiple mechanisms of human atrial arrhythmogenesis. *PLoS Comput. Biol.* 13:e1005587. doi: 10.1371/journal.pcbi.1005587

Committee for Medicinal Products for Human Use (2005). *ICH Note for Guidance on the Clinical Evaluation of QT/QTc Interval Prolongation and Proarrhythmic Potential for Non-antiarrhythmic Drugs (ICH E14) (CHMP/ICH/2/04).* London: EMEA. Available online at: http://www.ema.europa.eu/docs/en_GB/document_library/Scientific_guideline/2009/09/WC500002879.pdf

Committee for Medicinal Products for Human Use (2012). *ICH Topic E14: The Clinical Evaluation of QT/QTc Interval Prolongation and Proarrhythmic Potential for Non-antiarrhythmic Drugs Questions and Answers (EMA/CHMP/ICH/310133/2008).* London: EMEA. Available online at: http://

www.ema.europa.eu/docs/en_GB/document_library/Scientific_guideline/2009/09/WC500002878.pdf

Dobrev, D., Carlsson, L., and Nattel, S. (2012). Novel molecular targets for atrial fibrillation therapy. *Nat. Rev. Drug Discov.* 11, 275–291. doi: 10.1038/nrd3682

Dobrev, D., and Ravens, U. (2003). Remodeling of cardiomyocyte ion channels in human atrial fibrillation. *Basic Res. Cardiol.* 98, 137–148. doi: 10.1007/s00395-003-0409-8

Echt, D. S., Liebson, P. R., Mitchell, L. B., Peters, R. W., Obias-Manno, D., Barker, A. H., et al. (1991). Mortality and morbidity in patients receiving encainide, flecainide, or placebo. *N. Engl. J. Med.* 324, 781–788. doi: 10.1056/NEJM199103213241201

Ellinwood, N., Dobrev, D., Morotti, S., and Grandi, E. (2017). Revealing kinetics and state-dependent binding properties of IKur-targeting drugs that maximize atrial fibrillation selectivity. *Chaos Interdiscip. J. Nonlinear Sci.* 27:093918. doi: 10.1063/1.5000226

Fan, X., Wang, C., Wang, N., Ou, X., Liu, H., Yang, Y., et al. (2016). Atrial-selective block of sodium channels by acehytisine in rabbit myocardium. *J. Pharmacol. Sci.* 132, 235–243. doi: 10.1016/j.jphs.2016.03.014

Feng, J., Xu, D., Wang, Z., and Nattel, S. (1998a). Ultrarapid delayed rectifier current inactivation in human atrial myocytes: properties and consequences. *Am. J. Physiol. Heart Circ. Physiol.* 275, H1717–H1725.

Feng, J., Yue, L., Wang, Z., and Nattel, S. (1998b). Ionic mechanisms of regional action potential heterogeneity in the canine right atrium. *Circ. Res.* 83, 541–551. doi: 10.1161/01.RES.83.5.541

Ford, J., Milnes, J., El Haou, S., Wettwer, E., Loose, S., Matschke, K., et al. (2016). The positive frequency-dependent electrophysiological effects of the Ikur inhibitor Xen-D0103 are desirable for the treatment of atrial fibrillation. *Heart Rhythm.* 13, 555–564. doi: 10.1016/j.hrthm.2015.10.003.

Gima, K., and Rudy, Y. (2002). Ionic current basis of electrocardiographic waveforms a model study. *Circ. Res.* 90, 889–896. doi: 10.1161/01.RES.0000016960.61087.86

Gögelein, H., Brendel, J., Steinmeyer, K., Strübing, C., Picard, N., Rampe, D., et al. (2004). Effects of the atrial antiarrhythmic drug AVE0118 on cardiac ion channels. *Naunyn. Schmiedebergs Arch. Pharmacol.* 370, 183–192. doi: 10.1007/s00210-004-0957-y

Grandi, E., Pandit, S. V., Voigt, N., Workman, A. J., Dobrev, D., Jalife, J., et al. (2011). Human atrial action potential and Ca^{2+} model sinus rhythm and chronic atrial fibrillation. *Circ. Res.* 109, 1055–1066. doi: 10.1161/CIRCRESAHA.111.253955

Haan, S., de Greiser, M., Harks, E., Blaauw, Y., Hunnik, A., van Verheule, S., et al. (2006). AVE0118, blocker of the transient outward current (Ito) and ultrarapid delayed rectifier current (IKur), fully restores atrial contractility after cardioversion of atrial fibrillation in the goat. *Circulation* 114, 1234–1242. doi: 10.1161/CIRCULATIONAHA.106.630905

Hancox, J. C., James, A. F., Marrion, N. V., Zhang, H., and Thomas, D. (2016). Novel ion channel targets in atrial fibrillation. *Expert Opin. Ther. Targets* 20, 947–958. doi: 10.1517/14728222.2016.1159300

Hartmann, N., Mason, F. E., Braun, I., Pabel, S., Voigt, N., Schotola, H., et al. (2016). The combined effects of ranolazine and dronedarone on human atrial and ventricular electrophysiology. *J. Mol. Cell. Cardiol.* 94, 95–106. doi: 10.1016/j.yjmcc.2016.03.012

Hondeghem, L. M., and Snyders, D. J. (1990). Class III antiarrhythmic agents have a lot of potential but a long way to go. Reduced effectiveness and dangers of reverse use dependence. *Circulation* 81, 686–690. doi: 10.1161/01.CIR.81.2.686

Jarman, J. W. E., Wong, T., Kojodjojo, P., Spohr, H., Davies, J. E., Roughton, M., et al. (2012). Spatiotemporal behavior of high dominant frequency during paroxysmal and persistent atrial fibrillation in the human left atrium. *Circ. Arrhythm. Electrophysiol.* 5, 650–658. doi: 10.1161/CIRCEP.111.967992

Kirchhoff, J. E., Goldin Diness, J., Sheykhzade, M., Grunnet, M., and Jespersen, T. (2015). Synergistic antiarrhythmic effect of combining inhibition of Ca^{2+}-activated K^+ (SK) channels and voltage-gated Na+ channels in an isolated heart model of atrial fibrillation. *Heart Rhythm* 12, 409–418. doi: 10.1016/j.hrthm.2014.12.010

Koskinas, K. C., Fragakis, N., Katritsis, D., Skeberis, V., and Vassilikos, V. (2014). Ranolazine enhances the efficacy of amiodarone for conversion of recent-onset atrial fibrillation. *Europace* 16, 973–979. doi: 10.1093/europace/eut407

Li, G.-R., Lau, C.-P., and Shrier, A. (2002). Heterogeneity of sodium current in atrial vs. epicardial ventricular myocytes of adult guinea pig hearts. *J. Mol. Cell. Cardiol.* 34, 1185–1194. doi: 10.1006/jmcc.2002.2053

Li, G.-R., Wang, H.-B., Qin, G.-W., Jin, M.-W., Tang, Q., Sun, H.-Y., et al. (2008). Acacetin, a natural flavone, selectively inhibits human atrial repolarization potassium currents and prevents atrial fibrillation in dogs. *Circulation* 117, 2449–2457. doi: 10.1161/CIRCULATIONAHA.108.769554

Loose, S., Mueller, J., Wettwer, E., Knaut, M., Ford, J., Milnes, J., et al. (2014). Effects of IKur blocker MK-0448 on human right atrial action potentials from patients in sinus rhythm and in permanent atrial fibrillation. *Pharmacol. Ion Channels Channelopathies* 5:26. doi: 10.3389/fphar.2014.00026

Luo, C. H., and Rudy, Y. (1994). A dynamic model of the cardiac ventricular action potential. I. Simulations of ionic currents and concentration changes. *Circ. Res.* 74, 1071–1096. doi: 10.1161/01.RES.74.6.1071

Moreno, J. D., Zhu, Z. I., Yang, P.-C., Bankston, J. R., Jeng, M.-T., Kang, C., et al. (2011). A computational model to predict the effects of class i anti-arrhythmic drugs on ventricular rhythms. *Sci. Transl. Med.* 3:98ra83. doi: 10.1126/scitranslmed.3002588

Morotti, S., McCulloch, A. D., Bers, D. M., Edwards, A. G., and Grandi, E. (2016). Atrial-selective targeting of arrhythmogenic phase-3 early afterdepolarizations in human myocytes. *J. Mol. Cell. Cardiol.* 96, 63–71. doi: 10.1016/j.yjmcc.2015.07.030

Narayan, S. M., Bode, F., Karasik, P. L., and Franz, M. R. (2002). Alternans of atrial action potentials during atrial flutter as a precursor to atrial fibrillation. *Circulation* 106, 1968–1973. doi: 10.1161/01.CIR.0000037062.35762.B4

Narayan, S. M., Franz, M. R., Clopton, P., Pruvot, E. J., and Krummen, D. E. (2011). Repolarization alternans reveals vulnerability to human atrial fibrillation. *Circulation* 123, 2922–2930. doi: 10.1161/CIRCULATIONAHA.110.977827

Narayan, S. M., Shivkumar, K., Krummen, D. E., Miller, J. M., and Rappel, W.-J. (2013). Panoramic electrophysiological mapping but not electrogram morphology identifies stable sources for human atrial fibrillation. *Circ. Arrhythm. Electrophysiol.* 6, 58–67. doi: 10.1161/CIRCEP.111.977264

Nattel, S., and Dobrev, D. (2017). Controversies about atrial fibrillation mechanisms: aiming for order in chaos and whether it matters. *Circ. Res.* 120, 1396–1398. doi: 10.1161/CIRCRESAHA.116.310489

Nattel, S., Matthews, C., Blasio, E. D., Han, W., Li, D., and Yue, L. (2000). Dose-dependence of 4-aminopyridine plasma concentrations and electrophysiological effects in dogs potential relevance to ionic mechanisms *in vivo*. *Circulation* 101, 1179–1184. doi: 10.1161/01.CIR.101.10.1179

O'Hara, T., Virág, L., Varr,ó, A., and Rudy, Y. (2011). Simulation of the undiseased human cardiac ventricular action potential: model formulation and experimental validation. *PLoS Comput Biol* 7:e1002061. doi: 10.1371/journal.pcbi.1002061

Osaka, T., Itoh, A., and Kodama, I. (2000). Action potential remodeling in the human right atrium with chronic lone atrial fibrillation. *Pacing Clin. Electrophysiol.* 23, 960–965. doi: 10.1111/j.1540-8159.2000.tb00881.x

Pandit, S. V., and Jalife, J. (2013). Rotors and the dynamics of cardiac fibrillation. *Circ. Res.* 112, 849–862. doi: 10.1161/CIRCRESAHA.111.300158

Pavri, B. B., Greenberg, H. E., Kraft, W. K., Lazarus, N., Lynch, J. J., Salata, J. J., et al. (2012). Mk-0448, a specific Kv1.5 inhibitor safety, pharmacokinetics, and pharmacodynamic electrophysiology in experimental animal models and humans. *Circ. Arrhythm. Electrophysiol.* 5, 1193–1201. doi: 10.1161/CIRCEP.111.969782

Persson, F., Carlsson, L., Duker, G., and Jacobson, I. (2005). Blocking characteristics of hKv1.5 and hKv4.3/hKChIP2.2 after administration of the novel antiarrhythmic compound AZD7009. *J. Cardiovasc. Pharmacol.* 46, 7–17. doi: 10.1097/01.fjc.0000161405.37198.c1

Qi, X.-Y., Diness, J. G., Brundel, B. J. J. M., Zhou, X.-B., Naud, P., Wu, C.-T., et al. (2014). Role of small-conductance calcium-activated potassium channels in atrial electrophysiology and fibrillation in the dog. *Circulation* 129, 430–440. doi: 10.1161/CIRCULATIONAHA.113.003019

Rappel, W.-J., Zaman, J. A. B., and Narayan, S. M. (2015). Mechanisms for the termination of atrial fibrillation by localized ablation: computational and clinical studies. *Circ. Arrhythm. Electrophysiol.* 8, 1325–1333. doi: 10.1161/CIRCEP.115.002956

Ravens, U., and Wettwer, E. (2011). Ultra-rapid delayed rectifier channels: molecular basis and therapeutic implications. *Cardiovasc. Res.* 89, 776–785.

doi: 10.1093/cvr/cvq398

Reiffel, J. A., Camm, A. J., Belardinelli, L., Zeng, D., Karwatowska-Prokopczuk, E., Olmsted, A., et al. (2015). The HARMONY trial: combined ranolazine and dronedarone in the management of paroxysmal atrial fibrillation: mechanistic and therapeutic synergism. *Circ. Arrhythm. Electrophysiol.* 8, 1048–1056. doi: 10.1161/CIRCEP.115.002856

Roukoz, H., and Saliba, W. (2007). Dofetilide: a new class III antiarrhythmic agent. *Expert Rev. Cardiovasc. Ther.* 5, 9–19. doi: 10.1586/14779072.5.1.9

Schmidt, C., Wiedmann, F., Voigt, N., Zhou, X.-B., Heijman, J., Lang, S., et al. (2015). Upregulation of K2P3.1 K^+ current causes action potential shortening in patients with chronic atrial fibrillation. *Circulation* 132, 82–92. doi: 10.1161/CIRCULATIONAHA.114.012657

Scholz, E. P., Carrillo-Bustamante, P., Fischer, F., Wilhelms, M., Zitron, E., Dössel, O., et al. (2013). Rotor termination is critically dependent on kinetic properties of IKur inhibitors in an *in silico* model of chronic atrial fibrillation. *PLoS ONE* 8:e83179. doi: 10.1371/journal.pone.0083179

Schotten, U., Haan, S., de Verheule, S., Harks, E. G. A., Frechen, D., Bodewig, E., et al. (2007). Blockade of atrial-specific K^+-currents increases atrial but not ventricular contractility by enhancing reverse mode Na^+/Ca^{2+}-exchange. *Cardiovasc. Res.* 73, 37–47. doi: 10.1016/j.cardiores.2006.11.024

Sicouri, S., Burashnikov, A., Belardinelli, L., and Antzelevitch, C. (2010). Synergistic electrophysiologic and antiarrhythmic effects of the combination of ranolazine and chronic amiodarone in canine atria. *Circ. Arrhythm. Electrophysiol.* 3, 88–95. doi: 10.1161/CIRCEP.109.886275

Tamargo, J., Caballero, R., Gómez, R., and Delpón, E. (2009). IKur/Kv1.5 channel blockers for the treatment of atrial fibrillation. *Expert Opin. Investig. Drugs* 18, 399–416. doi: 10.1517/13543780902762850

Tsujimae, K., Murakami, S., and Kurachi, Y. (2008). *In silico* study on the effects of IKur block kinetics on prolongation of human action potential after atrial fibrillation-induced electrical remodeling. *Am. J. Physiol. Heart Circ. Physiol.* 294, H793–H800. doi: 10.1152/ajpheart.01229.2007

Voigt, N., and Dobrev, D. (2016). Atrial-selective potassium channel blockers. *Card. Electrophysiol. Clin.* 8, 411–421. doi: 10.1016/j.ccep.2016.02.005

Voigt, N., Li, N., Wang, Q., Wang, W., Trafford, A. W., Abu-Taha, I., et al. (2012). Enhanced sarcoplasmic reticulum Ca^{2+} leak and increased Na^+-Ca^{2+} exchanger function underlie delayed afterdepolarizations in patients with chronic atrial fibrillation. *Circulation* 125, 2059–2070. doi: 10.1161/CIRCULATIONAHA.111.067306

Wagoner, D. R. V., Pond, A. L., McCarthy, P. M., Trimmer, J. S., and Nerbonne, J. M. (1997). Outward K^+ current densities and Kv1.5 expression are reduced in chronic human atrial fibrillation. *Circ. Res.* 80, 772–781. doi: 10.1161/01.RES.80.6.772

Wettwer, E., Hála, O., Christ, T., Heubach, J. F., Dobrev, D., Knaut, M., et al. (2004). Role of ikur in controlling action potential shape and contractility in the human atrium influence of chronic atrial fibrillation. *Circulation* 110, 2299–2306. doi: 10.1161/01.CIR.0000145155.60288.71

Wettwer, E., and Terlau, H. (2014). Pharmacology of voltage-gated potassium channel Kv1.5—impact on cardiac excitability. *Curr. Opin. Pharmacol.* 15, 115–121. doi: 10.1016/j.coph.2014.02.001

Whittaker, D. G., Ni, H., Harchi, A. E., Hancox, J. C., and Zhang, H. (2017). Atrial arrhythmogenicity of KCNJ2 mutations in short QT syndrome: insights from virtual human atria. *PLoS Comput. Biol.* 13:e1005593. doi: 10.1371/journal.pcbi.1005593

Wilhelms, M., Maleckar, M. M., Koivumäki, J. T., Dössel, O., and Seemann, G. (2013). Benchmarking electrophysiological models of human atrial myocytes. *Front. Comput. Physiol. Med.* 3:487. doi: 10.3389/fphys.2012.00487

Wirth, K. J., Brendel, J., Steinmeyer, K., Linz, D. K., Rütten, H., and Gögelein, H. (2007). *In vitro* and *in vivo* effects of the atrial selective antiarrhythmic compound AVE1231. *J. Cardiovasc. Pharmacol.* 49, 197–206. doi: 10.1097/FJC.0b013e318032002f

Woods, C. E., and Olgin, J. (2014). Atrial fibrillation therapy now and in the future drugs, biologicals, and ablation. *Circ. Res.* 114, 1532–1546. doi: 10.1161/CIRCRESAHA.114.302362

Workman, A. J., Kane, K. A., and Rankin, A. C. (2001). The contribution of ionic currents to changes in refractoriness of human atrial myocytes associated with chronic atrial fibrillation. *Cardiovasc. Res.* 52, 226–235. doi: 10.1016/S0008-6363(01)00380-7

Wu, H.-J., Wu, W., Sun, H.-Y., Qin, G.-W., Wang, H.-B., Wang, P., et al. (2011). Acacetin causes a frequency- and use-dependent blockade of hKv1.5 channels by binding to the S6 domain. *J. Mol. Cell. Cardiol.* 51, 966–973. doi: 10.1016/j.yjmcc.2011.08.022

Yap, Y. G., and Camm, A. J. (2003). Drug induced QT prolongation and torsades de pointes. *Heart* 89, 1363–1372. doi: 10.1136/heart.89.11.1363

Yuan, Y., Bai, X., Luo, C., Wang, K., and Zhang, H. (2015). The virtual heart as a platform for screening drug cardiotoxicity. *Br. J. Pharmacol.* 172, 5531–5547. doi: 10.1111/bph.12996

Zhang, H., Garratt, C. J., Zhu, J., and Holden, A. V. (2005). Role of up-regulation of IK1 in action potential shortening associated with atrial fibrillation in humans. *Cardiovasc. Res.* 66, 493–502. doi: 10.1016/j.cardiores.2005.01.020

Zhu, Y., Kyle, J. W., and Lee, P. J. (2006). Flecainide sensitivity of a Na channel long QT mutation shows an open-channel blocking mechanism for use-dependent block. *Am. J. Physiol. Heart Circ. Physiol.* 291, H29–H37. doi: 10.1152/ajpheart.01317.2005

Zygmunt, A. C., Nesterenko, V. V., Rajamani, S., Hu, D., Barajas-Martinez, H., Belardinelli, L., et al. (2011). Mechanisms of atrial-selective block of Na^+ channels by ranolazine: I. Experimental analysis of the use-dependent block. *Am. J. Physiol. Heart Circ. Physiol.* 301, H1606–H1614. doi: 10.1152/ajpheart.00242.2011

6

Proton Pump Inhibitors and Serum Magnesium Levels in Patients with Torsades de Pointes

Pietro E. Lazzerini[1], Iacopo Bertolozzi[2], Francesco Finizola[1], Maurizio Acampa[3], Mariarita Natale[1], Francesca Vanni[1], Rosella Fulceri[4], Alessandra Gamberucci[4], Marco Rossi[1,5], Beatrice Giabbani[1], Michele Caselli[1], Ilaria Lamberti[1], Gabriele Cevenini[6], Franco Laghi-Pasini[1†] and Pier L. Capecchi[1†]*

[1] Department of Medical Sciences, Surgery and Neurosciences, University of Siena, Siena, Italy, [2] Cardiology Intensive Therapy Unit, Department of Internal Medicine, Hospital of Carrara, Carrara, Italy, [3] Stroke Unit, University Hospital of Siena, Siena, Italy, [4] Department of Molecular and Developmental Medicine, University of Siena, Siena, Italy, [5] Centre of Pharmacovigilance, University Hospital of Siena, Siena, Italy, [6] Department of Medical Biotechnologies, University of Siena, Siena, Italy

***Correspondence:**
Pietro E. Lazzerini
lazzerini7@unisi.it

† These authors have contributed equally to this work.

Background: Torsades de pointes (TdP) is a life-threatening ventricular tachycardia occurring in long QT-syndrome patients. It usually develops when multiple QT-prolonging factors are concomitantly present, more frequently drugs and electrolyte imbalances. Since proton–pump inhibitors (PPIs)-associated hypomagnesemia is an increasingly recognized adverse event, PPIs were recently included in the list of drugs with conditional risk of TdP, despite only few cases of TdP in PPI users have been reported so far.

Objectives: Aim of the present study is to evaluate whether PPI-induced hypomagnesemia actually has a significant clinical impact on the risk of TdP in the general population.

Methods: Forty-eight unselected patients who experienced TdP were consecutively enrolled (2008-2017). Shortly after the first TdP episode, in those patients who did not receive magnesium sulfate and/or potassium or calcium replacement therapy, serum electrolytes were measured and their relationship with PPI usage analyzed.

Results: Many patients (28/48, 58%) were under current PPI treatment when TdP occurred. Among TdP patients in whom serum electrolyte determinations were obtained before replacement therapy (27/48), those taking PPIs had significantly lower serum magnesium levels than those who did not. Hypomagnesemia occurred in ~40% of patients receiving PPIs (6/14), in all cases after an extended treatment (>2 weeks). In patients taking PPIs the mean QT-prolonging risk factor number was significantly higher than in those who did not, a difference which was mainly driven by lower magnesium levels.

Conclusions: In unselected TdP patients, PPI-induced hypomagnesemia was common and significantly contributed to their cumulative arrhythmic risk. By providing clinical support to current recommendations, our data confirm that more awareness is needed when a PPI is prescribed, specifically as regards the risk of life-threatening arrhythmias.

Keywords: proton-pump inhibitors, Torsades de pointes, serum magnesium levels, long-QT syndrome, sudden cardiac death

INTRODUCTION

Torsades de pointes (TdP) is a life-threatening polymorphic ventricular tachycardia that can degenerate into ventricular fibrillation (VF) and cause sudden cardiac death (SCD) (Drew et al., 2010). It is characterized by a pattern of twisting points and occurs in patients with long QT syndrome (LQTS), both acquired and congenital. Indeed, in congenital-LQTS the more the heart rate-corrected QT interval (QTc) prolongs, the greater the TdP risk exponentially increases (i.e., 5–7% risk increase each 10 ms prolongation in QTc) until being significant for QTc>500 ms; such a value associated with a 2–3-fold higher risk for TdP (Drew et al., 2010).

Since a marked QTc prolongation is usually required for TdP development, in most cases the simultaneous presence of multiple QTc-prolonging factors synergistically operating in impairing ion channels responsible for the ventricular repolarization process is necessary. Congenital factors are included, mainly resulting from mutations affecting genes encoding for potassium or sodium channels, as well as acquired risk factors (Viskin, 1999; El-Sherif and Turitto, 2003; Drew et al., 2010; Itoh et al., 2016). Among the latter factors, electrolyte imbalances (i.e., hypokaliemia, hypocalcemia, hypomagnesemia) and QT-prolonging drugs blocking the hERG potassium channel are those most frequently implicated in TdP development. Other established causes of acquired LQTS and TdP include structural heart diseases, bradyarrhythmias, endocrine disorders, liver diseases, nervous system injuries, HIV infection, starvation, hypothermia and toxins (El-Sherif and Turitto, 2003; Drew et al., 2010). In addition, autoimmunity (Lazzerini et al., 2017d) (particularly anti-Ro/SSA antibodies) (Yue et al., 2015; Lazzerini et al., 2016) and systemic inflammation (Lazzerini et al., 2015, 2017a,b) in the recent years are being increasingly recognized as novel acquired QT-prolonging risk factors significantly impacting TdP risk in the general population.

Proton-pump inhibitors (PPIs) are the most effective therapeutic agents for acid related disorders (ARD), including peptic ulcer disease and gastroesophageal reflux disease (Strand et al., 2017). Moreover, such drugs are also used for the prevention of non-steroidal anti-inflammatory drug-induced gastric injury and as a part of *Helicobacter pylori* eradication regimens (Strand et al., 2017). As a result, PPIs currently represent the fifth best-selling drug in the market with millions of chronic users worldwide (Patterson Burdsall et al., 2013). During the last years, concern has been raised because of PPIs long-term overutilization. In fact, in the clinical practice PPIs are often prescribed in patients without a specific ARD, and such a habit is leading to significant cost expenditure and possible adverse events (Moayyedi and Leontiadis, 2012).

Hypomagnesemia is a potentially serious side effect of PPIs, that could account for ~1% of all adverse events reported by drug users (Famularo et al., 2013; Luk et al., 2013). Although several data suggest an interference on intestinal magnesium absorption, the exact underlying mechanism is poorly understood (Famularo et al., 2013). In 2011 the US FDA warned that long-term use of PPI has the potential to reduce circulating magnesium levels, particularly in patients concomitantly receiving other drugs capable to cause magnesium depletion such as diuretics (2011)[1]. Accordingly, in 2016 the Arizona Center for Education and research on Therapeutics (AZCERT) included the PPIs omeprazole, esomeprazole, lansoprazole and pantoprazole in the list of drugs with conditional risk of TdP and to be avoided in patients with congenital LQTS (AZCERT, 2016), despite only few cases of QTc prolongation and TdP have been reported in patients with severe PPI-induced hypomagnesemia and/or taking a PPI concomitantly with drugs known to directly prolong QTc (Asajima et al., 2012; Bibawy et al., 2013; Hansen and Bruserud, 2016). As a result, it is now recommended that in patients taking a PPI for an extended period of time (>2 weeks) serum magnesium levels be monitored periodically, particularly if extended PPI therapy is used in association with drugs carrying a known risk of TdP (Asajima et al., 2012; 2016). Notably, a very recent longitudinal observational study performed in a large primary cohort of new users of acid suppression therapy followed for a median of 5.7 years, found a significant association between PPI use and risk of all-cause mortality. The risk was increased among those with no documented medical indications for PPI use and prolonged duration of use (Xie et al., 2017).

Regardless of official recommendations, available real-life information on this subject is relatively poor so far. The present study is specifically aimed at evaluating whether PPI-induced hypomagnesemia has a significant clinical impact on the risk of TdP in the general population. Thus, the actual usage of PPIs and its relationship with serum magnesium levels were analyzed in a cohort of TdP patients, prospectively and consecutively enrolled independent of ongoing therapies and concomitant diseases.

PATIENTS AND METHODS

Study Populations

Local Ethical Committee approved the study, and patients gave their oral and written informed consent in accordance with the Principles of the Declaration of Helsinki.

We prospectively enrolled (from January 2008 to May 2017) 48 consecutive hospitalized patients who presented with TdP, independent of ongoing therapies and concomitant diseases. Since the only inclusion criteria was the occurrence of TdP, all patients who came to our attention in that period of time were enrolled. No patients were excluded. Demographic, clinical and laboratory characteristics of study patients, as well as ongoing treatment with QTc-prolonging medications are provided in **Table 1**. In these patients, PPI usage was assessed, and a cut-off time of 2 weeks was used to define treatment duration as extended (>2 weeks) or not, according to current AZCERT recommendations to minimize the risk of TdP in patients treated with PPI (AZCERT, 2016).

ECG Recordings

Diagnosis of TdP was based on the presence of at least one episode of polymorphic ventricular arrhythmia at a rate ranging

[1]FDA Drug Safety Communication: Low magnesium levels can be associated with long-term use of proton pump inhibitor drugs (PPIs). Available at www.fda.gov/Drugs/DrugSafety/ucm245011.htm Accessed May 26 (2017).

TABLE 1 | Demographic, clinical and laboratory characteristics of patients with Torsades de pointes.

Patients, n	48
Age, median years (interquartile range)	81(73–85)
Females, n	31/48(65%)
Mean QTc, ms(range)	596.0 ± 80.7(490–910)
Electrolyte imbalances, n	37/47(79%)
Hypokaliemia	28/45(62%)
Hypocalcemia	22/37(59%)
Hypomagnesemia	7/27(26%)
Concomitant diseases*, n	45/48(94%)
Cardiac diseases	40/48(83%)
Left ventricular hypertrophy	19/48(40%)
Dilated cardiomyopathy/heart failure	13/48(27%)
II-III degree atrioventricular block	10/48(21%)
Acute coronary syndrome	9/48(19%)
Chronic coronary artery disease	7/48(15%)
Sinus bradycardia	6/48(13%)
Extra-cardiac diseases	20/48(42%)
Diabetes mellitus type II	13/48(27%)
Chronic kidney disease	8/48(17%)
Hypothyroidism	2/48(4%)
Subarachnoid hemorrhage	1/48(2%)
Cirrhosis	1/48(2%)
Anorexia nervosa	1/48(2%)
HIV infection	1/48(2%)
QTc prolonging-medications, n	34/48(71%)
Amiodarone	14/48(29%)
Citalopram	5/48(10%)
Sertraline	4/48(8%)
Fluconazole	3/48(6%)
Trazodone	3/48(6%)
Levofloxacin	2/48(4%)
Clarithromycin	2/48(4%)
Promazine	2/48(4%)
Quetiapine	2/48(4%)
Mean medication number per patient	1.1 ± 1.0
Anti-Ro/SSA positivity, n	18/32(56%)
Systemic inflammation, n†	38/48(79%)
C-reactive protein, mg/dl(range)	2.66(0.1–29.65)
Definite inflammatory diseases	22/48(46%)
Acute infections	15/48(31%)
Immuno-mediated diseases	5/48(10%)
Others	2/48(4%)
Mean QTc-prolonging risk factor number per patient§	5.3 ± 1.5

Except where indicated otherwise, data are expressed as mean ± standard deviation or median (range).

Appropriate serum potassium, calcium or magnesium measurements available in 45, 37, and 27 out of 48 patients, respectively; anti-Ro/SSA antibodies tested in 32 out of 48 patients.

**Diseases recognized to be a risk factor for QTc prolongation (Viskin, 1999; El-Sherif and Turitto, 2003; Drew et al., 2010).*

†Increased C-reactive protein level (>0.5 mg/dl) with or without a definite inflammatory disease. §Including electrolyte imbalances, diseases, QTc-prolonging medications, anti-Ro/SSA positivity, and systemic inflammation (Viskin, 1999; El-Sherif and Turitto, 2003; Drew et al., 2010; Yue et al., 2015; Lazzerini et al., 2016, 2017b).

from 160 to 240 beats/min, associated with QTc prolongation (Drew et al., 2010; **Figure 1**). The QT interval was manually measured on a standard 12-lead ECG, from the onset of the Q wave or the onset of the QRS complex to the end of the T wave, defined as the return to the T-P baseline. When present, prominent U waves (>1 mm) merging into T waves were included in QT measurement (Gupta et al., 2007). QTc, determined as the longest hand-measured QTc in any lead (Rautaharju et al., 2009) was corrected for heart rate by the Bazett formula (dividing the QT by the square root of the preceding R-R interval of each beat: $QT/\sqrt{RR}$) to yield the QTc value. QTc was measured from 3 non-consecutive beats (mean value) by a single investigator.

Laboratory Analysis

Shortly after the first TdP episode [no later than 24 h (median 6 h, range 1–22 h)], patients underwent a venous withdrawal to determine serum electrolyte levels, including potassium, sodium, calcium, and magnesium. Potassium and sodium were determined by indirect potentiometry (COBAS-6000 platform); values were expressed as mEq/L (reference values: potassium 3.5–5.5; sodium 132–148). Calcium and magnesium were assayed by a colorimetric method (COBAS-6000 platform); values were expressed as mg/dl (reference values: calcium 8.0-11.0; magnesium 1.5–2.5).

Only determinations obtained before the administration of intravenous magnesium sulfate and/or replacement therapy with potassium or calcium were considered appropriate to be included in the study. As a result, serum potassium, calcium or magnesium measurements were available in 45, 37, and 27 out of 48 patients, respectively.

Other laboratory parameters included circulating levels of anti-Ro/SSA antibodies (*see* Supplementary Methods for more details) and C-reactive protein (CRP), as well as pH, bicarbonates and serum glucose.

Statistical Analysis

To compare TdP patients subgroups, the following parametric or non-parametric statistical analyses were respectively carried out: the two-tail Student's unpaired *t*-test, or the two-tail Mann-Whitney test to evaluate differences in quantitative variables; the Pearson or Spearman rank correlation-test to verify possible statistical association between quantitative variables; the two-sided Fisher's exact test to evaluate statistical correlation between categorical variables. $p < 0.05$ were considered as significant. All statistical analyses were performed using GraphPad-InStat, version 3.06 for Windows 2000.

RESULTS

TdP Patients Characteristics

As detailed in **Table 1**, demographic, clinical and laboratory characteristics of our cohort were fully consistent with those expected in TdP patients based on established epidemiological data. In fact, the large majority of subjects were females (31/48, 65%) and older than 65 years (median age: ~80 years). Moreover, many recognized QTc-prolonging risk factors of acquired origin

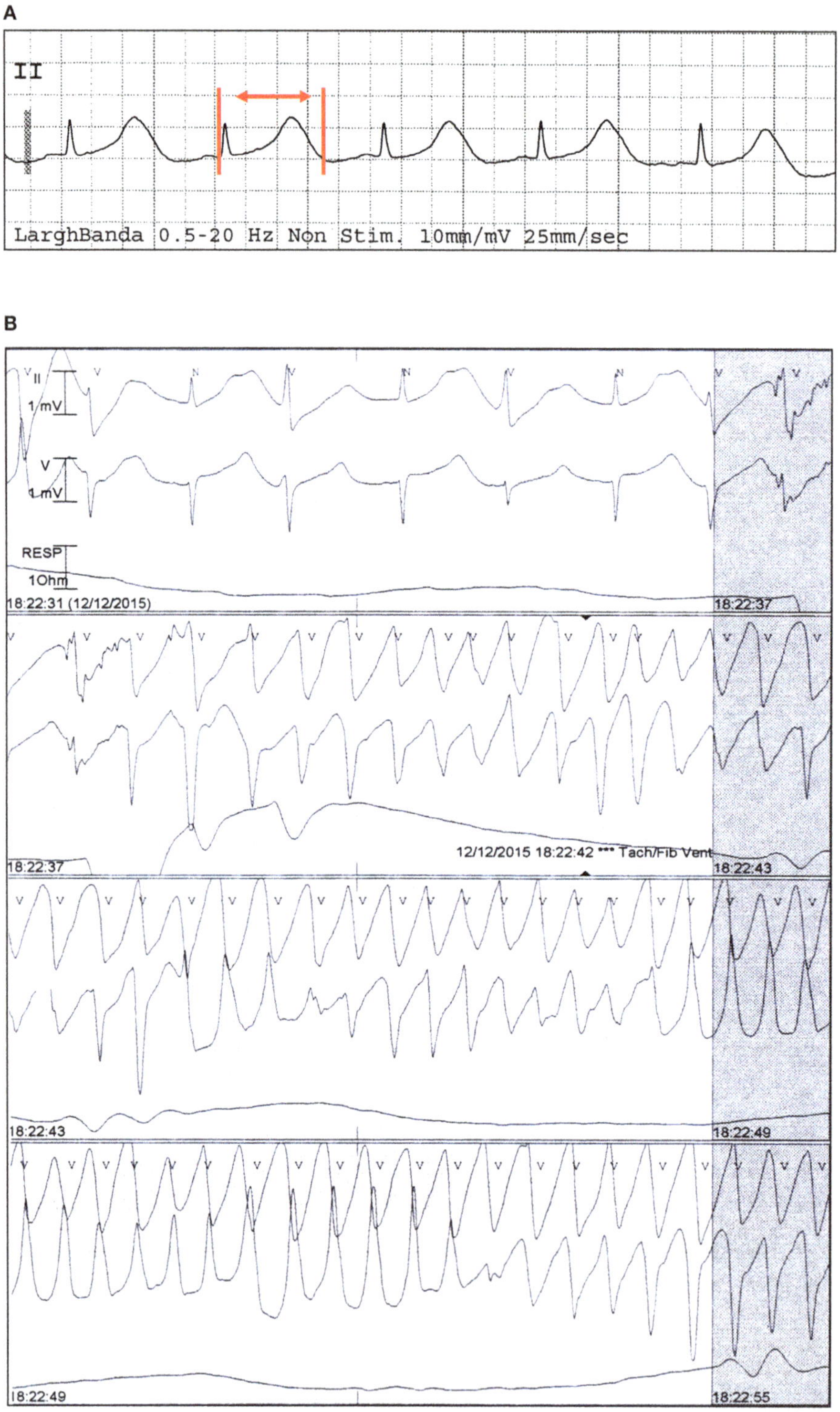

FIGURE 1 | Electrocardiographic findings of a patient with TdP and PPI-associated hypomagnesemia. ECG strip in sinus rhythm **(A)** and during TdP **(B)** from a patient who was under current and extended treatment with oral lansoprazole (15 mg/day), and had low magnesium levels (1.46 mg/dl) and a QTc of 670 ms. Red vertical lines and arrow in lead II show QT interval.

were identifiable, particularly an underlying cardiac disease (45/48, 83%, more frequently ventricular hypertrophy, dilated cardiomyopathy/heart failure and atrio-ventricular blocks), electrolyte imbalances (37/47, 79%) and QTc-prolonging medications (34/48, 71%). Hypokalemia occurred in 62% of patients (28/45), thereby representing the most common specific risk factor. Anti-Ro/SSA-52 kD antibodies were detected in 56% of the tested cases (18/32), although a history of autoimmune disease was present in two patients only (1 rheumatoid arthritis, 1 celiac disease). The majority of TdP patients (38/48, 79%) showed signs of systemic inflammation, as indicated by the increase in CRP levels (>0.5 mg/dl; median value 2.66 mg/dl). A definite inflammatory disease was present in 22/48 patients (46%), most commonly an acute infection (n = 15, particularly sepsis and pneumonia), but also chronic immune-mediated diseases (n = 5, including 3 chronic inflammatory arthritis), or acute aseptic inflammatory processes (n = 2). Among drugs, amiodarone was the most frequently administered (14/48, 29%). Notably, in almost all cases more than one known QTc-prolonging factor was simultaneously identifiable; on average ~5. In addition, a significant proportion of patients (25/48, 52%) experienced an adverse short-term arrhythmic outcome, i.e., VF/cardiac arrest (CA), and/or underwent electric shock (TdP rapidly degenerated to VF/CA; out-of-hospital VF/CA followed with DC-shock, only later revealing a manifestation of TdP episodes; sustained TdP not responsive to medical therapy).

Proton-Pump Inhibitors Usage in TdP Patients

In our cohort, a significant percentage of patients were under active treatment with PPI when TdP occurred (28/48, 58%). Many subjects (16/25, 64%) were taking a PPI for an extended period of time, i.e., >2 weeks. The most frequently administered PPI was pantoprazole, followed by lansoprazole, together accounting for ~85% of the cases (24/28). Remaining patients ($n = 4$), were administered with omeprazole ($n = 3$), or esomeprazole (n = 1). In three patients under extended home PPI therapy, the molecule was changed during hospitalization, before TdP development (from oral lansoprazole or pantoprazole to intravenous pantoprazole in two cases; from oral omeprazole to oral pantoprazole in the other one). The commonest route of administration was the oral one, but in 6/28 cases (21%) where the PPI was being given intravenously at the time of TdP occurrence (**Table 2**). Notably, none of the intravenously-treated patients showed hypomagnesemia.

TABLE 2 | Proton-pump inhibitors use in patients with Torsades de Pointes.

Patients under active treatment with PPIs, n	28/48(58%)
Specific PPI used, n	
Pantoprazole	18/28(64%)
Lansoprazole	6/28(21%)
Omeprazole	3/28(11%)
Esomeprazole	1/28(4%)
Treatment duration*	
Extended therapy (>2 weeks), n	16/25(64%)
Not extended therapy (<2 weeks), n	9/25(36%)
Daily dose, mg†	
Pantoprazole	33.3 ± 9.7
Lansoprazole	27.5 ± 6.1
Omeprazole	26.7 ± 11.5
Esomeprazole	20
Route of administration, n†	
Oral	22/28(79%)
Intravenous	6/28(21%)

Except where indicated otherwise, values are expressed as mean ± standard deviation.
**Data missing in 3 out of 28 patients.*
†At the moment of TdP occurrence.

Serum Electrolytes Levels and Other TdP Risk Factors in Patients Taking or Not Taking Proton-Pump Inhibitors

Consistently with the findings obtained in the whole TdP population, a high prevalence of electrolyte imbalances (collectively ~80%) was found in both patients taking (PPI+) or not taking PPI (PPI−). However, while the prevalence of hypokaliemia and hypocalcemia as well as serum potassium, calcium (and sodium) levels in the two groups were overalapping, circulating magnesium levels were significantly lower in PPI+ than in PPI− subjects (1.60 ± 0.21 vs. 1.84 ± 0.33 mg/dl, Δ = −0.24 mg/dl; $p = 0.03$) (**Figures 2, 3**). Hypomagnesemia (<1.5 mg/dl) occurred 5-times more frequently in the PPI+ vs. PPI- group (6/14, 43% vs. 1/13, 8%), although this difference did not reach statistical significance ($p = 0.07$) (**Table 3**). Notably, hypomagnesemia was found almost exclusively (6 out of 7 cases, 85%) in patients receiving PPI therapy; all cases of PPI-associated hypomagnesemia ($n = 6$) were observed in patients under extended PPI therapy (>2 weeks), involving all the 4 different PPIs used in the cohort (pantoprazole, $n = 3$; lansoprazole, $n = 1$; omeprazole, $n = 1$; esomeprazole, $n = 1$). Diuretics usage, which was not different in the PPI+ vs. PPI− group (**Table 3**), was not *per se* associated with significant magnesium changes in our cohort. In fact, by comparing patients taking ($n = 16$) and not taking diuretics ($n = 11$), neither serum magnesium levels (1.67 ± 0.31 vs. 1.78 ± 0.26 mg/dl; $p = 0.32$, two-tail unpaired t-test) nor the prevalence of hypomagnesemia (6/16, 37% vs. 1/11, 9%; $p = 0.18$, two-sided Fisher's exact test) were significantly different. Although these findings suggest that diuretics alone, differently to PPIs alone, were not sufficient to cause magnesium depletion, nevertheless diuretics may exacerbate PPI-associated magnesium reduction when administered in association. Indeed, in patients concomitantly receiving PPIs and diuretics ($n = 9$, vs. others $n = 18$) serum magnesium levels further decreased slightly (1.55 ± 0.21 vs. 1.80 ± 0.30 mg/dl, Δ = −0,25 mg/dl; $p = 0.02$, two-tail Mann-Whitney test), and the prevalence of hypomagnesemia increased, reaching statistical significance (5/9, 56% vs. 2/18, 11%; $p = 0.02$, two-sided Fisher's exact test). Despite a specific investigation, no any significant impact of other common causes of hypomagnesemia was found in our cohort of patients (see Supplementary Results for more details). Moreover, no significant correlation was present between magnesium levels and other continuous variables, particularly calcium ($r = 0.33$, $p = 0.10$; Pearson correlation-test) potassium ($r = 0.10$, $p = 0.57$; Pearson correlation-test), sodium ($r = 0.11$, $p = 0.58$; Spearman rank correlation-test) or CRP levels ($r = -0.14$, $p = 0.46$; Spearman rank correlation-test), or QTc duration ($r = -0.19$, $p = 0.32$; Pearson correlation-test).

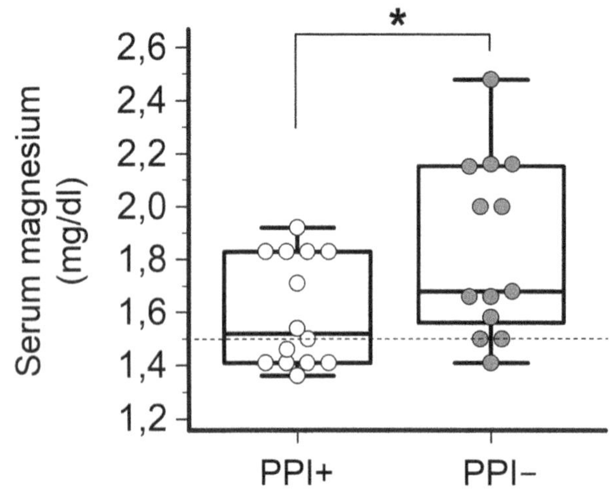

FIGURE 2 | Serum magnesium levels in TdP patients taking or not taking PPIs. Patients taking PPIs (PPI+), $n = 14$; patients not taking PPIs (PPI−), $n = 13$. Two-tail Student's unpaired t-test, *$p < 0.05$. Horizontal dotted line indicates the lower limit of reference values for serum magnesium levels, i.e., 1.5 mg/dl.

As regards the other QTc-prolonging risk factors of acquired origin, individually considered, no significant differences in terms of concomitant diseases, both cardiac and extra.-cardiac, QTc prolonging medications use, anti-Ro/SSA positivity or presence of systemic inflammation were observed by comparing PPI+ vs. PPI− patients (**Table 3**). Nevertheless, when all these factors were considered together, also including electrolyte imbalances, the mean QTc-prolonging risk factor number per patient was significantly higher in the PPI+ than the PPI- group (5.8 ± 1.6 vs. 4.9 ± 1.4, Δ: 0.9; $p = 0.04$). Notably, statistical significance of this difference was lost if hypomagnesemia, i.e., the only individual TdP risk factor discriminating the two groups, was selectively excluded by the total count (5.6 ± 1.5 vs. 4.9 ± 1.4, Δ: 0.7; $p = 0.07$; **Table 3**). It is important to underline that for a number of patients, some data on QT-prolonging risk factors were missing, particularly serum levels of potassium (available in 26/28 of PPI+ 19/20 of PPI− patients, respectively), calcium (27/28 of PPI+ and 18/20 of PPI− patients, respectively), magnesium (14/28 of PPI+ and 13/20 of PPI− patients, respectively), and anti-Ro/SSA positivity (18/28 of PPI+ and 14/20 of PPI− patients, respectively). Nevertheless, when we restricted the analysis to patients with full data only, i.e., 8 PPI+ and 10 PPI−, differences (Δ) in mean QTc-prolonging risk factor number per patient remained completely unchanged, both when all risk factors were considered (6.1 ± 1.7 vs. 5.2 ± 1.3, Δ: 0.9) and when hypomagnesemia was excluded (5.8 ± 1.4 vs. 5.1 ± 1.3, Δ: 0.7), thus indicating that the results were not influenced by missing data.

Conversely, PPI treatment did not seem to affect the short-term outcome in our cohort of patients. In fact, the percentage of subjects experiencing VF/CA, and/or that underwent electric shock was not significantly different by comparing PPI+ vs. PPI− patients (15/28, 54% vs. 10/20, 50%) (**Table 3**).

Finally, in order to specifically address the question of whether magnesium levels are different between PPI+ patients who developed TdP vs. PPI+ patients who did not, 21 hospitalized patients matched for age, gender and concomitant diseases (Supplementary Table 1), but without QTc prolongation or history of TdP were prospectively enrolled as a control group (C). Similarly to that observed in TdP subjects, more than a half of control patients were under current treatment with PPIs (12/21, 57%), in most cases for an extended period of time (10/12, 83%) (Supplementary Table 2). Among these patients, hypomagnesemia was found in 2 patients (2/21, 9%), one treated and one untreated with PPIs. As shown in **Figure 4A**, circulating magnesium levels were significantly lower in TdP vs. controls (1.72 ± 0.30 vs. 1.91 ± 0.40 mg/dl; $p = 0.0094$). Such a difference significantly increased when the comparison was restricted to PPI-treated patients from the two groups (TdP/PPI+: 1.60 ± 0.21 vs. C/PPI+: 1.93 ± 0.48 mg/dl; $p = 0.0007$; **Figure 4B**), while serum magnesium levels were not different in PPI-untreated TdP vs. control patients (TdP/PPI−: 1.84 ± 0.33 vs. C/PPI−: 1.88 ± 0.30 mg/dl; $p = 0.78$, two-tail Student's unpaired t-test).

As a confirmation of the results on subgroups, we also evaluated the interaction between magnesemia and PPI treatment (PPI+/PPI−), by combining (multiplying) the two variables in the whole population (TdP vs. C). We found that sample differences between TdP and C in such interaction-corrected levels of magnesium were not longer statistically significant ($p = 0.09$, two-tail Mann-Whitney test).

DISCUSSION

The key findings of the present study are the following: a large proportion of patients (>50%) who developed TdP were under current treatment with a PPI; TdP patients taking PPIs had significantly lower serum magnesium levels with respect to TdP patients not taking PPIs; hypomagnesemia frequently occurred in patients receiving PPIs (~40%, 6/14), in all cases after an extended period of time (>2 weeks) of administration; in subjects taking PPIs the mean QTc-prolonging risk factor number per patient was significantly higher than it was in those not taking PPIs, a difference which was mainly driven by lower magnesium levels.

Magnesium, representing the most abundant intracellular divalent cation, plays a key role in regulating potassium and calcium channels in the heart (Gupta et al., 2007). Experimental studies demonstrated that cytosolic magnesium promotes repolarization of myocardial cells via modulating effects on several potassium currents, including the rapid component of the delayed rectifier potassium current (IKr) and transient outward current (Ito) (Kelepouris et al., 1993; El-Sherif and Turitto, 2011). Moreover, magnesium markedly inhibits the L(long-lasting)-type calcium current (ICaL), possibly as a result of a direct block of the L-type-calcium channel pore by external magnesium or via modification of the activity of protein kinases or phosphoprotein phosphatases (Zhao et al., 2015). ICaL determines the plateau phase thereby critically contributing to action potential duration (APD) (Viskin, 1999; El-Sherif and Turitto, 2003). Moreover, ICaL is the main depolarizing current that generates early after depolarizations (EADs), in turn representing the primary

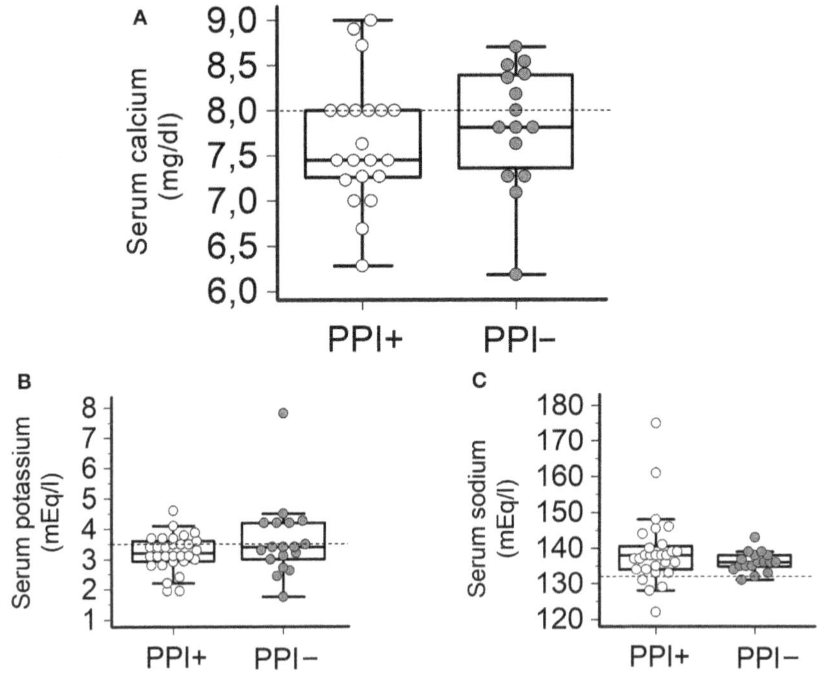

FIGURE 3 | Serum levels of calcium, potassium and sodium in TdP patients taking or not taking PPIs. **(A)** Serum calcium levels. Patients taking PPIs (PPI+), $n = 20$; patients not taking PPIs (PPI−), $n = 17$. Two-tail Student's unpaired t-test ($p > 0.05$). Horizontal dotted line indicates the lower limit of reference values for calcium levels, i.e., 8.0 mg/dl. **(B)** Serum potassium levels. PPI+, $n = 27$; PPI−, $n = 18$. Two-tail Student's unpaired t-test ($p > 0.05$). Horizontal dotted line indicates the lower limit of reference values for potassium levels, i.e., 3.5 mEq/L. **(C)** Serum sodium levels. PPI+, $n = 28$; PPI−, $n = 20$. Two-tail Student's unpaired t-test ($p > 0.05$). Horizontal dotted line indicates the lower limit of reference values for sodium levels, i.e., 132 mEq/L.

electrophysiological mechanism underlying TdP development (Viskin, 1999; El-Sherif and Turitto, 2003). This supports the fact that hypomagnesemia is a recognized risk factor for QTc prolongation and TdP (Viskin, 1999; El-Sherif and Turitto, 2003, 2011), as well as the clinical evidence that magnesium sulfate is very effective for the treatment of TdP thus being considered the standard of care for this arrhythmia (Drew et al., 2010).

PPI-induced hypomagnesemia, for the first time described in 2006, has been increasingly recognized in the last years as a potentially life-threatening adverse event whose actual incidence is probably largely underestimated (Famularo et al., 2013). Two recent systematic reviews and meta-analysis, each one including nine studies and over 100,000 patients, consistently found that PPI users have a ~40–80% higher risk of developing hypomagnesemia when compared to non-users (Park et al., 2014; Cheungpasitporn et al., 2015).

PPI-associated hypomagnesemia occurs after extended treatments (>2 weeks, but in most cases > 1 year), is not clearly dose-related, and was reported with different PPIs, thus suggesting a class effect. Until PPI interruption, hypomagnesemia is refractory to oral or parenteral magnesium replacement irrespective of high-dose supplementation; when the PPI is stopped, serum magnesium levels returned to normal in less than 2 weeks (2011; Famularo et al., 2013). However, hypomagnesemia may recur after re-challenge with the same or a different PPI. In these patients, when prolonged antiacid treatment is needed, prescription of a H_2 histamine receptor-blocker (H_2-blocker) may be an appropriate therapeutic alternative (Famularo et al., 2013). In fact, although mechanisms of PPI-induced hypomagnesemia are not clear, hypochlorhydria does not seem to be involved. Pathogenesis possibly includes both gastrointestinal and renal losses, via dysfunction of the Transient Receptor Potential Melastatin 6/7 (TRPM6/7) located in the intestine as well as in the distal convoluted tubule (Famularo et al., 2013). Accordingly, recent data suggest that carriers of TRPM6 polymorphisms are at increased risk (Hess et al., 2017).

To date only three reports of patients who developed TdP while they were taking a PPI (i.e., omeprazole, pantoprazole, or lansoprazole, respectively) (Asajima et al., 2012; Bibawy et al., 2013; Hansen and Bruserud, 2016) have been described in the literature, in two cases associated with hypomagnesemia (Bibawy et al., 2013; Hansen and Bruserud, 2016). The results of the present study suggest that the phenomenon is significantly more common than reported, being probably underestimated because in the clinical practice PPIs do not currently receive the due attention as a factor potentially contributing to QTc prolongation and TdP. Consistently with literature data (Famularo et al., 2013), PPI-associated hypomagnesemia seems to be a class effect which requires extended drug administration to occur. In fact, although in our TdP patients most subjects used pantoprazole, hypomagnesemia was found to be associated with all 4 PPIs included in the AZCERT list (AZCERT, 2016) (i.e., pantoprazole, omeprazole, esomeprazole, lansoprazole),

TABLE 3 | Demographic, clinical and laboratory characteristics in proton pump inhibitor users (PPI+) vs. non-proton pump inhibitor users (PPI−).

	PPI+	PPI−	p
Patients, n	28	20	
Age, median years (interquartile range)	80.5(73–85)	81.5(75–87.5)	0.40
Females, n	18/28(64%)	15/20(75%)	0.53
Mean QTc, ms	591.9 ± 88.8	601.5 ± 70.1	0.69
FV/CA/EcS	15/28(54%)	10/20(50%)	1
Electrolyte imbalances, n	22/28(79%)	15/19(79%)	1
Hypokaliemia	17/27(63%)	11/18(61%)	1
Hypocalcemia	12/20(60%)	10/17(59%)	1
Hypomagnesemia	6/14(43%)	1/13(8%)	0.07
Potassium, mEq/L (r.v.3.5–5.5)	3.25 ± 0.61	3.41 ± 0.74	0.47
Calcium, mg/dl (r.v.8.0–11.0)	7.71 ± 0.67	7.85 ± 0.65	0.44
Magnesium, mg/dl (r.v.1.5–2.5)	1.60 ± 0.21	1.84 ± 0.33	**0.03**
Sodium, mEq/L (r.v.132–148)	139.1 ± 10.0	136.1 ± 2.9	0.23
Diuretics use, n	19/28(68%)	10/20(50%)	0.24
Furosemide median daily dose, mg (range)	25(10–100)	72.5(20–500)	0.58
Glucose, mg/dl	171.2 ± 78.8	172.8 ± 80.4	0.96
pH	7.46 ± 0.11	7.50 ± 0.12	0.53
Bicarbonates, mmol/L	25.4 ± 1.8	25.3 ± 2.2	0.97
Concomitant diseases*, n	26/28(93%)	19/20(95%)	1
Cardiac diseases	23/28(82%)	17/20(85%)	1
Extra-cardiac diseases	14/28(50%)	6/20(30%)	0.23
QTc prolonging-medications, n	21/28(75%)	13/20(65%)	0.52
Amiodarone	8/28(29%)	6/20(30%)	1
Mean medication number per patient	1.3 ± 1.1	1.0 ± 0.9	0.17
Anti-Ro/SSA positivity, n	8/18(44%)	10/14(71%)	0.16
Systemic inflammation, n	23/28(82%)	13/20(80%)	1
Mean QTc-prolonging risk factor number per patient			
Per patient†	5.8 ± 1.6	4.9 ± 1.	**0.04**
Mean QTc-prolonging risk factor number			
Per patient† excluding hypomagnesemia	5.6 ± 1.5	4.9 ± 1.4	0.07

Wherever not specified, data are expressed as mean±standard deviation. Appropriate serum potassium, calcium or magnesium measurements available in 45, 37, and 27 out of 48 patients, respectively; anti-Ro/SSA antibodies tested in 32 out of 48 patients.
VF, ventricular fibrillation; CA, cardiac arrest; EcS, electric shock.
**Diseases recognized to be a risk factor for QTc prolongation (Viskin, 1999; El-Sherif and Turitto, 2003; Drew et al., 2010).*
†Including electrolyte imbalances, diseases, QTc-prolonging medications, anti-Ro/SSA positivity, and systemic inflammation (Viskin, 1999; El-Sherif and Turitto, 2003; Drew et al., 2010; Yue et al., 2015; Lazzerini et al., 2016, 2017b).
Differences were evaluated by the two-tailed unpaired t-test, or the two-tailed Mann-Whitney test. Difference in categorical variables were evaluated by the two-sided Fisher's exact test.
Statistically significant p values are reported in bold.

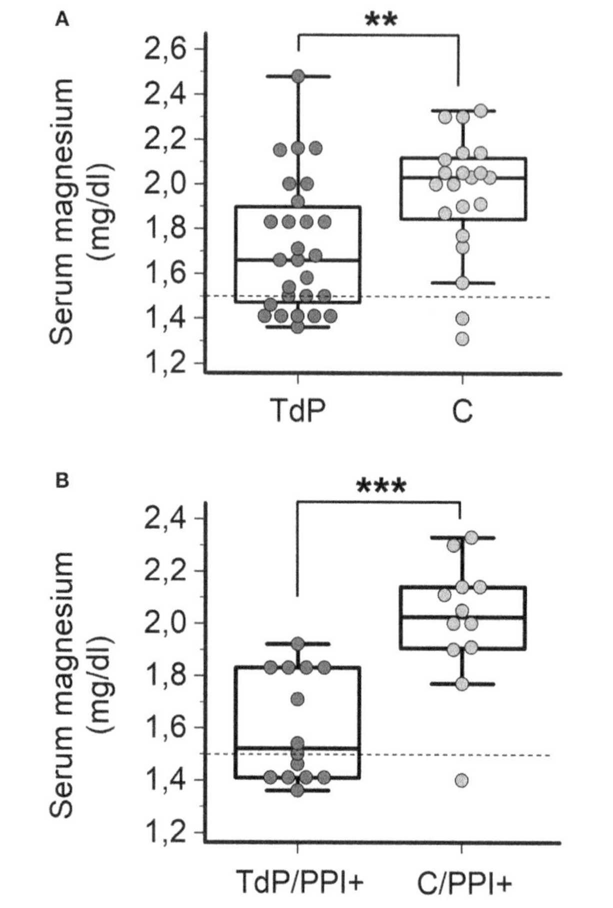

FIGURE 4 | Comparison of serum magnesium levels in TdP patients and controls. **(A)** Serum magnesium levels in all TdP patients ($n = 27$) vs. controls (C, $n = 21$), regardless of PPI therapy. Two-tail Mann-Whitney test, $^{**}p < 0.01$. **(B)** Serum magnesium levels in TdP patients under PPI therapy (TdP/PPI+) ($n = 14$) vs. controls under PPI therapy (C/PPI+, $n = 12$). Two-tail Student's unpaired t-test, $^{***}p < 0.001$. Horizontal dotted line indicates the lower limit of reference values for magnesium levels, i.e., 1.5 mg/dl.

in all cases administered for an extended period of time (>2 weeks). Our data seem also to confirm that the risk of PPI-induced hypomagnesemia further increases when PPIs are co-administered with diuretics, probably as a result of an enhancement of the renal loss of magnesium. Conversely, although in PPI users hypomagnesemia has been reported to be often accompanied by hypocalcemia and hypokalaemia (Famularo et al., 2013), the prevalence of these electrolyte imbalances as well as serum calcium, potassium and sodium levels were similar in PPI+ vs. PPI− TdP patients, thus indicating a rather selective effect of this class of drugs on magnesium levels.

Another important suggestion arising from the present study is that PPI-associated changes in magnesium levels have a relevant clinical impact by increasing the risk of developing TdP in these patients. In fact, PPI users showed a significantly higher mean total number of QTc-prolonging risk factors per patient when compared to non-users. Nevertheless, despite a comprehensive evaluation also taking into account recently recognized "non-classical" QT-prolonging factors, such as anti-Ro/SSA antibodies (Yue et al., 2015; Lazzerini et al., 2016, 2017d) and systemic inflammatory activation (Lazzerini et al., 2015, 2017a,b), serum magnesium levels represented the only specific TdP risk factor which was significantly different between the two groups. Accordingly, when hypomagnesemia was excluded from the total risk factor count, this difference was no longer statistically significant.

Notably, we also found that magnesium levels in TdP/PPI+ patients were significantly lower when compared to C/PPI+

matched for age, gender and concomitant diseases. It suggests that TdP may act as a "clustering factor" for those patients, among the general population, who are more susceptible to the magnesium-lowering effect of PPIs, possibly as a result of a genetic predisposition (Hess et al., 2017). This view, further supporting the role of PPI-induced hypomagnesemia as a risk factor for TdP, warrants specific investigation.

Although our data point to the conclusion that PPIs can increase the risk of TdP by inducing hypomagnesemia, the involvement of additional, possibly molecule-related mechanisms could not be ruled out. In particular, this may be the case of lansoprazole which has been recently associated to an increased risk of QTc prolongation and TdP when used in combination with ceftriaxone, via direct blocking effects of the drug association on the hERG potassium channel (Lorberbaum et al., 2016; Lazzerini et al., 2017c). Indeed, 2 patients in our cohort were under current treatment with lansoprazole + ceftriaxone when TdP occurred, in 1 case in the absence of hypomagnesemia. Notably, it has been demonstrated that also lansoprazole alone significantly inhibits hERG potassium channel and related current IKr (−14%), although to a lesser extent when compared to the drug combination (−58%) (Lorberbaum et al., 2016). This may help explain why serum magnesium level was normal in one out of three case reports of PPI-associated TdP, in which lansoprazole administration precipitated arrhythmia development in a patients under long-term treatment with a drug known to directly prolong QTc (disopyramide) (Asajima et al., 2012). Thus, it cannot be ruled out that also in our patients, particularly those without hypomagnesemia, lansoprazole (and possibly also the other PPIs involved, since to date no specific patch-clamp studies are available) could have contributed to promote TdP occurrence also via a direct electrophysiological interference.

Our data suggest a number of important recommendations to translate in the clinical practice. In particular, patients may experience TdP in the presence of hypomagnesemia while they were under active treatment with a PPI. Such patients may be required to stop PPI treatment as it could have significantly contributed to development and maintenance of the electrolyte imbalance. Since it is expected that PPI-induced hypomagnesemia is refractory to magnesium oral or parenteral supplementation despite high doses (Famularo et al., 2013), drug discontinuation is a key action to normalize serum magnesium levels and thereby reduce the associated risk of TdP recurrence. This measure may be of particular importance in patients concomitantly requiring diuretic therapy, given the role of this class of drugs in exacerbating magnesium depletion. Moreover, based on the evidence that PPI-induced hypomagnesemia may rapidly recur after re-challenge with the same or a different PPI (median time ~2 weeks; Famularo et al., 2013), the alternative use of a H_2-blocker may be appropriate in the case the patient needs prolonged antiacid treatment. Finally, since some data suggest that PPIs may also directly contribute to QTc prolongation via electrophysiological effects on the cardiomyocyte, it cannot be excluded that PPI discontinuation could be a useful therapeutic measure even in TdP patients without evidence of hypomagnesemia, particularly when the PPI involved is lansporazole and other known QT-prolonging drugs are concomitantly administered.

In conclusion, the present study demonstrates that PPI-induced hypomagnesemia is a more than expected common finding in unselected patients with TdP, significantly contributing to increase the cumulative risk of developing this life-threatening arrhythmia. Our real-life data provide important clinical evidence in support to AZCERT recommendations which cautiously already had warned about the potential role of PPI-induced hypomagnesemia in promoting TdP, despite only few cases were reported. Nevertheless, considering the relative small sample size as well as the main focus on magnesium levels, we did not perform any multivariate analysis on our population. Since this may represent a limitation of the study, larger sample studies are warranted to confirm our results. They should include non-TdP patients and/or younger populations, and could clarify whether PPIs significantly influence the QTc also regardless of hypomagnesemia.

In practice, more awareness is needed by the clinician when a PPI is prescribed since the safety profile of this class of drugs is probably not so neutral as commonly believed, specifically as regards the risk of life-threatening arrhythmias and SCD.

AUTHOR CONTRIBUTIONS

PL: Conception and design of the work; PL, IB, FF, MA, MN, FV, BG, MC, and IL: Substantial contributions to the acquisition of data for the work; PL, RF, AG, MR, GC, FL-P, and PC: Substantial contributions to the analysis of data for the work; PL, RF, AG, MR, GC, FL-P, and PC: Substantial contributions to the interpretation of data for the work; PL and PC: Drafting the work; PL, RF, AG, MR, FL-P, and PC: Revising the draft of the work critically for important intellectual content; PL, IB, FF, MA, MN, FV, RF, AG, MR, BG, MC, IL, GC, FL-P, and PC: Final approval of the version to be published; PL, IB, FF, MA, MN, FV, RF, AG, MR, BG, MC, IL, GC, FL-P, and PC: Agreement to be accountable for all aspects of the work in ensuring that questions related to the accuracy or integrity of any part of the work are appropriately investigated and resolved.

ACKNOWLEDGMENTS

This work has received funding from FAS-Salute ToRSADE project (FAS Salute 2014, Regione Toscana).

REFERENCES

(2011). In brief: PPI's and hypomagnesemia. *Med. Lett. Drugs Ther.* 53:25.

(2016). In brief: PPIs and Torsades de Pointes. *Med. Lett. Drugs Ther.* 58:153.

Asajima, H., Saito, N., Ohmura, Y., and Ohmura, K. (2012). Lansoprazole precipitated QT prolongation and torsade de pointes associated with disopyramide. *Eur. J. Clin. Pharmacol.* 68:331. doi: 10.1007/s00228-011-1119-z

AZCERT (2016). *New Drugs Added to CredibleMeds Drugs Lists.* Available online at: www.crediblemeds.org/blog/news-drugs-added-qtdrugs-lists (Accessed May 26, 2017).

Bibawy, J. N., Parikh, V., Wahba, J., Barsoum, E. A., Lafferty, J., Kowalski, M., et al. (2013). Pantoprazole (proton pump inhibitor) contributing to torsades de pointes storm. *Circ. Arrhythm. Electrophysiol.* 6:e17. doi: 10.1161/CIRCEP.112.000101

Cheungpasitporn, W., Thongprayoon, C., Kittanamongkolchai, W., Srivali, N., Edmonds, P. J., Ungprasert, P., et al. (2015). Proton pump inhibitors linked to hypomagnesemia: a systematic review and meta-analysis of observational studies. *Ren. Fail.* 37, 1237–1241. doi: 10.3109/0886022X.2015.1057800

Drew, B. J., Ackerman, M. J., Funk, M., Gibler, W. B., Kligfield, P., Menon, V., et al. (2010). Prevention of torsade de pointes in hospital settings: a scientific statement from the American Heart Association and the American College of Cardiology Foundation. *Circulation* 121, 1047–1060. doi: 10.1161/CIRCULATIONAHA.109.192704

El-Sherif, N., and Turitto, G. (2003). Torsade de pointes. *Curr. Opin. Cardiol.* 18, 6–13. doi: 10.1097/00001573-200301000-00002

El-Sherif, N., and Turitto, G. (2011). Electrolyte disorders and arrhythmogenesis. *Cardiol. J.* 18, 233–245.

Famularo, G., Gasbarrone, L., and Minisola, G. (2013). Hypomagnesemia and proton-pump inhibitors. *Expert Opin. Drug Saf.* 12, 709–716. doi: 10.1517/14740338.2013.809062

Gupta, A., Lawrence, A. T., Krishnan, K., Kavinsky, C. J., and Trohman, R. G. (2007). Current concepts in the mechanisms and management of drug-induced QT prolongation and torsade de pointes. *Am. Heart J.* 153, 891–899. doi: 10.1016/j.ahj.2007.01.040

Hansen, B. A., and Bruserud, Ø. (2016). Hypomagnesemia as a potentially life-threatening adverse effect of omeprazole. *Oxf. Med. Case Rep.* 2016:147. doi: 10.1093/omcr/omw062

Hess, M. W., de Baaij, J. H., Broekman, M. M., Bisseling, T. M., Haarhuis, B. J., Tan, A. C., et al. (2017). Common single nucleotide polymorphisms in transient receptor potential melastatin type 6 increase the risk for proton pump inhibitor-induced hypomagnesemia: a case-control study. *Pharmacogenet. Genomics* 27, 83–88. doi: 10.1097/FPC.0000000000000259

Itoh, H., Crotti, L., Aiba, T., Spazzolini, C., Denjoy, I., Fressart, V., et al. (2016). The genetics underlying acquired long QT syndrome: impact for genetic screening. *Eur. Heart J.* 37, 1456–1464. doi: 10.1093/eurheartj/ehv695

Kelepouris, E., Kasama, R., and Agus, Z. S. (1993). Effects of intracellular magnesium on calcium, potassium and chloride channels. *Miner. Electrolyte Metab.* 19, 277–281.

Lazzerini, P. E., Bertolozzi, I., Rossi, M., Capecchi, P. L., and Laghi-Pasini, F. (2017c). Combination therapy with ceftriaxone and lansoprazole, acquired long qt syndrome, and torsades de pointes risk. *J. Am. Coll. Cardiol.* 69:1876–1877. doi: 10.1016/j.jacc.2016.11.090

Lazzerini, P. E., Capecchi, P. L., and Laghi-Pasini, F. (2015). Long QT syndrome: an emerging role for inflammation and immunity. *Front. Cardiovasc. Med.* 2:26.doi: 10.3389/fcvm.2015.00026

Lazzerini, P. E., Capecchi, P. L., and Laghi-Pasini, F. (2017b). Systemic inflammation and arrhythmic risk: lessons from rheumatoid arthritis. *Eur. Heart J.* 38, 1717–1727. doi: 10.1093/eurheartj/ehw208

Lazzerini, P. E., Capecchi, P. L., Laghi-Pasini, F., and Boutjdir, M. (2017d). Autoimmune channelopathies as a novel mechanism in cardiac arrhythmias. *Nat. Rev. Cardiol.* 14, 521–535. doi: 10.1038/nrcardio.2017.61

Lazzerini, P. E., Laghi-Pasini, F., Bertolozzi, I., Morozzi, G., Lorenzini, S., Simpatico, A., et al. (2017a). Systemic inflammation as a novel QT-prolonging risk factor in patients with torsades de pointes. *Heart* 103, 1821–1829. doi: 10.1136/heartjnl-2016-311079

Lazzerini, P. E., Yue, Y., Srivastava, U., Fabris, F., Capecchi, P. L., Bertolozzi, I., et al. (2016). Arrhythmogenicity of anti-Ro/SSA antibodies in patients with torsades de pointes. *Circ. Arrhythm. Electrophysiol.* 9:e003419. doi: 10.1161/CIRCEP.115.003419

Lorberbaum, T., Sampson, K. J., Chang, J. B., Iyer, V., Woosley, R. L., Kass, R. S., et al. (2016). Coupling data mining and laboratory experiments to discover drug interactions causing QT prolongation. *J. Am. Coll. Cardiol.* 68, 1756–1764. doi: 10.1016/j.jacc.2016.07.761

Luk, C. P., Parsons, R., Lee, Y. P., and Hughes, J. D. (2013). Proton pump inhibitor-associated hypomagnesemia: what do FDA data tell us? *Ann. Pharmacother.* 47, 773–780. doi: 10.1345/aph.1R556

Moayyedi, P., and Leontiadis, G. I. (2012). The risks of PPI therapy. *Nat. Rev. Gastroenterol. Hepatol.* 9, 132–139. doi: 10.1038/nrgastro.2011.272

Park, C. H., Kim, E. H., Roh, Y. H., Kim, H. Y., and Lee, S. K. (2014). The association between the use of proton pump inhibitors and the risk of hypomagnesemia: a systematic review and meta-analysis. *PLoS ONE* 9:e112558. doi: 10.1371/journal.pone.0112558

Patterson Burdsall, D., Flores, H. C., Krueger, J., Garretson, S., Gorbien, M. J., Iacch, A., et al. (2013). Use of proton pump inhibitors with lack of diagnostic indications in 22 Midwestern US skilled nursing facilities. *J. Am. Med. Dir. Assoc.* 14, 429–432. doi: 10.1016/j.jamda.2013.01.021

Rautaharju, P. M., Surawicz, B., Gettes, L. S., Bailey, J. J., Childers, R., Deal, B. J., et al. (2009). AHA/ACCF/HRS recommendations for the standardization and interpretation of the electrocardiogram: part IV: the ST segment, T and U waves, and the QT interval: a scientific statement from the American Heart Association Electrocardiography and Arrhythmias Committee, Council on Clinical Cardiology; the American College of Cardiology Foundation; and the Heart Rhythm Society. Endorsed by the International Society for Computerized Electrocardiology. *J. Am. Coll. Cardiol.* 53, 982–991. doi: 10.1016/j.jacc.2008.12.014

Strand, D. S., Kim, D., and Peura, D. A. (2017). 25 Years of proton pump inhibitors: a comprehensive review. *Gut Liver* 11, 27–37. doi: 10.5009/gnl15502

Viskin, S. (1999). Long QT syndromes and torsade de pointes. *Lancet* 354, 1625–1633. doi: 10.1016/S0140-6736(99)02107-8

Xie, Y., Bowe, B., Li, T., Xian, H., Yan, Y., and Al-Aly, Z. (2017).Risk of death among users of Proton Pump Inhibitors: a longitudinal observational cohort study of United States veterans. *BMJ Open* 7:e015735. doi: 10.1136/bmjopen-2016-015735

Yue, Y., Castrichini, M., Srivastava, U., Fabris, F., Shah, K., Li, Z., et al. (2015). Pathogenesis of the novel autoimmune-associated long QT syndrome. *Circulation* 132, 230–240. doi: 10.1161/CIRCULATIONAHA.115.009800

Zhao, M., Feng, R., Shao, D., Liu, S., Lei, M., Wang, H., et al. (2015). $Mg^{(2+)}$-dependent facilitation and inactivation of L-type $Ca^{(2+)}$ channels in guinea pig ventricular myocytes. *J. Pharmacol. Sci.* 129, 143–149. doi: 10.1016/j.jphs.2015.08.001

7

Digging into Lipid Membrane Permeation for Cardiac Ion Channel Blocker d-Sotalol with All-Atom Simulations

*Kevin R. DeMarco[1,2,3], Slava Bekker[1,4], Colleen E. Clancy[1,2], Sergei Y. Noskov[5] and Igor Vorobyov[1,2]**

[1] Department of Physiology and Membrane Biology, University of California, Davis, Davis, CA, United States, [2] Department of Pharmacology, University of California, Davis, Davis, CA, United States, [3] Biophysics Graduate Group, University of California, Davis, Davis, CA, United States, [4] Hartnell College, Salinas, CA, United States, [5] Centre for Molecular Simulations, Department of Biological Sciences, Faculty of Science, University of Calgary, Calgary, AB, Canada

***Correspondence:**
Igor Vorobyov
ivorobyov@ucdavis.edu

Interactions of drug molecules with lipid membranes play crucial role in their accessibility of cellular targets and can be an important predictor of their therapeutic and safety profiles. Very little is known about spatial localization of various drugs in the lipid bilayers, their active form (ionization state) or translocation rates and therefore potency to bind to different sites in membrane proteins. All-atom molecular simulations may help to map drug partitioning kinetics and thermodynamics, thus providing in-depth assessment of drug lipophilicity. As a proof of principle, we evaluated extensively lipid membrane partitioning of d-sotalol, well-known blocker of a cardiac potassium channel $K_V11.1$ encoded by the hERG gene, with reported substantial proclivity for arrhythmogenesis. We developed the positively charged (cationic) and neutral d-sotalol models, compatible with the biomolecular CHARMM force field, and subjected them to all-atom molecular dynamics (MD) simulations of drug partitioning through hydrated lipid membranes, aiming to elucidate thermodynamics and kinetics of their translocation and thus putative propensities for hydrophobic and aqueous hERG access. We found that only a neutral form of d-sotalol accumulates in the membrane interior and can move across the bilayer within millisecond time scale, and can be relevant to a lipophilic channel access. The computed water-membrane partitioning coefficient for this form is in good agreement with experiment. There is a large energetic barrier for a cationic form of the drug, dominant in water, to cross the membrane, resulting in slow membrane translocation kinetics. However, this form of the drug can be important for an aqueous access pathway through the intracellular gate of hERG. This route will likely occur after a neutral form of a drug crosses the membrane and subsequently re-protonates. Our study serves to demonstrate a first step toward a framework for multi-scale *in silico* safety pharmacology, and identifies some of the challenges that lie therein.

Keywords: hERG, long QT syndrome, cardiotoxicity, CHARMM force field, molecular dynamics, umbrella sampling, lipophilicity, water-membrane partitioning

INTRODUCTION

The continuing failure to accurately predict the risk of drug toxicity is the primary reason for drug candidates being abandoned or approved drugs being removed from the market (Chi, 2013), illustrating the critical need for a more rational approach to drug development. One example of such a need is the longstanding failure of drug-based treatment of cardiac arrhythmias. The SWORD clinical trial (Waldo et al., 1996) famously showed that the antiarrhythmic drug d-sotalol, which we focus on in this work, actually *increased* mortality and risk of sudden cardiac death in patients, leading to its removal from the marketplace. Similarly, the gastrokinetic agent cisapride has been removed from the market in many countries due to its arrhythmogenic potential (Quigley, 2011), and a number of such cases for drugs and drug candidates with diverse pharmacological action has been growing over the years. Each year, over 360,000 people die in the US die from cardiac arrhythmias that are often drug-induced, demonstrating that the pharmacological assessment of cardiotoxicity still remains significantly hindered (Benjamin et al., 2017). The proposed Comprehensive *in vitro* Proarrhythmia Assay (CiPA) initiative is intended to address this shortcoming by improving predictions of pro-arrhythmic drug proclivities through the combination of *in vitro* assays on several cardiac ion channels and multi-scale modeling and simulation (Colatsky et al., 2016; Fermini et al., 2016). Atomistic MD simulations have the potential to serve as part of such *in silico* screen (Clancy et al., 2016) for the development of cardiac-safe medicines, and can be used to identify molecular determinants of acquired arrhythmogenesis.

On the molecular level, drug-induced arrhythmogenesis is typically associated with the binding of drugs to cardiac ion channels, membrane proteins responsible for the propagation of electrical signal in cardiomyocytes. It is known that multiple environmental factors, including drug blockade, can modulate the gating and permeation of many ion channels. More specifically, experimental studies aimed at understanding ion channel blockade by drugs often focus on mapping binding sites at or around the intra-cellular cavity of the ion channel. This assumes, either explicitly or implicitly, that a drug (often weakly cationic) is able to diffuse from the intra-cellular space and physically occlude ion permeation. Such a mechanism is supported, for example, by the role of two intra-cavity residues (F656 and Y652) in the drug-induced current block of the voltage gated potassium channel $K_V11.1$ (also known as hERG), which is considered a major drug anti-target due to its promiscuous binding of many drug-like molecules (Vandenberg et al., 2012).

Many of the common ion channel blockers are weak bases with a pK_a of ~7.8–8.5. Thus, at a physiological pH of 7.4, up to ~7–28% of drug molecules remain uncharged, and therefore potentially capable of interacting with the channel by traversing a lipophilic pathway in the plasma membrane toward a binding site, either on the lipid-facing exterior of the channel or within the channel pore via passage through lipid-facing fenestrations. A possible lipophilic access route has been established for ivabradine blockade of hERG in a recent study that implicated a lipid-facing residue (M651) as critical for drug-induced blockade (Lees-Miller et al., 2015). This finding was further substantiated by the recent publication of Cryo-EM structures of hERG (putatively open), and related EAG (putatively closed) channels, suggesting that F656 and M651 can be exposed to lipids in either channel state (Whicher and MacKinnon, 2016; Wang and MacKinnon, 2017). Furthermore, hERG block by the endogenous components of cardiac membranes has also been well-established, with various lipophilic molecules including hormones (Yang et al., 2017), ceramides (Ganapathi et al., 2010; Sordillo et al., 2015), sphingosine-1-phosphate (Sordillo et al., 2015), and polyunsaturated fatty acids (Guizy et al., 2005; Moreno et al., 2012) blocking hERG but without obvious intra-cellular access to the intra-cavity site. Therefore, mapping the lipophilic pathways for common ion channel blockers and understanding the chemistry of drug-lipid interactions remains an unmet pharmacological challenge.

The complexity in understanding the lipophilic access pathways of many blockers arises from their chemical structure. Most drug molecules can coexist in multiple ionization states with different membrane permeabilities or localization on the bilayer surface and consequent access to binding sites in hERG. Hence, significant challenges exist in developing a framework for atomic-scale *in silico* screening and predictive pharmacology. One example is *the lack of robust topologies and parameters defined for most drugs in popular MD force fields*, necessitating their *de novo* development. This task requires computationally expensive calculations of quantum mechanical (QM) optimized molecular geometries and atomic charge distributions, and the time-consuming process of fitting molecular mechanical (MM) parameters to the optimal computed QM data. Here we have developed CHARMM generalized force field (CGENFF) (Vanommeslaeghe et al., 2010) parameters for the hERG blocker d-sotalol, which has high cardiotoxic risk (Colatsky et al., 2016) for the ventricular tachycardia characterized by Torsades de Pointes (TdP) arrhythmias (Waldo et al., 1996; Yap and Camm, 2003). Preliminary parameters for the intermediate-TdP risk compound cisapride (Colatsky et al., 2016), and low-risk compound moxifloxacin (Haverkamp et al., 2012) were developed for the purpose of comparing their membrane affinities, and will be briefly discussed as well.

Computing the free energy cost required for drugs to partition from bulk solution across the cell membrane represents a critical test for drug model viability used in MD simulations. This is because the membrane permeability of a drug not only determines its bioavailability, but is also linked to its medically

Abbreviations: aLQTS, acquired Long QT syndrome; CGENFF, CHARMM generalized force field; CHARMM, Chemistry at Harvard Molecular Mechanics; CiPA, comprehensive *in vitro* pro-arrhythmic assay; CisC, cationic cisapride; COM, center of mass; Cryo-EM, cryo-electron microscopy; DMPC, dimyristoylphosphatidylcholine; ECG, electro-cardiogram; GPU, Graphics Processing Unit; hERG, human *Ether-à-go-go*-Related Gene; K_v, voltage gated potassium channel; LQTS, Long QT syndrome; MD, molecular dynamics; MM, molecular mechanics; MoxZ, zwitterionic moxifloxacin; PBC, periodic boundary conditions; PMF, potential of mean force; POPC, 1-palmitoyl-2-oleoyl-phosphatidylcholine; POPS, 1-palmitoyl-2-oleoyl-phosphatidylserine; QM, quantum mechanics; SotA, anionic d-sotalol; SotC, cationic d-sotalol; SotN, neutral d-sotalol; SotZ, zwitterionic d-sotalol; US, umbrella sampling; VSD, voltage sensing domain; WHAM, weighted histogram analysis method.

relevant concentration, and pathway to its target. Many drugs are delivered to their targets via a lipophilic pathway, and drug permeation across lipid membranes is crucial for their absorption by tissue, metabolism, extraction from the body, and toxicity (ADME-Tox) (Yu and Adedoyin, 2003). This is especially relevant for predicting propensity for off-target effects of a drug, which is necessarily linked to its tissue permeability. Empirically derived ADME-Tox drug profiles, however, are inherently limited, lacking transferability to different drug classes, and providing no information regarding the structural determinants of membrane-drug distribution or kinetics (Swift and Amaro, 2013). Obtaining these measurements through MD simulation represents a final major challenge: namely, *obtaining sufficient sampling of the configurational space in a modeled system to calculate accurate thermodynamic quantities of interest.* Ideally, unbiased all-atom MD simulations of drug permeation across large, explicit lipid membranes would provide the most accurate kinetic and thermodynamic profiles for membrane-drug interactions (Swift and Amaro, 2013), however the sampling (or simulation time) mandated by such an exhaustive approach makes it computationally prohibitive. Fortunately, more computationally tractable techniques for enhanced sampling exist that allow for the robust calculation of membrane distribution coefficients and permeability measurements of an isolated drug across a small membrane patch. We have employed one such technique, umbrella sampling (US) (Torrie and Valleau, 1977), in this report in order to compute the free energies and diffusion coefficients required for drugs to pass through the cell membrane. Similar approaches have been used for various drug molecules in a number of other studies (Carpenter et al., 2014; Di Meo et al., 2016; Bennion et al., 2017), including previous works by our groups (Boiteux et al., 2014; Yang et al., 2016). The approaches and data presented here serve as preliminary steps in overcoming the many challenges that arise in the messy task of atomistic *in silico* predictive cardiovascular pharmacology.

MATERIALS AND METHODS

Drug Force Field Parameterization

We obtained starting molecular structures from either PubChem (Kim et al., 2016) (CID 5253 for d-sotalol) or the ZINC (Irwin and Shoichet, 2005) (3775140 for cisapride, 3826253 for moxifloxacin) databases, and used them to generate initial guesses for partial atomic charges and other force field parameters (i.e., bond lengths, bond angles, dihedral angles) using CGENFF program, version 1.0 (Vanommeslaeghe and MacKerell, 2012; Vanommeslaeghe et al., 2012).

Initial topology and parameters for SotC and SotN, were subsequently validated and optimized using QM target data following the suggested CGENFF force field methodology (Vanommeslaeghe et al., 2010). High-quality parameters not already present in CGENFF are assigned from existing parameters based on chemical analogy, with poor chemical analogy corresponding to a high penalty score for use in MD simulation (Vanommeslaeghe et al., 2012). Our optimizations focused on such high-penalty, poorly analogous parameters generated by the CGENFF program. Quantum mechanical (QM) target data for parameter optimization were obtained utilizing Møller–Plesset (MP2) and Hartree-Fock (HF) electronic structure methods and the 6–31(d) basis set using the Gaussian 09 program (Frisch et al., 2009).

MP2/6-31G(d) molecular dipole magnitude and orientation as well as scaled HF/6-31G(d) interaction energies with water were used for partial atomic charge optimization for compatibility with the CHARMM atomistic biomolecular force fields (MacKerell, 2004). The gas-phase MP2/6-31G(d) dipole, along with HF/6-31G(d) interaction energies, should be overestimated by CHARMM (by ~16% for the latter) in order to account for polarization in aqueous media (MacKerell, 2004; Vanommeslaeghe et al., 2010). Internal bond and angle parameters were validated or modified based on comparison of MP2/6-31G(d) and CHARMM optimized geometries and scaled vibrational frequencies. For bond lengths and angles, respective differences within 0.01 Å and 1° between QM and CHARMM values were sought. Dihedral angle parameters were optimized to reproduce MP2/6-31G(d) potential energy scans for rotation around a particular bond. We used the Force Field Toolkit plugin (fftk) (Mayne et al., 2013) for the Visual Molecular Dynamics program (VMD) (Humphrey et al., 1996) in order to generate files for QM reference calculations and to perform parameter optimizations. We were able to achieve substantial improvement over the initial CGENFF generated parameters (highlighted in **Figure 3C** for a selected dihedral angle energy profile), with markedly better agreement between CHARMM and QM geometries, vibrational frequencies, and interactions with water. Final topology and parameters for SotC and SotN are provided in the Supplementary Information. Optimized parameters for charged cisapride and zwitterionic moxifloxacin, obtained using the same methodology, will be subsequently published after additional validation and any necessary improvement.

Drug Membrane Partitioning: Molecular Systems

Partitioning of charged (SotC) and neutral d-sotalol (SotN), charged cisapride (CisC), and a zwitterionic form of moxifloxacin (MoxZ) were assessed using CHARMM (Brooks et al., 1983, 2009) and NAMD (Phillips et al., 2005) programs. CHARMM-GUI tool (Jo et al., 2008) was used in order to build the simulation systems, which consisted of 128 1-palmitoyl-2-oleoylphosphatidylcholine (POPC) lipids, ~7,000 water molecules, 21 or 22 K^+ and 22 Cl^- ions to ensure 0.15 M electrolyte concentration and overall electrical neutrality, and one drug molecule, totaling ~38,250 atoms.

A separate set of simulations that investigated membrane composition was equilibrated with NAMD and run on Anton 2 supercomputer (Shaw et al., 2014). In these simulations lipid membranes were composed of either pure POPC or a mixture of 85% POPC and 15% of 1-palmitoyl-2-oleoylphosphatidylserine (POPS) lipids. These systems were larger and contained ~103,000 atoms with 256 lipids, 15 SotC or 16 SotN molecules, ~22,800 water molecules, 50–88 K^+ and 50–65 Cl^- ions.

CHARMM biomolecular, and compatible CGENFF forcefields were used throughout all simulations. In particular, C36 lipid

(Klauda et al., 2010) and standard CHARMM ion parameters (Beglov and Roux, 1994), newly developed CGENFF drug parameters (see above) along with the TIP3P water model (Jorgensen et al., 1983) were utilized.

Drug Membrane Partitioning: Molecular Dynamics Simulations

CHARMM simulations of SotC, SotN, CisC, and MoxZ, and NAMD simulations of SotC and SotN in a hydrated 128 lipid POPC membrane were carried out in *NPT* ensemble with 1 atm of pressure maintained by Langevin piston barostat (Feller et al., 1995) and 310 K temperature controlled by Nosé-Hoover thermostat (Nosé, 1984; Hoover, 1985). Tetragonal cells with periodic boundary conditions (PBC) were used in all the simulations, with $P2_1$ space group (Dolan et al., 2002) utilized in CHARMM runs. SHAKE algorithm (Ryckaert et al., 1977) was employed to fix the bonds to all hydrogen atoms, allowing a time step of 2 fs for all our simulations. Electrostatic interactions were computed via Particle Mesh Ewald (Darden et al., 1993), with a mesh grid of 1 Å.

For partitioning calculations of each drug we used the US method (Torrie and Valleau, 1977) with 81 independent simulation windows, placing the center of mass (COM) of the drug in 1 Å intervals from −40 Å to 40 Å with respect to COM of the membrane. The COM of the drug was restrained along the z axis with a force constant of 2.5 kcal/mol/Å^2 to provide sufficient sampling with an additional 5 kcal/mol/Å^2 cylindrical constraint applied to prevent the drift of the molecule in the xy plane (Li et al., 2008). Free energy or potential of mean force (PMF) profiles was computed using weighted histogram analysis method (WHAM) (Kumar et al., 1992).

SotC and SotN simulations ran for 15 ns with NAMD and 10 ns with CHARMM per window. To improve sampling, for NAMD runs we used additional US windows from −20 Å to 20 Å, whereas 7 central windows (i.e., for $|z| \leq 3$ Å) were used for CHARMM SotC simulations, all running for the same simulation time as the original runs (see Supplementary text). Based on solvation analysis of SotC and SotN (Figure S5), we discarded the first 4 ns to account for equilibration. For consistency, similar procedure was followed for CHARMM simulations of CisC and MoxZ, both of which ran 10 ns/window plus additional 10 ns for the 5 central windows ($|z| \leq 2$ Å) of CisC.

Unbiased MD simulations were run for larger membrane systems with several SotC or SotN molecules. First, systems were equilibrated for 50 ns using NAMD and the simulation parameters mentioned above. Then, production simulations were run for 500 or 1000 ns (for SotN system with POPC/POPS mixed membrane) using Anton 2 software (Shaw et al., 2014) version 1.31.0. These simulations were carried out using tetragonal PBC in the *NPT* ensemble at 310 K, a 2 fs time step with non-bonded long range interactions computed every 6 fs using the RESPA multiple time step algorithm (Tuckerman et al., 1992). The multi-integrator (multigrator) algorithm (Lippert et al., 2013) was used for temperature and semi-isotropic pressure coupling, whereas a novel u-series method (Shaw et al., 2014) was used for handling long-range electrostatic interactions. An electric field in the z direction was applied, gradually increasing from 0 to 160 mV during the first 100 ns of the simulation. A long-range Lennard-Jones (LJ) correction (beyond cutoff) was not used as was suggested for C36 lipid force field (Klauda et al., 2010).

Drug Membrane Partitioning: Simulation Analyses

Solvation numbers were computed as number of oxygen atoms of water, lipid phosphate or ester functional groups within 4.25 Å of drug non-hydrogen atoms, with this distance cutoff obtained from an analysis of corresponding radial distribution functions (see Figure S6). Drug orientation was computed based on a polar angle θ between z axis corresponding to a bilayer normal and drug N1···S vector, which is almost anti-parallel to its dipole orientation (see **Figure 3**). Average angles were computed as:

$$<\theta_{N1...S}>= \text{atan2}(<\sin\theta>,<\cos\theta>) \quad (1)$$

whereas corresponding order parameters were computed as (Vorobyov et al., 2012)

$$S_{N1...S} = ½(3 < \cos^2\theta > -1) \quad (2)$$

Drug water-membrane partition coefficients were calculated as (Vorobyov et al., 2012):

$$K(\text{wat} \rightarrow \text{mem}) = \frac{1}{z_2 - z_1}\int_{z_1}^{z_2} e^{-\frac{\{W(z)-W(z_1)\}}{k_BT}}dz \quad (3)$$

where $W(z)$ is the PMF, z_1 and z_2 are points in aqueous solution on opposite sides of the membrane, k_B is Boltzmann constant, and T is the absolute temperature. Partitioning free energies were calculated as

$$\Delta G(\text{wat} \rightarrow \text{mem}) = -k_BT\, ln\, K(\text{wat} \rightarrow \text{mem}) \quad (4)$$

Error bars were estimated from PMFs by propagation of uncertainties.

To estimate the 1D diffusion constant in the z direction, $D(z_i)$, we analyzed the corresponding US windows with Hummer's method (Hummer, 2005):

$$D(z_i) = \frac{\langle \delta z^2 \rangle_i}{\tau_i} \quad (5)$$

where $\langle \delta z^2 \rangle_i$ and τ_i are the mean square deviation from the average position and the position correlation time for US window i.

$$\tau_i = \lim_{s\rightarrow 0} \tau_i(s) = \lim_{s\rightarrow 0} \frac{\hat{C}_z(s; z_i)}{\langle \delta z^2 \rangle_i} = \lim_{s\rightarrow 0} \frac{\int_0^\infty e^{-st}\langle \delta z(t)\delta z(0) \rangle_i dt}{\langle \delta z^2 \rangle_i} \quad (6)$$

$\hat{C}_z(s; z_i)$ is the Laplace transform of the position autocorrelation function $C_z(t; z_i)$:

$$\hat{C}_z(s; z_i) = \int_0^\infty e^{-st} C_z(t; z_i)\, dt \quad (7)$$

where $C_z(t; z_i) = \langle \delta z(t)\delta z(0)\rangle_i$, s is the inverse time and $\delta z = z - \langle z\rangle_i$ is the drug COM position displacement.

Values of $\tau_i(s)$ were calculated at s-values 0.01, 0.02, ..., 0.1, 0.2, ..., 1.0, 2.0, ..., 10.0 ps^{-1}. $\tau_i(s)$ were extrapolated to $s = 0$ by fitting the function $a/(s+b)$, where a and b are parameters, in the s range from 0.02 to 1.00 ps^{-1}. See our previous study (Vorobyov et al., 2014) for more details.

Based on PMF and diffusion coefficient profiles we computed water-membrane drug permeability rate as,

$$P = \left(\int_{-L/2}^{L/2} \frac{\exp(W_z/k_B T)}{D(z)}\, dz \right)^{-1} \tag{8}$$

an integral over the local bilayer resistance (Marrink and Berendsen, 1994), spanning $-14 \le z \le 14$ Å for SotN and $-20 \le z \le 20$ Å for SotC (with PMF-values adjusted to be 0 at the borders), where the drug is expected to cross a central barrier; essential for modeling permeation via a single molecule PMF (Roux and Karplus, 1991). This description assumes we are in the diffusion limit, where the mean velocity is proportional to the mean force, which is valid if the drug displacement correlation length is short compared to the spatial variations in the force (Marrink and Berendsen, 1994).

RESULTS

Comparative Ionized Drug Membrane Partitioning

First, we studied membrane partitioning of SotC and compared it to the partitioning of CisC and MoxZ, each drug form representing the dominant protonation state in aqueous solution at the physiological pH. We studied their translocation across POPC membranes using US MD simulations, which allow for more efficient sampling of energetically unfavorable drug distributions across a lipid membrane compared to conventional unbiased MD simulations. US works by restraining drug positions at different values of z across the membrane using a harmonic potential. Thus, we can compute free energy for drug positions along the bilayer normal, with $z = 0$ corresponding to membrane center.

When all 3 drugs are located near $z = 0$ (see **Figure 1A**), we observed substantial membrane deformations, where they are coordinated by water molecules and lipid headgroups from one (for CisC) or both (for SotC and especially for MoxZ) membrane interfaces. Not surprisingly, such membrane deformations lead to substantial energetic penalties for ionized drugs to move across the membrane with the peak values at $z = 0$: around 18 kcal/mol for MoxZ, 10 kcal/mol for SotC and just 5 kcal/mol for CisC. Interestingly, such differences in peak free energy values correlate with computed MM drug dipole moments, which are 41.3 Debye for MoxZ, 15.5 Debye for SotC and 6.8 Debye for CisC for the same drug molecule "standard" positions and orientation (as defined by Gaussian software). For MoxZ, extensive membrane deformation exhibited by both leaflets are due to the positively charged ammonium and negatively charged carboxylate moieties at opposite ends of the molecule (**Figure 1C**). For SotC, a cationic secondary ammonium and polar sulfonamide groups can also attract water molecules or lipid headgroups. Both SotC and MoxZ can stretch along the membrane normal to interact with both bilayer interfaces. However, the situation is different for CisC, which also has several polar functional groups and a positively charged tertiary ammonium functionality at the center of the molecule, but it is floppier than those drugs and seems to be attracted to one membrane interface (see **Figure 1**). Also, CisC has a pronounced binding trough of around −3 kcal/mol at $14 \le |z| \le 17$ Å. This suggests, that unlike SotC and MoxZ it will accumulate at water—membrane interface. The presence of the binding trough will also inadvertently increase a barrier a drug will need to overcome to cross a membrane from ~5 to 8 kcal/mol (see **Figure 1B**). These calculations suggest fairly high but surprisingly different energetic costs to cross the membrane for this collection of ionized molecules.

Models of d-Sotalol

We performed a more detailed analysis of different protonation states of d-sotalol, focusing on the energetics of its membrane crossing. Like many other drugs in aqueous solution, d-sotalol can exist in several protonation states depending on solution pH and other factors, such as proximity to specific protein residues. Data from the literature indicate that aqueous pK_a-values for d-sotalol are 8.3 and 9.8 attributed to deprotonation of sulfonamide and secondary ammonium functionalities, respectively (Foster and Carr, 1992; Hancu et al., 2014). This indicates that at physiological pH 7.4, SotC is the predominant form (around 89%), while deprotonation of the sulfonamide functionality leads to a second dominant SotZ form (around 11%). At more basic pH, the secondary ammonium functionality will deprotonate as well, leading to a negatively charged, anionic form SotA (**Figure 2**).

However, there is yet another possibility, in which deprotonation of secondary ammonium group occurs first, leading to a neutral d-sotalol form (SotN). In fact, there is likely an equilibrium, and possibly interconversion, between SotN and SotZ forms, in which either one is favored depending on the polarity of the surrounding medium. We expect that a substantially less polar SotN form would be favored in the hydrophobic environment of the lipid membrane interior based on our MoxZ simulations discussed above, whereas a more polar SotZ might be favored in aqueous solution. Unfortunately, there are no experimental data to address this issue for d-sotalol. We performed a series of implicit solvent QM calculations, which seem to indicate slight preference for SotN even in bulk water (see Supplementary text for more information), but their accuracy is very uncertain. However, a recent experimental study using a combination of potentiometric titration and spectrophotometry measurements has suggested around 90% of zwitterionic and 10% of neutral form of moxifloxacin is present at physiological pH range, and that only a neutral form contributes to drug partitioning into a non-polar environment of lipid membranes or 1-octanol often used as a membrane mimetic (Langlois et al., 2005). This suggests that a neutral form of a drug is likely the one to undergo an unassisted membrane translocation.

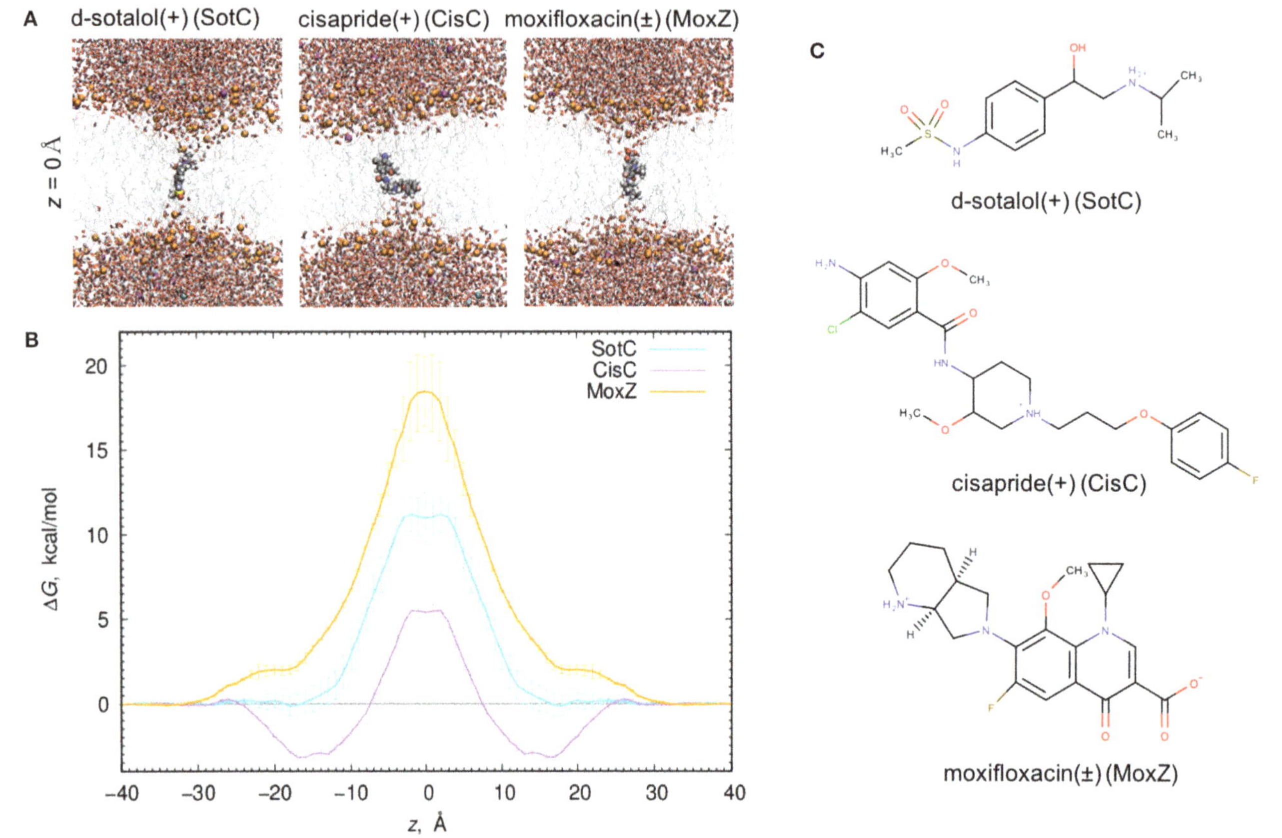

FIGURE 1 | Ionized drug translocation across a POPC membrane. **(A)** Representative snapshots from a central ($z = 0$) umbrella sampling windows for cationic d-sotalol (SotC), cationic cisapride (CisC), and zwitterionic moxifloxacin (MoxZ). Drug molecules along with lipid P atoms (orange), K^+ (purple) and Cl^- (cyan) ions are shown in a space-filling representation. Other elements are colored as follows: C—gray, H—white, O—red, N—blue, S—yellow. Water molecules are shown as tubes and lipid tails as wireframes. **(B)** PMF profiles for POPC membrane crossing for 3 drugs shown in **(A)**. Error bars represent measures of asymmetry. **(C)** Chemical structures of those drugs drawn using MarvinSketch program.

Since we are particularly interested in lipophilic access of cardiotoxic drugs known to block hERG, we have developed standard CHARMM (Klauda et al., 2010) compatible models of d-sotalol in charged (SotC) and neutral (SotN) forms. The QM and MM dipole moments for those d-sotalol forms and drug—water interactions probed for the model optimizations are shown in **Figures 3A,B** for SotN and SotC, respectively. Optimized CHARMM charges (Table S3) provide good agreement with QM target dipole values. The optimized MM dipole moments point in same direction (<1° difference in angle between QM and MM for both SotC and SotN) and are each within 20% difference in magnitude (SotN 6%, and SotC 14%). The water interaction distances were all within 0.4 Å of QM target values (see Tables S4, S5). The dipole moment is significantly higher for SotC (17.64 Debye), than for SotN (5.98 Debye), as is to be expected for charged vs. neutral species and in agreement with QM-values. Interaction energies with water were also in good agreement with QM-values with root mean square (RMS) and maximum errors of 0.8 and 1.5 kcal/mol for SotN (Table S5) as well as 1.6 and 3.0 kcal/mol (see Table S4) for SotC, respectively. No internal (bond, angle, dihedral angle) parameters needed to be optimized for SotC, whereas for SotN there was a high penalty score for the C2-N1-C3 bond angle (shown by blue arrow in **Figure 3C**), and optimization yielded a difference of 0.86° (i.e., <1° as required) between MM and QM values. Also for SotN, 7 dihedral angle parameter optimizations yielded marked improvement over CGENFF initial guesses (illustrated in **Figure 3C** for SotN C8-C3-N1-C2 dihedral angle highlighted in pink, with all the dihedral scan profiles shown in Figure S2), with optimized torsional energy minima within ~0.5 kcal/mol of QM values. For comparison, raw CGENFF dihedral parameters with high penalties yielded QM energy minima differences sometimes as high ~2 kcal/mol. These optimized parameters represent a significant improvement over initial guesses and should yield more accurate computed energetics from MD simulations.

At this time, we were not able to develop empirical models of the SotZ and SotA forms of the drug (**Figure 2**), since a negatively charged sulfonamide nitrogen atom type does not exist in either CHARMM biomolecular, or generalized (CGENFF) force fields. The fraction of these forms in aqueous solution or other media is uncertain, but based on a very high free energy barrier for zwitterionic moxifloxacin translocation (**Figure 1** and discussion

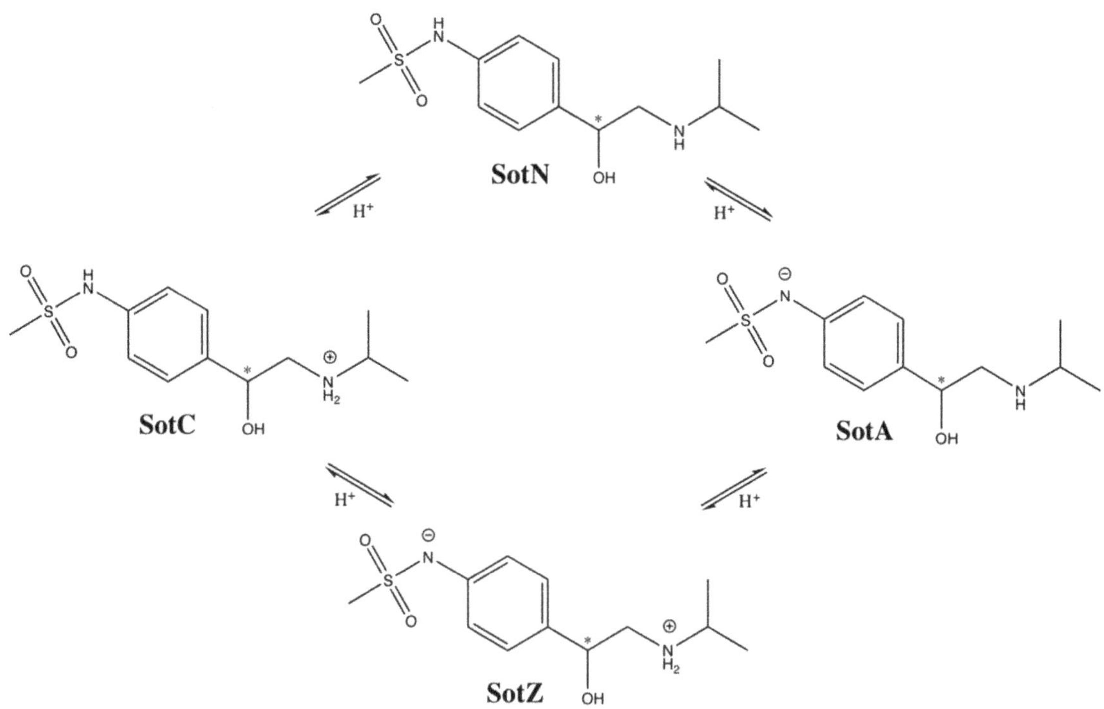

FIGURE 2 | Protonation states of d-sotalol. Chemical structures were drawn using ChemDraw program. Asterisk (*) indicates chiral C atom.

above) as well as the very large dipole moments for SotZ and SotA (see Table S1 and Supplementary text), we do not expect them to contribute substantially to the passive diffusion of d-sotalol across a lipid membrane, or the lipophilic access of this drug to hERG or other protein targets.

We should also mention that sotalol has a chiral center at C1 atom (shown by an asterisk in **Figures 2**, **3C**), and in this study we only focused on S-enantiomer, d-sotalol. However, the developed force field parameters can be also used for R-enantiomer, l-sotalol, which will be also considered in our subsequent studies.

d-Sotalol Solvation and Orientation across the Membrane

We used our SotC and SotN models to investigate their interactions with a lipid membrane as they move across using US MD simulations. For those simulations we applied extensive sampling, especially important for hindered drug reorientation in the membrane interior (see Supplementary text for more information). We also performed those simulations with two popular biomolecular modeling packages, NAMD and CHARMM, with the former being more computationally efficient on our GPU (Graphics Processing Unit) cluster. However, CHARMM allows using $P2_1$ symmetry to take into account likely changes in the areas of top and bottom bilayer leaflets as a drug moves through the membrane by shuffling lipid molecules between them as it happens. We established that the lipid membrane properties of our simulated systems are in agreement with experimental data in this case (See Supplemental text).

We then started to investigate membrane—drug interactions, first, by looking at equilibrated system snapshots at the membrane center ($z = 0$ Å) and water/membrane interfacial region $|z| = 14$ Å, corresponding to free energy minimum for SotN (see **Figure 4**). It can clearly be seen that both charged and neutral drug molecules can adapt different orientations with respect to the membrane normal and can be solvated by both water molecules and lipid head groups even deep in the membrane interior for SotC in agreement with our CHARMM multiple-drug simulations shown in **Figure 1** and discussed above. Interestingly, that in NAMD simulation snapshots shown in **Figure 4**, we observed that SotC while held around membrane center ($z = 0$) can adopt different long-lasting (see below) orientations "grabbing" water molecules and lipid head groups from either top or bottom membrane interface, but did not observe them making interfacial connections to both leaflets, as was observed in our CHARMM simulations (**Figure 1**).

Next, we performed a quantitative analysis of drug solvation shown in **Figure 5.** While SotC and SotN are found in bulk water regions, for $|z| > 25$ Å ($\sim$5 Å beyond phosphate groups), they are solvated by $\sim$5.5 and 5 water molecules, respectively. We defined the interfacial region as $15 < |z| < 25$ Å, where 15 Å boundary was established based on an experimentally determined POPC hydrophobic thickness of 28.8 $\pm$ 0.6 Å (Kucerka et al., 2011). The water coordination remains the same as in bulk, until the drug reaches inside the core of the membrane, where we observe a bigger drop in the number of water molecules solvating SotN. In the center of the bilayer, at $z = 0$ Å, almost no water molecules are found coordinating the neutral drug, while at

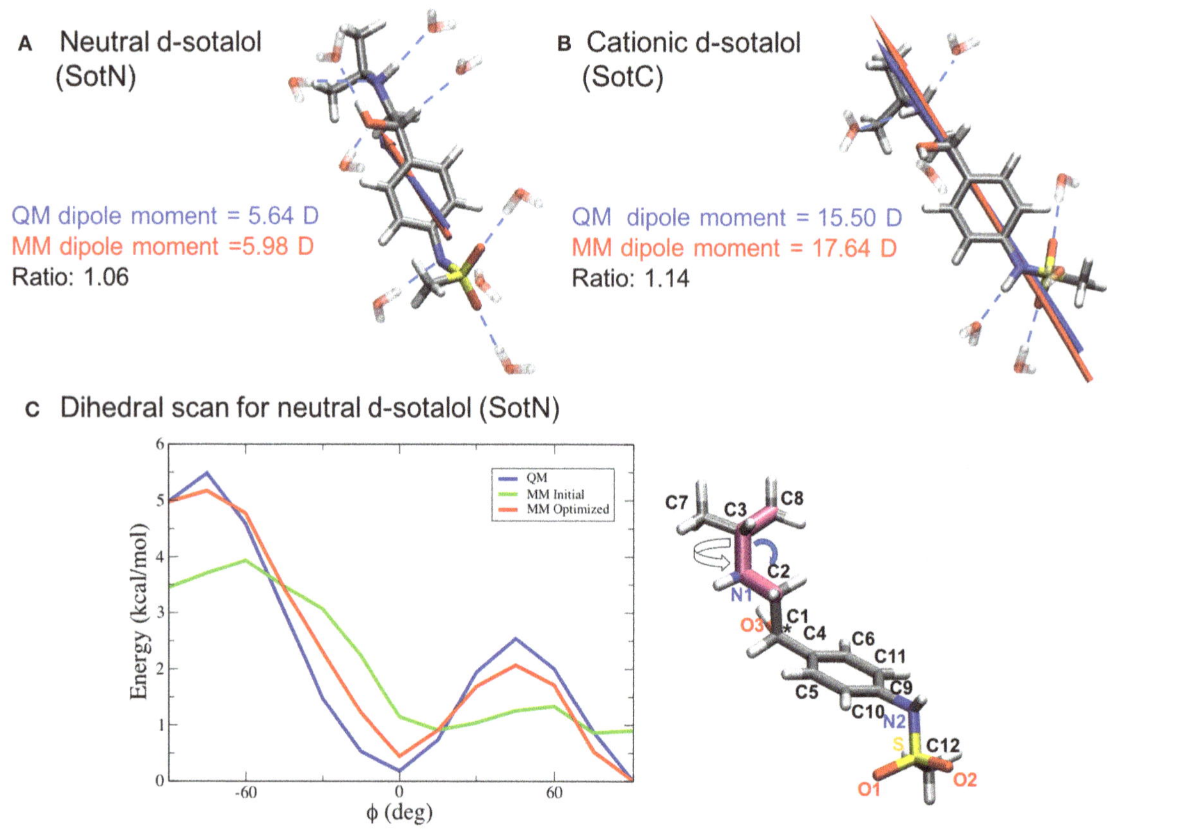

FIGURE 3 | CHARMM force field parameter optimization of d-sotalol. The QM (blue arrow) and MM (red arrow) dipole moments for neutral, SotN **(A)**, and charged, SotC **(B)**, forms of d-sotalol are compared, and their QM optimized water interactions are shown by dashed blue lines. A sample dihedral angle C8-C3-N1-C2 optimization (bonds are highlighted in purple on SotN molecule) is shown in **(C)**, with reference QM computed energy scan in blue, non-optimized CGENFF energy scan in green, and optimized MM energy scan in red, demonstrating marked improvement. Asterisk (*) indicates chiral C atom (C1).

least 1.2 water molecules continue to coordinate the charged species. Additionally, when SotC is found at the interface or the hydrophobic core of the membrane, it is coordinated by lipid phosphate and carbonyl groups, while SotN remains virtually uncoordinated by these functional groups in the membrane core and has a similar coordination by carbonyl O and smaller by phosphate O atoms in the interfacial region (**Figure 5**).

Such solvation results in the preferential orientation of both SotC and SotN with respect to bilayer normal (coinciding with the z axis) as shown in **Figure 6**. There is no preferred orientation of both drugs in bulk water as expected, which is exemplified by average θ being around 90° and order parameter being 0 (see **Figure 6** and top right panels in Figures S7, S8 for time series). There is a strong preference for N1···S vector of both drugs to be aligned with the z axis in the outer interfacial region i.e., at $20 < |z| < 25$ Å, whereas there is some tendency for drugs to lie perpendicular to the membrane normal i.e., in the membrane plane (with order parameter $S < 0$) in the inner interfacial and outer core regions at $10 < |z| < 20$ Å (see Figures S7, S8 for time series). In the inner core region ($|z| < 10$ Å) the drugs again become aligned or anti-aligned with the z-axis. Interestingly, the orientation of SotN and SotC in the inner interfacial and core regions seem to be opposite—with SotC favoring parallel orientation and SotN—antiparallel with the membrane normal for the drug positions with the negative z-values (**Figure 6**). This results from different relative affinities of SotC and SotN functional groups: the cationic ammonium group in SotC strongly attracts water molecules and lipid head groups, whereas its deprotonation makes its sulfonamide functionality a better attractor leading to this functional group re-orientation to be closer to the membrane interface. These interactions lead to hindered rotation (see Figures S7, S8) on the time scale of MD simulations we performed here (10–15 ns for each drug z) leading to difficulties sampling thermodynamics of drug–membrane interactions discussed below (see Supplemental text for more details).

d-Sotalol Energetics and Protonation across the Membrane

We computed free energy profiles for SotC and SotN moving across a POPC membranes based on analysis of drug position fluctuations around restrained z positions in US MD simulations as described above. Those profiles are shown in **Figure 7A** for both NAMD and CHARMM simulations. For SotN, differences between NAMD and CHARMM free energies are within

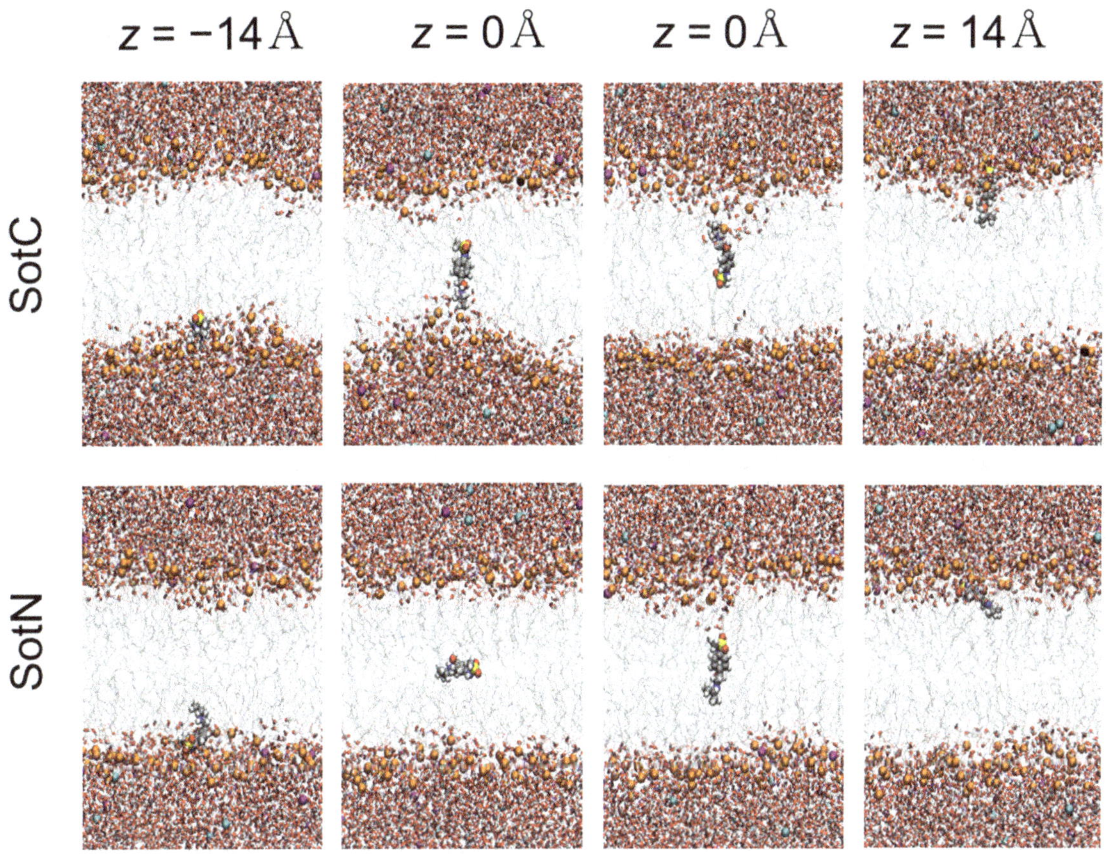

FIGURE 4 | Representative snapshots of charged (SotC) and neutral (SotN) d-sotalol moving across a POPC membrane from umbrella sampling MD simulations. Reference d-sotalol center of mass (COM) z positions with respect to membrane COM are shown on the top. See **Figure 1** caption for molecular representation and coloring information. Two structures for $z = 0$ for each drug represent final system snapshots from two independent simulations with a different initial drug orientation (see Supplementary text for more information).

uncertainties (shown as error bars in **Figure 7A**), obtained as measures of profile asymmetries (see Figure S9 and Supplemental text). However, for SotC the free energy barrier is ~3 kcal/mol smaller for CHARMM (11.2 ± 1.1 kcal/mol) compared to NAMD (14.4 ± 0.1 kcal/mol). Such free energy decrease along with a flat free energy profile for $|z| < 3$ Å can be due to $P2_1$ point group transformations used in CHARMM simulations. This is also in line with interfacial connections to both bilayer interfaces seen in these simulations (see **Figure 1** and discussion above). However, relatively large asymmetries of up to ~2 kcal/mol (Figure S9) preclude us from an unambiguous assignment of this difference.

If we compare SotC and SotN free energy profiles shown in **Figure 7A**, we will see differences such as substantially higher central peak for SotC, e.g., 14.4 vs. 5.4 kcal/mol for SotN from NAMD simulations, as well as presence of a deep interfacial minimum of −2.8 kcal/mol for SotN at $|z| = 14$ Å, similar to one seen for cationic cisapride (**Figure 1** and discussion above). Such minimum indicates a substantial neutral drug accumulation at the water-membrane interface. Interestingly, there is practically no such minimum for SotC, although, a shallow ~-1 kcal/mol trough can be seen on a not-symmetrized PMF profile in Figure S9. The substantial difference in peak heights for SotC and SotN is not unexpected, however, and was also observed for basic amino acid side chains in our previous simulations (Li et al., 2008, 2013). It can be explained by different molecular mechanisms governing SotC and SotN permeation: substantial membrane deformations for the former and nearly complete drug dehydration for the latter (Vorobyov et al., 2010, 2014; Li et al., 2012, 2013). Based on free energy difference between charged and neutral drug forms we can also approximate pK_a shift and thus preferred protonation form of a drug across the membrane:

$$\Delta pK_a = 1/(2.303 k_B T) \quad \{\Delta W_{\mathrm{SotN}}(z) - \Delta W_{\mathrm{SotC}}(z)\} \tag{9}$$

where k_B is Boltzmann constant, T—absolute temperature and $\Delta W(z)$ are position-specific free energies for charged and neutral d-sotalol. Corresponding ΔpK_a profiles are shown in **Figure 7B** and indicate rapid downward ΔpK_a shifts soon after the drug gets into contact with membrane. Near the membrane center ΔpK_a reaches about −6.5 for NAMD and −4.5 for CHARMM based calculations, with the latter estimate being smaller due to a ~3 kcal/mol smaller SotC free energy barrier discussed above. Qualitatively, both results are similar and indicate rapid drug deprotonation soon after a drug starts moving across a

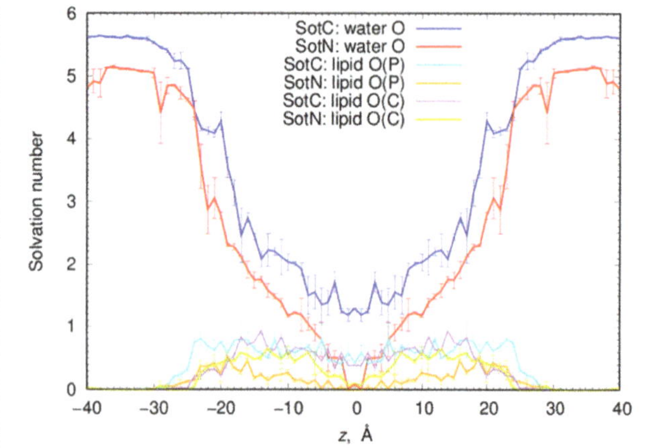

FIGURE 5 | Analysis of d-sotalol solvation from umbrella sampling MD simulations. Solvation numbers of water or lipid oxygen atoms within 4.25 Å cutoff distance from non-hydrogen atoms of SotC or SotN were computed based on integrated radial distribution function (RDF) profiles. See Figure S6 for a few representative RDF profiles. Error bars shown in all the graphs are computed from profile asymmetries.

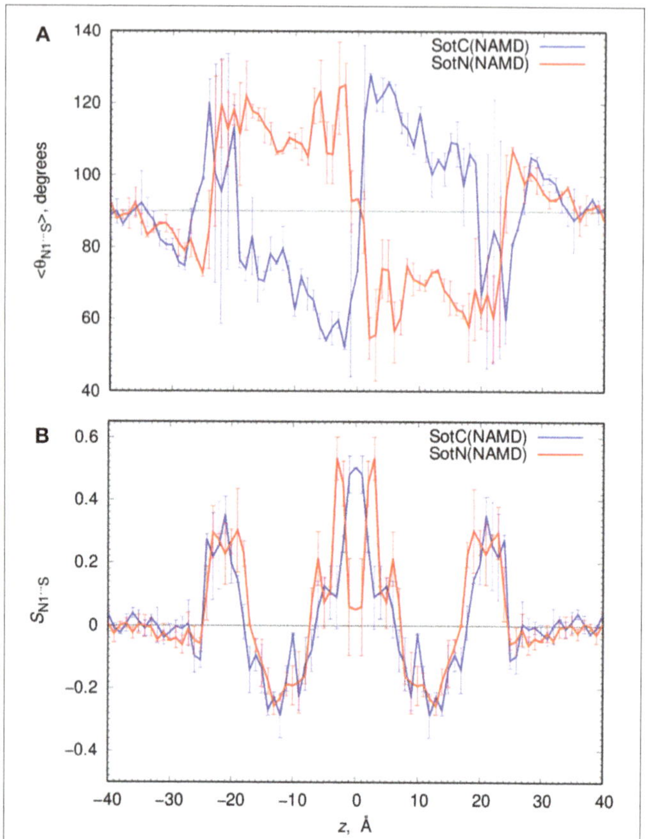

FIGURE 6 | Analysis of d-sotalol tumbling during umbrella sampling MD simulations. **(A)** Average polar angle θ distribution for N1···S d-sotalol vector with respect to the *z* axis for charged (SotC, blue) and neutral (SotN, red) drug moving across POPC membrane. **(B)** Corresponding order parameter profiles for this vector with respect to the *z* axis. Error bars shown in all the graphs are computed from profile asymmetries. See Figures S7, S8 for a few representative θ(N1···S) time series.

membrane. In fact, considering its first aqueous pK_a of 8.3, even getting as close as 20 Å to the membrane center will already lead to drug deprotonation. However, it should be noted that we have not considered a possible role of a zwitterionic d-sotalol form, SotZ, in this equilibrium.

d-Sotalol Water-Membrane Partitioning and Permeations: Connection to Experiments

Next, we need to attempt connecting our findings to experimental observables such as water—membrane partitioning coefficient K and permeability rate P. All the relevant data are summarized in **Table 1**. There is an experimental estimate for water—dimyristoylphosphatidylcholine (DMPC) membrane $K'(\text{wat}\rightarrow\text{mem})$ of 2.50 obtained at 303 K (Redman-Furey and Antinore, 1991). This is an apparent value, which takes into account a pH-dependent fraction of membrane-active drug species at those conditions. However, since we know that only SotN is expected to accumulate in the membrane we can compute an intrinsic K-value at experimental pH = 7.2 using drug aqueous $pK_a = 8.37$ and Henderson-Hasselbach equation to obtain $K(\text{wat}\rightarrow\text{mem}) = 2.50 * 10^{(8.37-7.20)} = 37.0$. And corresponding partitioning free energy is $\Delta G(\text{wat}\rightarrow\text{mem}) = -RT \ln K(\text{wat}\rightarrow\text{mem}) = -2.17$ kcal/mol. These estimates, again, do not take into account a presence of SotZ form in the drug protonation equilibrium, which will likely further increase K-value and decrease corresponding ΔG. Nevertheless, we can compare experimental estimates with values we computed from NAMD US free energy profiles using Equations (3) and (4). Estimated $K(\text{wat}\rightarrow\text{mem})$ and $\Delta G(\text{wat}\rightarrow\text{mem})$ values for SotN of 13.4 ± 8.6 and −1.6 ± 0.4 kcal/mol (see also **Table 1**), respectively, are in good agreement with experiment also considering a different lipid (POPC vs. DMPC) and temperature (310 vs. 303 K) used in simulations and experiment. Estimates from CHARMM simulations (Table S6) are similar, within an error of NAMD values. As expected, SotC does not accumulate in the membrane, with $K(\text{wat}\rightarrow\text{mem})$ and $\Delta G(\text{wat}\rightarrow\text{mem})$ of 0.69 ± 0.36 and 0.23 ± 0.0.28 kcal/mol, respectively (**Table 1**).

MD simulations of water-membrane partitioning are a good test of the drug model accuracy, and can predict how much drug accumulates in the membrane compared to bulk water. However, it does not consider the kinetics of drug movement across a membrane, which is also essential for predicting its pharmacology and toxicology. Permeability rates, P, provide corresponding estimates and are measured experimentally using different cell lines such as caco-2 or artificial membrane systems such as PAMPA (Parallel Artificial Membrane Permeability Assay) (Bermejo et al., 2004). Experimental estimates for d-sotalol P are available from a recent study (Liu et al., 2012) with a PAMPA P-value of 3.2×10^{-7} cm/s. A direct comparison between experimental and computed P values is known to be challenging, with many complicating factors precluding direct quantitative assessment of absolute values (Carpenter et al., 2014;

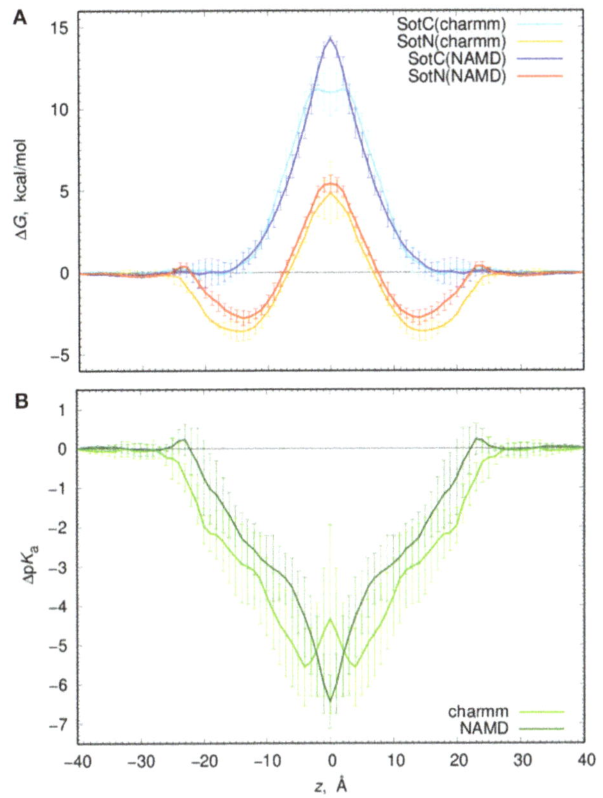

FIGURE 7 | Analysis of d-sotalol thermodynamics from umbrella sampling MD simulations. **(A)** Free energy or potential of mean force (PMF) profiles for charged (SotC, blue and cyan) and neutral (SotN, red and orange) d-sotalol moving across a POPC membrane. In CHARMM simulations (cyan for SotC and orange for SotN) $P2_1$ symmetry was used. See text for more details. **(B)** d-sotalol pK_a shifts computed from PMFs in **(A)**.

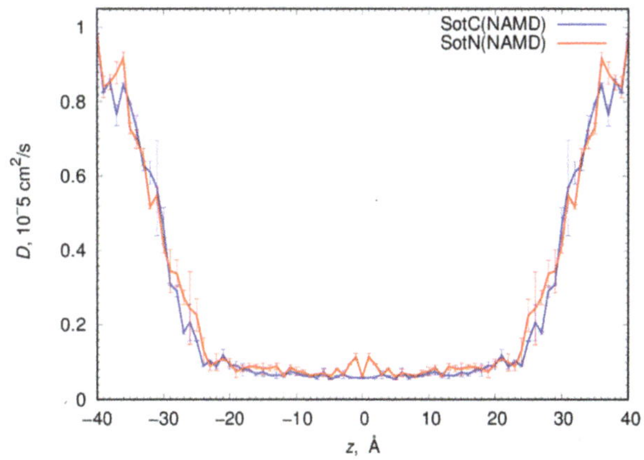

FIGURE 8 | Analysis of d-sotalol diffusion from umbrella sampling MD simulations. Diffusion coefficient profiles are computed as described in the text. Error bars shown are computed from profile asymmetries.

TABLE 1 | Water-membrane partitioning and permeability data from umbrella sampling MD simulations for charged (SotC) and neutral (SotN) d-sotalol translocation across a POPC membrane using NAMD.

	Experiment	Umbrella sampling MD simulations	
		SotC	SotN
W(peak), kcal/mol		14.38 ± 0.14	5.43 ± 0.53
|*z*(peak)|, Å		0.0	0.0
W(well), kcal/mol		−0.16 ± 0.10	−2.79 ± 0.47
|*z*(well)|, Å		32.5	14.0
W(barrier), kcal/mol		14.54 ± 0.17	8.22 ± 0.71
ΔG(wat->mem), kcal/mol	−2.17[a]	0.23 ± 0.28	−1.60 ± 0.37
K(wat->mem)	37[a]	0.69 ± 0.36	13.41 ± 8.58
D(wat), 10^{-5} cm^2/s		0.99 ± 0.14	0.98 ± 0.06
D(mem), 10^{-5} cm^2/s		0.061 ± 0.039	0.087 ± 0.020
log *P*(wat->mem), [log cm/s]	−6.50[b]	−8.57	−4.43

[a] *Redman-Furey and Antinore (1991) using pK_a = 8.3 to compute intrinsic values based on observed apparent K′(wat→mem) of 2.50.*
[b] *Liu et al. (2012) using measured PAMPA permeability rate.*

Di Meo et al., 2016; Bennion et al., 2017). Nevertheless, we computed *P* estimates for both SotC and SotN using Equation (8) as was done in our previous study (Vorobyov et al., 2014) based on free energy and diffusion coefficient profiles. The latter, shown in **Figure 8**, were obtained based on correlation times and mean fluctuations of drug COM in *z* direction using Equation (5) as was also done previously (Vorobyov et al., 2014). The computed diffusion coefficient profiles indicate a rapid 10-fold drop of diffusion coefficients for both SotC and SotN as drug molecules start interacting with lipid membranes, similar to many previous observations (Carpenter et al., 2014; Vorobyov et al., 2014). Interestingly, diffusion coefficients for SotC and SotN are similar, both in water and in the membrane interior (**Figure 8** and **Table 1**), despite difference in net charge and very different drug—membrane interactions. Computed *P*-values, presented in **Table 1** as log *P* of −8.57 for SotC, and −4.43 for SotN encompass an experimental estimate of −6.50. Based on those values alone, we cannot comment on accuracy of our prediction, and comparison with values for other drug molecules (desirably, with similar functionalities) as was done in a recent study (Bennion et al., 2017) would be the best. What our computed values indicate though, that a neutral drug is about 4-orders of magnitude more permeable compared to a cationic one, and that both values are within few orders of magnitude of an experimentally observed permeability.

d-Sotalol—Membrane Interactions: Effect of Anionic Lipids

Thus far, we only considered d-sotalol partitioning across a POPC membrane using US MD simulations for a single drug molecule. However, we also tested if lipid membrane composition affects drug—lipid interactions. In fact, cardiomyocyte lipid membrane is known to host multiple lipid types: in addition to dominant zwitterionic phosphatidylcholine and phosphatidylethanolamine, it also has a substantial fraction of anionic lipids—phosphatidylserine, phosphatidylinositol and phosphatidic acid [6–13% in human (Post et al., 1995) or 17–18% in feline cardiac cells (Leskova and Kryzhanovsky, 2011) based on total phospholipid content]. Anionic lipids are expected to increase membrane binding affinity for cationic drug forms and other cations, as was evidenced by our previous study where we saw increase in the interfacial binding for a positively charged arginine side chain analog, methyl guanidinium, in the presence of an anionic lipid phosphatidylglycerol (Vorobyov and Allen, 2011). The possible effect of anionic lipids on neutral drug binding is less clear and is worth testing as well. Therefore, we performed simulations of both SotC and SotN in lipid membranes containing 15% POPS and 85% POPC, respectively, and compared the results to corresponding drug simulations with pure POPC membranes.

We used 500 or 1000 ns long unbiased MD simulations with multiple (15–16) drug molecules initially placed in bulk aqueous solution, corresponding to ~40 mM drug concentration. Most SotN molecules become bound to the lipid membrane within 200 ns for the simulation with pure POPC and around 400 ns with a POPC/POPS mixture (see Figure S11). The equilibrium aqueous concentration of SotN drops to ~8 mM for POPC/POPS and ~5 mM for a POPC only system. For systems containing SotC, most drug molecules remain in aqueous solution throughout the simulations with only ~4 (out of 15) interacting with membrane regardless of the lipid composition (Figure S11). Equilibrated systems are shown in **Figure 9C** demonstrating substantial membrane binding of SotN but not of SotC. Drug probability distributions from those simulations, computed based on simulation data after equilibration (which was achieved in 200 or 400 ns), are shown in **Figure 9A.** These data confirm the picture demonstrating substantial interfacial binding for SotN with well-defined probability maxima around $|z|$ = 15 Å for both POPC and POPC/POPS systems. No interfacial binding was detected for systems containing SotC (**Figure 9A**). In the cationic sotalol system with POPS present, there is a slightly increased accumulation of the drug density in $|z|$ range of 15–30 Å compared to a system with POPC only. This can be due to expected attraction between anionic lipid head groups of POPS and positively charged SotC moieties. However, the effect is small and is thus unlikely to be physiologically significant in this case.

The probability distributions shown in **Figure 9A** can be converted to free energy profiles as $\Delta G(z) = -k_B T \ln \rho(z)$, where ρ is probability density, k_B is Boltzmann constant, and T is the absolute temperature (see also analogous Equation 4 above). Those profiles are shown in **Figure 9B** and are in general agreement with those from US MD simulations shown in **Figure 7A** previously. As expected, we did not observe SotC located near the membrane center during 500 ns of unbiased MD simulations, and therefore free energy profiles are not defined in this region. However, we observe that the slope of the profile is steeper in the presence of POPS, suggesting a higher translocation barrier and hence slower translocation in this case. SotN molecules were distributed throughout the membrane, and thus we could compute complete free energy profiles including central peaks. Interestingly, there are shallower interfacial binding troughs (by 0.5–0.6 kcal/mol at $|z|$ = 14–15 Å), higher central peak (by ~1.1 kcal/mol) and thus larger translocation barriers in the presence of POPS, indicating less favorable membrane binding and slower translocation rates for SotN. Upon comparison of SotN free energy profiles from US and unbiased MD simulations, shown in **Figure 7A**, **9B**, respectively, we observed a substantially smaller central free energy peak (by 3.7 kcal/mol) and shallower interfacial binding (by 0.6 kcal/mol) in unbiased simulations. There are several factors which can contribute to such differences, including multiple drug molecules, larger membrane patch, and presence of applied electric field in unbiased MD simulations, all of which can possibly lead to smaller permeation barriers. A detailed elucidation of these and other factors is beyond the scope of this study and will be investigated in our subsequent works.

DISCUSSION

Exploring Ionized Drug Membrane Partitioning

At physiological pH many cardiac channel blockers exist in aqueous solution mostly in their cationic form for d-sotalol and cisapride, and zwitterionic form for moxifloxacin (ionized, but with net zero charge). Our MD simulations have demonstrated that all of them cause substantial membrane deformations, with lipid head groups and water molecules coordinating them deep into the hydrophobic membrane core. Large free energy barriers occur at the center of the membrane as a result of the deformations, making such mode of drug translocation unlikely. Moreover, ionized d-sotalol and moxifloxacin do not demonstrate any interfacial membrane binding, indicating that they will not be accumulating there, and thus limiting their protein target accessibility through this route. Interfacial membrane binding is, however, possible for cationic cisapride, and its accumulation there could play a role in its pharmacological profile. However, to provide a more complete picture for drug membrane translocation and membrane-mediated protein target affinity, additional less-polar drug protonation states should be considered. This is what we did for d-sotalol; a prominent example of high-arrhythmia risk hERG blocker. At a physiological pH of 7.4, 89% of this drug exists in a cationic form, indicating a ~1.3 kcal/mol energetic penalty for its deprotonation, which can be easily overcome by the hydrophobic environment of lipid membranes that provide a barrier for charged and polar species (Gennis, 1989).

Computing Charged and Neutral d-Sotalol Membrane Partitioning

In addition to a cationic d-sotalol force field model, we developed parameters for one of the neutral forms of d-sotalol. SotN is substantially more lipophilic, as expected, with a free energy penalty near the membrane center of ~5 kcal/mol, compared to ~15 kcal/mol barrier for the cationic species, which, interestingly, correlates with the ratio of their dipole moments. Moreover, unlike SotC, SotN accumulates at the water-membrane interface, making it accessible for binding to protein targets through the lipophilic

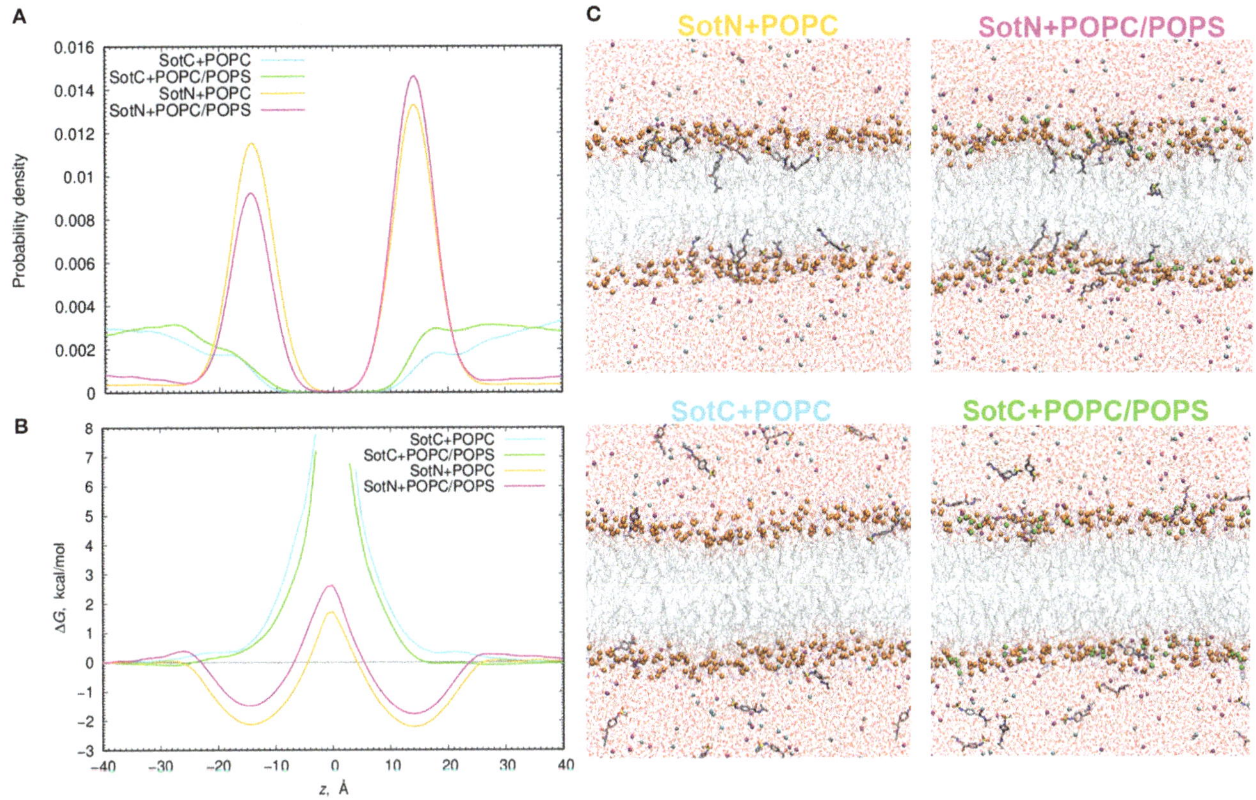

FIGURE 9 | Analysis of d-sotalol partitioning in the presence of anionic lipids from unbiased MD simulations. **(A)** Probability density and **(B)** free energy or potential of mean force (PMF) profiles for charged (SotC) and neutral (SotN) d-sotalol moving across a 100% POPC lipid bilayer (cyan and yellow for SotC and SotN, respectively) or a bilayer composed of an 85% POPC and 15% POPS lipid mixture (green and magenta for SotC and SotN, respectively). **(C)** Molecular snapshots of equilibrated SotN+POPC, SotC+POPC, SotC+POPC/POPS systems after 500 ns, and SotN+POPC/POPS system after 1000 ns of unbiased MD simulations on the Anton 2 supercomputer. P atoms of POPC and POPS lipids are shown as orange and green balls, respectively. See **Figure 1** caption for other molecular representation and coloring information.

pathway. Such accumulation, which can be quantified by water-membrane partitioning coefficient, $K(\text{wat}\rightarrow\text{mem})$, is in agreement with experiment (within an uncertainty, see **Table 1**), suggesting a good quality of the developed empirical model.

Also, SotN does not lead to substantial membrane perturbations; it transiently coordinates with only a few water molecules as it moves across a hydrophobic core of a membrane, unlike SotC. This entails different molecular mechanisms of membrane translocation: a traditional "solubility-diffusion" for SotN governed by drug dehydration, and so called "ion induced defect" for a cationic form, where a cost of membrane deformation plays a major role as was suggested in our previous studies on charged amino acid side chain and small hydrophilic ion translocation (Li et al., 2012; Vorobyov et al., 2014). Thus, we can expect very different dependence of their membrane translocation energetics on lipid membrane composition, such as a strong decrease with a corresponding reduction in membrane thickness for SotC, but not for SotN. This is why we expect good agreement with experiment for SotN water-membrane partitioning despite using a different lipid bilayer (POPC vs. DMPC). Translocation of SotC, however, is expected to be very sensitive to the mechanical properties of membrane such as thickness, as well as the presence of cholesterol, or polyunsaturated fatty acid tails, which can increase or reduce membrane rigidity, respectively (Feller et al., 2002; Pitman et al., 2004). Our computed membrane translocation energetics for charged cisapride and neutral d-sotalol across POPC membrane are very similar, but we expect a larger barrier for cisapride in thicker and/or cholesterol-containing membranes. This will lead to different modulation of drug accessibility for intracellular and membrane-located protein targets. As a first step toward the investigation of lipid composition dependence, we briefly examined the role of anionic lipids in water-membrane d-sotalol partitioning energetics. Despite expected more favorable drug membrane binding in the presence of POPS, we observed an opposite trend with shallower interfacial troughs for SotN and larger translocation barriers for both SotN and SotC. This indicates that such modulation can be due to specific drug—membrane interactions rather than a general electrostatic attraction.

Estimating d-Sotalol Membrane Permeation Kinetics

For SotC and SotN, we also provide estimates of membrane translocation kinetics, expressed as permeability rates (P). SotN has a translocation rate that is four orders of magnitude faster than SotC (see **Table 1**), which is as expected from the difference in their membrane translocation energetics, and similarly reduced diffusion coefficients in the membrane interior. This is in agreement with our previous estimations for ions (Vorobyov et al., 2014) and other drugs (Boiteux et al., 2014). Based on the computed P-values and the membrane thickness considered in those calculations, we estimate that a single SotN molecule can translocate between interfacial binding sites on opposite sides of the membranes in about 7.5×10^{-3} s (millisecond time range), whereas for SotC crossing membrane will take around 150 s. SotN is expected to be accumulated in the membrane over 10-fold compared to its equilibrium concentration in bulk aqueous solution, which is why we are considering its permeation, even though it is a minor component in the bulk aqueous solution at the physiological pH, regardless of its unknown ratio to a membrane-impermeable zwitterionic form. An experimental P estimate for d-sotalol based on measurements using PAMPA is in between our computed values for SotC and SotN (see **Table 1** and Liu et al., 2012). Yet, a direct numerical comparison of our computed and experimental P estimates is extremely challenging, as has been indicated in many previous studies (Orsi et al., 2009; Carpenter et al., 2014; Di Meo et al., 2016; Bennion et al., 2017). This is largely because experimentally measured quantities mostly represent so-called apparent values, which typically include contributions from different drug protonation forms at experimental pH, depend on water layer thickness and condition, and may encompass different drug permeation routes (Bermejo et al., 2004; Avdeef et al., 2005; Ottaviani et al., 2006; Orsi et al., 2009). More standardized intrinsic P-values for neutral drug forms are typically harder to get (Bermejo et al., 2004; Orsi et al., 2009), and even then, quantitative agreement with MD computed values remains challenging due to substantial differences between an experimental macroscopic system, and a microscopic molecular model. Therefore, an agreement between relative P-values for different drugs is typically sought (Orsi et al., 2009; Carpenter et al., 2014; Bennion et al., 2017), which will be explored in our future studies.

Predicting Possible Membrane-Mediated Ion Channel Accessibility Pathways

One mode of ion channel block by drugs is through an intracellular aqueous pathway, where a drug in the cytosol passes through a channel lower gate, when it is open, and occludes a channel pore (Hille, 2001). Another possible mechanism for ion channel block is through a lipophilic route, which was observed in a recent MD study for a local anesthetic, benzocaine, entering a central pore of sodium voltage-gated channel Na_VAb via lipid-facing channel openings (fenestrations) (Boiteux et al., 2014). In the case of the hERG blocker d-sotalol studied here, SotN would likely to be a dominant drug form binding to the channel via this route, but it could become protonated again once it is in the pore.

Our recent combined experimental/computational studies of pH- and state-dependent hERG block by another high-risk pro-arrhythmic drug dofetilide (sharing the same functional groups as d-sotalol, but more potent) suggested that drug protonation equilibrium plays a crucial role in its channel binding affinity (Wang et al., 2016). To the best of our knowledge, no such studies have been done for d-sotalol yet. The experimentally measured on-rate of d-sotalol binding to hERG is quite slow, in the range of several minutes (Numaguchi et al., 2000). This is consistent with our computed membrane permeation rate for cationic d-sotalol form. Recent experimental studies using cells pre-equilibrated with sotalol, i.e., after the drug crossing cell membranes, demonstrate faster than 200 ms hERG block (Li et al., 2017; Windley et al., 2017), indicating that drug membrane permeation could be a rate-limiting step considering preferential drug channel access via the intracellular aqueous pore. However, other reasons for such outcome, such as a preponderance of a lipophilic channel access pathway from of a local membrane bound pool of the drug, suggested by our neutral d-sotalol simulations, are possible and can be tested by additional experiments as well as comprehensive drug—channel MD simulations. This along with pH-dependent measurements can help elucidating roles of different drug protonation states and their contribution to channel block.

Moreover, experimental drug—channel on-rates, which are crucial components of functional scale kinetic models used for *in silico* evaluation of pro-arrhythmia proclivities (as in the CiPA initiative), can be corroborated using atomistic MD simulations, such as those presented in this study. Moreover, atomistic MD simulations can be used to identify different drug—channel interaction pathways not easily discernable via experiment alone. For instance, through comparison of computed rates for drug membrane translocation and binding to the channel via aqueous and lipophilic pathways, we can predict likely rate limiting step, and relative contributions of all those processes to experimentally measured rates, thus informing kinetic models and likely improving their accuracy and predictive power. The spatially resolved ionization-state-specific drug localization profiles and water—membrane permeation rates computed here represent the first crucial step toward this goal.

Further insight into structural determinants of drug-induced channel blockade, including possible drug access pathways, can be provided by comprehensive mutagenesis studies, similar to one done recently for a large set of congenital long QT syndrome 2 associated hERG mutations (Anderson et al., 2014). Though not directly related to drug-induced hERG block, several mutations that were implicated in directly affecting channel gating or permeation were for hERG residues facing the water-membrane interface (Lees-Miller et al., 2015; Saxena et al., 2016), and therefore would be easily accessible by drugs like neutral d-sotalol, and cationic cisapride, that we explored in this study.

Even more importantly, similar computational approaches can be used as one of the steps to design drugs, which have similar membrane binding affinities and bind around mutated protein residues that result in altered channel function. Such an approach focusing on a desired drug lipophilicity and spatial arrangement of crucial functional groups was used, for instance, to design selective sodium channel blockers (Muraglia et al., 2007; De Luca et al., 2012; De Bellis et al., 2017). Such a structure-function based approach was shown to improve drug safety profile through mitigation of off-target effects, including hERG block (De Bellis et al., 2017).

Limitations and Future Directions

Our study represents just a first step in atomistic-level elucidation of thermodynamics and kinetics of cardiac channel blocking drug translocation across a lipid membrane. We obtained reasonable free energy profiles and water-membrane partitioning coefficients with a moderate amount of sampling (10–15 ns per umbrella sampling window or 0.8–1.2 μs for entire simulations). In some cases, we had to run additional simulations with alternative initial drug orientations to compensate for their slow reorientation in the membrane interior observed in our study. More extensive simulations for other drug membrane partitioning using a different empirical force field and molecular modeling software were reported recently (Bennion et al., 2017). They can potentially provide improved accuracy provided a high quality of an underlying empirical model and sufficient sampling of drug tumbling, and thus can be considered as a viable alternative of our approach. In our future studies we will also test several alternative options for enhanced sampling (Bernardi et al., 2015) such as metadynamics (Barducci et al., 2011), which has been recently used in membrane partitioning simulations to properly sample degrees of freedom orthogonal to the reaction coordinate and thus provide a more accurate energetics (Jambeck and Lyubartsev, 2013).

Alternatively, replica exchange simulations can be employed, which can be especially useful for modeling mixed membrane systems (Huang and Garcia, 2014). In our study, we mostly used a one component lipid membrane containing POPC, whereas lipid composition of cellular membranes is much more complex. For instance, plasma membranes of cardiomyocytes (where hERG channels are mostly located) has substantial fractions of zwitterionic posphatidylcholine, phosphatidyethanolamine, and sphingomyelin, negatively charged phosphatidylserine and non-polar cholesterol with substantial differences in their distribution between inner and outer leaflets (Post et al., 1995). This is without taking into account lateral membrane heterogeneity and existence of functional microdomains such as lipid rafts and caveolae, suggested to influence cardiac ion channel function (Maguy et al., 2006). At this time, however, we are not yet in position to study such complex heterogeneous systems via atomistic simulations, but coarse-grained models, such as a popular MARTINI force field (Marrink and Tieleman, 2013), are well-suited for such investigations and can be potentially used for studying cardiac drug interactions with realistic lipid membranes. In terms of atomistic simulations, we are planning to extend our studies to simulate drug partitioning to binary mixtures of phospholipids and cholesterol, which is expected to substantially influence ionizable drug partitioning and permeation, as discussed above. Another direction, which we already started exploring here, are binary mixtures of two phospholipids with different head groups, possibly influencing drug permeation kinetics and thermodynamics via specific interactions and/or altering membrane physical-chemical properties.

Estimated drug permeation rates and their relation to experimentally measured quantities remain uncertain as was mentioned above. In this study we could only compare relative values for cationic and neutral d-sotalol, which encompass an experimental estimate. However, it is not clear if we can simply relate those values to a measured apparent permeability via computing effective resistances to permeation as was done in a recent study (Carpenter et al., 2014). Another pertinent issue is computing permeability rates for drug molecules with pronounced interfacial binding (such as neutral d-sotalol in this study), which will clearly increase a barrier height a drug will need to hop over to permeate as was noted previously (Orsi et al., 2009). Therefore, an expression for permeability rates (Marrink and Berendsen, 1994) traditionally used for their calculations for polar and ionic species, where free energies are referenced to bulk aqueous solution, might not work anymore. In this study for SotN we used a variant of this expression with free energy set to 0 at the interfacial binding site and computing permeability just across a central barrier. A validity of such approximation remains to be seen in more thorough investigations, e.g., by comparing results with drug translocation rates computed from long unbiased MD simulations. Moreover, this approach does not take into account drug translocation between the interfacial binding site and bulk water. This contribution becomes dominant for hydrophobic drugs such as general anesthetics (Vorobyov et al., 2012), not considered in this study.

For d-sotalol and other hERG blockers with sulfonamide functional group (e.g., dofetilide, ibutilide, E4031), an unresolved issue is its anionic, deprotonated drug fraction, such as one in the zwitterionic d-sotalol (SotZ). A neutral sulfonamide group has been thoroughly parameterized recently and is included in the generalized CHARMM force field (Yu et al., 2012), whereas no atom type for anionic N or any associated parameters are available to the best of our knowledge. For d-sotalol in water at the physiological pH, a cationic form with a neutral sulfonamide group is a dominant form, with SotZ and/or SotN having a ~11% contribution. Based on our prediction, only SotN can move across a membrane, but we need to know SotZ and SotN ratios in order to relate computed membrane partitioning energetics to experimental observables. Moreover, SotZ can be potentially an important contributor to hERG binding through the interactions of its negatively charged sulfonamide functionality with basic residues in the voltage-sensing domain (VSD) of a channel, for example. Such interactions were revealed in a recent crystallographic/electrophysiological study in a VSD of a voltage gated $Na_V1.7/Na_VAb$ chimera channel, where an anionic sulfonamide "warhead" directly and selectively interacts with a gating charge carrying arginine residue, immobilizing a voltage sensor in its activated state (Ahuja et al., 2015). Whether a similar binding motif is possible for hERG remains to be seen, but it should not be discounted, and thus accurate empirical force field for an anionic sulfonamide functionality will need to be developed and can be validated on predicting an aforementioned drug—channel interaction.

Sotalol is a chiral molecule, and in this work we only studied one enantiomer: d-sotalol, which was used in an infamous SWORD clinical study (Waldo et al., 1996) mentioned above. Sotalol enantiomers can be synthesized and separated (Carr et al., 1991; Foster and Carr, 1992; Brodfuehrer et al., 1997), however, a racemic mixture of d- and l-isomers has been used in many biophysical, physiological and pharmacological experimental studies up to date. l-sotalol is known to have some beta-blocking activities, whereas d-sotalol seems to be inert (Gomoll and Bartek, 1986) (a reason why it was used for SWORD study), but they share very similar electrophysiological properties, including QT prolongation (Touboul, 1993; Manoach and Tribulova, 2001). Even though interaction between two chiral molecules, e.g., sotalol and lipid, can be different for stereoisomers (and used for their separation), we do not expect substantial changes for l-sotalol—membrane interactions as they are mostly governed by dehydration for a neutral drug or membrane deformation by a charged drug electric field. Therefore, simulations with d-sotalol should be sufficient, however, a more complex situation will arise for drug—channel interaction simulations, where both stereoisomers might need to be tested.

Nevertheless, despite the limitations of this study, related to tested drug and membrane models, our work demonstrated good agreement between computed and experimental data, and can definitely be used to predict the molecular mechanisms, energetics and kinetics of drug-membrane interactions, and potentially ion channel binding pathways. Moreover, the presented study can be used, for instance, for informing multi-scale kinetic models of cardiovascular (and other) drug effects on cellular, tissue and organ levels (Clancy et al., 2016), as was done in our recent study, where we modeled charged and neutral flecainide (cardiac sodium channel blocker with some pro-arrhythmic proclivity) effects (Yang et al., 2016). We are planning a similar extension of the current study along with atomistic structure based investigations of sotalol interactions with hERG using a combination of molecular docking and all-atom molecular dynamics simulations. Several other drugs with different hERG affinities and pro-arrhythmia proclivities will be investigated as well for both lipid membrane and hERG binding assays.

AUTHOR CONTRIBUTIONS

IV, CC, and SN: designed the research; KD, SB, and IV: performed the research and analyzed data; All authors prepared the manuscript and approved the final submitted version.

FUNDING

This work was supported by American Heart Association Predoctoral Fellowship 16PRE27260295 (to KD), the National Institutes of Health NHLBI R01HL128537-02 (to CC, SN, SB, and IV), NHLBI U01HL126273-02 (to CC, SB, and IV), NHLBI R01HL128170-03 (to CC), R01GM101928-04 (to CC), the Canadian Institutes of Health Research [Grant 201103MOP-CSA-244888] (to SN). The computational support for this work was provided by University of California, Davis and WestGrid/Compute Canada through a Resource Allocation Award to SN. Anton 2 computer time was provided by the Pittsburgh Supercomputing Center (PSC) through Grant R01GM116961 from the National Institutes of Health. The Anton 2 machine at PSC was generously made available by D.E. Shaw Research.

ACKNOWLEDGMENTS

We would like to thank Profs. Heike Wulff, Vladimir Yarov-Yarovoy, and Jon Sack for helpful discussions.

REFERENCES

Ahuja, S., Mukund, S., Deng, L., Khakh, K., Chang, E., Ho, H., et al. (2015). Structural basis of Nav1.7 inhibition by an isoform-selective small-molecule antagonist. *Science* 350:aac5464. doi: 10.1126/science.aac5464

Anderson, C. L., Kuzmicki, C. E., Childs, R. R., Hintz, C. J., Delisle, B. P., and January, C. T. (2014). Large-scale mutational analysis of Kv11.1 reveals molecular insights into type 2 long QT syndrome. *Nat. Commun.* 5, 5535. doi: 10.1038/ncomms6535

Avdeef, A., Artursson, P., Neuhoff, S., Lazorova, L., Grasjo, J., and Tavelin, S. (2005). Caco-2 permeability of weakly basic drugs predicted with the double-sink PAMPA pKa(flux) method. *Eur. J. Pharm. Sci.* 24, 333–349. doi: 10.1016/j.ejps.2004.11.011

Barducci, A., Bonomi, M., and Parrinello, M. (2011). Metadynamics. *WIREs Comput. Mol. Sci.* 1, 826–843. doi: 10.1002/wcms.31

Beglov, D., and Roux, B. (1994). Finite representation of an infinite bulk system: solvent boundary potential for computer simulations. *J. Chem. Phys.* 100, 9050–9063. doi: 10.1063/1.466711

Benjamin, E. J., Blaha, M. J., Chiuve, S. E., Cushman, M., Das, S. R., Deo, R., et al. (2017). Heart Disease and Stroke Statistics-2017 update: a report from the american heart association. *Circulation* 135, e146–e603. doi: 10.1161/CIR.0000000000000485

Bennion, B. J., Be, N. A., McNerney, M. W., Lao, V., Carlson, E. M., Valdez, C. A., et al. (2017). Predicting a drug's membrane permeability: a computational model validated with *in vitro* permeability assay data. *J. Phys. Chem. B* 121, 5228–5237. doi: 10.1021/acs.jpcb.7b02914

Bermejo, M., Avdeef, A., Ruiz, A., Nalda, R., Ruell, J. A., Tsinman, O., et al. (2004). PAMPA–a drug absorption *in vitro* model 7. Comparing rat *in situ*, Caco-2, and PAMPA permeability of fluoroquinolones. *Eur. J. Pharm. Sci.* 21, 429–441. doi: 10.1016/j.ejps.2003.10.009

Bernardi, R. C., Melo, M. C. R., and Schulten, K. (2015). Enhanced sampling techniques in molecular dynamics simulations of biological systems. *Biochim. Biophys. Acta* 1850, 872–877. doi: 10.1016/j.bbagen.2014.10.019

Boiteux, C., Vorobyov, I., French, R. J., French, C., Yarov-Yarovoy, V., and Allen, T. W. (2014). Local anesthetic and antiepileptic drug access and binding to a bacterial voltage-gated sodium channel. *Proc. Natl. Acad. Sci. U.S.A.* 111, 13057–13062. doi: 10.1073/pnas.1408710111

Brodfuehrer, P. R., Smith, P., Dillon, J. L., and Vemishetti, P. (1997). Asymmetric synthesis of the antiarrhythmia agent d-sotalol. *Organ. Process Res. Dev.* 1, 176–178. doi: 10.1021/op960043t

Brooks, B. R., Brooks, C. L., MacKerell, A. D., Nilsson, L., Petrella, R. J., Roux, B., et al. (2009). CHARMM: the biomolecular simulation program. *J. Comput. Chem.* 30, 1545–1614. doi: 10.1002/jcc.21287

Brooks, B. R., Bruccoleri, R. E., Olafson, B. D., States, D. J., Swaminathan, S. A., and Karplus, M. (1983). CHARMM: a program for macromolecular energy, minimization, and dynamics calculations. *J. Comput. Chem.* 4, 187–217. doi: 10.1002/jcc.540040211

Carpenter, T. S., Kirshner, D. A., Lau, E. Y., Wong, S. E., Nilmeier, J. P., and Lightstone, F. C. (2014). A method to predict blood-brain barrier permeability of drug-like compounds using molecular dynamics simulations. *Biophys. J.* 107, 630–641. doi: 10.1016/j.bpj.2014.06.024

Carr, R. A., Foster, R. T., and Bhanji, N. H. (1991). Stereospecific high-performance liquid chromatographic assay of sotalol in plasma. *Pharm. Res.* 8, 1195–1198. doi: 10.1023/A:1015870805757

Chi, K. R. (2013). Revolution dawning in cardiotoxicity testing. *Nat. Rev. Drug Discov.* 12, 565–567. doi: 10.1038/nrd4083

Clancy, C. E., An, G., Cannon, W. R., Liu, Y., May, E. E., Ortoleva, P., et al. (2016). Multiscale modeling in the clinic: drug design and development. *Ann. Biomed. Eng.* 44, 2591–2610. doi: 10.1007/s10439-016-1563-0

Colatsky, T., Fermini, B., Gintant, G., Pierson, J. B., Sager, P., Sekino, Y., et al. (2016). The Comprehensive *in vitro* proarrhythmia assay (CiPA) initiative - update on progress. *J. Pharmacol. Toxicol. Methods* 81, 15–20. doi: 10.1016/j.vascn.2016.06.002

Darden, T., York, D., and Pedersen, L. (1993). Particle mesh Ewald: an N·log(N) method for Ewald sums in large systems. *J. Chem. Phys.* 98, 10089–10092. doi: 10.1063/1.464397

De Bellis, M., Carbonara, R., Roussel, J., Farinato, A., Massari, A., Pierno, S., et al. (2017). Increased sodium channel use-dependent inhibition by a new potent analogue of tocainide greatly enhances *in vivo* antimyotonic activity. *Neuropharmacology* 113, 206–216. doi: 10.1016/j.neuropharm.2016.10.013

De Luca, A., De Bellis, M., Corbo, F., Franchini, C., Muraglia, M., Catalano, A., et al. (2012). Searching for novel anti-myotonic agents: pharmacophore requirement for use-dependent block of skeletal muscle sodium channels by N-benzylated cyclic derivatives of tocainide. *Neuromusc. Disord.* 22, 56–65. doi: 10.1016/j.nmd.2011.07.001

Di Meo, F., Fabre, G., Berka, K., Ossman, T., Chantemargue, B., Paloncyova, M., et al. (2016). *In silico* pharmacology: drug membrane partitioning and crossing. *Pharmacol. Res.* 111, 471–486. doi: 10.1016/j.phrs.2016.06.030

Dolan, E. A., Venable, R. M., Pastor, R. W., and Brooks, B. R. (2002). Simulations of membranes and other interfacial systems using P21 and Pc periodic boundary conditions. *Biophys. J.* 82, 2317–2325. doi: 10.1016/S0006-3495(02)75577-X

Feller, S. E., Gawrisch, K., and MacKerell, A. D. Jr. (2002). Polyunsaturated fatty acids in lipid bilayers: intrinsic and environmental contributions to their unique physical properties. *J. Am. Chem. Soc.* 124, 318–326. doi: 10.1021/ja0118340

Feller, S. E., Zhang, Y., Pastor, R. W., and Brooks, B. R. (1995). Constant pressure molecular dynamics simulation: the Langevin piston method. *J. Chem. Phys.* 103, 4613–4621. doi: 10.1063/1.470648

Fermini, B., Hancox, J. C., Abi-Gerges, N., Bridgland-Taylor, M., Chaudhary, K. W., Colatsky, T., et al. (2016). A new perspective in the field of cardiac safety testing through the comprehensive *in vitro* proarrhythmia assay paradigm. *J. Biomol. Screen.* 21, 1–11. doi: 10.1177/1087057115594589

Foster, R. T., and Carr, R. A. (1992). Sotalol. *Anal. Profiles Drug Subst. Excipients* 21, 501–533. doi: 10.1016/S0099-5428(08)60400-1

Frisch, M., Trucks, G., Schlegel, H., Scuseria, G., Robb, M., Cheeseman, J., et al. (2009). *Gaussian 09*. Wallingford, CT: Gaussian Inc.

Ganapathi, S. B., Fox, T. E., Kester, M., and Elmslie, K. S. (2010). Ceramide modulates HERG potassium channel gating by translocation into lipid rafts. *Am. J. Physiol. Cell Physiol.* 299, C74–86. doi: 10.1152/ajpcell.00462.2009

Gennis, R. B. (1989). *Biomembranes: Molecular Structure and Function*. New York, NY: Springer-Verlag.

Gomoll, A. W., and Bartek, M. J. (1986). Comparative beta-blocking activities and electrophysiologic actions of racemic sotalol and its optical isomers in anesthetized dogs. *Eur. J. Pharmacol.* 132, 123–135. doi: 10.1016/0014-2999(86)90597-2

Guizy, M., Arias, C., David, M., Gonzalez, T., and Valenzuela, C. (2005). ω-3 and ω-6 polyunsaturated fatty acids block *HERG* channels. *Am. J. Physiol. Cell Physiol.* 289, C1251–1260. doi: 10.1152/ajpcell.00036.2005

Hancu, G., Samarghitan, C., Rusu, A., and Mircia, E. (2014). Sotalol chiral separation by capillary electrophoresis. *J. Chilean Chem. Soc.* 59, 2559–2563. doi: 10.4067/S0717-97072014000300007

Haverkamp, W., Kruesmann, F., Fritsch, A., Van Veenhuyzen, D., and Arvis, P. (2012). Update on the cardiac safety of moxifloxacin. *Curr. Drug Saf.* 7, 149–163. doi: 10.2174/157488612802715735

Hille, B. (2001). *Ion Channels of Excitable Membranes*. Sunderland, MA: Sinauer.

Hoover, W. G. (1985). Canonical dynamics: equilibrium phase-space distributions. *Phys. Rev. A* 31, 1695–1697. doi: 10.1103/PhysRevA.31.1695

Huang, K., and Garcia, A. E. (2014). Acceleration of lateral equilibration in mixed lipid bilayers using replica exchange with solute tempering. *J. Chem. Theory Comput.* 10, 4264–4272. doi: 10.1021/ct500305u

Hummer, G. (2005). Position-dependent diffusion coefficients and free energies from Bayesian analysis of equilibrium and replica molecular dynamics simulations. *New J. Phys.* 7, 34. doi: 10.1088/1367-2630/7/1/034

Humphrey, W., Dalke, A., and Schulten, K. (1996). VMD: visual molecular dynamics. *J. Mol. Graph* 14, 33–38, 27–38. doi: 10.1016/0263-7855(96)00018-5

Irwin, J. J., and Shoichet, B. K. (2005). ZINC–a free database of commercially available compounds for virtual screening. *J. Chem. Inf. Model.* 45, 177–182. doi: 10.1021/ci049714+

Jambeck, J. P., and Lyubartsev, A. P. (2013). Exploring the free energy landscape of solutes embedded in lipid bilayers. *J. Phys. Chem. Lett.* 4, 1781–1787. doi: 10.1021/jz4007993

Jo, S., Kim, T., Iyer, V. G., and Im, W. (2008). CHARMM-GUI: a web-based graphical user interface for CHARMM. *J. Comput. Chem.* 29, 1859–1865. doi: 10.1002/jcc.20945

Jorgensen, W. L., Chandrasekhar, J., Madura, J. D., Impey, R. W., and Klein, M. L. (1983). Comparison of simple potential functions for simulating liquid water. *J. Chem. Phys.* 79, 926–935. doi: 10.1063/1.445869

Kim, S., Thiessen, P. A., Bolton, E. E., Chen, J., Fu, G., Gindulyte, A., et al. (2016). PubChem Substance and Compound databases. *Nucleic Acids Res.* 44, D1202–D1213. doi: 10.1093/nar/gkv951

Klauda, J. B., Venable, R. M., Freites, J. A., O'connor, J. W., Tobias, D. J., Mondragon-Ramirez, C., et al. (2010). Update of the CHARMM all-atom additive force field for lipids: validation on six lipid types. *J. Phys. Chem. B* 114, 7830–7843. doi: 10.1021/jp101759q

Kucerka, N., Nieh, M. P., and Katsaras, J. (2011). Fluid phase lipid areas and bilayer thicknesses of commonly used phosphatidylcholines as a function of temperature. *Biochim. Biophys. Acta* 1808, 2761–2771. doi: 10.1016/j.bbamem.2011.07.022

Kumar, S., Rosenberg, J. M., Bouzida, D., Swendsen, R. H., and Kollman, P. A. (1992). THE weighted histogram analysis method for free-energy calculations on biomolecules. I. The method. *J. Comput. Chem.* 13, 1011–1021. doi: 10.1002/jcc.540130812

Langlois, M. H., Montagut, M., Dubost, J. P., Grellet, J., and Saux, M. C. (2005). Protonation equilibrium and lipophilicity of moxifloxacin. *J. Pharm. Biomed. Anal.* 37, 389–393. doi: 10.1016/j.jpba.2004.10.022

Lees-Miller, J. P., Guo, J., Wang, Y., Perissinotti, L. L., Noskov, S. Y., and Duff, H. J. (2015). Ivabradine prolongs phase 3 of cardiac repolarization and blocks the hERG1 (KCNH2) current over a concentration-range overlapping with that required to block HCN4. *J. Mol. Cell. Cardiol.* 85, 71–78. doi: 10.1016/j.yjmcc.2015.05.009

Leskova, G. F., and Kryzhanovsky, G. N. (2011). Changes in phospholipid composition of cardiomyocyte plasma membranes during hemorrhagic shock. *Bull. Exp. Biol. Med.* 151, 284–287. doi: 10.1007/s10517-011-1310-3

Li, L. B., Vorobyov, I., and Allen, T. W. (2012). The role of membrane thickness in charged protein-lipid interactions. *Biochim. Biophys. Acta* 1818, 135–145. doi: 10.1016/j.bbamem.2011.10.026

Li, L., Vorobyov, I., and Allen, T. W. (2008). Potential of mean force and pKa profile calculation for a lipid membrane-exposed arginine side chain. *J. Phys. Chem. B* 112, 9574–9587. doi: 10.1021/jp7114912

Li, L., Vorobyov, I., and Allen, T. W. (2013). The different interactions of lysine and arginine side chains with lipid membranes. *J. Phys. Chem. B* 117, 11906–11920. doi: 10.1021/jp405418y

Li, Z., Dutta, S., Sheng, J., Tran, P. N., Wu, W., Chang, K., et al. (2017). Improving the *in silico* assessment of proarrhythmia risk by combining hERG (Human Ether-à-go-go-Related Gene) channel–drug binding kinetics and multichannel pharmacology. *Circulation* 10:e004628. doi: 10.1161/CIRCEP.116.004628

Lippert, R. A., Predescu, C., Ierardi, D. J., MacKenzie, K. M., Eastwood, M. P., Dror, R. O., et al. (2013). Accurate and efficient integration for molecular dynamics simulations at constant temperature and pressure. *J. Chem. Phys.* 139:164106. doi: 10.1063/1.4825247

Liu, W., Okochi, H., Benet, L. Z., and Zhai, S. D. (2012). Sotalol permeability in cultured-cell, rat intestine, and PAMPA system. *Pharm. Res.* 29, 1768–1774. doi: 10.1007/s11095-012-0699-3

MacKerell, A. D. Jr. (2004). Empirical force fields for biological macromolecules: overview and issues. *J. Comput. Chem.* 25, 1584–1604. doi: 10.1002/jcc.20082

Maguy, A., Hebert, T. E., and Nattel, S. (2006). Involvement of lipid rafts and caveolae in cardiac ion channel function. *Cardiovasc. Res.* 69, 798–807. doi: 10.1016/j.cardiores.2005.11.013

Manoach, M., and Tribulova, N. (2001). Sotalol: the mechanism of its antiarrhythmic-defibrillating effect. *Cardiovasc. Drug Rev.* 19, 172–182. doi: 10.1111/j.1527-3466.2001.tb00062.x

Marrink, S. J., and Tieleman, D. P. (2013). Perspective on the Martini model. *Chem. Soc. Rev.* 42, 6801–6822. doi: 10.1039/c3cs60093a

Marrink, S.-J., and Berendsen, H. J. (1994). Simulation of water transport through a lipid membrane. *J. Phys. Chem.* 98, 4155–4168. doi: 10.1021/j100066a040

Mayne, C. G., Saam, J., Schulten, K., Tajkhorshid, E., and Gumbart, J. C. (2013). Rapid parameterization of small molecules using the Force Field Toolkit. *J. Comput. Chem.* 34, 2757–2770. doi: 10.1002/jcc.23422

Moreno, C., Macias, A., Prieto, A., De La Cruz, A., and Valenzuela, C. (2012). Polyunsaturated fatty acids modify the gating of kv channels. *Front. Pharmacol.* 3:163. doi: 10.3389/fphar.2012.00163

Muraglia, M., Franchini, C., Corbo, F., Scilimati, A., Tortorella, V., Sinicropi, M. S., et al. (2007). Synthesis of beta-proline like derivatives and their evaluation as sodium channel blockers. *J. Heterocycl. Chem.* 44, 1099–1103. doi: 10.1002/jhet.5570440519

Nosé, S. (1984). A unified formulation of the constant temperature molecular dynamics methods. *J. Chem. Phys.* 81, 511–519. doi: 10.1063/1.447334

Numaguchi, H., Mullins, F. M., Johnson, J. P. Jr., Johns, D. C., Po, S. S., Yang, I. C., et al. (2000). Probing the interaction between inactivation gating and Dd-sotalol block of HERG. *Circ. Res.* 87, 1012–1018. doi: 10.1161/01.RES.87.11.1012

Orsi, M., Sanderson, W. E., and Essex, J. W. (2009). Permeability of small molecules through a lipid bilayer: a multiscale simulation study. *J. Phys. Chem. B* 113, 12019–12029. doi: 10.1021/jp903248s

Ottaviani, G., Martel, S., and Carrupt, P. A. (2006). Parallel artificial membrane permeability assay: a new membrane for the fast prediction of passive human skin permeability. *J. Med. Chem.* 49, 3948–3954. doi: 10.1021/jm060230+

Phillips, J. C., Braun, R., Wang, W., Gumbart, J., Tajkhorshid, E., Villa, E., et al. (2005). Scalable molecular dynamics with NAMD. *J. Comput. Chem.* 26, 1781–1802. doi: 10.1002/jcc.20289

Pitman, M. C., Suits, F., MacKerell, A. D. Jr., and Feller, S. E. (2004). Molecular-level organization of saturated and polyunsaturated fatty acids in a phosphatidylcholine bilayer containing cholesterol. *Biochemistry* 43, 15318–15328. doi: 10.1021/bi048231w

Post, J. A., Verkleij, A. J., and Langer, G. A. (1995). Organization and function of sarcolemmal phospholipids in control and ischemic/reperfused cardiomyocytes. *J. Mol. Cell. Cardiol.* 27, 749–760. doi: 10.1016/0022-2828(95)90080-2

Quigley, E. M. M. (2011). Cisapride: what can we learn from the rise and fall of a prokinetic? *J. Dig. Dis.* 12, 147–156. doi: 10.1111/j.1751-2980.2011.00491.x

Redman-Furey, N. L., and Antinore, M. J. (1991). Determination of partition coefficients between dimyristoylphosphatidylcholine and water using differential scanning calorimetry. *Anal. Chim. Acta* 251, 79–81. doi: 10.1016/0003-2670(91)87118-Q

Roux, B., and Karplus, M. (1991). Ion transport in a model gramicidin channel. Structure and thermodynamics. *Biophys. J.* 59, 961–981. doi: 10.1016/S0006-3495(91)82311-6

Ryckaert, J.-P., Ciccotti, G., and Berendsen, H. J. C. (1977). Numerical integration of the cartesian equations of motion of a system with constraints: molecular dynamics of n-alkanes. *J. Comput. Phys.* 23, 327–341. doi: 10.1016/0021-9991(77)90098-5

Saxena, P., Zangerl-Plessl, E. M., Linder, T., Windisch, A., Hohaus, A., Timin, E., et al. (2016). New potential binding determinant for hERG channel inhibitors. *Sci. Rep.* 6:24182. doi: 10.1038/srep24182

Shaw, D. E., Grossman, J. P., Bank, J. A., Batson, B., Butts, J. A., Chao, J. C., et al. (2014). "Anton 2: RAISING the bar for performance and programmability in a special-purpose molecular dynamics supercomputer," in *Sc14: International Conference for High Performance Computing, Networking, Storage and Analysis* (New Orleans, LA), 41–53.

Sordillo, P. P., Sordillo, D. C., and Helson, L. (2015). Review: the prolonged QT interval: role of pro-inflammatory cytokines, reactive oxygen species and the ceramide and sphingosine-1 phosphate pathways. *In Vivo* 29, 619–636. Available online at: http://iv.iiarjournals.org/content/29/6/619.full

Swift, R. V., and Amaro, R. E. (2013). Back to the future: can physical models of passive membrane permeability help reduce drug candidate attrition and move us beyond QSPR? *Chem. Biol. Drug Des.* 81, 61–71. doi: 10.1111/cbdd.12074

Torrie, G. M., and Valleau, J. P. (1977). Nonphysical sampling distributions in Monte Carlo free-energy estimation: umbrella sampling. *J. Comput. Phys.* 23, 187–199. doi: 10.1016/0021-9991(77)90121-8

Touboul, P. (1993). Electrophysiologic properties of sotalol and d-sotalol. A current view. *Eur. Heart J.* 14(Suppl. H), 24–29.

Tuckerman, M., Berne, B. J., and Martyna, G. J. (1992). Reversible multiple time scale molecular dynamics. *J. Chem. Phys.* 97, 1990–2001. doi: 10.1063/1.463137

Vandenberg, J. I., Perry, M. D., Perrin, M. J., Mann, S. A., Ke, Y., and Hill, A. P. (2012). hERG K+ channels: structure, function, and clinical significance. *Physiol. Rev.* 92, 1393–1478. doi: 10.1152/physrev.00036.2011

Vanommeslaeghe, K., and MacKerell, A. D. (2012). Automation of the CHARMM general force field (CGenFF) I: bond perception and atom typing. *J. Chem. Inf. Model.* 52, 3144–3154. doi: 10.1021/ci300363c

Vanommeslaeghe, K., Hatcher, E., Acharya, C., Kundu, S., Zhong, S., Shim, J., et al. (2010). CHARMM general force field: a force field for drug-like molecules compatible with the CHARMM all-atom additive biological force fields. *J. Comput. Chem.* 31, 671–690. doi: 10.1002/jcc.21367

Vanommeslaeghe, K., Raman, E. P., and MacKerell, A. D. (2012). Automation of the CHARMM general force field (CGenFF) II: assignment of bonded parameters and partial atomic charges. *J. Chem. Inf. Model.* 52, 3155–3168. doi: 10.1021/ci3003649

Vorobyov, I., and Allen, T. W. (2011). On the role of anionic lipids in charged protein interactions with membranes. *Biochim. Biophys. Acta* 1808, 1673–1683. doi: 10.1016/j.bbamem.2010.11.009

Vorobyov, I., Bekker, B., and Allen, T. W. (2010). Electrostatics of deformable lipid membranes. *Biophys. J.* 98, 2904–2913. doi: 10.1016/j.bpj.2010.03.046

Vorobyov, I., Bennett, W. F., Tieleman, D. P., Allen, T. W., and Noskov, S. (2012). The role of atomic polarization in the thermodynamics of chloroform partitioning to lipid bilayers. *J. Chem. Theory Comput.* 8, 618–628. doi: 10.1021/ct200417p

Vorobyov, I., Olson, T. E., Kim, J. H., Koeppe, R. E. II., Andersen, O. S., and Allen, T. W. (2014). Ion-induced defect permeation of lipid membranes. *Biophys. J.* 106, 586–597. doi: 10.1016/j.bpj.2013.12.027

Waldo, A. L., Camm, A. J., Deruyter, H., Friedman, P. L., MacNeil, D. J., Pauls, J. F., et al. (1996). Effect of d-sotalol on mortality in patients with left ventricular dysfunction after recent and remote myocardial infarction. The SWORD Investigators. Survival With Oral d-Sotalol. *Lancet* 348, 7–12. doi: 10.1016/S0140-6736(96)02149-6

Wang, W., and MacKinnon, R. (2017). Cryo-EM Structure of the Open Human *Ether-à-go-go*-Related K^+ Channel hERG. *Cell* 169, 422.e410–430.e410. doi: 10.1016/j.cell.2017.03.048

Wang, Y., Guo, J., Perissinotti, L. L., Lees-Miller, J., Teng, G., Durdagi, S., et al. (2016). Role of the pH in state-dependent blockade of hERG currents. *Sci. Rep.* 6:32536. doi: 10.1038/srep32536

Whicher, J. R., and MacKinnon, R. (2016). Structure of the voltage-gated K(+) channel Eag1 reveals an alternative voltage sensing mechanism. *Science* 353, 664–669. doi: 10.1126/science.aaf8070

Windley, M. J., Abi-Gerges, N., Fermini, B., Hancox, J. C., Vandenberg, J. I., and Hill, A. P. (2017). Measuring kinetics and potency of hERG block for CiPA. *J. Pharmacol. Toxicol. Methods* 87, 99–107. doi: 10.1016/j.vascn.2017.02.017

Yang, P. C., Moreno, J. D., Miyake, C. Y., Vaughn-Behrens, S. B., Jeng, M. T., Grandi, E., et al. (2016). *In silico* prediction of drug therapy in catecholaminergic polymorphic ventricular tachycardia. *J. Physiol.* 594, 567–593. doi: 10.1113/JP271282

Yang, P. C., Perissinotti, L. L., Lopez-Redondo, F., Wang, Y., Demarco, K. R., Jeng, M. T., et al. (2017). A multiscale computational modelling approach predicts mechanisms of female sex risk in the setting of arousal-induced arrhythmias. *J. Physiol.* 595, 4695–4723. doi: 10.1113/JP273142

Yap, Y. G., and Camm, A. J. (2003). Drug induced QT prolongation and torsades de pointes. *Heart* 89, 1363–1372. doi: 10.1136/heart.89.11.1363

Yu, H., and Adedoyin, A. (2003). ADME-Tox in drug discovery: integration of experimental and computational technologies. *Drug Discov. Today* 8, 852–861. doi: 10.1016/S1359-6446(03)02828-9

Yu, W., He, X., Vanommeslaeghe, K., and MacKerell, A. D. Jr. (2012). Extension of the CHARMM General Force Field to sulfonyl-containing compounds and its utility in biomolecular simulations. *J. Comput. Chem.* 33, 2451–2468. doi: 10.1002/jcc.23067

8

Optimization of an *In silico* Cardiac Cell Model for Proarrhythmia Risk Assessment

Sara Dutta, Kelly C. Chang, Kylie A. Beattie, Jiansong Sheng, Phu N. Tran, Wendy W. Wu, Min Wu, David G. Strauss, Thomas Colatsky† and Zhihua Li*

Division of Applied Regulatory Science, Office of Clinical Pharmacology, Office of Translational Sciences, Center for Drug Evaluation and Research, U.S. Food and Drug Administration, Silver Spring, MD, United States

***Correspondence:**
Zhihua Li
zhihua.li@fda.hhs.gov

†Present Address:
Thomas Colatsky,
Marshview Life Science Advisors,
Seabrook Island, SC, United States

Drug-induced Torsade-de-Pointes (TdP) has been responsible for the withdrawal of many drugs from the market and is therefore of major concern to global regulatory agencies and the pharmaceutical industry. The Comprehensive *in vitro* Proarrhythmia Assay (CiPA) was proposed to improve prediction of TdP risk, using *in silico* models and *in vitro* multi-channel pharmacology data as integral parts of this initiative. Previously, we reported that combining dynamic interactions between drugs and the rapid delayed rectifier potassium current (IKr) with multi-channel pharmacology is important for TdP risk classification, and we modified the original O'Hara Rudy ventricular cell mathematical model to include a Markov model of IKr to represent dynamic drug-IKr interactions (IKr-dynamic ORd model). We also developed a novel metric that could separate drugs with different TdP liabilities at high concentrations based on total electronic charge carried by the major inward ionic currents during the action potential. In this study, we further optimized the IKr-dynamic ORd model by refining model parameters using published human cardiomyocyte experimental data under control and drug block conditions. Using this optimized model and manual patch clamp data, we developed an updated version of the metric that quantifies the net electronic charge carried by major inward and outward ionic currents during the steady state action potential, which could classify the level of drug-induced TdP risk across a wide range of concentrations and pacing rates. We also established a framework to quantitatively evaluate a system's robustness against the induction of early afterdepolarizations (EADs), and demonstrated that the new metric is correlated with the cell's robustness to the pro-EAD perturbation of IKr conductance reduction. In summary, in this work we present an optimized model that is more consistent with experimental data, an improved metric that can classify drugs at concentrations both near and higher than clinical exposure, and a physiological framework to check the relationship between a metric and EAD. These findings provide a solid foundation for using *in silico* models for the regulatory assessment of TdP risk under the CiPA paradigm.

Keywords: Torsade-de-Pointes (TdP), Comprehensive *in vitro* Proarrhythmia Assay (CiPA), rapid delayed rectifier potassium current (IKr), *in silico* cardiac cell model, drug block, proarrythmia risk, model optimization

INTRODUCTION

Drug-induced Torsade-de-Pointes (TdP) is a lethal arrhythmia that has caused removal of several drugs from the market (Gintant, 2008). The current cardiac safety paradigm (described by the ICH E14 and S7B guidelines) focuses on two markers to assess TdP risk: *in vitro* block of the hERG (human Ether-à-go-go-Related Gene) channel (representing the rapidly activating delayed rectifier potassium current, or IKr), and prolongation of the QTc interval in clinical studies (Sager et al., 2014). However, while eliminating the incidence of TdP in marketed drugs, this testing regime primarily aims at detecting delayed ventricular repolarization rather than the clinical end point TdP, and may be assigning proarrhythmia liability to drugs that could in fact be safe (Sager et al., 2014). Therefore, the Comprehensive *in vitro* Proarrhythmia Assay (CiPA) was proposed as a new regulatory paradigm that assesses drug TdP risk by combining measurements of drug effects on multiple cardiac ionic currents *in vitro* with *in silico* modeling of drug effects on the ventricular myocyte (Sager et al., 2014). The O'Hara Rudy cardiac cell model (ORd) (O'Hara et al., 2011) was chosen as the consensus base *in silico* model and a set of 28 drugs with known levels of clinical TdP risk (high, intermediate, low/none) were identified for the development and evaluation of the CiPA paradigm (Colatsky et al., 2016; Fermini et al., 2016). The three TdP risk categories were assigned by a Clinical Translation Working Group comprised of clinical cardiologists, safety pharmacologists, and clinical electrophysiologists according to published and publically available data and expert opinion. The 28 CiPA drugs were separated into a training set of 12 compounds to be used for calibration of the *in silico* model and the remaining 16 compounds are to be used later for validating the model. Both the training and validation compound sets comprise drugs that cover the full range of TdP risk categories and demonstrate varied electrophysiological profiles.

Previous studies have presented computational frameworks to assess TdP risk (Mirams et al., 2011; Kramer et al., 2013; Lancaster and Sobie, 2016), but their use within the CiPA framework is limited due to their differing TdP risk categories from those defined in CiPA. In addition, prior studies simulated drug effects using the half-maximal blocking concentration (IC50) for different drugs, which assumes simple pore block of the ion channels and neglects any intricacies of drug-ion channel interactions that may be important factors in predicting relative TdP risk. The importance of incorporating a kinetic representation of drug-ion channel interactions has been demonstrated in previous publications (Di Veroli et al., 2013, 2014; Li et al., 2017). In the Li et al. (2017) study we recently reported the development of a novel IKr dynamic model that can capture drug-channel dynamic interactions, and the integration of this IKr model into the ORd cardiac model with multi-channel pharmacology data. This IKr-dynamic ORd model (hereinafter referred to as the original IKr-dyn ORd model) was calibrated based on the original ORd model so that it can reproduce experimentally recorded adult human left ventricular cardiomyocyte action potential (AP) morphology and rate dependency under control (drug-free) conditions. However, this model calibration process in our previous work did not include experimental AP changes under the influence of different channel blocking drugs. This may negatively affect the model's predictive power as this model is intended for simulating drug effects under channel blocking conditions.

In this study we further optimized the original IKr-dyn ORd model by adjusting channel conductance values of major ionic currents according to human ventricular cardiomyocyte experimental data in the presence and absence of various drugs with different channel blocking activities. We show that this optimization procedure allowed the model (hereinafter referred to as optimized IKr-dyn ORd model) to quantify more accurately the impact of each individual current on the AP. We then screened a series of published and novel metrics computed by this model based on their capability of stratifying CiPA training compounds into their corresponding TdP risk categories using drug-IKr binding kinetics and multi-channel pharmacology data collected earlier through manual patch clamp systems (Li et al., 2017). The best metric identified to date is based on drug-induced changes to the net charge carried by ionic currents (qNet) during the AP, which can stratify the 12 CiPA training drugs into three TdP risk levels across various conditions. We also show that the increased predictive power of this metric is mechanistically linked to the incorporation of IKr-drug binding dynamics and the improved representation of the block effects of individual currents, two important features of the optimized IKr-dyn ORd model. Finally, we developed a framework to evaluate a cell's robustness against EAD generation, and demonstrated that the new qNet metric is correlated with the system's repolarization robustness to external pro-EAD perturbations that could reduce the membrane density of the hERG channel (IKr conductance).

METHODS

Optimization of the IKr-Dynamic ORd Model

The original IKr-dyn ORd model (described in Li et al., 2017 and Expanded Methods in the Supplemental Material) was further modified (optimized IKr-dyn ORd) by scaling five ionic current conductances [IKr, the slow rectifier potassium current (IKs), inwardly rectifying potassium current (IK1), the L-type calcium current (ICaL) and the late sodium current (INaL)] so that the model provides a good fit to published APD rate dependence experimental data for control and five channel blockers (O'Hara et al., 2011). The optimization was performed using the model parameterization algorithm described in Li et al. (2014). Briefly, an initial set of scaling factors was defined within a certain range (between 0.001 and 9) and their goodness of fit was assessed using an objective cost function defined as the weighted sum of the squared errors between model simulations

Abbreviations: CiPA, Comprehensive *in vitro* proarrhythmia assay; TdP, Torsade-de-Pointes; ORd, O'Hara Rudy dynamic cell model (O'Hara et al., 2011); IKr-dyn ORd, ORd model with dynamic IKr; Inet, net current (sum of currents ICaL, INaL, IKr, IKs, IK1, Ito); qNet, charge passed by Inet from the beginning to the end of the AP beat (same for qCaL and ICaL, qNaL and INaL...); cqInward, change in charge passed by ICaL and INaL; Cmax, free maximum plasma clinical drug exposures.

and experimental measurements. The set of scaling factors then underwent iterative changes (i.e., mutation and recombination) to create new generations of parameters and this process was continued until the convergence criterion was met (when the change in the minimum error of the new parameters is less than 5% over the last 30 generations). The experimental data used for fitting were taken from Figure 8 of the ORd model paper (O'Hara et al., 2011) and comprise APD rate dependence data for control and 5 drug blocking conditions: 1 μM E-4031 (70% IKr block), 1 μM HMR-1556 (90% IKs block), 1 μM nisoldipine (90% ICaL block), 100 μM BaCl2 (90% IK1 block), 10 μM mexiletine (54% INaL, 9% IKr, and 20% ICaL block). The simulated percentage of block for all drugs was kept the same as in the ORd model paper (O'Hara et al., 2011), apart from mexiletine, which used new pharmacology data from manual patch clamp systems at physiological temperatures (Crumb et al., 2016). The algorithm was run using in-house developed R scripts (R Core Team, 2014) and C programs using the Snow, Rmpi and deSolve packages (lsoda solver with a 10^{-6} relative and absolute tolerance) (Yu, 2002; Soetaert et al., 2010; Tierney et al., 2015) on the FDA High Performance Computer (HPC) with 160 cores.

Simulation Protocol for Metric Evaluation

All simulations were run from control steady state conditions (after 1,000 beats) at varying cycle lengths (CLs) 1,000, 2,000, and 4,000 ms and stimulus of −80 μA/μF for 0.5 ms (as in the original model). Block of ion channels at various concentrations were simulated and run for another 1,000 beats to reach a new steady state with drug. The last two beats were analyzed to check for alternans, which was observed in the presence of early afterdepolarizations (EADs), defined as having a positive derivative during the repolarization phase of the AP. The pharmacology data for the 12 CiPA training compounds (the full list and their corresponding risk categories can be found in Supplemental Table 1) were the same as in our previous report (Li et al., 2017), where drug-IKr binding kinetic parameters were estimated using an *in vitro* IKr dynamic protocol and IC50/Hill coefficients based on Crumb et al. (2016) were used for the remaining channels [the peak sodium current (INa), INaL, ICaL, IK1, IKs and transient outward potassium current (Ito); all the parameters can be found in the Supplemental Tables 2 and 3]. Simulations were run for a range of drug concentrations: from 0.5x up to 25x free maximum plasma clinical drug exposures (Cmax). Simulations were run in R and C using the deSolve package (Soetaert et al., 2010).

We assessed a range of standard metrics as also considered in Mirams et al. (2011), Lancaster and Sobie (2016): resting membrane potential (resting Vm), maximum upstroke velocity (dV/dtmax), peak membrane potential (peak Vm), APD at 50% of the amplitude (APD50), APD at 90% of the amplitude (APD90), APD triangulation (APDtri) defined as APD90-APD50, diastolic intracellular calcium concentration ($[Ca^{2+}]_i$) (diastolic Ca), peak $[Ca^{2+}]_i$ (peak Ca), calcium transient duration at 50% (CaD50) and 90% (CaD90) of the amplitude, calcium transient triangulation (Catri) defined as CaD90-CaD50, as well as the cqInward metric that quantifies the change in the amount of charge carried by INaL and ICaL, which demonstrated good separation between risk categories in our previous report (Li et al., 2017). In addition, we considered a new metric (qNet) calculated as the net charge constituting (the integral or area under the curve of) the net current (Inet) from the beginning to the end of the simulated beat (defined as Inet = ICaL + INaL + IKr + IKs + IK1 + Ito). The currents making up Inet within our study play an important role in modulating arrhythmic risk and have been chosen based on input from pharmaceutical company scientists and safety pharmacology experts as the main currents of interest within the CiPA paradigm, as outlined in Fermini et al. (2016).

To assess the robustness of a cell against EAD generation, we simulated an added perturbation by reducing the maximum conductance of IKr and reporting the minimum IKr reduction needed to trigger an EAD. Simulations were run for varying degrees of IKr conductance reduction (using a binary search algorithm) at a CL of 2,000 ms with a precision of 0.01%. For each IKr reduction tested, EADs were defined as having a positive differential (dV/dt) during the plateau phase of the AP (between APD30 and APD90) after 100 beats. The cell model was pulsed for a 100 beats before checking for EADs to allow the system to reach quasi-steady state, as in Kurata et al. (2017). The minimum IKr conductance reduction needed to trigger an EAD was named IKr reduction threshold, which reflects the system's repolarization robustness against, or distance from, EADs. To assess the relationship between the metric and the repolarization robustness, we calculated the correlation coefficients (using the pearson method) between the metric at steady state after 1,000 beats (without added IKr reduction) and the IKr reduction threshold for each drug across a series of concentrations (0.5x–25x Cmax). Situations where no IKr reduction threshold could be calculated (no EADs could be induced for the highest IKr reduction tested) or IKr reduction threshold is 0 (an EAD occurred without any added perturbation) were excluded from the correlation calculation.

Classification Methods

To assess the ability of the metrics to identify each drug's TdP risk level, we performed a proportional odds logistic regression classification and a leave-one-out validation, as in Mirams et al. (2011). If EADs were observed, the metric value at the concentration prior to EAD generation was used for the classification. We used the R lrm function from the rms package (https://CRAN.R-project.org/package=rms) and calculated the classification training error for each metric as follows: the mean (across 12 drugs) of the absolute error (difference between predicted and known risk categories), with the risk categories defined as 1 = low risk, 2 = intermediate risk and 3 = high risk. The proportional odds logistic regression model is a regression model for ordinal dependent variables, and accounts for the ordering by using cumulative probabilities defined as the odds of $(Y \leq i) = P(Y \leq i)/(1 - P(Y \leq i))$ for each risk category i, where Y is the variable that represents a drug's risk category and P(X) is the probability of X. The function uses maximum likelihood estimates to calculate the probability of each drug being a member of each risk category, and the drug is assigned to the risk category corresponding to its highest probability. We then performed a leave-one-out validation by removing one drug from the data set and then predicting its risk category based on the classification of the remaining drugs. This was performed in turn for each drug within the data set and its leave-one-out prediction error was calculated the same way as the training error.

RESULTS

Optimized IKr-dyn ORd Model

The optimized IKr-dyn ORd model was built by scaling the conductance of the main ion currents (IKr, IK1, IKs, INaL, ICaL) of the original IKr-dyn ORd model (presented in Li et al., 2017) to fit the APD rate dependence experimental data in control and drug block conditions from O'Hara et al. (2011). The set of scaling factors that gives the best fit for the optimized model is as follows: scaling IKr by 1.013, IKs by 1.870, IK1 by 1.698, ICaL by 1.007, and INaL by 2.661, as summarized in **Table 1**. A comparison of the simulation results from both the original and optimized models to the experimental data is shown in **Figure 1** and the corresponding sum of squares errors (between simulation and experimental data) are shown in **Table 2**. Sum of squares error for the original ORd model as presented in their paper (O'Hara et al., 2011) are also shown in **Table 2** for comparison purposes. We see that although for control and some current blocking conditions the original IKr-dyn ORd model has errors similar to the original ORd model, for other conditions the errors were worsened (IK1 and ICaL blocking experiments), resulting in an average error bigger than the original ORd model (72.33 vs. 57.77). However, the discrepancy between simulations and experiments was significantly reduced in the new optimized IKr-dyn ORd model.

As can be seen in **Figure 1A**, under control conditions both the original IKr-dyn ORd and optimized IKr-dyn ORd models display similar behavior. Although for control data points, the optimized IKr-dyn ORd model fitting is slightly worse than the original IKr-dyn ORd model (fitting error 22.63 vs. 18.82 in **Table 2**), the average fit across both control and all drug block conditions is much better for the optimized IKr-dyn ORd model compared to the original IKr-dyn ORd model (fitting error 30.81 vs. 72.33). The main improvements in the quality of fit to the experimental data are observed for drug blocking conditions, especially with mexiletine (INaL blocker) and E-4031 (IKr blocker) (**Figures 1B,E** respectively). In the case of mexiletine, a reduction in the fitting error from 91.09 (original IKr-dyn ORd model) to 18.36 (optimized IKr-dyn ORd model) was achieved (**Table 2**). **Figure 1B** shows that, with the original IKr-dyn ORd model, the simulated APD prolongation with mexiletine is significantly longer than experimental data. A similar pattern can be seen for the IKr blocker E-4031 (**Table 2** and **Figure 1E**). Due to the opposite roles of INaL and IKr in prolonging AP (Johannesen et al., 2016), this suggests that block of INaL is underestimated and that of IKr is overestimated in the original IKr-dyn ORd model. The optimized model corrected these inaccuracies with better fitting to the experimental data, which is important for TdP risk assessment as it is known that INaL block plays an important role in counteracting pro-arrhythmic APD prolongation of IKr block (Orth et al., 2006; Johannesen et al., 2016).

To further understand the contribution of various ionic currents to AP profile after the optimization process, we compared the simulated AP traces and the ionic currents over the time course of the steady state AP between the original and our optimized IKr-dyn ORd model at different cycle lengths. As described earlier in this section all of the current conductances are increased in the optimized IKr-dyn ORd model (**Table 1**). However, the AP shapes from both models under control conditions are very similar, as shown in **Figure 2A**. This is consistent with the fact that both models fit the control AP morphology parameters (**Figure 1A**) reasonably well. On the other hand, while only a small change in current amplitude is observed for ICaL (**Figure 2C**), which only has a 0.7% change in conductance (**Table 1**), clear differences are observed for all other currents (IKr, INaL, IKs and IK1) with the biggest changes occurring for INaL (conductance is increased by 166.1% between the optimized and original models as shown in **Table 1**). This further demonstrates that INaL plays a bigger role in the optimized model than the original IKr-dyn ORd model.

TABLE 1 | Conductance scaling factors for the original and optimized IKr-dynamic O'Hara-Rudy models (original and optimized IKr-dyn ORd): current conductances of the rapid (IKr) and slow (IKs) rectifier potassium current, inwardly rectifying potassium current (IK1), L-type calcium current (ICaL) and late sodium current (INaL) in the model are multiplied by the corresponding scaling factor.

Scaled currents	Original IKr-dyn ORd model	Optimized IKr-dyn ORd model
IKr	0.9	1.013
IKs	1.0	1.870
IK1	1.0	1.698
ICaL	1.0	1.007
INaL	1.0	2.661

Note that the IKr conductance in the original IKr-dyn ORd model was scaled as described in Li et al. (2017).

Candidate Metrics

We then investigated whether the optimized IKr-dyn ORd model could be used to stratify proarrhythmia risk levels. As a first step we explored the changes in AP and individual currents induced by three representative drugs (one taken from each one of the CiPA TdP risk categories), using pharmacology data as used in Li et al. (2017). Since it is known that the subtle balance between inward (such as INaL and ICaL) and outward (such as IKr, IKs, IK1, and Ito) currents underlies the generation of EADs, a mechanistic precursor to TdP (Vos et al., 1995; Volders et al., 2000; Wu et al., 2002; Weiss et al., 2010), we also examined the net current between inward and outward currents (Inet) in addition to individual currents. **Figure 3** shows simulations of AP, Inet, ICaL, INaL, IKr, IKs, IK1, and Ito for ranolazine (low risk), cisapride (intermediate risk) and dofetilide (high risk), for a CL of 2,000 ms and a dose of 25x Cmax

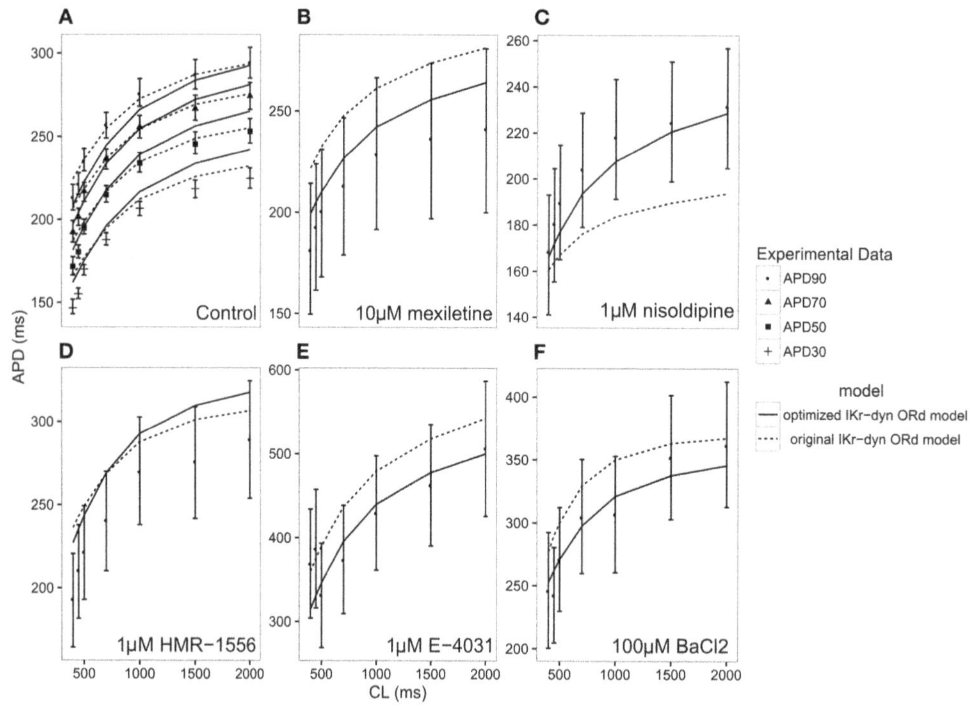

FIGURE 1 | Steady state action potential duration (APD) rate dependency under the conditions of control **(A)**, 10 μM mexiletine [late sodium current INaL block **(B)**], 1 μM nisoldipine [L-type calcium current ICaL block **(C)**], 1 μM HMR-1556 [slow rectifier potassium current IKs block **(D)**], 1 μM E-4031 [rapid rectifier potassium current IKr block **(E)**] and 100 μM $BACl_2$ [inwardly rectifying potassium current IK1 block **(F)**] at varying cycle lengths (CLs) for the original dynamic IKr O'Hara Rudy model (original IKr-dyn ORd; dashed lines) and the optimized dynamic IKr O'Hara Rudy model (optimized IKr-dyn ORd model; solid line). Experimental data mean (symbol) and standard deviation (error bars) are from O'Hara et al. (2011). Control **(A)** shows APD at 90% (APD90; filled circles), 70% (APD70; filled triangles), 50% (APD50; filled squares) and 30% (APD30; plus sign) repolarization. All other panels show APD90.

TABLE 2 | Sum of squares error (divided by 100) between experimental action potential duration (APD) rate dependence mean data (from Figure 8 in O'Hara et al., 2011) and the original O'Hara Rudy model (original ORd) (O'Hara et al., 2011), the original IKr-dyn ORd (Li et al., 2017) as well as the optimized IKr-dyn ORd under different conditions: control, mexiletine (blocks mainly INaL), HMR 1556 (blocks IKs), E-4031 (blocks IKr), BaCl2 (blocks IK1) and nisoldipine (blocks ICaL).

Experiment	Sum of squares error		
	Original ORd	Original IKr-dyn ORd	Optimized IKr-dyn ORd
Control	17.20	18.82	22.63
Mexiletine (INaL)	92.92*	91.09	18.36
HMR 1556 (IKs)	56.35	57.08	55.34
E4031 (IKr)	145.03	144.87	72.33
Bacl2 (IK1)	29.83	67.47	11.41
Nisoldipine (ICaL)	5.29	54.62	4.76
Average	57.77	72.33	30.81

**Error was calculated using the updated mexiletine IC50 data (Crumb et al., 2016); using the block suggested in the ORd paper of 90% INaL block (O'Hara et al., 2011), the sum of squares error is of 38.48, changing the average error to 48.70.*

using our optimized model. A slow pacing rate (CL 2,000 ms) is used here because bradycardia is a known risk factor for TdP (Kurita et al., 1992; Kallergis et al., 2012), and a high concentration (25x Cmax) is used to highlight the potential differences between various risk levels. The amount of electronic charge carried by each current is calculated as the area under the curve (AUC) of the individual current trace and is plotted for Inet in **Figure 3C**.

We see in **Figure 3A** that all three drugs cause prolongation of APD and the low risk drug, ranolazine, shows a greater prolongation of APD compared to the intermediate risk drug, cisapride (266.78 vs. 176 ms). The performance of APD90 as a metric for all the drugs from 0.5 to 25x Cmax, can be seen in Supplemental Figure 1. In fact, verapamil and ranolazine (both low risk) display APDs greater than most intermediate risk drugs over a wide range of doses. Therefore, the amount of APD prolongation is not a good indicator of the TdP risk of a drug, demonstrating the unsuitability of APD alone as a marker for TdP risk. However, we notice that Inet (**Figure 3B**), calculated as the sum of the five main currents that modulate the plateau phase of the action potential (ICaL, INaL, IK1, IKr, IKs, and Ito, shown in **Figures 3D–I**), does correlate with the TdP risk category. As shown in **Figure 3C**, the order of qNet (charge carried by Inet integrated from the beginning to the end of the AP beat) is consistent with the rank order of TdP risk levels for the three drugs. At the end of the CL, ranolazine has a qNet of 0.061 μC/μF while cisapride and dofetilide have a qNet of 0.037 μC/μF and 0.013 μC/μF, respectively. A detailed

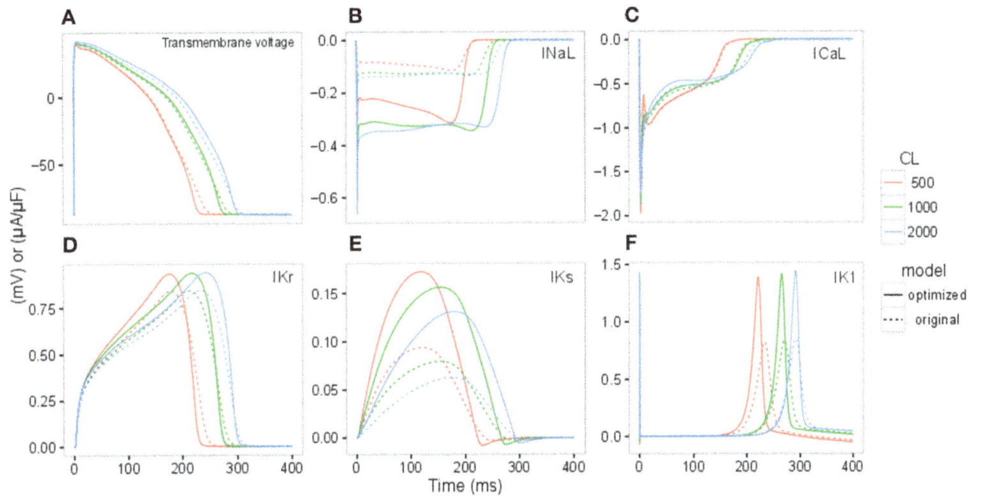

FIGURE 2 | Action potential (AP) **(A)**, INaL **(B)**, ICaL **(C)**, IKr **(D)**, IKs **(E)**, IK1 **(F)** traces under control conditions for the original IKr-dyn ORd (dashed line) and the optimized IKr-dyn ORd (solid line) for CLs of 500 (red), 1,000 (green) and 2,000 (blue) ms.

examination of the individual current profiles reveals why ranolazine caused the least amount of qNet decrease. As shown in **Figures 3D, G**, ranolazine (green lines) caused a marked decrease of the absolute amount of charge carried by IKr (qKr decrease of 0.119 μC/μF) and INaL (qNaL decrease of 0.07 μC/μF) at the end of the AP beat compared to control (black lines). Because the outward current IKr and inward current INaL have opposite directions, ranolazine-induced reduction (in absolute values) of the two currents balanced each other and resulted in only a small change of the net charge at the end of the AP (qNet, **Figure 3C**). In contrast, dofetilide (**Figure 3D**, red lines) and cisapride (**Figure 3D**, blue lines) caused a significant reduction of qKr (0.135 and 0.063 μC/μF respectively) through direct channel blocking, and a slight increase of qNaL through prolonged APD. These two effects changed Inet in the same direction and worked together to decrease qNet significantly, with dofetilide causing the biggest decrease due to more significant blocking of IKr. Note that these drugs have some effects on other currents (Ito, IKs, and IK1) as well, but those changes are relatively small and will not change the rank order of qNet values significantly for the three drugs tested here. However, these other currents may become important for drugs that directly block them. For example, the effects on ICaL may be critical in determining the qNet change and risk level for a calcium blocker.

These initial promising results prompted us to calculate this new Inet-based metric, qNet, for all 12 CiPA training compounds and systematically compare its capability of separating the three TdP risk levels to a range of commonly tested metrics (described in the Methods section). The risk categories, IC50 and IKr dynamic parameters for each drug are listed in Supplemental Tables 1–3. Included in the comparison is also the cqInward metric, described in our previous study and defined as the normalized drug-induced change of the charge carried by the inward currents INaL and ICaL (Li et al., 2017). As shown in **Figure 4**, we calculated the classification training error for each metric over a range of doses (0.5–25x Cmax) and a range of CLs (1,000, 2,000, and 4,000 ms) for the 12 CiPA training compounds. This error quantifies the mean (across the 12 CiPA drugs) difference between known and predicted risk levels for each metric. We can see that across the full range of concentrations and all CLs the qNet metric shows the smallest classification training error. Notably, the qNet metric shows a classification training error of 0 for concentrations greater than or equal to 1x Cmax, meaning it consistently classifies each of the 12 CiPA training compounds into the correct TdP risk category. The cqInward metric performance is comparable to that of qNet at low pacing rates (4,000 ms) and high drug concentrations. All of the other standard metrics we considered show training errors that never come down to 0, which fluctuate across the range of doses.

The results presented in **Figure 4** are consistent with the leave-one-out validation described in **Table 3** performed on a subset of the doses tested (1, 10, and 20x Cmax) for a CL of 2,000 ms; the cqInward and qNet show the smallest prediction errors with values of 0.33 and 0.08 respectively at 20x Cmax. The other next best performing metrics are peak Vm with an error of 0.42 and APD50, APD90 with errors of 0.5 at Cmax 20x. Of note, at 1x Cmax, qNet and APD90 all have the same prediction error of 0.17. This is because at lower concentrations (1x Cmax) the effects of each drug are harder to differentiate due to there often being only subtle effects on the AP morphology. However, the CiPA paradigm assumes that the assessment of TdP risk may occur at any time during drug discovery and development, even prior to the time the clinical effective drug concentrations are known with any certainty. In addition, the incidence of clinical TdP is limited and not necessarily related strictly to normal (1x) clinical exposure (i.e., concomitant factors may play a role in expressing clinical TdP events). Therefore, we propose that a metric should be evaluated under multiple physiological and pharmacological conditions. The overall evidence suggest

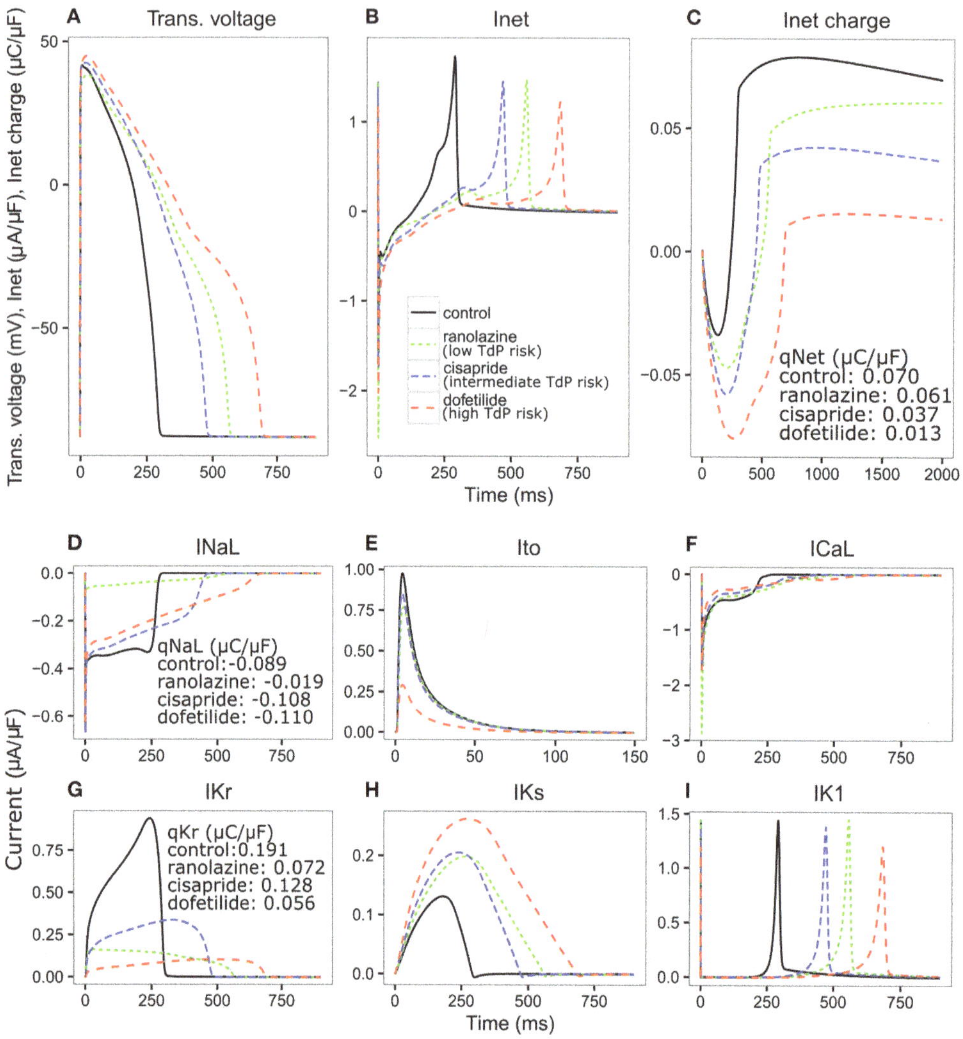

FIGURE 3 | Transmembrane voltage [Trans. voltage **(A)**], net current [Inet **(B)**], charge carried by Inet **(C)**, INaL **(D)**, Ito **(E)**, ICaL **(F)**, IKr **(G)**, IKs **(H)**, IK1 **(I)** traces for control (black solid line), ranolazine, a low TdP risk drug (green dashed line narrow spacing), cisapride, an intermediate TdP risk drug (blue dashed line normal spacing), and dofetilide, a high TdP risk drug (red dashed line wide spacing), at 25x Cmax for 2,000 ms CL using the optimized IKr-dyn ORd. Charge carried by Inet, INaL and IKr integrated from the beginning to the end of the AP beat (qX) are displayed on the graph.

that qNet is the best among all the metrics tested, because it has a training error of 0 across a wide range concentrations (1–25x Cmax) at various pacing frequencies (2,000 and 4,000 ms), and the lowest leave-one-out error at all concentrations tested.

The Impact of IKr-Drug Binding Kinetics and Channel Conductance Optimization on Risk Level Stratification

Compared to the original ORd (i.e., the consensus base model for CiPA), the optimized IKr-dyn ORd model presented in this work has two important changes: the incorporation of a dynamic IKr model to capture drug binding kinetics (Li et al., 2017), and an improved set of channel conductances to better represent the contribution of individual currents to AP (**Figures 1, 2**). In order to shed light on possible mechanistic differences among the drugs tested, we used the best candidate metric qNet as a benchmark, and compared the performance of the optimized IKr-dyn ORd model with model variations where each of the changes was removed in turn. **Figure 5** shows computed qNet values for the 12 CiPA training drugs calculated over a range of drug doses from 0.5x to 25x Cmax when using the optimized IKr-dyn ORd model (**Figure 5A**), a model variation without incorporating the IKr dynamic model (**Figure 5B**) and a model variation incorporating the IKr dynamic model but without optimizing channel conductances (**Figure 5C**). In line with results from **Figure 4** and **Table 3**, the metric qNet shows clear separation between the 3 TdP risk categories across the range of doses tested with the optimized IKr-dyn ORd model (**Figure 5A**); however, this is not the case for the other two model variations (**Figures 5B,C**).

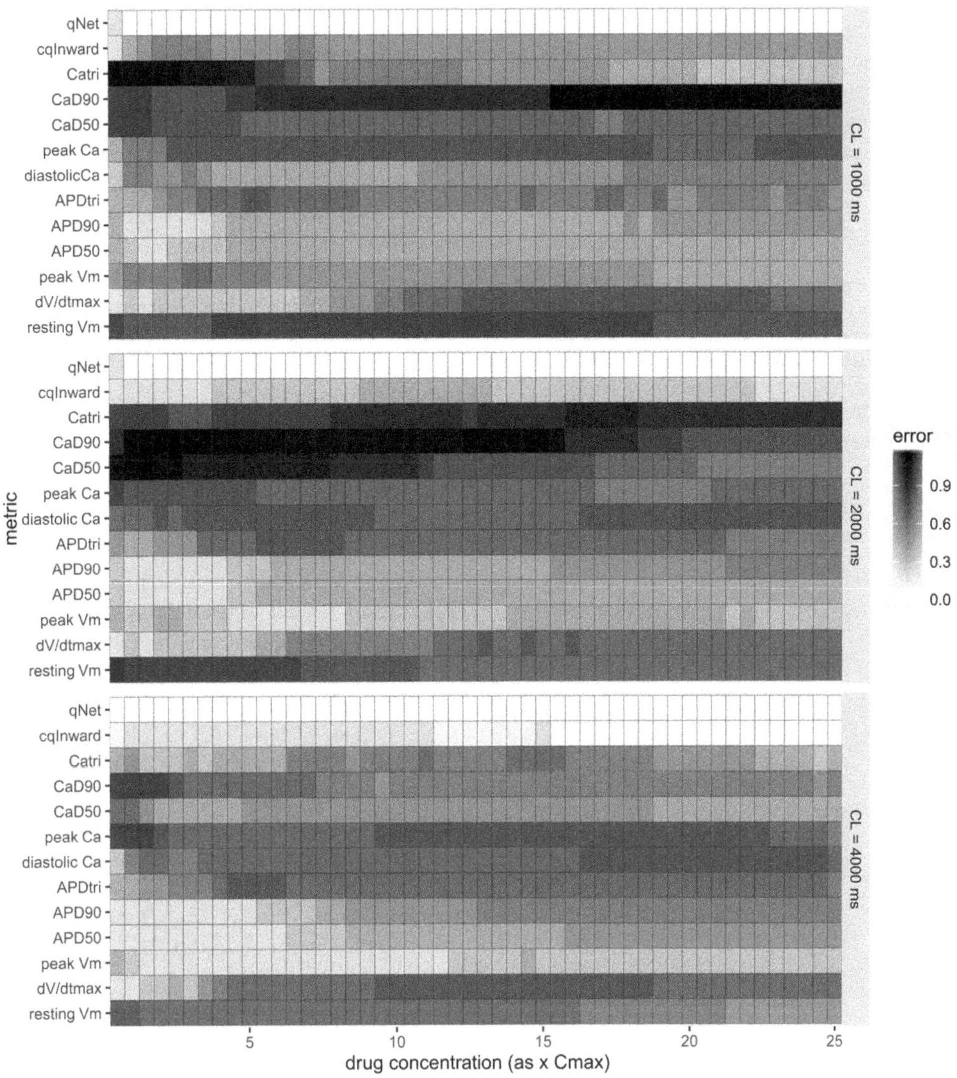

FIGURE 4 | Classification training error for a range of metrics [resting membrane potential (resting Vm), maximum upstroke velocity (dV/dtmax), peak membrane potential (peak Vm), APD50, APD90, action potential (AP) triangulation (APDtri), diastolic intracellular calcium concentration ($[Ca^{2+}]_i$) (diastolic Ca), peak $[Ca^{2+}]_i$ (peak Ca), calcium transient duration at 50 and 90% of the amplitude (CaD50 and CaD90), calcium transient triangulation (Catri), change in amount of charge carried by INaL and ICaL (cqInward) and the charge carried by Inet at the end of the AP beat normalized to control (qNet)] for varying drug doses (0.5–25x Cmax) and varying CLs (1,000, 2,000, and 4,000 ms). Each box represents the mean (across 12 drugs) error (between predicted and known risk levels) for each metric at each concentration (0.5–25X Cmax). A training error of 0 represents perfect separation between the risk categories.

The first model variation we tested does not have the IKr dynamic model incorporated but instead uses simple IC50s to represent channel block (**Figure 5B**). Note that this model variant has gone through a channel conductance optimization process similar to that presented in this article, as described in Dutta et al. (2016), so the difference observed between this model variant (**Figure 5B**) and the full optimized IKr-dyn ORd model (**Figure 5A**) is mainly due to the different representation of IKr block (dynamic vs. IC50s). From **Figure 5B** we can see that there are two intermediate risk drugs that are not correctly categorized: cisapride that is mixed with the high risk drugs, and chlorpromazine that is mixed with the low risk drugs. Cisapride is a potent and selective IKr blocker (IC50 10.1 nM and Cmax 2.6 nM see Supplementary Material), with a safety margin (IKr IC50/Cmax) of 3.8 (Redfern et al., 2003), which is close to that of the high risk drug dofetilide (IC50 4.87 nM and Cmax 2 nM, safety margin 2.4) for example. So if IC50 data are used with an assumption of simple pore drug block, cisapride is grouped with the high risk drugs. However, when we consider the IKr-drug binding dynamic data (Li et al., 2017), cisapride, but not high risk drugs like dofetilide, can rapidly dissociate from the hERG channel during diastolic intervals because it is not trapped in the closed channel. Consequently, cisapride has an actual block potency lower than high risk drugs despite similar IKr IC50/Cmax ratio, which may explain why it belongs to the intermediate rather than high risk level. On the other hand, chlorpromazine is not a potent IKr blocker (safety margin 24.4, similar to other low risk drugs) so when we look at IC50 only it is classified closer to the low risk drugs. But when IKr dynamic data are considered, chlorpromazine is highly trapped in the closed hERG channel and very slow in unbinding during diastolic intervals (Li et al., 2017). This makes it more dangerous than its IKr IC50 suggests and thus classified as an intermediate rather than low risk drug. This demonstrates that including a dynamic representation of IKr-ion channel interactions is important for categorizing TdP risk of drugs and IC50 data alone are not sufficient.

TABLE 3 | Leave-one-out prediction error for a range of metrics at a CL of 2,000 ms and 3 doses (1, 10, and 20x Cmax): resting membrane potential (resting Vm), maximum upstroke velocity (dV/dtmax), peak membrane potential (peak Vm), APD at 50 and 90% of the amplitude (APD50 and APD90), action potential (AP) triangulation (APDtri), diastolic intracellular calcium concentration ($[Ca^{2+}]_i$) (diastolic Ca), peak $[Ca^{2+}]_i$ (peak Ca), calcium transient duration at 50 and 90% of the amplitude (CaD50 and CaD90), calcium transient triangulation (Catri), change in amount of charge carried by INaL and ICaL (cqInward) (Li et al., 2017) and charge carried by the net current (qNet).

Metric	Leave-one out prediction error		
	1x Cmax	10x Cmax	20x Cmax
qNet	0.17	0.08	0.08
cqInward	0.25	0.33	0.33
Catri	1.25	1.08	1.08
CaD90	1.42	1.42	0.83
CaD50	1.42	1.0	0.83
peak Ca	0.92	0.75	0.83
diastolic Ca	0.92	0.83	0.83
APDtri	0.5	0.67	0.58
APD90	0.17	0.5	0.5
APD50	0.33	0.33	0.5
peak Vm	0.42	0.42	0.42
dV/dtmax	0.42	0.83	1.17
resting Vm	1.00	0.75	0.75

The second model variation we tested has the IKr dynamic model included, but without optimized channel conductances to reproduce AP changes under channel blocking conditions (**Figure 5C**). Note that this model variant is the same as the original IKr-dyn ORd model (Li et al., 2017) and, as demonstrated in **Figure 1**, has an inaccurate quantification of the block effects of individual currents compared to experimental data. In this scenario the low risk drug ranolazine is misclassified as a high risk compound (**Figure 5C**). Ranolazine is a potent IKr and INaL current blocker and these two effects can balance each other to reduce ranolazine's TdP risk (Antzelevitch et al., 2004; Johannesen et al., 2016; Saad et al., 2016). Because the INaL effect is underestimated and the IKr effect is overestimated without channel conductance optimization (**Figure 1**), ranolazine has a dominant IKr block effects when simulated by this model variant and thus will be mistakenly put in the high risk category (**Figure 5C**). Taken together, this suggests that the two added features are both important for TdP risk stratification and may mechanistically explain why a certain drug belongs to a specific TdP risk level.

Physiological Significance of qNet

In order to assess the physiological significance of the metric, we borrowed some concepts from non-linear dynamic theory, where EADs appear as membrane voltage oscillations when the equilibrium state at the plateau phase (membrane voltage between 0 and −40 mV) changes its stability via bifurcation (Qu et al., 2013; Kurata et al., 2017). The robustness of the system could be evaluated by applying a specific perturbation with a series of strengths and measuring the range of the perturbation

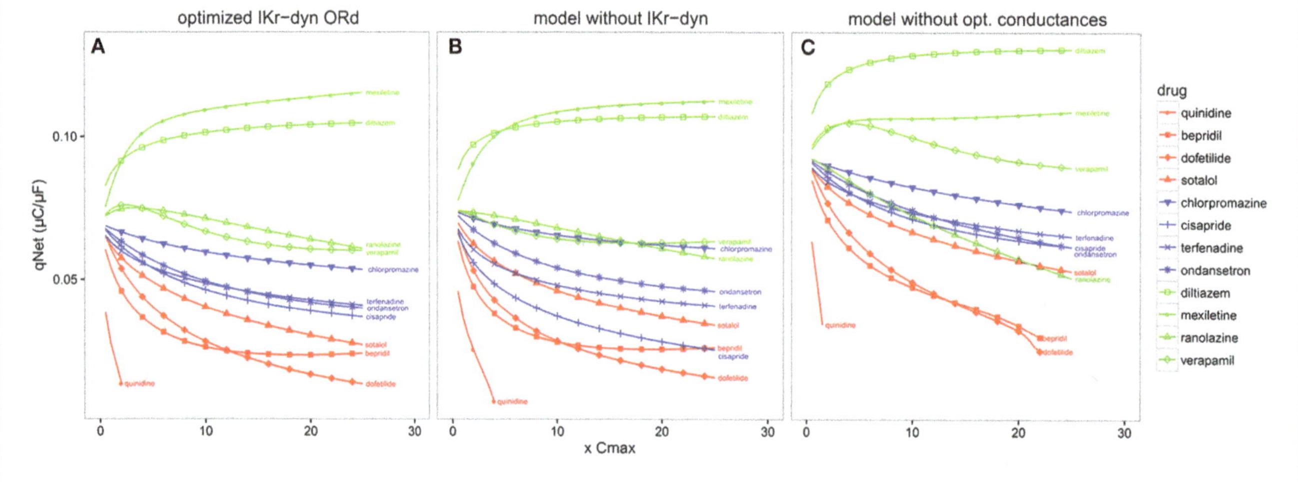

FIGURE 5 | qNet for the 12 CiPA training compounds for a range of doses (0.5–25x Cmax) at a pacing rate of 2,000 ms. **(A)** Optimized IKr-dyn ORd; **(B)** A model variation without the incorporation of the IKr dynamic model (note this is the same model as in Dutta et al., 2016) and; **(C)** A model variation without the optimized channel conductances to accurately quantify block effects of individual currents (note this is the same model as in Li et al., 2017). Different TdP risk levels are color coded (high risk in red, intermediate risk in blue and low/no risk in green). Results are not shown once drug concentrations are high enough to induce early after depolarizations (EADs) (i.e., quinidine).

the system can tolerate without changing stability (i.e., emergence or annihilation of oscillations) (Kurata et al., 2008). We applied this concept to our model using IKr maximum conductance reduction as a perturbation. In this case the minimum IKr reduction required to induce an EAD (IKr reduction threshold) reflects the system's robustness against, or distance from, EADs.

Therefore, for each drug over a range of concentrations from 0.5 to 25x Cmax we calculated the IKr reduction thresholds, and checked their correlation with the metrics qNet, APD90, and cqInward respectively. Detailed correlation plots for each metric can be found in the Supplemental Figures 2–4. **Table 4** shows the correlation coefficients for each drug across all concentrations for IKr reduction threshold vs. qNet, APD90 and cqInward respectively. We see that qNet shows a strong correlation across all drugs (close to 1). As qNet increases the IKr reduction threshold (and the system's robustness against EAD) increases and vice versa as qNet decreases. The bigger the qNet value the safer the system is and the harder it is to induce EAD.

For APD90, in most cases there is a strong negative correlation with IKr reduction threshold (close to −1) as expected, indicating the longer the APD the lower the repolarization robustness (i.e., the closer to EAD) and vice versa (**Table 4**). However, this trend reverses completely for some drugs like verapamil and mexiletine, where the correlation is positive (**Table 4**), suggesting the longer the APD90 the higher the repolarization robustness (the further away from EAD). This is contradictory to the general perception that longer APD90 (and QTc) signals a higher EAD/TdP liability. These unexpected relationships between APD and EAD can be seen more clearly in **Figure 6**, where the AP traces before and after the perturbation are shown. As can be seen from **Figure 6A** (left panel), using APD90 as a metric a cell under mexiletine at 1x Cmax seems safer (APD less prolonged) than at 10x Cmax, while qNet suggests otherwise (1x Cmax is more dangerous due to a smaller qNet value). When the same perturbation was applied (95% IKr reduction), the cell with 1x Cmax of mexiletine but not 10x, generated an EAD (**Figure 6A** right panel), indicating the cell with lower mexiletine concentration is actually closer to EAD generation, consistent with the prediction of qNet but not APD90. The same pattern can be seen in **Figure 6B**, where verapamil at 1x Cmax is shown to be closer to EAD than at 3x Cmax through perturbation assays (right panel), contradictory to the prediction using APD90 but not qNet (left panel). This pattern holds true when comparing ranolazine and cisapride as compared in **Figure 3**. As described earlier, a cell under ranolazine has a longer APD90 (indicating higher risk) and also a higher qNet value (indicating lower risk) than cisapride at 25x Cmax (**Figure 6C** left panel). An added perturbation of 75% IKr reduction will trigger an EAD with cisapride but not ranolazine (**Figure 6C** right panel), supporting the prediction of qNet but not APD90. Note that here we used 25x Cmax to match the concentrations used in **Figure 3**. When 1x Cmax was used, the same pattern was seen for the two drugs (see Supplemental Figure 5). This suggests under most circumstances qNet is a better metric than APD90 in marking the repolarization robustness to added perturbation of IKr reduction.

Finally, cqInward does not correlate well with robustness against EAD generation, measured as IKr reduction threshold (**Table 4**), despite a good performance (next to only qNet) on separating the risk categories for the training compounds (**Figure 4**). This suggests cqInward does not indicate the repolarization robustness to a perturbation of hERG channel density decrease. Whether cqInward is correlated with the robustness to another perturbation, or its separating power on the 12 training drugs is a non-physiological artifact, remains to be investigated. If the latter this highlights the importance to assess a metric in not only a pre-defined drug classification system, but also a physiological framework to quantitatively evaluate the correlation between the metric and EAD.

TABLE 4 | Correlation (using pearson method) between qNet, APD90 and cqInward and IKr reduction threshold for the 11 drugs (diltiazem is not included because EADs could not be induced for the highest IKr reduction tested 99.99%) for a CL of 2,000 ms across all doses from 0.5 to 25x Cmax. Simulations where the IKr reduction threshold is 0 (EADs occur without added IKr reduction, as for quinidine ≥ 2.3x Cmax) and results where the IKr reduction threshold could not be calculated (the maximum IKr reduction tested, 99.99%, did not trigger an EAD, as for diltiazem at all Cmax, verapamil ≥ 1.7x Cmax, and mexiletine ≥ 3.8x Cmax) were excluded.

Drug	Correlation with IKr reduction threshold		
	qNet	APD90	cqInward
Quinidine	0.996	−0.994	−0.197
Bepridil	0.948	−0.992	0.432
Sotalol	0.979	−0.992	−0.971
Dofetilide	0.96	−0.993	−1
Cisapride	0.988	−0.996	−0.994
Ondansetron	0.997	−0.999	−0.595
Terfenadine	0.968	−0.944	0.804
Chlorpromazine	0.995	−1	0.895
Ranolazine	0.87	−0.992	0.961
Verapamil	0.977	0.998	−0.991
Mexiletine	0.974	0.989	−0.983

DISCUSSION

In this study we present an optimized version of the ORd model (O'Hara et al., 2011), which incorporates a dynamic representation of IKr to allow modeling of drug-IKr channel interactions (Li et al., 2017) as well as providing a better fit to experimental data in both control and drug blocking conditions by rescaling ionic current conductances. Most notably, INaL current is increased compared to the original model. We also demonstrate that our optimized model, used in combination with a mechanistic net charge metric (qNet), enables good separation of 12 CiPA training compounds into their respective risk categories over a range of drug concentrations and pacing rates. Furthermore, we show that this is because qNet is correlated with a system's repolarization robustness to external perturbation of hERG channel density decrease, or IKr maximum conductance reduction.

Optimization of the O'Hara Rudy Model

To optimize the model we rescaled ionic current conductances in the model presented by Li et al. (2017). We demonstrate in

Figure 2 that recalibration of the model conductances leads to very little changes in the AP in control conditions across a range of pacing frequencies. It did however shift the effect of some of the different currents in the cardiac cell model, most notably increasing the role of INaL in contributing to AP. A recent study also optimized the ORd model to fit various LQTS profiles (Mann et al., 2016). Mann et al. present an optimized version of the ORd model by scaling the conductances of IKs (by 5.75), IKr (by 1.00), ICaL (by 2.01), INaL (by 1.00), INaCa (by 2.95), and INaK (by 9.12). The scaling factors are different to the ones observed in our model: IKs is increased in both models although ours is increased by a smaller amount 1.87, in their model IKr is unchanged while it is slightly increased in our model, ICaL is increased significantly in their model but only very slightly in ours and INaL is unchanged in their model while it is scaled by 2.661 in our model. The differences in INaL can be explained by the differences in context of use of the model: Mann et al. investigate the effects of increased INaL (LQTS3) as opposed to drug block of INaL, as in this study. Furthermore, a key difference between our model optimization process and Mann et al. is that we used human cardiomyocyte experimental data with various channel blockers, while they used clinical LQTS data. However, one of their findings was that the ORd model over predicts the effect of IKr block (50% IKr block produced a 42% increase in APD90 as opposed to the 16.5% observed clinically), which is concurrent with our findings. An awareness of this property of the ORd model is important as the model is often considered a consensus gold standard model for simulating drug effects on cardiac cells, and properties such as the over prediction of block of IKr may lead to inaccurate predictions of drug effects on cardiac electrophysiology. Our manuscript further highlights this point and provides an alternative model with improved balance of the effect of the different ionic currents in drug block conditions.

Performance of the qNet Metric Using the Optimized Model

Using pharmacology data for the 12 CiPA training compounds (Li et al., 2017), we assessed the suitability of a range of standard metrics based on AP morphology properties, as well as the recently published cqInward metric (Li et al., 2017) and our new qNet metric. We demonstrated that the commonly used AP-based metrics are poor indicators of TdP risk and found that our qNet metric allowed best separation of the CiPA training compounds into their risk categories. Our new metric outperformed the cqInward metric presented in Li et al. which may be a consequence of optimized channel conductances to better quantify the block effects of individual currents.

Our optimized IKr-dyn ORd model has two important features compared to the original ORd model: incorporation of modeling drug-IKr interaction kinetics based on dynamic hERG binding data (Li et al., 2017) and better characterization of individual currents' role in AP based on channel blocking data. We demonstrate the importance of simulating drug-IKr dynamics and accurate drug block conditions by providing rationale for misclassification of compounds when either one of the features were removed during TdP risk classification (**Figure 5**). This highlights the need for more precise model representation to simulate drug effects and stratify TdP risk levels. Additional human cardiomyocyte data may help to further refine this model.

qNet Correlates with the System's Robustness against EADS

Based on ideas from non-linear dynamic theory and studies demonstrating mechanisms of EAD generation (Guo et al., 2007; Weiss et al., 2010; Xie et al., 2010; Chang et al., 2013; Kurata et al., 2017), we established a theoretical framework to quantitatively evaluate the physiological consequences of the change of the qNet (and in principle any) metric. A key concept here is the system robustness (Kurata et al., 2008), which is defined as the level of a specific perturbation the system can tolerate without a qualitative change of stability (e.g., emergence or annihilation of oscillations). We applied that concept here using IKr maximum conductance reduction as a perturbation. Note that in our model all drugs' hERG/IKr block is modeled as binding to different channel states without changing the IKr conductance. Thus the IKr conductance decrease applied here reflects extra pro-EAD perturbations independent of each drug's direct ion channel block activities, for example inter-subject variability (hERG channel density variation due to genetic background), intra-subject variability (regional difference in hERG channel density), chronic drug effects (to block hERG maturation), or drug-drug interaction. We found that qNet is correlated with the cell's repolarizing robustness to the perturbation of IKr conductance reduction. When qNet increases, the cell's IKr reduction threshold also increases, meaning the cell is moving away from EAD and needs a more severe perturbation of IKr conductance reduction to trigger an EAD. The opposite happens when qNet decreases. This positive correlation is consistent across all the compounds tested in this study. In contrast, APD90 does not show a consistent correlation with the repolarization robustness across all the drugs, suggesting for some drugs (mainly compounds with balanced inward and outward current blocking activities) APD90 may not be a good indicator of distance from EAD.

The concept of robustness to pro-EAD perturbations is highly related to that of repolarization reserve, developed by Roden (1998) to describe the redundant cellular mechanisms to effect orderly and rapid repolarization, which can be disrupted by an added stressor (perturbation), resulting in APD prolongation and/or EAD. We chose to use the term robustness instead of repolarization reserve because the latter has been widely used to describe a cell's repolarization mechanism against both delayed repolarization (APD prolongation) and voltage oscillation (EAD), which we show in **Figure 6** are not necessarily correlated with each other. In contrast, robustness of a system, a concept borrowed from non-linear dynamic theory (Kurata et al., 2008), is directly related to emergence or annihilation of oscillations (EADs) in the presence of perturbations. There are different types of perturbations that could be used to test a system's robustness, for instance an applied bias current (Gray and Huelsing, 2008; Kurata et al., 2008), or an increased conductance for ICaL and/or INaL. We chose IKr conductance

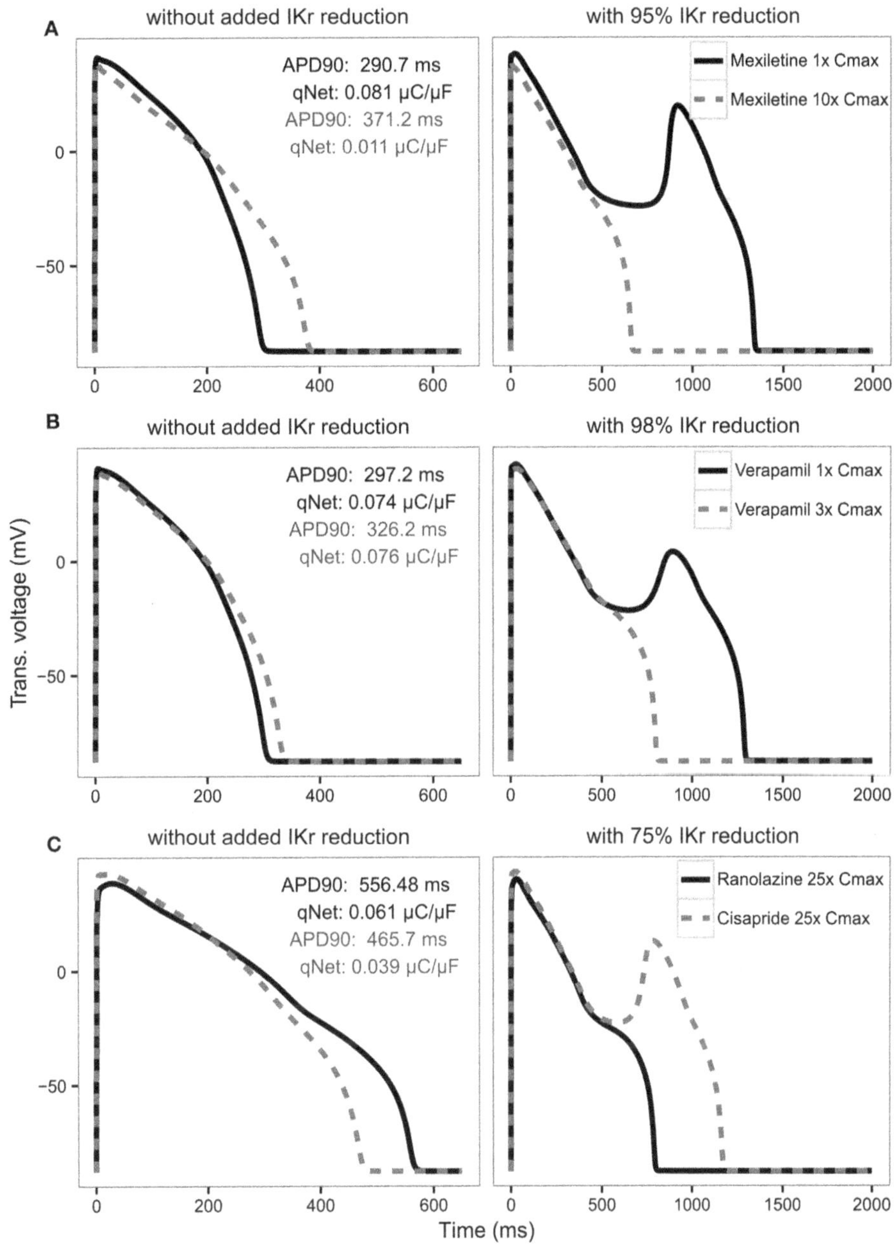

FIGURE 6 | AP traces for mexiletine **(A)** at 1x Cmax (black solid line) and 10x Cmax (gray dashed line) without (left panel) and with 95% IKr reduction (right panel); verapamil **(B)** at 1x Cmax (black solid line) and 3x Cmax (gray dashed line) without (left panel) and with 98% IKr reduction (right panel); and ranolazine (black solid line) and cisapride (dashed gray line) **(C)** at 25x Cmax without (left panel) and with 75% IKr reduction (right panel) for a CL of 2,000 ms. Corresponding APD90 (ms) and qNet (μC/μF) values are reported in black for mexiletine 1x Cmax, verapamil 1x Cmax and ranolazine 25x Cmax and in gray for mexiletine 10x Cmax, verapamil 3x Cmax and cisapride 25x Cmax. Note the IKr reduction (simulated by scaling the IKr maximum conductance) is applied in addition to the drug block effect and is used to assess the system's robustness against EADs (see Results section).

reduction as a perturbation because it is independent of the direct drug effects (the dynamic IKr model allows us to model IKr blockers without changing IKr conductance), and also it naturally reflects many physiological and pharmacological factors (hERG channel density variability, hERG channel trafficking block, etc.). It is possible that using different perturbations the same system can show different robustness against EADs. For example, the second best metric cqInward in terms of risk category separation does not correlate with the robustness to IKr conductance reduction, but could potentially correlate with the robustness to other perturbations. We also note that even qNet is not perfectly correlated with the robustness to IKr reduction. The correlation between qNet and IKr reduction threshold was checked only for 12 drugs at selected concentrations (0.5–25x Cmax), and it is not known if the strong correlation holds true beyond the drugs and concentrations tested. Even within the concentrations tested, some drugs (for instance ranolazine) do not have a consistent correlation across all the concentrations (Supplemental Figure 2). This suggests it may be beneficial to use the repolarization robustness (for instance IKr reduction threshold) directly as a metric so that it has clear and direct physiological meaning. However, this method is much more computationally intensive: for each drug at each concentration, the computing time for the IKr reduction threshold is more than 10 times that for qNet, as multiple levels of perturbations are needed to find the threshold. In addition, it is hard to define the metric if different perturbations to the same system lead to different thresholds (robustness). Thus, using a highly correlated surrogate metric qNet is a practical choice currently.

Limitations and Ongoing Work

While the model and metric combination presented here have been able to separate all the CiPA training compounds into their respective TdP risk categories, we have yet to test this approach on the CiPA validation compounds or any compounds that were not used in the training of the model, which would provide an independent validation of this framework. A key limitation of this approach that prevents an independent validation study is that we have not provided thresholds for the qNet metric, which could be used to place an unknown compound within a specific TdP risk category. Instead we would only be able to group together compounds which would be expected to pose similar TdP risk.

As suggested in previous studies the sodium potassium pump (Lancaster and Sobie, 2016; Britton et al., 2017) and the sodium calcium exchanger (Armoundas et al., 2003; Nagy et al., 2004) play an important role in EAD generation. Simulations of hypothetical drugs by Lancaster and Sobie (2016) show that both the sodium potassium pump and sodium calcium exchanger were ranked as having the greatest influence on TdP risk, above IKs, IK1, and Ito (but excluding IKr, ICaL, and INa). Further experiments and simulations are needed to assess how CiPA drugs affect these currents and whether they should be directly taken into account in our net current calculation to improve TdP risk prediction.

Another key factor to consider is that while we have demonstrated the success of our approach using gold standard manual patch clamp data. At least in a pre-regulatory setting, the CiPA framework will likely rely on the use of high-throughput ion channel screening data acquired from different platforms routinely used within the pharmaceutical industry. We would therefore need to further refine this model to fit to high-throughput system generated data and demonstrate that the model and metric combination identified perform equally well in this case. Furthermore, dynamic modeling of other channels (such as ICaL) may be needed as the project moves forward; however, at this stage detailed kinetic drug block data for other channels is not available, nor are the protocols to extract the necessary parameters. A priority of CiPA is to keep the framework simple and constrain the cost of data generation; therefore, we use only IC50 data for other channels as, based on our current knowledge, they provide enough information to correctly separate drugs into their TdP risk categories. Additionally, calcium transient properties in the ORd model differ from other models, such as the Grandi et al. model (Grandi et al., 2010); therefore, changes to the calcium transient could improve prediction of TdP risk. In fact, Cummins et al. incorporated the Grandi et al. model [along with the ORd and the ten Tusscher et al. model (ten Tusscher and Panfilov, 2006)] in their TdP risk classification and found diastolic intracellular calcium and APD to be good markers of TdP risk (Cummins et al., 2014). However, as mentioned earlier in this study Cummins et al. define a binary TdP risk stratification that does not follow the same categorization as defined by CiPA.

A number of different avenues for further improvement of the model and TdP risk prediction approach presented here are currently being explored. We are examining the use of thresholds for TdP risk level classification, as well as incorporating both variability and uncertainty within the model predictions. In conclusion, in this manuscript we present an optimized version of the IKr-dyn ORd model presented in Li et al. (2017) that is able to accurately separate the CiPA training compounds into their respective risk categories and correlates well with the system's robustness against EADs. An independent validation of this approach is limited, but more ongoing work will see further refinement of this model and increasing its suitability to be used routinely within the CiPA paradigm.

AUTHOR CONTRIBUTIONS

JS, PT, MW, and WW contributed to the acquisition of data and provided experimental data guidance. SD and ZL contributed to designing the work and carried out simulations. TC and DS contributed to revising the manuscript. SD, ZL, KC, and KB contributed to the analysis and interpretation of the data and writing of the manuscript.

ACKNOWLEDGMENTS

We would like to thank Drs. Thomas O'Hara, Norman Stockbridge, Richard Gray, Leonid Livshitz, Jules Hancox, Najah Abi-Gerges, Jamie Vandenberg, Gary Mirams, Bernard Fermini, Adam Hill, Meisam Hosseini and Jose Vicente for useful discussions and input.

REFERENCES

Antzelevitch, C., Belardinelli, L., Zygmunt, A., Burashnikov, A., Di Diego, J., Fish, J., et al. (2004). Electrophysiological effects of ranolazine, a novel antianginal agent with antiarrhythmic properties. *Circulation* 110, 904–910. doi: 10.1161/01.CIR.0000139333.83620.5D

Armoundas, A., Hobai, I., Tomaselli, G., Winslow, R., and O'Rourke, B. (2003). Role of sodium-calcium exchanger in modulating the action potential of ventricular myocytes from normal and failing hearts. *Circ. Res.* 93, 46–53. doi: 10.1161/01.RES.0000080932.98903.D8

Britton, O. J., Bueno-Orovio, A., Virág, L., Varró, A., and Rodriguez, B. (2017). The Electrogenic Na^{+}/K^{+} pump is a key determinant of repolarization abnormality susceptibility in human ventricular cardiomyocytes: a population-based simulation study. *Front. Physiol.* 8:278. doi: 10.3389/fphys.2017.00278

Chang, M., de Lange, E., Calmettes, G., Garfinkel, A., Qu, Z., and Weiss, J. (2013). Pro- and antiarrhythmic effects of ATP-sensitive potassium current activation on reentry during early afterdepolarization-mediated arrhythmias. *Heart Rhythm* 10, 575–582. doi: 10.1016/j.hrthm.2012.12.017

Colatsky, T., Fermini, B., Gintant, G., Pierson, J., Sager, P., Sekino, Y., et al. (2016). The Comprehensive *in Vitro* Proarrhythmia Assay (CiPA) initiative—Update on progress. *J. Pharmacol. Toxicol. Methods* 81, 15–20. doi: 10.1016/j.vascn.2016.06.002

Crumb, W., Vicente, J., Johannesen, L., and Strauss, D. (2016). An evaluation of 30 clinical drugs against the comprehensive *in vitro* proarrhythmia assay (CiPA) proposed ion channel panel. *J. Pharmacol. Toxicol. Methods.* 81, 251–262. doi: 10.1016/j.vascn.2016.03.009

Cummins, M., Dalal, P., Bugana, M., Severi, S., and Sobie, E. (2014). Comprehensive analyses of ventricular myocyte models identify targets exhibiting favorable rate dependence. *PLoS Comput. Biol.* 10:e1003543. doi: 10.1371/journal.pcbi.1003543

Di Veroli, G., Davies, M., Zhang, H., Abi-Gerges, N., and Boyett, M. (2013). High-throughput screening of drug-binding dynamics to HERG improves early drug safety assessment. *Am. J. Physiol. Heart Circ. Physiol.* 304, H104–H117. doi: 10.1152/ajpheart.00511.2012

Di Veroli, G., Davies, M., Zhang, H., Abi-Gerges, N., and Boyett, M. (2014). hERG inhibitors with similar potency but different binding kinetics do not pose the same proarrhythmic risk: implications for drug safety assessment. *J. Cardiovasc. Electrophysiol.* 25, 197–207. doi: 10.1111/jce.12289

Dutta, S., Strauss, D., Colatsky, T., and Li, Z. (2016). "Optimization of an *in silico* cardiac cell model for proarrhythmia risk assessment," in *2016 Computing in Cardiology Conference (CinC)* (Vancouver, BC), 869–872.

Fermini, B., Hancox, J., Abi-Gerges, N., Bridgland-Taylor, M., Chaudhary, K., Colatsky, T., et al. (2016). A new perspective in the field of cardiac safety testing through the comprehensive *in vitro* proarrhythmia assay paradigm. *J. Biomol. Screen.* 21, 1–11. doi: 10.1177/1087057115594589

Gintant, G. (2008). Preclinical torsades-de-pointes screens: advantages and limitations of surrogate and direct approaches in evaluating proarrhythmic risk. *Pharmacol. Ther.* 119, 199–209. doi: 10.1016/j.pharmthera.2008.04.010

Grandi, E., Pasqualini, F., and Bers, D. (2010). A novel computational model of the human ventricular action potential and Ca transient. *J. Mol. Cell. Cardiol.* 48, 112–121. doi: 10.1016/j.yjmcc.2009.09.019

Gray, R., and Huelsing, D. (2008). Excito-oscillatory dynamics as a mechanism of ventricular fibrillation. *Heart Rhythm* 5, 575–584. doi: 10.1016/j.hrthm.2008.01.011

Guo, D., Zhao, X., Wu, Y., Liu, T., Kowey, P., and Yan, G.-X. (2007). L-type calcium current reactivation contributes to arrhythmogenesis associated with action potential triangulation. *J. Cardiovasc. Electrophysiol.* 18, 196–203. doi: 10.1111/j.1540-8167.2006.00698.x

Johannesen, L., Vicente, J., Mason, J. W., Erato, C., Sanabria, C., Waite-Labott, K., et al. (2016). Late sodium current block for drug-induced long QT syndrome: results from a prospective clinical trial. *Clin. Pharmacol. Ther.* 99, 214–223. doi: 10.1002/cpt.205

Kallergis, E., Goudis, C., Simantirakis, E., Kochiadakis, G., and Vardas, P. (2012). Mechanisms, risk factors, and management of acquired long QT syndrome: a comprehensive review. *ScientificWorldJournal.* 2012:212178. doi: 10.1100/2012/212178

Kramer, J., Obejero-Paz, C., Myatt, G., Kuryshev, Y., Bruening-Wright, A., Verducci, J., et al. (2013). MICE models: superior to the HERG model in predicting torsade de pointes. *Sci. Rep.* 3:2100. doi: 10.1038/srep02100

Kurata, Y., Matsuda, H., Hisatome, I., and Shibamoto, T. (2008). Regional difference in dynamical property of sinoatrial node pacemaking: role of na+ channel current. *Biophys. J.* 95, 951–977. doi: 10.1529/biophysj.107.112854

Kurata, Y., Tsumoto, K., Hayashi, K., Hisatome, I., Tanida, M., Kuda, Y., et al. (2017). Dynamical mechanisms of phase-2 early afterdepolarizations in human ventricular myocytes: insights from bifurcation analyses of two mathematical models. *Am. J. Physiol. Heart Circ. Physiol.* 312, H106–H127. doi: 10.1152/ajpheart.00115.2016

Kurita, T., Ohe, T., Marui, N., Aihara, N., Takaki, H., Kamakura, S., et al. (1992). Bradycardia-induced abnormal QT prolongation in patients with complete atrioventricular block with torsades de pointes. *Am. J. Cardiol.* 69, 628–633. doi: 10.1016/0002-9149(92)90154-Q

Lancaster, C., and Sobie, E. A. (2016). Improved prediction of drug-induced torsades de pointes through simulations of dynamics and machine learning algorithms. *Clin. Pharmacol. Ther.* 100, 371–379. doi: 10.1002/cpt.367

Li, Z., Dutta, S., Sheng, J., Tran, P. N., Wu, W., Chang, K., et al. (2017). Improving the *in silico* assessment of proarrhythmia risk by combining herg (human ether-à-go-go-related gene) channel–drug binding kinetics and multichannel pharmacology. *Circ. Arrhythm. Electrophysiol.* 10:e004628. doi: 10.1161/CIRCEP.116.004628

Li, Z., Zhou, H., Lu, Y., and Colatsky, T. (2014). A critical role for immune system response in mediating anti-influenza drug synergies assessed by mechanistic modeling. *CPT Pharmacometrics Syst. Pharmacol.* 3, 1–9. doi: 10.1038/psp.2014.32

Mann, S., Imtiaz, M., Winbo, A., Rydberg, A., Perry, M., Couderc, J.-P., et al. (2016). Convergence of models of human ventricular myocyte electrophysiology after global optimization to recapitulate clinical long QT phenotypes. *J. Mol. Cell. Cardiol.* 100, 25–34. doi: 10.1016/j.yjmcc.2016.09.011

Mirams, G., Cui, Y., Sher, A., Fink, M., Cooper, J., Heath, B., et al. (2011). Simulation of multiple ion channel block provides improved early prediction of compounds' clinical torsadogenic risk. *Cardiovasc. Res.* 91, 53–61. doi: 10.1093/cvr/cvr044

Nagy, Z., Virág, L., Tóth, A., Biliczki, P., Acsai, K., Bányász, T., et al. (2004). Selective inhibition of sodium–calcium exchanger by SEA-0400 decreases early and delayed afterdepolarization in canine heart. *Br. J. Pharmacol.* 143, 827–831. doi: 10.1038/sj.bjp.0706026

O'Hara, T., Virág, L., Varró, A., and Rudy, Y. (2011). Simulation of the undiseased human cardiac ventricular action potential: model formulation and experimental validation. *PLoS Comput. Biol.* 7:e1002061. doi: 10.1371/journal.pcbi.1002061

Orth, P., Hesketh, C., Mak, C., Yang, Y., Lin, S., Beatch, G., et al. (2006). RSD1235 blocks late INa and suppresses early afterdepolarizations and torsades de pointes induced by class III agents. *Cardiovasc. Res.* 70, 486–496. doi: 10.1016/j.cardiores.2006.01.026

Qu, Z., Xie, L. H., Olcese, R., Karagueuzian, H. S., Chen, P. S., Garfinkel, A., et al. (2013). Early afterdepolarizations in cardiac myocytes: beyond reduced repolarization reserve. *Cardiovasc. Res.* 99, 6–15. doi: 10.1093/cvr/cvt,104

R Core Team (2014). *R: A Language and Environment for Statistical Computing.* Vienna: R Foundation for Statistical Computing. Available online at: http://www.R-project.org/.

Redfern, W. S., Carlsson, L., Davis, A. S., Lynch, W. G., MacKenzie, I., Palethorpe, S., et al. (2003). Relationships between preclinical cardiac electrophysiology, clinical QT interval prolongation and torsade de pointes for a broad range of drugs: evidence for a provisional safety margin in drug development. *Cardiovasc. Res.* 58, 32–45. doi: 10.1016/S0008-6363(02)00846-5

Roden, D. M. (1998). Taking the "idio" out of "idiosyncratic": predicting torsades de pointes. *Pacing Clin. Electrophysiol.* 21, 1029–1034. doi: 10.1111/j.1540-8159.1998.tb00148.x

Saad, M., Mahmoud, A., Elgendy, I., and Richard Conti, C. (2016). Ranolazine in cardiac arrhythmia. *Clin. Cardiol.* 39, 170–178. doi: 10.1002/clc.22476

Sager, P., Gintant, G., Turner, R., Pettit, S., and Stockbridge, N. (2014). Rechanneling the cardiac proarrhythmia safety paradigm: a meeting report from the Cardiac Safety Research Consortium. *Am. Heart J.* 167, 292–300. doi: 10.1016/j.ahj.2013.11.004

Soetaert, K., Petzoldt, T., and Setzer, R. W. (2010). Solving differential equations in R: package deSolve. *J. Stat. Softw.* 33, 1–25. doi: 10.18637/jss.v033.i09

9

Novel Two-Step Classifier for Torsades de Pointes Risk Stratification from Direct Features

*Jaimit Parikh, Viatcheslav Gurev and John J. Rice**

IBM T. J. Watson Research Center, Yorktown Heights, NY, United States

***Correspondence:**
John J. Rice
johnrice@us.ibm.com

While pre-clinical Torsades de Pointes (TdP) risk classifiers had initially been based on drug-induced block of hERG potassium channels, it is now well established that improved risk prediction can be achieved by considering block of non-hERG ion channels. The current multi-channel TdP classifiers can be categorized into two classes. First, the classifiers that take as input the values of drug-induced block of ion channels (direct features). Second, the classifiers that are built on features extracted from output of the drug-induced multi-channel blockage simulations in the *in-silico* models (derived features). The classifiers built on derived features have thus far not consistently provided increased prediction accuracies, and hence casts doubt on the value of such approaches given the cost of including biophysical detail. Here, we propose a new two-step method for TdP risk classification, referred to as Multi-Channel Blockage at Early After Depolarization (MCB@EAD). In the first step, we classified the compound that produced insufficient hERG block as non-torsadogenic. In the second step, the role of non-hERG channels to modulate TdP risk are considered by constructing classifiers based on direct or derived features at critical hERG block concentrations that generates EADs in the computational cardiac cell models. MCB@EAD provides comparable or superior TdP risk classification of the drugs from the direct features in tests against published methods. TdP risk for the drugs highly correlated to the propensity to generate EADs in the model. However, the derived features of the biophysical models did not improve the predictive capability for TdP risk assessment.

Keywords: Torsades de Pointes, machine-learning, classification and prediction, cardiac modeling, early afterdepolarization

1. INTRODUCTION

In-vitro examination of drug effects on multiple cardiac ion channels and *in-silico* reconstruction of cardiac electrical activity from *in-vitro* experiments are two coupled components in the new paradigm of TdP risk assessment (Sager et al., 2014). At the molecular/ionic level, pharmacological TdP genesis is associated with drug-induced reduction in the net repolarizing current (Antzelevitch, 2007), which is manifested in prolongation of the QT interval in the body-surface ECGs. Drug-induced block of hERG (human Ether-à-go-go-Related Gene) channels, which gate the primary repolarizing current I_{Kr}, is an acknowledged marker for TdP risk prediction. However, recent studies have shown that the classification that is based on the safety margins from the hERG channel assays has moderate concordance with QTc prolongation (Gintant, 2011) and TdP risk (Mirams et al., 2011; Kramer et al., 2013). Drug-induced modulation of non-hERG channels either mitigates (i.e., block of L-type voltage regulated calcium channel current I_{CaV} and inward late sodium current I_{NaL}) or enhances (i.e., block of slow activating potassium current I_{Ks} or increase of I_{NaL}) the pro-arrhythmic effects of hERG channel block (Bril et al., 1996; Antzelevitch, 2004; Lacerda et al., 2008; Towart et al., 2009; Fermini et al., 2016). Several multi-channel TdP risk classifiers have already been created (Mirams et al., 2011; Christophe, 2013, 2015; Kramer et al., 2013; Mistry et al., 2015; Okada et al., 2015; Lancaster and Sobie, 2016; Abbasi et al., 2017). **Table 1** lists previously published classifiers that are based on several *in-vitro* ion channel assays.

The drug-induced changes in the ionic currents result in altering of action potential and calcium transient at the cellular level. These modulations can further trigger events in the cardiac cells, such as early or delayed afterdepolarizations (EADs or DADs), and increase heterogeneity in the electrical activity across the myocardium [i.e., increase in transmural dispersion of repolarization (TDR)]; both effects are thought to be the key determinants for TdP genesis (Wu et al., 2002; Antzelevitch, 2007). *In-silico* reconstruction of drug-induced responses of action potential and calcium transient at cellular or electrical activity at tissue levels could potentially provide better mechanistic insight. The classifiers that use the features from the *in-silico* simulations (derived features) have shown the capability to make good predictions (**Table 1**) of torsadogenic risk (Mirams et al., 2011, 2014; Christophe, 2013, 2015; Okada et al., 2015; Lancaster and Sobie, 2016; Abbasi et al., 2017; Li et al., 2017). However, in spite of providing better biological insights for TdP genesis, the role of computational models in improving TdP risk prediction is controversial as machine-learning/statistical analysis of the *in-vitro* ion channel measurements (direct features) have been shown to produce equally accurate TdP risk assessment (Kramer et al., 2013; Mistry et al., 2015).

The amount of drug-induced block of the channels depends on the compound's effective free therapeutic plasma concentration (EFTPC). Unfortunately, reported EFTPC values are highly variable (Redfern et al., 2003). The maximum EFTPC values, which is used to determine the ion channel block, also vary across the datasets (e.g., Moxifloxacin 3.5 μM in Crumb et al., 2016, 10.9 μM in Kramer et al., 2013). In addition, the actual free plasma concentrations of drugs in subjects could also differ because of inter-individual variations, impaired metabolism, and interactions with other drugs. In fact, drug concentrations could potentially be much larger than reported maximum EFTPC values. Researchers have employed different strategies to address the uncertainty in EFTPC. Direct and derived features have been evaluated at the drug's EFTPC, at supra-therapeutic drug concentrations (which is several times above maximum EFTPC), or across a wide range of drug concentrations (Christophe, 2013, 2015; Kramer et al., 2013; Mirams et al., 2014; Mistry et al., 2015; Okada et al., 2015; Lancaster and Sobie, 2016; Abbasi et al., 2017; Ando et al., 2017; Li et al., 2017). The range is obtained by titrating up the drug concentrations until a fixed threshold, until a predetermined increase in action potential prolongation is reached, or until EADs are triggered.

Here, we propose a new two-step method for TdP risk classification, referred to as Multi-channel Blockage at Early After Depolarization (MCB@EAD). The MCB@EAD classifier employs as inputs direct or derived features obtained at drug concentrations that produce critical hERG block (~60% block that generates pause-induced EADs in the biophysical models). We test the proposed classifier on several previously published datasets derived from *in-vitro* screening of the ion channels and on a large composite dataset comprising of all datasets. Finally, we examine the connection between TdP risk of the drugs and drug propensity to induce pause-dependent EADs. Our results show that MCB@EAD classification from the direct features performs better or equivalently to previously suggested methods including the classifiers built on derived features from biophysical models. We also highlight the link between the direct and derived feature based classifiers and demonstrate that TdP risk for the drugs highly correlates to the likelihood to produce EADs in the model.

2. METHODS

Table 2 provides a brief summary for each of the analyzed datasets. More extensive descriptions of the datasets is provided in the Supplemental Material.

2.1. Torsadogenicity Definition

The definition of drug groups according to their torsadogenic risk is critical for the development of the TdP risk classifiers. Different torsadogenic definitions from previous classification studies are listed below.

Redfern et al. assigned drugs to five categories based on the number of reports of TdP in humans, QT prolongation and TdP associated withdrawal from the market (Redfern et al., 2003). The five categories are:

- R1: Class Ia and III antiarrhythmics with QT prolongation as intended effect.
- R2: Drugs that have been withdrawn from the market due to unacceptable risk of TdP for condition being treated.
- R3: Drugs with numerous case reports of TdP in humans.
- R4: Drugs with isolated reports of TdP in humans.
- R5: Drugs with no published reports of TdP in humans when used alone.

Arizona Center for Education and Research on Therapeutics (AZCERT) maintains a list of drugs associated with QT prolongation/TdP risk (Woosley et al., 2017) (https://crediblemeds.org/) and has categorized the drugs into three groups:

- CM1: Drugs with known risk of TdP. These drugs prolong the QT interval and are clearly associated with a known risk of TdP, even when taken as recommended.
- CM2: Drugs with possible risk of TdP. These drugs can cause QT prolongation but currently there is lack of evidence for a risk of TdP associated with them when taken as recommended.

TABLE 1 | TdP classifiers based on *in-vitro* ion channel assays.

Feature	*In-silico* model	Classification		References	N_{Total}	$N_{Correct}$
		TDP+	TDP−			
$\frac{IC_{50,hERG}}{EFTPC}$	NA	Feature < 30	Feature > 30	Redfern et al., 2003	52	NA
APD_{90}	Ventricular myocyte models of rabbit, rat and human	LDA		Mirams et al., 2011	31	30
$-log(\frac{IC_{50,hERG}}{IC_{50,CaV}})$	NA	LR		Kramer et al., 2013	55	50
$\frac{1+a_0BP_{CaV}+a_1BP_{Na,fast}}{1+a_2BP_{hERG}}$	NA	LR		Mistry et al., 2015	31 from (Mirams et al., 2011) 55 from (Kramer et al., 2013)	28
TDR	Human ventricular myocyte model	TDR profiles		Christophe, 2015	55 from (Kramer et al., 2013)	NA
$\frac{C_{Drug,Arrhythmia}}{EFTPC}$	3D FEM model of human heart	Feature < 200	Feature > 200	Okada et al., 2015	12	12
EADs	Human ventricular myocyte model	Waveform appearance		Abbasi et al., 2017	12 from (Okada et al., 2015)	11
APD_{50} & Diastolic Ca^{2+}	Human ventricular myocyte models	SVM and PCA		Lancaster and Sobie, 2016	86 from (Kramer et al., 2013) and (Mirams et al., 2011)	75
$\frac{AUCI_{NaL,drug}}{AUCI_{NaL,control}} + \frac{AUCI_{CaV,drug}}{AUCI_{CaV,control}}$	Human ventricular myocyte model	LDA		Li et al., 2017	12	12

LDA, Linear Determinant Analysis; LR, Logistic Regression; SVM, Support Vector Machine; PCA, Principal Component Analysis; $C_{drug,EAD}$, concentration of the drug that produces EAD; BP_x, % block of the x (x = Na, fast, CaV, hERG) ion channels; TDR, transmural dispersion of repolarization; $C_{drug,Arrhythmia}$, concentration of the drug that produces arrhythmia in the model; EAD, early after depolarizations; $AUCI_{x,drug/control}$, area under the curve of the x (x = CaV, NaL) current transient at steady state action potential in the presence (drug) or absence of the drug (control). Table also lists the number of compounds analyzed in the study (N_{Total}) and the number of correctly classified compounds ($N_{correct}$).

- CM3: Drugs with conditional risk of TdP. These drugs are associated with TdP but only under certain conditions of their use.

Champeroux et al. assigned drugs into three categories based on the number of reports of TdP cases associated with the drug (Champeroux et al., 2005):

- CH1: Drugs with numerous reports of TdP.
- CH2: Drugs causing QT prolongation and/or TdP at very low frequency.
- CH3: Drugs without reports of TdP or QT prolongation.

Based on a general consensus, a working group formed under the Comprehensive *in vitro* Proarrhythmia Assay (CiPA) initiative picked 28 compounds and categorized them into three groups (Colatsky et al., 2016; Fermini et al., 2016) for testing/training of the classifiers under the new CiPA paradigm:

- CP1: Drugs with high risk.
- CP2: Drugs with intermediate risk.
- CP3: Drugs with low risk.

To consistently compare with other methods we attempt to use the binary TdP definitions [i.e., a drug is either torsadogenic (TdP+) or non-torsadogenic (TdP−)] as in the original publications (see **Table 2** and the Supplemental Material for further details regarding the exact risk definition used for the particular datasets). For dataset 7 where tertiary definition is reported, binary TdP definition was defined by placing CP1 and CP2 drugs into torsadogenic (TdP+) and CP3 drugs to non-torsadogenic (TdP−) categories. In the case of the merged dataset or the datasets that lacked binarized TdP definitions (Crumb et al., 2016), we assigned drugs as TdP+ or TdP− using a similar approach as in Lancaster and Sobie (2016). The drugs which fell in the known risk category (CM1) in the CredibleMeds database, R1, R2, and R3 category in Redfern et al. (2003) or drugs with several reports for TdP (CH1) (Champeroux et al., 2005) were assigned to TdP+. For the remaining drugs we categorized the drug as TdP+ if a warning for TdP associated with QT prolongation appeared on its package label (http://dailymed.nlm.nih.gov/). The risk categorization for the drugs are provided in the Supplemental Material. Paroxetine has a warning for TdP in the label and Imipramine was assigned to CH1 category in Champeroux et al. (2005). These two drugs were also assigned as TdP+ in Lancaster and Sobie (2016). Here, we defined them as TdP− as these two compounds are not directly associated

TABLE 2 | Datasets analyzed for TdP risk. The total number of drugs in each dataset is listed in the "Number compounds" column.

Datasets	Number compounds	Risk categorization tested	Figure/Table
Dataset 1 (Mirams et al., 2011)	31	TdP+: R1, R2, R3 categories (RCOD)	**Figure 3**, **Table 4**
Dataset 2 (Kramer et al., 2013)	55	TdP+: R1, R2, R3, CM1, CM2, CM3 categories or label warning (RCOD)	**Figure 3**, **Table 4**
Dataset 3 (Okada et al., 2015)	12	TdP+: R1, R2, R3 categories (RCOD)	**Figure 3**, **Table 4**
Dataset 4 (Lancaster and Sobie, 2016)	86	TdP+: CM1 and CH1 categories, Drugs in CM2 and CM3 if label warning (RCOD)	**Figure 3**, **Table 4**
Dataset 5 (Crumb et al., 2016)	30	TdP+: R1, R2, R3, CH1, CM1 category or label warning TdP+: CM1 and CM2 TdP+: CM1 TdP+: CM1 and CM3	**Figures 2A,B**, left panel, **Figure 4** **Tables 4**, **5** **Figures 2A,B**, right panel, **Figure 4**, **Table 5** **Table 5** **Table 5**
Dataset 6 (Ando et al., 2017)	57	TdP+: CM1	**Figure 3**, **Table 4**
Dataset 7 (Li et al., 2017)	12	TdP+: CP1 and CP2 category High: CP1 Intermediate: CP2 Low: CP3 (RCOD)	**Figure 3**, **Table 4** **Figure 6**
Dataset 8 (Combined Datasets 1, 2, 3, 5, 6, and 7)	197	TdP+ R1, R2, R3, CH1, CM1 category or label warning TdP+: CM1 and CM2 TdP+: CM1 TdP+: CM1 and CM3	**Figure 5** **Table 6** **Table 6** **Table 6**
Dataset 9 (Fermini et al., 2016) ($IC_{50,channel}$ extracted from Datasets 1, 2, 3, 5, 6, and 7)	26	High: CP1 Intermediate: CP2 Low: CP3 (RCOD)	**Figure 6**

"Risk categorization tested" column refers to the TdP risk definition (see more info on definitions in the text) used to test/train the particular datasets, and the "Figure/Table" column list the corresponding Figure and Table numbers where the results of the particular dataset and risk categorization pair are reported. The IC_{50} values and risk category of individual drug for each datasets are also reported in the Supplemental Material.

with QT prolongation or TdP. These drugs inhibit CYP2D6 and increase plasma concentrations of TdP positive drugs such as Thioridazine (http://dailymed.nlm.nih.gov/). Sometimes alternative definitions were also considered and are explicitly defined in the manuscript.

2.2. Drug-Induced Ion Channel Block

The *in-vitro* ion channel assay data is converted to drug-induced block of ion channel (direct features) using

$$Block_{channel} = 100 \times \left(\frac{{C_{Drug}}^h}{{IC_{50,channel}}^h + {C_{Drug}}^h}\right), \quad (1)$$

where $IC_{50,channel}$ is the drug concentrations at which the whole-cell current through particular channels is reduced by half, C_{Drug} is the concentration of the drug and h is the Hill-coefficient. The Hill coefficient values were taken as reported in the original datasets. The IC_{50}, Hill coefficients, and EFTPC values for each of the datasets are given in the Supplemental Material. Note that Hill coefficient values had little impact, and even fixing Hill coefficient to 1 for all the drugs did not significantly alter the observed classification accuracies (results not shown). The drug-induced blocks of ion channels are used as input features for the machine-learning based classifiers or utilized to scale the maximum conductance ($g_{channel}$) of the particular ion channels in the *in-silico* models, assuming that drug-induced effect on multiple ion-channels are well represented by a simple conductance-block model (Mirams et al., 2011),

$$g_{channel,drug} = (1 - Block_{channel}/100) \times g_{channel}. \quad (2)$$

The effects of drug-induced modulation of multi-channel conductance (Equation 2) on the action potentials (AP) and calcium transients are simulated for all of the compounds using two versions of human ventricular myocyte models (O'Hara et al., 2011; Dutta et al., 2016). Ohara et al. model (OHR) (O'Hara et al., 2011) was picked as it has been chosen as the consensus base model for proarrhythmic risk assessment (Colatsky et al., 2016). OHR model was also shown to have the best predictive capability for TdP risk classification among the few tested models in Lancaster and Sobie (2016). We also utilized the modified version of the OHR model (OHRmv) which has been shown to better fit APD-rate dependence experimental data under drug block conditions, particularly improving the effect of I_{NaL} block on action potential prolongation (Dutta et al., 2016). Several derived features are extracted from AP and calcium transients, and TdP risk classifiers are constructed using these derived features. The details on the simulation protocols and the computations of the derived features are reported in section 2.6 that describes *in-silico* simulations.

2.3. Two-Step Classifier—Multi-Channel Blockage at hERG EAD(MCB@EAD)

We propose a two-step approach for TdP risk prediction. In the first step, we classified the drugs into non-torsadogenic and potentially torsadogenic categories. We performed the classification in the first step considering solely the block of hERG channels. Using a Redfern-like criteria (Redfern et al., 2003), we obtained the ratio between the drug concentration that produces 60% block of the hERG channel current ($IC_{60,hERG}$) and the drug EFTPC (i.e., $hERGratio = \frac{IC_{60,hERG}}{EFTPC}$). The motivation for using $IC_{60,hERG}$ was that the 60% block of hERG channel currents triggers pause-induced EAD in the mid cell type of OHR and OHRmv models (2 Hz pacing rate) at a quiescent interval greater than 700 ms. For example, a drug with hERG IC_{60} of 500 nM and EFTPC of 1 nM would yield a threshold of 500. Since this drug's EFTPC would be far from the critical hERG block concentration, we would classify this compound as non-torsadogenic. Previous classifiers based on EAD appearance for different datasets have shown a wide range of thresholds (approximately 30× −200× EFTPC) for achieving best TdP risk predictions (Christophe, 2013; Okada et al., 2015). Hence, we tested four different thresholds for hERG ratio of 50, 100, 150, and 200 for all the datasets and chose the one that gives the best classification accuracy. For the remaining drugs with EFTPC above the critical hERG block concentrations (hERG ratio less than the threshold), the role of multi-channel block was examined in the second step using logistic regression classifiers ignoring the EFTPC values of the drugs. The regression classifiers employed as inputs either the $Block_{channel}$ of additional non-hERG ion channels (direct features) or the features derived from the simulated calcium transient and the AP in the ventricular myocyte models, at drug concentrations equal to $IC_{60,hERG}$. Such two-step classifier partially solves the problem of EFTPC variability, restricting EFTPC usage only to the first step to primarily discard the drugs that produce insufficient hERG block at extremely high concentrations by classifying them as non-torsadogenic. Therefore, the moderate variations in EFTPC values of the drugs would only matter for a very small population of the drugs with hERG ratio close to the threshold in the classification. A summary of the two-step approach is given in **Figure 1**.

In order to compare the performance of the classifiers based on the two-step approach to the performance of the classifiers based on features obtained at actual drug EFTPC concentrations, we also constructed TdP risk classifiers using the direct and derived features at reported maximum EFTPC of the drugs. They are referred in the current paper as one-step classifiers (hERG ratio is not utilized for these classifiers).

2.4. Classifiers

We utilized statistical/machine-learning models for binary classification of the drugs into TdP+ or TdP− categories. The binarized torsadogenic definitions for each drug were used to train/test the classifier models. Here, we used Logistic regression model. SVM and neural network models were also tested and resulted in comparable classification accuracies (results are shown in the Supplemental Material). Python's scikit-learn package (Pedregosa et al., 2011) (http://scikit-learn.org/stable/) was used to train/test different models. Here, we present results for logistic regression models only as other methods produced similar results. The generalized model equation is described as

$$logit(TdP) = \frac{1}{1 + exp^{-(\beta_0 + \sum_i^n \beta_i Feature_i)}}, \tag{3}$$

where *Feature* represents the input metrics to the model (either direct feature or the derived feature), n is the number of input features used to train/test the model, and β_0 and βi $(i = 1, 2, .., n)$ are the parameters to be determined. The predictive power of the model was evaluated by the leave-one-out (LOO) cross validation technique.

2.5. Two-Dimensional TdP Risk Map

A two-dimensional TdP risk map with hERG ratio ($\frac{IC_{60,hERG}}{EFTPC}$) on the x-axis and summation of one or more features (block of I_{CaV} and I_{NaL}) on the y-axis were constructed for visualization of the two-step (MCB@EAD) classifier. The hERG ratio threshold and regression coefficients from the two-step classifier are used to generate the two-dimensional risk maps. The hERG ratio (step 1 in the two-step classifier) that provides the best classification in the two-step classifier is used to set the threshold along the x-axis. Drugs that fall in the region above the hERG ratio threshold are considered to be non-torsadogenic. For the drugs with hERG ratio less than the threshold, the coefficients of the logistic regression model in step 2 of the two-step classifier are used to determine the threshold along the y-axis of the risk map. An example of separating hyperplane that would be obtained from the second step of the two-step classifier is given by

$$\beta_{I_{CaV}} block_{I_{CaV}} + \beta_{I_{NaL}} block_{I_{NaL}} + \sum_{i=3}^{n} \beta_{feature,i} feature_i + \beta_{intercept} = 0 \tag{4}$$

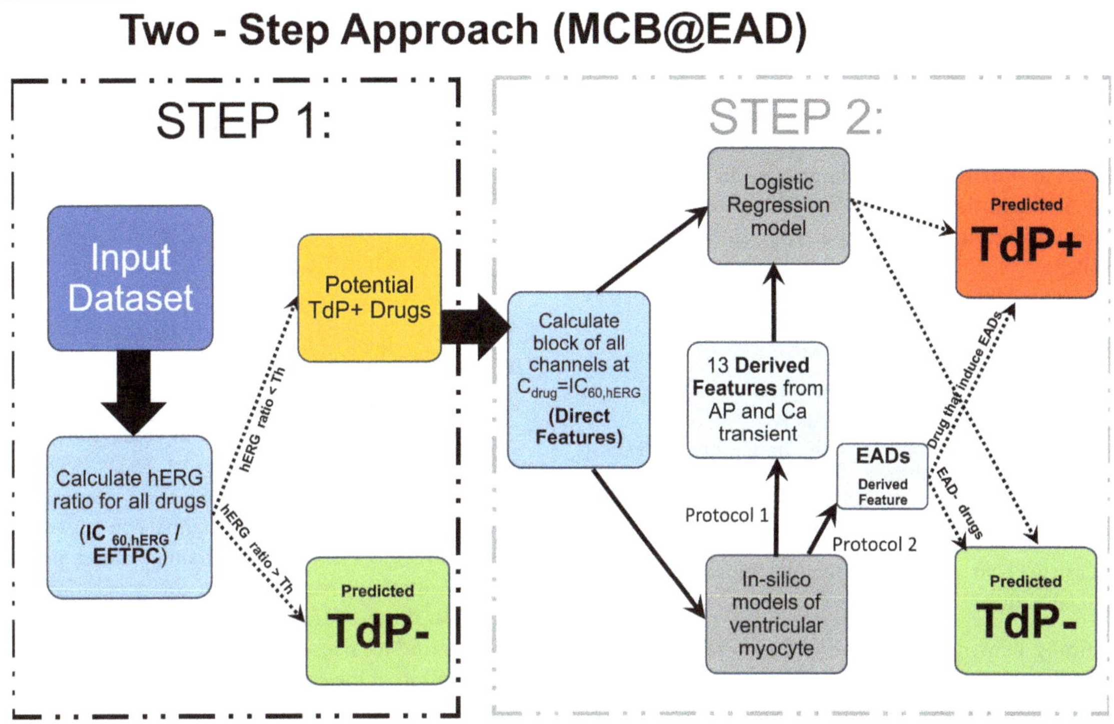

FIGURE 1 | Schematic representation of the MCB@EAD two-step approach. *In-vitro* assay datasets are used to obtain the drug-induced blocks of multiple ion-channels at drug concentrations equal to $IC_{60,hERG}$. hERG ratio ($\frac{IC_{60,hERG}}{EFTPC}$) is used as the classification criteria in the first step. Drugs that do not result in 60% hERG block at concentrations well above their maximum EFTPC are classified as non-torsadogenic (TdP−). hERG ratio thresholds of 50, 100, 150, and 200 were tested, and the one that provides the best TdP risk discrimination was chosen for the particular datasets. The remaining drugs are considered to be potentially torsadogenic and analyzed in the second step. The drug-induced blocks of multiple ion-channels at 60% hERG block concentrations (direct features) are used as inputs to the logistic regression model for TdP risk classification or used to simulate drug-induced changes in action potential (AP) and calcium (Ca) transients using different protocols. The derived features are extracted from the AP and Ca transients. These derived features are then used to train the logistic-regression model for TdP risk classification or used directly (e.g., in case of EADs) to classify drugs to TdP+ and TdP− categories.

where $block_{I_{CaV}}$ and $block_{I_{NaL}}$ are the blocks of I_{CaV} and I_{NaL}, respectively. $feature_i$ are additional input features of the model, such as drug trapping parameters. $\beta_{I_{CaV}}$, $\beta_{I_{NaL}}$, and $\beta_{feature,i}$ represent the regression coefficients. The regression coefficients obtained from the step 2 are normalized to the coefficient $\beta_{I_{CaV}}$ for the I_{CaV} block. This gives

$$block_{I_{CaV}} + \frac{\beta_{I_{NaL}}}{\beta_{I_{CaV}}} block_{I_{NaL}} + \sum_{i=3}^{n} \frac{\beta_{feature,i} feature_i}{\beta_{I_{CaV}}} = -\frac{\beta_{intercept}}{\beta_{I_{CaV}}}. \quad (5)$$

Thus, the left hand side of Equation (5) is plotted on the y-axis, and the ratio $\frac{\beta_{intercept}}{\beta_{I_{CaV}}}$ determines the threshold along this axis. For example, if only block of I_{CaV} is taken into consideration, the risk map has the values of I_{CaV} along the y-axis and hERG ratio along the x-axis.

Ternary classification for Dataset 7 requires multiple hyperplanes with different regression coefficients to separate the high, low and intermediate risk drugs. To represent the ternary classification in a two-dimensional risk map similar to the binary classification, we summed the different features ($Feature_{sum}$) assuming identical weights for each of the features (i.e., $\beta_1 = \beta_2 = .. = \beta_n$ equal to β_f) reducing the classification model to $\frac{1}{1+exp^{-(\beta_0+\beta_f Feature_{sum})}}$. For Dataset 7, assuming identical weights for different features resulted in similar accuracy to a multinomial logistic regression classifier while providing a simpler visualization in one two-dimensional plot as in the binary classification. The ratio $\frac{-\beta_0}{\beta_f}$ obtained after training the model is used to set the two thresholds along the y-axis. Along the x-axis arbitrary hERG ratio of 25, the value slightly greater than the maximum hERG ratio observed for high risk drugs in Li et al. (2017) and Fermini et al. (2016), was utilized to separate low and intermediate risk drugs from the high risk drugs. The hERG ratio of 150 obtained from the merged dataset was utilized to separate the high and intermediate risk drugs from the low risk drugs.

2.6. *In-Silico* Simulations

The alteration in the action potential and calcium transients at the cellular level arising from drug-induced multi-channel block were simulated for all the compounds (Dataset 8) using the OHR model. Using a similar approach as in Lancaster and Sobie (2016), simulations were carried out at three pacing rates (0.5, 1, and 2 Hz) for each of the endo, mid and epi cell types resulting in 9 simulations per drug, and 13 metrics were obtained from the

AP and Ca^{2+} transients. Simulations were carried out for 1,000 beats to allow the models to reach the steady state. The 13 metrics obtained from the *in-silico* models are listed below:

- Upstroke velocity
- Peak voltage
- Action potential at half maximum duration (APD50)
- Action potential duration at −60 mV (APD @ −60 mV)
- Action potential duration at 90% repolarization (APD90)
- Resting voltage
- Action potential triangulation (AP triangulation), calculated as APD90 - APD30
- Diastolic calcium level (diastolic $[Ca^{2+}]_i$)
- Amplitude of the calcium transient (amplitude of CaT)
- Peak value of intracellular calcium (peak $[Ca^{2+}]_i$)
- Calcium transient duration at half maximum duration (CaTD50)
- Calcium transient duration at 90% repolarziation (CaTD90)
- Triangulation of the calcium transient (CaT triangulation), calculated as CaTD90 - CaTD30 (calcium transient duration at 30% repolarization)

We systematically construct the classifiers on each of the 13 derived features extracted from the action potentials and calcium transients at two different drug concentrations (i.e., at $C_{Drug} = EFTPC$ and $C_{Drug} = hERG\ IC_{60}$).

The onset of TdP is usually preceded by a sudden reduction of the heart rate (i.e., by pauses or long cycle lengths) (Neal Kay et al., 1983; Viskin et al., 2000). Here, we test the generation of pause-induced EADs, that are implicated as triggers of TdP (Viswanathan and Rudy, 1999; Liu and Laurita, 2005), in simulations of drug-induced multi-channel blockage in the ventricular myocytes models (O'Hara et al., 2011; Dutta et al., 2016). The basic protocol was similar to that in Viswanathan and Rudy (1999), where stimulation of the cell is carried out 200 times at a constant cycle length of 500 ms. After 200 stimuli, an additional stimulus was applied following a pause of 1,000 ms. Drug-induced EAD development was tested at drug concentrations $= IC_{60,hERG}$ in the mid cell type. EAD analysis was also performed at $C_{drug} = IC_{60,hERG}$ for combinations of I_{CaV}, I_{NaL}, and I_{Ks} blocks ranging from 0–100% with step of 10% resulting in a set of 1,000 simulations. TdP risk prediction was carried out using ability of drugs to induce EADs as a classification criteria (EAD+: drugs that induce EADs at 60% hERG block concentrations, EAD−: drugs that do not induce EADs at 60% hERG block concentrations). **Figure 1** illustrates the classification based on the drug EAD risk. The drugs with hERG ratio greater than the hERG ratio threshold determined for the particular dataset (using the two-step approach on the direct features) were considered EAD−. For the remaining drugs the block of ion-channels was calculated at drug concentration equal to $IC_{60,hERG}$ and overlaid on the parametric space obtained from EAD analysis at varying combinations of I_{CaV}, I_{NaL} and I_{Ks} blocks (**Figure 2A**), for both the OHR and OHRmv models, to determine whether a drug will induce EAD or not at 60% hERG block concentrations.

The system of ordinary differential equations were solved using the rapid integration scheme (a combination of forward Euler, Rush-Larsen method, Rush and Larsen, 1978 and adaptive time-step) proposed in the original model (O'Hara et al., 2011). For the EAD simulations rapid integration scheme proposed in O'Hara et al. (2011) yielded different results to gold standard simulations with fixed time step of 0.001 ms. Hence, for the EAD simulations we utilized forward Euler method with a time step of 0.001 ms. Execution scripts were written in C++.

3. RESULTS

3.1. Drugs TdP Risk Highly Correlates to EAD Propensity

A short-long cycle length (i.e., pause) often precedes the onset of TdP (Neal Kay et al., 1983; Viskin et al., 2000). The pause is known to facilitate the formations of EADs (Viswanathan and Rudy, 1999; Liu and Laurita, 2005). Here, we test the effects of drug-induced block of different channels on triggering of pause-induced EADs. Block of hERG channel causes prolongation of action potential and can result in the generation of EADs. In the OHR and the OHRmv models, the amount of hERG block required to induce pause-induced EADs is reduced with increase in the duration of the pause. hERG block by 57 and 55% induced EADs in the mid-cell paced at 2 Hz (500 ms pacing cycle length) following a 700 ms pause in the OHR and OHRmv models, respectively. The amount of hERG block required to induce EADs in the OHR and OHRmv model following 1,000 ms pause is reduced to a 47 and 46% block, respectively. Under these critical blocks of hERG channel, modifications of other channels may promote or inhibit the EADs. First, we tested individually the effects of block of six ion-channel currents (I_{CaV}, I_{NaL}, I_{Ks}, I_{K1}, $I_{Na,fast}$, and I_{to}) in promoting or inhibiting pause-induced EADs at fixed blocks of hERG channels that are marginally above (60%) and below (40%) the critical value (48%) of hERG block that is required to induced EADs in the models. At 60% hERG block, block of I_{CaV} (> 30% for both the OHR and OHRmv models) and I_{NaL} (> 60% for the OHRmv model) resulted in suppression of EADs. The remaining five channels had no inhibitory effects. At 40% hERG block, blocks of I_{Ks} and I_{K1} led to induction of EADs with lower block of I_{Ks} currents promoting triggering of EADs compared to I_{K1}. The block of remaining five channels did not result in EADs at 40% hERG block.

For visualization of combined effects of the channels on EAD induction, we performed EAD analysis for varying combinations of block of the three most sensitive non-hERG channels (I_{CaV}, I_{NaL}, and I_{Ks}) regulating EAD generation, each ranging from 0 to 100% at $C_{drug} = IC_{60,hERG}$. **Figure 2A** represents the EAD test for the models. The red region represents the set of combinations of blocks for these currents that resulted in the EADs in the OHR model (EAD+ region). The region in green covers the parameter subspace where no EADs were observed in the OHR model (EAD− region). Separation of the EAD+ region and EAD− region is outlined by the blue and yellow surfaces for the OHR and OHRmv model, respectively (**Figure 2A**). Among the non-hERG channels, block of I_{CaV} had the highest modulatory effects on EAD generation under normal

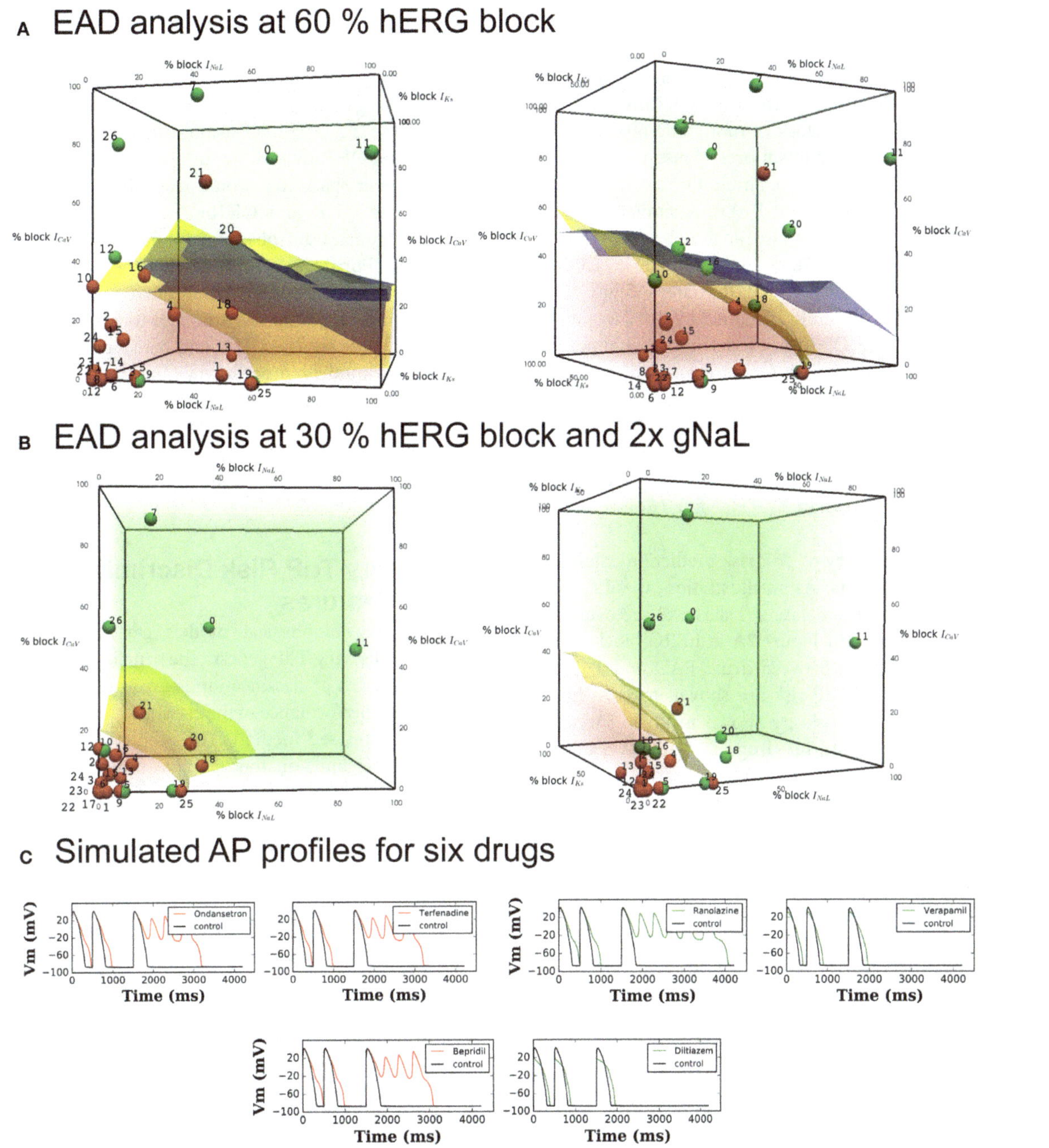

FIGURE 2 | Pause-induced EAD generation: combination of 0–100% I_{CaL}, I_{NaL}, and I_{Ks} blocks tested at **(A)** 60% hERG block in the OHR and OHRmv **(B)** 30% hERG block in the OHRmv that is modified to simulate LQT3 through increase in late sodium current conductance by 2-fold. Red regions cover the set of combinations of the blocks of the three channels that induced EADs in the model. Green region covers the set of combinations where EADs did not appear. Blue and yellow surfaces represent the separation between the EAD+ and EAD− region in OHR and OHRmv, respectively. The blue and yellow surfaces are plotted together in both plots in **(A)** to allow for easy comparision, but note that the red and green regions corresponds to the results for the OHR model. Block of I_{CaL}, I_{NaL}, and I_{Ks} at drug concentrations equal to 60 and 30% hERG block are calculated from *in-vitro* patch-clamp data in Crumb et al. (2016) using (Equation 1) and represented as dots in the parameter space of **(A,B)**, respectively. The drugs with torsadogenic potential were plotted as the red dots, while drugs with no known torsadogenicity risk are plotted as the green dots for two different TdP definitions. Definition 1 (left panels) - TdP+: Drugs in R1, R2, R3, CH1, CM1 or torsade label. Definition 2 (right panels) - TdP+: Drugs in CM1 and CM2. The data points for the Dataset 5: 0-Amitriptyline, 1-Azithromycin, 2-Bepridil, 3-Chloroquine, 4-Chlorpromazine, 5-Cibenzoline, 6-Cisapride, 7-Diltiazem, 8-Dofetilide, 9-Flecainide, 10-Lopinavir, 11-Mexiletine, 12-Mibefradil, 13-Moxifloxacin, 14-Nilotinib, 15-Ondansetron, 16-Propafenone, 17-Quinidine, 18-Quinine, 19-Ranolazine, 20-Ritonavir, 21-Saquinavir, 22-Sertindole, 23-Sotalol, 24-Terfenadine, 25-Toremifene, 26-Verapamil. Three drugs (Amiodarone, Lidocaine and Rufinamide) with hERG ratio greater than 200 were not included in the plot. **(C)** Transient AP profiles at 200th beat obtained from simulation of six drugs in the OHR model. Red and green traces show that the drug is defined as TdP+ and TdP−, respectively.

conditions. Under critical hERG block (60%), block of I_{CaV} by more than 30% resulted in suppression of the EADs in both the OHR and OHRmv models (**Figure 2A**). Block of I_{NaL} in the absence of the block of I_{CaV} did not result in suppression of the EADs in the OHR model. Even in the OHRmv model with improved I_{NaL} formulation, block of more than 60% of the late sodium current was required to suppress pause-induced EADs. Block of I_{Ks} currents increased the amount of block of I_{NaL} and I_{CaV} currents required to prevent EADs. A similar parametric space for EAD generation was also analyzed under enhanced late sodium currents (**Figure 2B**), associated with LQT3. In the OHRmv model the conductance of the late sodium current was doubled. Block of the hERG channel by 30% was enough to induce EADs in the OHRmv model under enhanced late sodium currents. EAD generation was examined at this 30% hERG block and is shown in **Figure 2B**. For the simulations with enhanced late sodium currents, the difference in the effects of I_{NaL} and I_{CaV} was significantly reduced. At 30% hERG block in the OHRmv model, block of greater than 20 and 30% was required for EAD suppression by I_{CaV} and I_{NaL}, respectively (**Figure 2B**).

Table 3 lists the accuracy of TdP risk prediction using EADs as the classification criteria. As an illustration, the data points for the drugs in one of the datasets (Dataset 5) are overlaid on the the parametric space in **Figure 2A** at hERG blocks of 60% to visualize the agreement between drugs EAD and TdP risks. The drugs with positive TdP risk are shown in red, while the drugs with negative TdP risk are shown in green. Actual AP profiles were also simulated for drugs in Datasets 5 and 7 at 60% hERG block concentrations taking into account the block of all seven channels. **Figure 2C** gives representative examples of the AP profiles for the multi-channel block of six of the drugs from Dataset 7 simulated in the OHR model. Our results show a good concordance between drugs torsadogenic risk and its propensity to induce EADs (i.e., most of the torsadogenic drugs resulted in pause-induced EADs in the models while no EADs are observed for majority of the non-torsadogenic drugs at 60% hERG block drug concentrations) across all the datasets. Majority of the datasets (Datasets 1, 2, 4, 6) contains values of blocks for two non-hERG channels (I_{CaV}, $I_{Na,fast}$) of which only I_{CaV} had an impact on EAD occurrence in the OHR and OHRmv models. Hence, for these datasets, OHR and OHRmv models give identical accuracies as the drugs with greater than 30% I_{CaV} block would result in EAD suppression in both of these models. For the Datasets 3, 5, and 7, drug-induced blocks of multiple ion channels are reported. However, very few drugs among these datasets are located in the region between the EAD risk decision surfaces for the OHR (blue surface) and OHRmv (yellow surface) models (i.e., the region in the parameter space that would result in a different prediction between the OHR and OHRmv models, **Figure 2A**). Hence, similar accuracies are observed for both of the models across all datasets. For the Dataset 7, Ranolazine (TdP−) was the only drug that was located on the negative side of the EAD risk decision surface for the OHRmv and to the positive side of the decision surface for the OHR, and hence predicted correctly by the OHRmv model but not by the OHR model. On the contrary for Dataset 5, Quinine (TdP+) ended up on the negative side of the EAD risk separating surface for the OHRmv and to the positive side of the EAD risk decision surface of the OHR model resulting in its incorrect prediction using the OHRmv model (**Figure 2A**).

TABLE 3 | Accuracy of drug classification based on EAD.

Datasets	Accuracy: OHR	Accuracy: Modified OHR
Dataset 1 (Mirams et al., 2011)	97	97
Dataset 2 (Kramer et al., 2013)	87	87
Dataset 3 (Okada et al., 2015)	84	84
Dataset 4 (Lancaster and Sobie, 2016)	87	87
Dataset 5 (Crumb et al., 2016)	83	80
Dataset 6 (Ando et al., 2017)	83	83
Dataset 7 (Li et al., 2017)	92	100
Dataset 8 (Merged Dataset)	83	83

3.2. Binary TdP Risk Discrimination from Direct Features

Although the biophysical models can provide mechanistic insights underlying TdP genesis, the benefits of using biophysical models in terms of classification is unclear. Here, we wanted to examine the performance of the classifiers built on direct features using the proposed method. The predictive power of the TdP risk classifiers built on the direct features using the proposed method (MCB@EAD) is shown in **Table 4** (two-step classifier column). Classification scores on the direct features at EFTPC are reported for comparison (one-step classifier column). The predictive ability of the two-step classifier was comparable or better than those for the classifiers built on the various features in the original datasets and also better than those for the one-step classifier. Most datasets comprise *in-vitro* assay data for drug-induced block of I_{Kr}, $I_{Na,fast}$, and I_{CaV} (Datasets 1, 2, 4, and 6). Drug-induced blocks of additional channels were reported in three datasets (Datasets 3, 5, and 7). The classifiers built using the block of I_{Kr} and I_{CaV} as inputs provided high TdP risk prediction scores (**Table 4**). Utilizing the block of I_{NaL} as an additional input feature improved the prediction for the two datasets (Dataset 3 and Dataset 7) by classifying correctly one more drug, Ranolazine, as TdP−. On the contrary, in Dataset 5, addition of the block of I_{NaL} to the features reduced the number of correctly classified drugs by one (classifying Ritonavir incorrectly as TdP−). Taking into account the block of additional ion channels ($I_{Na,fast}$ for Datasets 1, 2, 4, 6 and $I_{Na,fast}$, I_{Ks}, I_{to}, I_{K1} for Datasets 3, 5 ,7) did not provide any further improvement in the performance of the classifier for all datasets.

For visualization of our two-step approach we presented two-dimensional risk maps. Drug-induced block of the I_{CaV} or the sum of I_{CaV} and I_{NaL} blocks is plotted against the hERG ratio ($\frac{IC_{60,hERG}}{EFPTC_{drug}}$) for each drug in a two-dimensional risk map (**Figure 3**). The values of the hERG ratio (x-axis) and the block of I_{CaV} (y-axis) that provide the best discrimination vary widely

TABLE 4 | Binary TdP classifier scores of one-step and two-step classification on the direct features for the eight datasets.

Datasets			One step classifier	Two step classifier	Channel currents
Datasets	N_{Drugs}	**Original model Accuracy (Feature)**	$C_{drug} = EFTPC$	$C_{drug} = IC_{60,hERG}$	
Dataset 1 (Mirams et al., 2011)	31	97 (APD_{90})	90 (97)	100 (100)	I_{Kr} & I_{CaV}
Dataset 2 (Kramer et al., 2013)	55	91 ($-log(\frac{IC_{50,hERG}}{IC_{50,CaV}})$)	89 (82)	95 (95)	I_{Kr} & I_{CaV}
Dataset 3 (Okada et al., 2015)	12	100 ($\frac{C_{Drug,Arrhythmia}}{EFTPC}$)	58 (66)	92 (92)	I_{Kr} & I_{CaV}
			66 (66*)	100 (92*)	I_{Kr}, I_{CaV} & I_{NaL}
Dataset 4 (Lancaster and Sobie, 2016)	86	87 (APD_{50} & Diastolic Ca^{2+})	85 (85)	89 (90)	I_{Kr} & I_{CaV}
Dataset 5 (Crumb et al., 2016)	30		83 (83)	83 (83)	I_{Kr} & I_{CaV}
			80 (83*)	80 (83*)	I_{Kr}, I_{Cav} & I_{NaL}
Dataset 6 (Ando et al., 2017)	36	83 (APD prolongation and EAD (iPSCs))	86 (83)	86 (86)	I_{Kr} & I_{CaV}
Dataset 7 (Li et al., 2017)	12	100 $\left(\frac{AUCI_{NaL,drug}}{AUCI_{NaL,control}} + \frac{AUCI_{CaV,drug}}{AUCI_{CaV,control}}\right)$	92 (92)	92 (92)	I_{Kr} & I_{CaV}
			100 (92*)	100 (100*)	I_{Kr}, I_{CaV} & I_{NaL}
Dataset 8	197		79 (79)	85 (86)	I_{Kr} & I_{CaV}

*The total number of drugs in the particular dataset are reported in the N_{Drugs} column. Table also lists the feature used for classification in the original methods and corresponding scores if applicable. The last column shows a list of channel currents used to construct the classifiers. For comparision with the classification accuracy obtained with the direct features, we reported the highest accuracy obtained for the classifiers from the 13 derived features in isolation at different pacing rate/cell type in the bracket in One step and Two step classifier columns. *The derived features were extracted from simulations of the drug-induced block of all the reported ion channel currents in the in-vitro assay datasets.*

across the datasets (**Figure 3**). Using the threshold of 22 and 100 for the block of I_{CaV} and hERG ratio, respectively, resulted in the perfect classification for Dataset 1 (Mirams et al., 2011). However, for Dataset 2 the hERG ratio threshold of 200 and threshold for I_{CaV} of 57 provided the best classification. Looking at the risk maps in **Figure 3** we can see that the thresholds that provide best classification accuracy vary across datasets resulting in variations in the obtained high risk zones across datasets. For datasets 3, 5, 7 where we also considered block of I_{NaL} as one of the input feature in addition to the block of I_{CaV} the value on y-axis of the risk map were reported using Equation (5). A two-dimensional risk map for Dataset 5 for two alternate TdP definitions is shown in **Figure 4**. On the two-dimensional risk map with only I_{CaV} block on the y-axis, we also highlight, using a blue rectangular outline, the separation between the region with EAD presence and absence observed in the *in-silico* simulation at varying I_{CaV} blocks. For example, at critical hERG block simulations in the model at block of I_{CaV} less than 30% would result in EADs. Block of I_{CaV} by more than 30% results in suppression of the observed EADs. There is approximate correspondence between the EAD observance region in the *in-silico* model and the high torsadogenic region obtained from classifying the direct-features using machine learning.

3.3. Derived vs. Direct Features as Predictors for TdP Risk

We examine the performance of classifiers from various derived features extracted from the simulated action potential and calcium transient in predicting TdP risk. Drug-induced multi-channel block was simulated in the OHR model for all the compounds in the merged dataset (Dataset 8) considering the block I_{Kr} and I_{CaV} channels. Simulations were also carried out taking into account drug-induced block of all the channels with available IC_{50} values. Taking into account the block of additional channels resulted in similar accuracies and are reported in the Supplemental Material. **Figure 5** shows the performance of the logistic-regression classifier to discriminate TdP+ and TdP− drugs (**Figures 5A,B**) and to predict drug-induced EADs (**Figures 5C,D**). The classifiers were built on 13 features extracted from the steady-state APs and Ca^{2+} transients (for 3 cell types at 3 pacing rates). The derived features were extracted at either EFTPC of the drugs (**Figures 5A,C**) or at concentrations at which each drug would produce 60% hERG block ($C_{drug} = IC_{60,hERG}$) (**Figures 5B,D**). Among the various derived features obtained at $C_{drugs} = EFTPC$, diastolic Ca^{2+} levels provided the best discrimination score between the TdP+ and TdP− drugs (~79% accuracy at 1 Hz in epi cell type, **Figure 5A**) in agreement with a

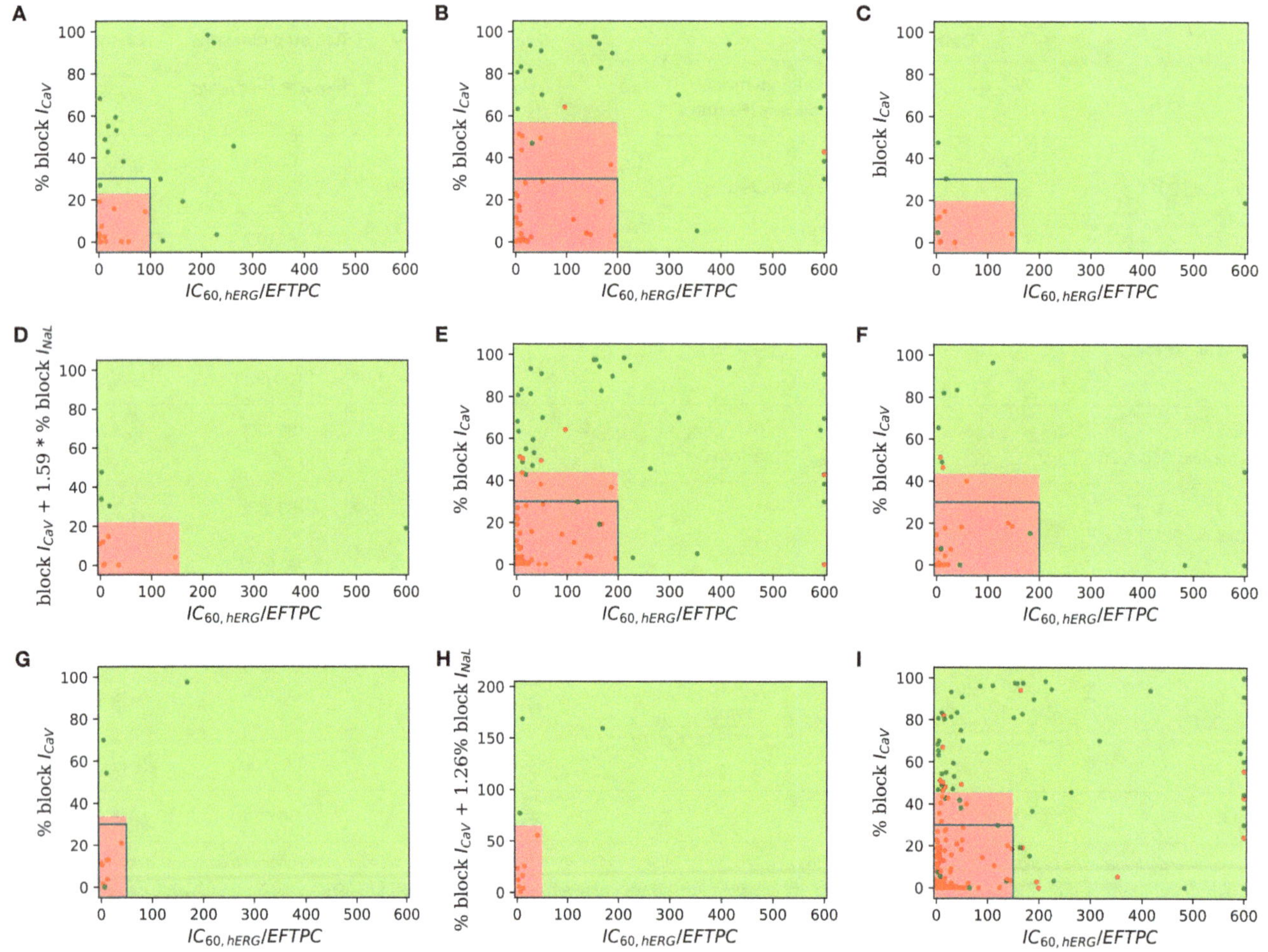

FIGURE 3 | Two-dimensional TdP risk map; blocks of channels are on y-axes and hERG ratio on x-axes for **(A)** Dataset 1 (Mirams et al., 2011), **(B)** Dataset 2 (Kramer et al., 2013), **(C)** Dataset 3 (Okada et al., 2015), **(D)** Dataset 3 (I_{Kr}, I_{CaV}, I_{NaL}) (Okada et al., 2015), **(E)** Dataset 4 (Lancaster and Sobie, 2016), **(F)** Dataset 6 (Ando et al., 2017), **(G)** Dataset 7 (I_{Kr}, I_{CaV}) (Li et al., 2017), **(H)** Dataset 7 (I_{Kr}, I_{CaV}, I_{NaL}) (Li et al., 2017), and **(I)** Dataset 8 (merged dataset). The regions in green are low risk regions and the regions in red are high risk areas. Red dots (•) indicate TdP+ drugs and green dots (•) indicate TdP− drugs. For comparsion purposes, we superimpose a blue rectangular outline that shows the separation between EAD+ and EAD− regions of parameter space. For binary classification the high and intermediate risk drugs in Dataset 7 were assigned TdP+ and the low risk drugs were assigned to TdP−.

previous report (Lancaster and Sobie, 2016). Classifier was also built using APD_{50} and Diastolic Ca^{2+} together as inputs (the combination that provided the best prediction in Lancaster and Sobie, 2016) but did not give an improved classification for the merged dataset. Several derived features performed well (>90% accuracy) for EAD risk prediction (**Figure 5**). However, at drug concentrations equal to $IC_{60,hERG}$ ($C_{drug} = IC_{60,hERG}$), each of the 13 features from the Ca^{2+} transient and AP provided high classification scores (~85% maximum) for TdP risk assessment (**Figure 5C**). The highest accuracy for each of the features was obtained at different pacing rates (0.5, 1, and 2 Hz) and for different cell types (endo, mid and epi). The maximum classification scores to discriminate the drugs that induced EAD in the model from the drugs that did not induce EADs was 100% (**Figure 5D**) for each of the features. Our results suggest that at fixed hERG block concentrations where trigger events such as EADs arise, several derived features obtained from the model including features from the Ca^{2+} transient can provide good TdP risk prediction. These derived features also highly correlate with EADs (**Figure 5**). However, the derived features extracted from simulations of the drug-induced effects in ventricular myocyte model did not result in much improvement in TdP risk assessment over the classifiers built on the direct-features using the proposed method (**Table 4**). Moreover, combining the direct and derived features to build the TdP risk classifiers also did not improve the classification performance (results are not shown).

3.4. Direct Features Perform Well to Allow Tertiary Risk Classification

Our results show that classifiers built on the direct features serve as excellent predictors of TdP risk of the drugs categorized into binary risk groups. However, a working committee under the CiPA initiative led by FDA has recently categorized 28 drugs into

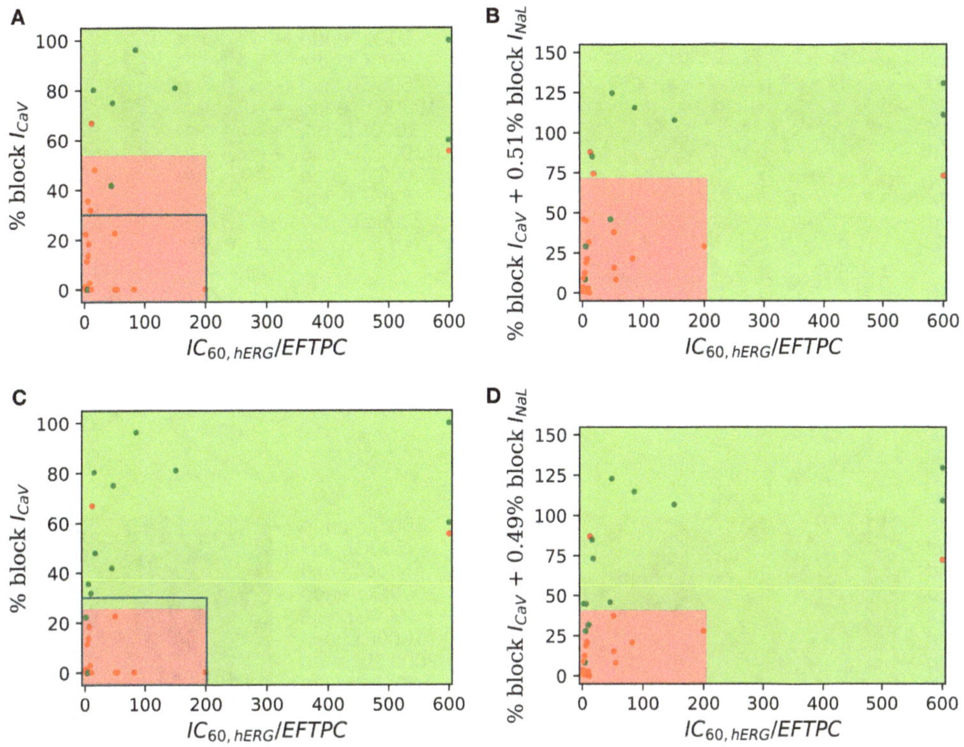

FIGURE 4 | Two-dimensional TdP risk map for Dataset 5 (Crumb et al., 2016). The region in green is a low risk region and the region in red is a high risk area. Red dots (•) indicate TdP+ drugs and green dots (•) indicate TdP− drugs. Blue rectangle outlines the separation of EAD+ (<30% CaV block) and EAD− (> 30% CaV block) regions. The misclassified drugs are **(A)** Ranolazine (CM3, CP3), Cibenzoline (R5), Mibefradil (R4), Saquinavir (CM2) and Amiodarone (CM1, R1); **(B)** Cibenzoline, Ranolazine, Mibefradil, Ritonavir (CM3), Saquinavir and Amiodarone; **(C)** Cibenzoline, Ranolazine, Quinine (CM3), Saquinavir and Amiodarone; and **(D)** Cibenzoline, Ranolazine, Chlorpromazine (CM1), Saquinavir and Amiodarone. **(A,B)** TdP Definition 1: TdP+: Drugs belonging to R1,CM1,CH1 category or drug label has TdP warning. **(C,D)** TdP Definition 2: TdP+: Drugs belonging to CM1 or CM2 category.

tertiary risk categories (low, medium, and high risk compounds) (Colatsky et al., 2016; Fermini et al., 2016). Hence, we test the predictive capabilities of the classifier based on direct features to classify the drugs categorized into tertiary risk categories. **Figures 6A,B** show a two-dimensional risk map for the 12 drugs in Li et al. (2017). These drugs have been analyzed previously using modified OHR model that incorporate dynamic hERG channel interactions. The 12 drugs are a subset of the 28 drugs categorized into three risk categories (CP1, CP2, and CP3) under the CiPA initiative. As a first step, we developed a TdP risk map using only the block of I_{CaV} channel. The hERG ratio threshold of 150 and the threshold of I_{CaV} block of 45%, the values that provided best classification for the merged dataset, were utilized for classifying the low high and intermediate risk drugs from low risk drugs **Figure 6A**. Arbitrary value of hERG ratio and I_{CaV} block of 25 and 15, respectively (a value greater than the maximum hERG ratio and maximum block of I_{CaV} among the high risk drugs in Datasets 7 and 9) was utilized to separate high risk drugs from the low and intermediate risk drugs. Three of the four drugs in low risk (CP3) category were classified correctly. Ranolazine was the only misclassified drug. The boundaries of red zone were defined to include all high risk drugs and hence all the drugs from CP1 category were correctly classified. However, several drugs in intermediate risk were incorrectly classified. Next, we built regression classifier using as input metric the sum of block of I_{CaV}, I_{NaL} channels and the degree of drug-trapping parameter which was shown to be essential to improve risk prediction of intermediate risk drugs in the original dataset. **Figure 6B** shows the risk map built using this metric. The threshold along the y-axis was obtained from the regression coefficients. The hERG ratio threshold of 25 and 150 were utilized as before. Including the degree of drug trapping characterized by open-bound/closed-bound ratio for the drugs at steady-state (Li et al., 2017) as one of the features in addition to the blocks of CaV and NaL channels, resulted in the perfect separation of the 12 drugs in 3 categories (**Figure 6B**).

We employed the same approach to test all of the 28 drugs (Fermini et al., 2016) categorized in CP1, CP2, and CP3 categories under the CiPA initiative. *In-vitro* assays for 12 of these 28 drugs were reported in Crumb et al. (2016) and analyzed in Li et al. (2017). To augment this dataset, we extract the IC_{50} values for hERG and CaV blocks from Datasets 1, 2, 3, 5, 6, 7 resulting in characterization of 26 of the 28 drugs categorized under the CiPA initiative. Two drugs (Azimilide and Loratidine) were absent in all of the datasets analyzed here and hence were not taken into consideration. We used the mean value of the block if the drug was present in more than one

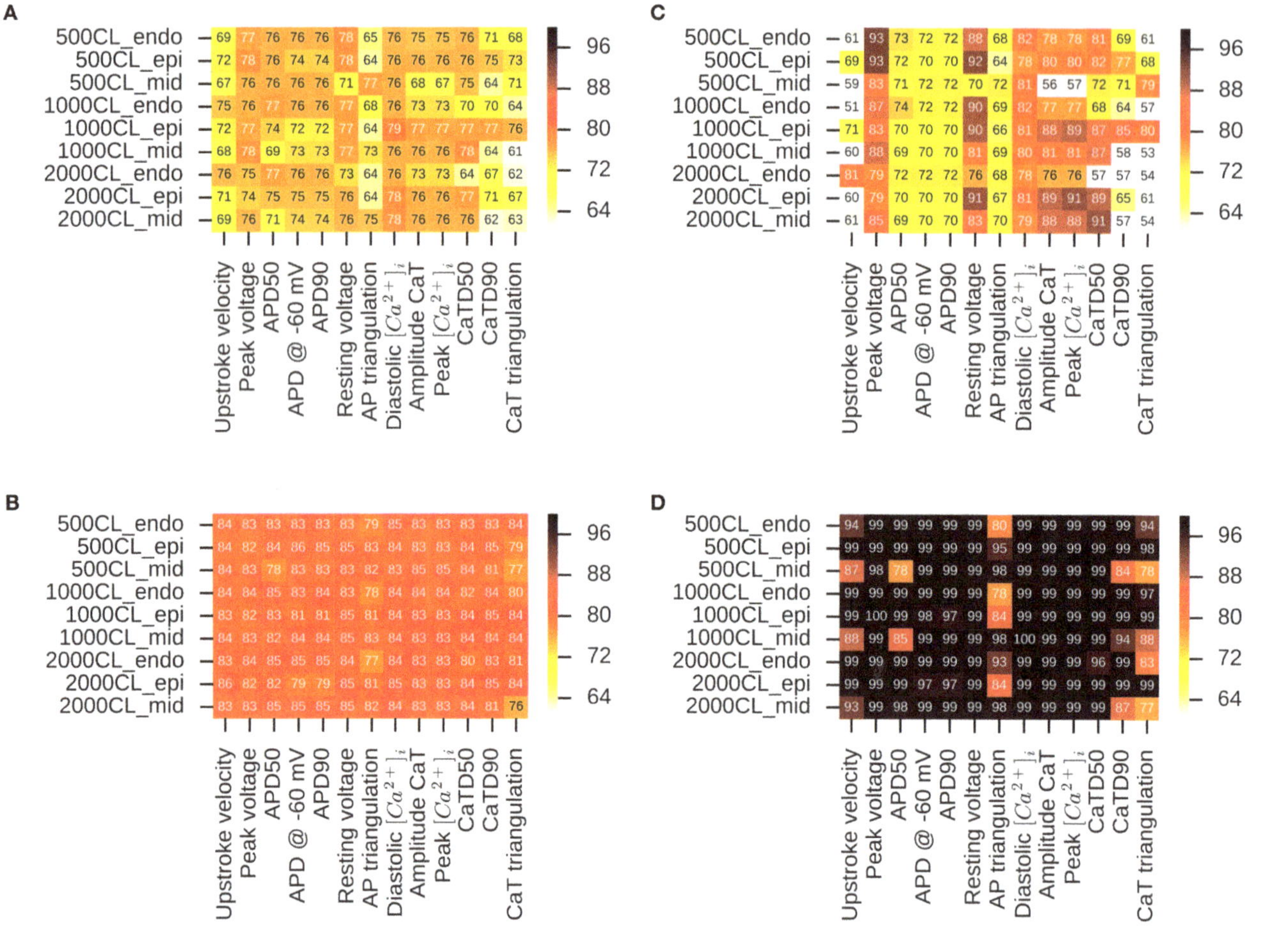

FIGURE 5 | Heat maps of leave-one-out cross validation scores for logistic regression classifiers built on 13 features extracted from the APs and Ca^{2+} transients in OHR model simulations. Drug-induced multi-channel block evaluated in the mid, endo and epi cell types at 500, 1,000, and 2,000 ms pacing rates. TdP risk classification at **(A)** EFTPC drug concentrations and **(B)** drug concentrations equal to hERG IC_{50}. EAD induction classification at **(C)** EFTPC drug concentrations **(D)** drug concentrations equal to hERG IC_{50}.

dataset. The final dataset of the 26 drugs is reported in the Supplemental Material. **Figure 6C** show the two-dimensional risk maps for the 26 drugs with hERG ratio on the x-axis and the block of CaV on the y-axis. The 45% I_{CaV} block threshold and hERG ratio threshold of 150 yielded almost perfect binary classification (high and intermediate vs. low risk drugs) with only 2 (Ranolazine and Tamoxifen) drugs of the 8 from the CP3 category and one drug (Clozapine) of the 16 drugs from CP1 and CP2 cateogry (high and intermediate risk drugs) classifying incorrectly. However, no clear separation was observed amoung the drugs in CP1 and CP2 categories, with several drugs from CP2 category ending up in the high risk region. Considering additional features such as I_{NaL} and the degree of drug trapping (if either of the features were not available their value was set to zero) and utilizing the threshold obtained from training the Dataset 7 (**Figure 6B**) resulted in only 3 intermediate risk drugs (Clarithromycin, Domperidone, Droperidol) and 1 low risk drug (Tamoxifen) of the 26 drugs to be misclassified (**Figure 6D**). The classifier already performs well in spite of testing data from heterogeneous sources with some missing values. Further refinement of the method may be possible when a dataset is available with all 28 drugs characterized with a consistent methodology.

3.5. Diverse Definition of Drugs Torsadogenicity Lead to Different Prediction Accuracies

Different binary definitions for the drug's torsadogenic risk have been used across the literature (Lancaster and Sobie, 2016; Ando et al., 2017; Wiśniowska and Polak, 2017). **Tables 5, 6** list the different classification accuracy scores obtained for four different binary TdP definitions (Datasets 5 and 8, respectively). Classifiers were constructed on the block of one or multiple-ion channels as inputs at critical hERG block concentrations ($C_{drug} = IC_{60,hERG}$). The various definitions not only resulted in variability of classification scores (**Tables 5, 6**), but also changed the role of different ion channels in accurate TdP risk classification

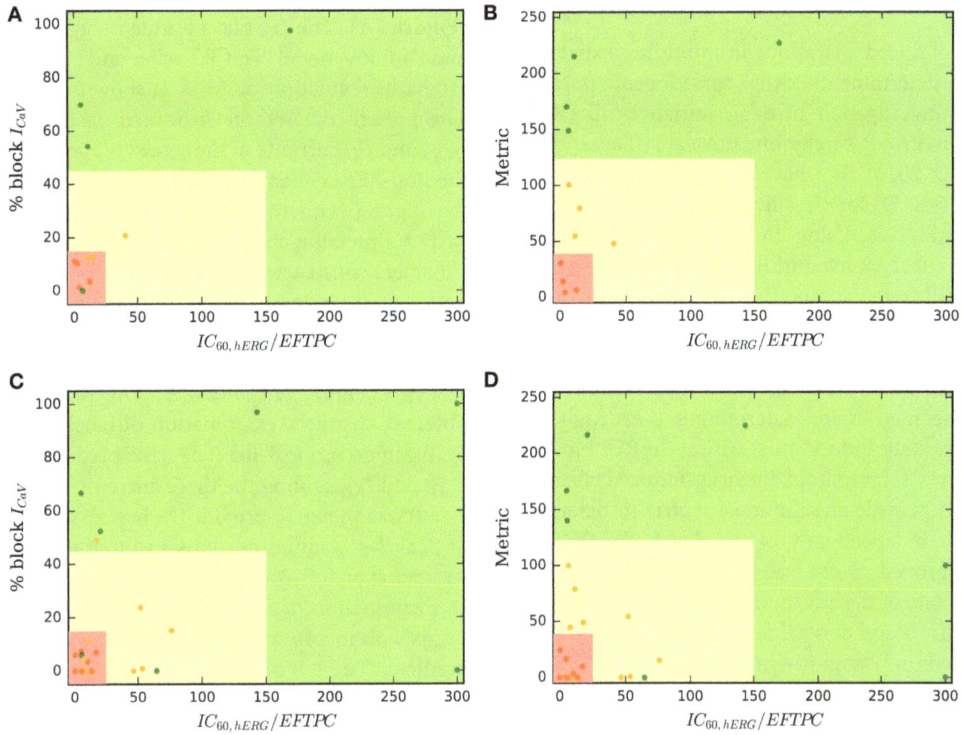

FIGURE 6 | Two-dimensional TdP risk map for Dataset 7 (Li et al., 2017) **(A,B)**, and drugs in Fermini et al. (2016) **(C,D)**. The region in green is a low risk region. Yellow region is an intermediate risk region, and the region in red is a high risk area. Red dots (•) indicate high risk drugs, green dots (•) indicate low risk drugs and orange dots (•) indicate intermediate risk drugs. Metric = % block CaV + % block NaL + degree of drug trapping.

TABLE 5 | Accuracy scores of TdP classifiers on the direct features for Dataset 5 under four different TdP definitions.

Crumb et al., 2016	Target 1	Target 2	Target 3	Target 4
	2-step $C_{drug} = IC_{60,hERG}$, direct features			
Step1:$IC_{60,hERG}/EFTPC$	73	60	60	60
Step1:$IC_{60,hERG}/EFTPC$ Step2:% block I_{CaV}	83	83	70	70
Step1:$IC_{60,hERG}/EFTPC$ Step2:% block I_{CaV} & I_{NaL}	80	83	83	76
Step1:$IC_{60,hERG}/EFTPC$ Step2:% block I_{CaV}, I_{NaL} & I_{Ks}	80	83	83	76
	2-step $C_{drug} = IC_{60,hERG}$, Derived Features			
Step1:$IC_{60,hERG}/EFTPC$ Step2: Derived features	83	83	83	76

Target1: TdP+ = CM1, CH1, R1, R2, R3, and FDA label QT prolongation and torsade warnings. Target 2: TdP+ = CM1 and CM2. Target 3: TdP+ = CM1. Target 4: TdP+ = CM1 and CM3. Row reporting the maximum accuracies obtained using the derived features is reported for comparision with the direct features.

(**Table 5**). Using the block of I_{CaV} currents provided the best accuracy scores under two of the four definitions (Target 1 and Target 2) for Dataset 5. Including the effects on additional ion-channels did not improve classification scores for these two definitions. Taking into account the block of late sodium currents in addition to CaV channels, provided the best classification accuracy for remaining two of the four TdP definitions (Target 3 and 4) (**Table 5**).

TABLE 6 | Accuracy scores of TdP classifiers on the direct features for Dataset 8 under four different TdP definitions.

Dataset 8	Target 1	Target 2	Target 3	Target 4
	2-step $C_{drug} = IC_{60,hERG}$, direct features			
Step1:$IC_{60,hERG}/EFTPC$	77	69	64	66
Step1:$IC_{60,hERG}/EFTPC$ Step2:% block I_{CaV}	85	77	74	73
Step1:$IC_{60,hERG}/EFTPC$ Step2:% block I_{CaV} & $I_{Na,fast}$	85	76	74	72
	2-step $C_{drug} = IC_{60,hERG}$, derived features			
Step1:$IC_{60,hERG}/EFTPC$ Step2: Derived features	86	76	74	73

Target1: TdP+ = CM1, CH1, R1, R2, R3, and FDA label QT prolongation and torsade warnings. Target 2: TdP+ = CM1 and CM2. Target 3: TdP+ = CM1. Target 4: TdP+ = CM1 and CM3. Row reporting the maximum accuracies obtained using the derived features is reported for comparision with the direct features.

4. DISCUSSION

Evaluation of drug-induced alterations in multiple cardiac ion-channel currents to determine the drug's torsadogenic potential is currently under investigation through initiatives like CiPA (Comprehensive *In-vitro* Proarrhythmia Assay) (Sager et al., 2014; Fermini et al., 2016). We have developed a novel two-step method (MCB@EAD) for classification of drugs according to their torsadogenic risk. Using the proposed method, we examined the drug effects at fixed hERG block (i.e., 60% block) concentrations for all tested compounds. This approach allows to isolate the effects of hERG and non-hERG channels in the classification problem. The proximity of the drug's EFTPC to the concentration that results in the critical hERG block provides one of the metrics for determining the drug's TdP risk. For the drugs that induce this critical hERG block at concentrations below a set threshold, the drug-induced effects on non-hERG channels provide an additional metric to determine pro-arrhythmic risk independently of the drug's EFTPC. Our classifier shows improved or equivalent prediction to existing methods. However, one of the advantages compared to previous studies is that the direct and derived features based MCB@EAD classifiers were tested on several *in-vitro* assay datasets reported previously, as well as on a large composite dataset obtained by merging the different datasets together. One of the important findings of the study was that MCB@EAD TdP classifiers from the direct features provides excellent TdP risk prediction and performs identical to the TdP classifiers from the derived features, which are extracted from complex biophysical models. Although the derived features provided by the biophysical models did not improve the predictive capability for TdP risk assessment, the biophysical models helped determine the amount of block that generates EADs (i.e., the concentration at which the direct features are analyzed using the MCB@EAD classifier). The proposed method not only performs comparably or better than the previous classifiers (**Table 4**) across various *in-vitro* assay datasets published previously, but also highlights the link between direct and derived feature based classifiers. The results also show strong correlation between the drugs that generate EADs and the drugs with positive TdP risk.

4.1. Ion-Channels Critical for TdP Risk Prediction

Although the role of multiple ion-channels have been suggested for improved TdP risk prediction, classifiers have been primarily built on the blocks of I_{Kr}, I_{CaV}, and $I_{Na,peak}$ currents (Mirams et al., 2011; Christophe, 2013, 2015; Kramer et al., 2013; Lancaster and Sobie, 2016). A recent assay reports the drug-induced effects on seven ion channels (Crumb et al., 2016) providing an opportunity to identify the ion channels that are important for pro-arrhythmic risk assessment. The results of our parametric simulations of EAD indicate a potential role of block of I_{CaV}, I_{NaL}, and I_{Ks} currents, in addition to I_{Kr}, for determination of torsadogenic risk of the drugs (**Figure 2**). It should be noted that the EAD simulations results are highly dependent on the ventricular myocyte model. For example, block of late sodium current in the OHRmv plays a more prominent role in regulation of AP sensitivity to EADs as compared to the OHR model (**Figure 2A**). The I_{Ks} plays a much bigger role in Ten Tusscher and Panfilov model (Ten Tusscher and Panfilov, 2006) than OHR model in regulation of APD as shown in Mirams et al. (2014). The present datasets have limited examples of block of I_{CaV}, I_{NaL}, and I_{Ks} currents in the same compounds. Moreover, among the non-hERG channels, the regulatory effect of I_{CaV} block was the highest with the block of I_{CaV} by only 30% resulting in EAD suppression at critical hERG current block (**Figure 2**). The classifiers constructed on the block of I_{Kr} and I_{CaL} provided the best discrimination between torsadogenic and non-torsadogenic drugs for the majority of the datasets tested here, including the dataset where drug-induced effects on seven ion channels were reported (**Figure 2**, **Tables 4**, **5**). Our results suggest that among different channels, examination of block of I_{CaV} and I_{Kr} might be the most critical for TdP risk prediction. Relative block of I_{CaV} and I_{Kr} (among the three currents measured in the *in-vitro* assay) was shown to provide the best risk prediction, with no role of peak/fast sodium currents in improving the classification in Kramer et al. (2013).

Examination of late sodium block can be important for the drugs with low to moderate I_{CaV} block as these drugs would be predicted TdP+ if only I_{Kr} and I_{CaV} block are considered for risk prediction. Moderate to high block of I_{NaL} by these drugs can result in suppression of EADs (**Figure 2**) indicating lower TdP risk. Earlier datasets did not report values for I_{NaL} block. Dataset 5 reports the value of drug-induced block of seven ion-channels, including the block of I_{NaL}. Among the drugs with low to moderate I_{CaV} in Dataset 5, only three drugs [Ranolazine(CM3), Toremifene(CM2) and Quinine(CM3)] have greater than 30% I_{NaL} block at critical hERG block concentrations. For the limited data with inconsistent risk categorization, taking into account the I_{NaL} block did not improve predictive power of the classifiers (**Tables 4**, **5**). A small improvement in TdP prediction was observed for Datasets 3 and 7 (Okada et al., 2015; Li et al., 2017) when considering drug-induced block of I_{NaL} as one of the input features by correctly classifying Ranolazine (the only drug with high late sodium block in absence of I_{CaV} block) in both the datasets (**Table 4** and **Figure 3**). The limited data and inconclusive/minor improvement in torsadogenic risk classification make it difficult to ascertain the role of ion channels such as I_{NaL} and I_{Ks} in predicting TdP risk.

4.2. Predictive Power of Direct vs. Derived Features

In-silico biophysical models can be thought of as a complex non-linear transfer function, which translates the drug-induced multi-channel block effects at channel level (input) to alterations in APs and calcium transients at cellular/tissue levels (output). Several *in-silico* electrical biophysical models of human ventricular cell models have been published over the last decade (e.g.,Ten Tusscher and Panfilov, 2006; Grandi et al., 2010; O'Hara et al., 2011; Himeno et al., 2015). TdP risk classification on features extracted from the drug-induced responses in isolated cell (Mirams et al., 2011; Christophe, 2013, 2015; Lancaster and Sobie, 2016), tissue (Trenor et al., 2013; Kubo et al., 2017) or organ level (Okada et al., 2015) computational models can provide physiological/mechanistic insights. Moreover, *in-silico* models serve as an excellent tool for evaluation of drug-safety in diseased conditions (Trenor et al., 2013; Kubo et al., 2017). Our simulations in the OHRmv model under pathological conditions (enhanced late sodium currents) reveal that EAD can appear at significantly lower drug concentrations as only 30% hERG block was required to induce pause-induced EADs under pathological conditions compared to 60% hERG block under normal conditions. Moreover, the modulatory effects of non-hERG channels on EAD induction was also significantly different for simulations under pathological conditions (**Figure 2**). On the other hand, biophysical models show considerable differences in their formulations and can lead to different predictions based on the chosen model. Simulations of EAD generation show a significant difference between the surfaces separating EAD+ region from EAD− region, that are obtained from the OHR and OHRmv models (**Figure 2**). Recently, several efforts have been carried out for optimization of *in-silico* cardiac cell models for pro-arrhythmia risk assessment (Dutta et al., 2016; Mann et al., 2016; Li et al., 2017).

Statistical/machine learning classifiers that use measured *in-vitro* block of multiple cardiac channels (direct features) as their input (Kramer et al., 2013; Mistry et al., 2015) demonstrated comparable accuracy as compared to TdP risk classifiers built on derived features, questioning the need of additional complexity provided by the *in-silico* models. On the contrary, the study by Okada et al. suggested the need of highly detailed three-dimensional cardiac models for pro-arrhythmic risk assessment and showed relatively low predictive ability using the direct features and also certain derived features from the *in-silico* lumped parameter (zero-dimensional) cellular models (Okada et al., 2015). Derived features from *in-silico* simulations that incorporate dynamic drug-hERG channel interactions were shown to improve prediction of TdP risk (Li et al., 2017). For all the datasets tested here, including the datasets in Okada et al. (2015) and Li et al. (2017), we showed that the classifiers built on the direct features performed equally or better than the previously developed classifiers on the derived features (**Table 4**). Our results show that for currently available *in-vitro* assay datasets simple models based on the direct features can provide similar accuarcy to more complex models based on derived features. It should be noted that our two-dimensional risk classifiers on the direct features also utilized insights gained from the computational models (the direct features are examined at critical hERG block concentrations where EAD can arise in the *in-silico* models). Our parametric simulation for EAD induction highlights one of the possible reasons for the insignificant improvement in predictive power of classifiers built on the derived features from the *in-silico* models. Although a non-linear surface is obtained from the *in-silico* models separating the EAD+ and EAD− regions (**Figure 2**), a hyperplane

$$a \times block_{I_{CaV}} + b \times block_{I_{NaL}} + c \times block_{I_{Ks}} + d = 0 \quad (6)$$

constructed using direct features can result in nearly identical separation, where a, b, c, and d are the parameters of the hyperplane and $block_{I_{CaV}}$, $block_{I_{NaL}}$, and $block_{I_{Ks}}$ are the values of block of I_{CaV} I_{NaL}, and I_{Ks}, respectively. Moreover, with most of the datasets comprising values for block of few channels (Mirams et al., 2011; Kramer et al., 2013) and the much higher incidence of drug-induced block of particular ion channels (I_{NaL}, I_{CaV}, and I_{Kr}) even when drug-induced modulation of several channels are examined (Crumb et al., 2016), the result is a congregation of majority of the data in a small region of the plausible high-dimensional risk space (e.g., see **Figure 2**). For example, the data in Mirams et al. (2011) and Kramer et al. (2013) would fall on a single edge of the 3D EAD space in **Figure 2** in the absence of values for drug-induced block on I_{NaL} and I_{Ks} in these datasets. This allows risk classification to be performed by a hyperplane with a single parameter, such as $block_{I_{CaV}}$. Here, we utilized an additional metric, i.e., the hERG ratio, to further improve the classification performance of the direct-feature based classifiers (**Figures 3**, **4**, **6**). For the limited data currently available, risk classification using simple statistical models built on the direct features as the one presented here may suffice.

4.3. Diversity in the Proposed Derived Features

The classifiers built on derived features obtained from the *in-silico* models are based on certain underlying physiological phenomenon (APD, increase in calcium levels, etc.). Hence, derived features are thought to allow better extrapolation to examine drug targets other than those in the training set. However, diverse derived features from the *in-silico* models have been suggested as possible candidate metrics. Several features from the biophysical models, such as APD_{50}, APD_{90}, calcium level peak, and CaD_{90} provided the best classification depending on the selected *in-silico* model (Mirams et al., 2011). Other derived features (EADs, TDR, change in I_{CaV} & I_{NaL}) extracted from the AP and calcium transient (Christophe, 2013, 2015; Li et al., 2017) have also been suggested as possible candidate metrics for TdP risk prediction. Rather than examining the individual features separately, a recent study performed a comprehensive feature selection among 331 metrics and determined that two metrics, APD_{50} and diastolic Ca^{2+} in the OHR model at 1 Hz pacing, provided the best discrimination between torsadogenic and non-torsadogenic drugs (Lancaster and Sobie, 2016). The overall diversity in reported plausible candidate metrics for TdP risk classification can be attributed to different simulation protocols, drug concentrations and biophysical models. We showed that several derived features obtained from the *in-silico* models may track together and provide equal predictive power for risk classification when examined independent of drug EFTPC (**Figure 5C**). Equal predictive ability of several features makes it difficult to determine the underlying causal mechanism. In addition, the identical performance of several derived features limits the extensibility of the classifier to untrained targets, as classification results depend on the specific set of features chosen to perform the classification. For example, examination of untrained ion-channel targets using a classifier with diastolic Ca^{2+} level as the primary risk discriminating feature predicts a decrease in torsadogenic risk for increased $Na^+ - Ca^{2+}$ currents (Lancaster and Sobie, 2016). On the contrary, TdP risk prediction under $Na^+ - Ca^{2+}$ modulation using a classifier with APD_{50} or APD_{90} as the primary discriminating feature would predict opposite effects, with decreased $Na^+ - Ca^{2+}$ exchanger current being associated with decreased TdP risk. Moreover, the derived features obtained from the highly complex biophysical models did not result in improved prediction over the classfiers built on the direct features using the proposed method.

4.4. Limitations

One of the primary limitations is the quality of the datasets itself. The variability in the IC_{50} values among the several datasets can be one of the reasons for the observation of different thresholds for the hERG ratio and I_{CaV} block that resulted in the best discrimination between TdP+ and TdP− drugs (**Figure 3**). Quantification of the uncertainties in the *in-vitro* channel screening data and their effects on risk prediction are presented in Johnstone et al. (2016). Inconsistencies in risk definition presents another important challenge for torsadogenic risk assessment. Wiśniowska and Polak (2017) reports a comprehensive list of compounds that have been inconsistently defined as TdP+ or TdP− in different studies to develop torsadogenic risk classifiers. The different categorizations can lead to different interpretations and accuracy scores for TdP risk determination (**Table 5**). Standardization of torsadogenicity definition, which would allow comparison of the performance of different classifiers/features, is required. Certain steps in this direction have been started. Based on a general consensus, a working group formed under CiPA initiative picked 28 compounds and categorized each into three groups (Colatsky et al., 2016; Fermini et al., 2016) for testing/training of the classifiers. *In-silico* simulations of dynamic drug-channel interactions might be essential to further improve the TdP risk assessment (Li et al., 2017). Inclusion of the drug-binding parameter, in addition to the amount of block of ion-channels, resulted in 100% prediction using our approach. Sufficient I_{Kr} block was assumed to be necessary for TdP generation in our method. The effects of non-hERG channels are thought to enhance or mitigate the torsadogenic effects of I_{Kr} block. The method resulted in excellent predictive performance across several datasets that report drug-induced block of various ion channels only. However, drug-induced enhancement of ion-channel currents such as I_{NaL} can result in increased TdP risk in the absence of hERG block (Lacerda et al., 2008; Yang et al., 2014). The method could be further extended to examine such effects when more data are available. The present work not only provides a new method for *in-vitro* ion-channel screening based TdP risk classification but also highlights several important issues in regards to the use of drug-induced multi-channel blockage for torsadogenic risk prediction.

AUTHOR CONTRIBUTIONS

JP, VG, and JR wrote the manuscript. JP, VG, and JR designed the research. JP and VG performed the simulations. JP, VG, and JR analyzed the data.

REFERENCES

Abbasi, M., Small, B. G., Patel, N., Jamei, M., and Polak, S. (2017). Early assessment of pro-arrhythmic risk of drugs using the *in vitro* data and single cell based *in silico* models: proof of concept. *Toxicol. Mech. Methods* 27, 88–99. doi: 10.1080/15376516.2016.1256460

Ando, H., Yoshinaga, T., Yamamoto, W., Asakura, K., Uda, T., Taniguchi, T., et al. (2017). A new paradigm for drug-induced torsadogenic risk assessment using human iPS cell-derived cardiomyocytes. *J. Pharmacol. Toxicol. Methods* 84, 111–127. doi: 10.1016/j.vascn.2016.12.003

Antzelevitch, C. (2004). Electrophysiological effects of ranolazine, a novel antianginal agent with antiarrhythmic properties. *Circulation* 110, 904–910. doi: 10.1161/01.CIR.0000139333.83620.5D

Antzelevitch, C. (2007). Ionic, molecular, and cellular bases of QT-interval prolongation and torsade de pointes. *Europace* 9(Suppl. 4), iv4–iv15. doi: 10.1093/europace/eum166

Bril, A., Gout, B., Bonhomme, M., Landais, L., Faivre, J. F., Linee, P., et al. (1996). Combined potassium and calcium channel blocking activities as a basis for antiarrhythmic efficacy with low proarrhythmic risk: experimental profile of BRL-32872. *J. Pharmacol. Exp. Therapeut.* 276, 637–646.

Champeroux, P., Viaud, K., El Amrani, A. I., Fowler, J. S., Martel, E., Le Guennec, J.-Y., et al. (2005). Prediction of the risk of Torsade de Pointes using the model of isolated canine Purkinje fibres. *Br. J. Pharmacol.* 144, 376–385. doi: 10.1038/sj.bjp.0706070

Christophe, B. (2013). Simulation of early after-depolarisation in non-failing human ventricular myocytes: can this help cardiac safety pharmacology? *Pharmacol. Rep.* 65, 1281–1293. doi: 10.1016/S1734-1140(13)71486-5

Christophe, B. (2015). *In silico* study of transmural dispersion of repolarization in non-failing human ventricular myocytes: contribution to cardiac safety pharmacology. *Br. J. Pharmaceut. Res.* 7, 88–101. doi: 10.9734/BJPR/2015/17850

Colatsky, T., Fermini, B., Gintant, G., Pierson, J. B., Sager, P., Sekino, Y., et al. (2016). The comprehensive *in vitro* proarrhythmia assay (CiPA) initiative–update on progress. *J. Pharmacol. Toxicol. Methods* 81, 15–20. doi: 10.1016/j.vascn.2016.06.002

Crumb, W. J., Vicente, J., Johannesen, L., and Strauss, D. G. (2016). An evaluation of 30 clinical drugs against the comprehensive *in vitro* proarrhythmia assay (CiPA) proposed ion channel panel. *J. Pharmacol. Toxicol. Methods* 81, 251–262. doi: 10.1016/j.vascn.2016.03.009

Dutta, S., Strauss, D., Colatsky, T., and Li, Z. (2016). Optimization of an *in silico* cardiac cell model for proarrhythmia risk assessment. *Comput. Cardiol.* 43, 2–5. doi: 10.22489/CinC.2016.253-483

Fermini, B., Hancox, J. C., Abi-Gerges, N., Bridgland-Taylor, M., Chaudhary, K. W., Colatsky, T., et al. (2016). A new perspective in the field of cardiac safety testing through the comprehensive *in vitro* proarrhythmia assay paradigm. *J. Biomol. Screen.* 21, 1–11. doi: 10.1177/1087057115594589

Gintant, G. (2011). An evaluation of hERG current assay performance: translating preclinical safety studies to clinical QT prolongation. *Pharmacol. Therapeut.* 129, 109–119. doi: 10.1016/j.pharmthera.2010.08.008

Grandi, E., Pasqualini, F. S., and Bers, D. M. (2010). A novel computational model of the human ventricular action potential and Ca transient. *J. Mol. Cell. Cardiol.* 48, 112–121. doi: 10.1016/j.yjmcc.2009.09.019

Himeno, Y., Asakura, K., Cha, C. Y., Memida, H., Powell, T., Amano, A., et al. (2015). A human ventricular myocyte model with a refined representation of excitation-contraction coupling. *Biophys. J.* 109, 415–427. doi: 10.1016/j.bpj.2015.06.017

Johnstone, R. H., Bardenet, R., Gavaghan, D. J., and Mirams, G. R. (2016). Hierarchical Bayesian inference for ion channel screening dose-response data. *Wellcome Open Res.* 1:6. doi: 10.12688/wellcomeopenres.9945.1

Kramer, J., Obejero-Paz, C. A., Myatt, G., Kuryshev, Y. A., Bruening-Wright, A., Verducci, J. S., et al. (2013). MICE Models: superior to the HERG model in predicting torsade de pointes. *Sci. Rep.* 3, 1–7. doi: 10.1038/srep02100

Kubo, T., Ashihara, T., Tsubouchi, T., and Horie, M. (2017). Significance of integrated *in silico* transmural ventricular wedge preparation models of human non-failing and failing hearts for safety evaluation of drug candidates. *J. Pharmacol. Toxicol. Methods* 83, 30–41. doi: 10.1016/j.vascn.2016.08.007

Lacerda, A. E., Kuryshev, Y. A., Chen, Y., Renganathan, M., Eng, H., Danthi, S. J., et al. (2008). Alfuzosin delays cardiac repolarization by a novel mechanism. *J. Pharmacol. Exp. Therapeut.* 324, 427–433. doi: 10.1124/jpet.107.128405

Lancaster, M. C., and Sobie, E. A. (2016). Improved prediction of drug-induced torsades de pointes through simulations of dynamics and machine learning algorithms. *Clin. Pharmacol. Therapeut.* 100, 371–379. doi: 10.1002/cpt.367

Li, Z., Dutta, S., Sheng, J., Tran, P. N., Wu, W., Chang, K., et al. (2017). Improving the *in silico* assessment of proarrhythmia risk by combining hERG (human ether-?-go-go-related gene) channel? Drug binding kinetics and multichannel pharmacology. *Circulation* 10:e004628.

Liu, J., and Laurita, K. R. (2005). The mechanism of pause-induced torsade de pointes in long QT syndrome. *J. Cardiovasc. Electrophysiol.* 16, 981–987. doi: 10.1111/j.1540-8167.2005.40677.x

Mann, S. A., Imtiaz, M., Winbo, A., Rydberg, A., Perry, M. D., Couderc, J. P., et al. (2016). Convergence of models of human ventricular myocyte electrophysiology after global optimization to recapitulate clinical long QT phenotypes. *J. Mol. Cell. Cardiol.* 100, 25–34. doi: 10.1016/j.yjmcc.2016.09.011

Mirams, G. R., Cui, Y., Sher, A., Fink, M., Cooper, J., Heath, B. M., et al. (2011). Simulation of multiple ion channel block provides improved early prediction of compounds' clinical torsadogenic risk. *Cardiovasc. Res.* 91, 53–61. doi: 10.1093/cvr/cvr044

Mirams, G. R., Davies, M. R., Brough, S. J., Bridgland-Taylor, M. H., Cui, Y., Gavaghan, D. J., et al. (2014). Prediction of thorough QT study results using action potential simulations based on ion channel screens. *J. Pharmacol. Toxicol. Methods* 70, 246–254. doi: 10.1016/j.vascn.2014.07.002

Mistry, H. B., Davies, M. R., and Di Veroli, G. Y. (2015). A new classifier-based strategy for *in-silico* ion-channel cardiac drug safety assessment. *Front. Pharmacol.* 6:59. doi: 10.3389/fphar.2015.00059

Kay, G. N., Plumb, V. J., Arciniegas, J. G., Henthorn, R. W., and Waldo, A. L. (1983). Torsade de pointes: the long-short initiating sequence and other clinical features: observations in 32 patients. *J. Am. College Cardiol.* 2, 806–817. doi: 10.1016/S0735-1097(83)80226-5

O'Hara, T., Virág, L., Varró, A., and Rudy, Y. (2011). Simulation of the undiseased human cardiac ventricular action potential: model formulation and experimental validation. *PLoS Comput. Biol.* 7:e1002061. doi: 10.1371/journal.pcbi.1002061

Okada, J., Yoshinaga, T., Kurokawa, J., Washio, T., Furukawa, T., Sawada, K., et al. (2015). Screening system for drug-induced arrhythmogenic risk combining a patch clamp and heart simulator. *Sci. Adv.* 1:e1400142. doi: 10.1126/sciadv.1400142

Pedregosa, F., Varoquaux, G., Gramfort, A., Michel, V., Thirion, B., Grisel, O., et al. (2011). Scikit-learn: machine learning in Python. *J. Mach. Learn. Res.* 12, 2825–2830.

Redfern, W. S., Carlsson, L., Davis, A. S., Lynch, W. G., Mackenzie, I., Palethrope, S., et al. (2003). Relationships between preclinical cardiac electrophysiology, clinical QT interval prolongation and torsade de pointes for a broad range of drugs: evidence for a provisional safety margin in drug development. *Cardiovasc. Res.* 58, 32–45. doi: 10.1016/S0008-6363(02)00846-5

Rush, S., and Larsen, H. (1978). A practical algorithm for solving dynamic membrane equations. *IEEE Trans. Biomed. Eng.* BME-25, 389–392. doi: 10.1109/TBME.1978.326270

Sager, P. T., Gintant, G., Turner, J. R., Pettit, S., and Stockbridge, N. (2014). Rechanneling the cardiac proarrhythmia safety paradigm: a meeting report from the Cardiac Safety Research Consortium. *Am. Heart J.* 167, 292–300. doi: 10.1016/j.ahj.2013.11.004

Ten Tusscher, K. H., and Panfilov, A. V. (2006). Cell model for efficient simulation of wave propagation in human ventricular tissue under normal and pathological conditions. *Phys. Med. Biol.* 51, 6141–6156. doi: 10.1088/0031-9155/51/23/014

Towart, R., Linders, J. T., Hermans, A. N., Rohrbacher, J., van der Linde, H. J., Ercken, M., et al. (2009). Blockade of the IKs potassium channel: an overlooked cardiovascular liability in drug safety screening? *J. Pharmacol. Toxicol. Methods* 60, 1–10. doi: 10.1016/j.vascn.2009.04.197

Trenor, B., Gomis-Tena, J., Cardona, K., Romero, L., Rajamani, S., Belardinelli, L., et al. (2013). *In silico* assessment of drug safety in human heart applied to late sodium current blockers. *Channels* 7, 249–262. doi: 10.4161/chan.24905

Viskin, S., Fish, R., Zeltser, D., Belhassen, B., Heller, K., Brosh, D., et al. (2000). Arrhythmias in the congenital long QT syndrome: how often is torsade de pointes pause dependent? *Heart.* 83, 661–666. doi: 10.1136/heart.83.6.661

Viswanathan, P. C., and Rudy, Y. (1999). Pause induced early afterdepolarizations in the long QT syndrome: a simulation study. *Cardiovasc. Res.* 42, 530–542. doi: 10.1016/S0008-6363(99)00035-8

Wiśniowska, B., and Polak, S. (2017). Am I or am I not proarrhythmic? Comparison of various classifications of drug TdP propensity. *Drug Discov. Today* 22, 10–16. doi: 10.1016/j.drudis.2016.09.027

Woosley, R., Heise, C., and Romero, K. (2017). *QTdrugs List.* Oro Valley, AZ: AZCERT, Inc. Available online at: https://www.crediblemeds.org

Wu, J., Wu, J., and Zipes, D. P. (2002). Early afterdepolarizations, U waves, and torsades de pointes. *Circulation* 105, 675–676.

Yang, T., Chun, Y. W., Stroud, D. M., Mosley, J. D., Knollmann, B. C., Hong, C., et al. (2014). Screening for acute ikr block is insufficient to detect torsades de pointes liability: role of late sodium current. *Circulation* 130, 224–234. doi: 10.1161/CIRCULATIONAHA.113.007765

10

Mechanistic Systems Modeling to Improve Understanding and Prediction of Cardiotoxicity Caused by Targeted Cancer Therapeutics

*Jaehee V. Shim[1], Bryan Chun[2], Johan G. C. van Hasselt[1], Marc R. Birtwistle[1], Jeffrey J. Saucerman[2] and Eric A. Sobie[1]**

[1] *Department of Pharmacological Sciences, Icahn School of Medicine at Mount Sinai, New York, NY, United States,*
[2] *Department of Biomedical Engineering, University of Virginia, Charlottesville, VA, United States*

Correspondence:
Eric A. Sobie
eric.sobie@mssm.edu

Tyrosine kinase inhibitors (TKIs) are highly potent cancer therapeutics that have been linked with serious cardiotoxicity, including left ventricular dysfunction, heart failure, and QT prolongation. TKI-induced cardiotoxicity is thought to result from interference with tyrosine kinase activity in cardiomyocytes, where these signaling pathways help to control critical processes such as survival signaling, energy homeostasis, and excitation–contraction coupling. However, mechanistic understanding is limited at present due to the complexities of tyrosine kinase signaling, and the wide range of targets inhibited by TKIs. Here, we review the use of TKIs in cancer and the cardiotoxicities that have been reported, discuss potential mechanisms underlying cardiotoxicity, and describe recent progress in achieving a more systematic understanding of cardiotoxicity via the use of mechanistic models. In particular, we argue that future advances are likely to be enabled by studies that combine large-scale experimental measurements with Quantitative Systems Pharmacology (QSP) models describing biological mechanisms and dynamics. As such approaches have proven extremely valuable for understanding and predicting other drug toxicities, it is likely that QSP modeling can be successfully applied to cardiotoxicity induced by TKIs. We conclude by discussing a potential strategy for integrating genome-wide expression measurements with models, illustrate initial advances in applying this approach to cardiotoxicity, and describe challenges that must be overcome to truly develop a mechanistic and systematic understanding of cardiotoxicity caused by TKIs.

Keywords: tyrosine kinase inhibitors, quantitative systems pharmacology, mathematical modeling, drug-induced adverse events

INTRODUCTION

Tyrosine kinase inhibitors (TKIs) constitute a class of cancer therapeutics, many of which are known to cause cardiotoxicity as a major adverse event. Reported cardiotoxicities include heart failure, cardiomyopathy, conduction abnormalities, QT prolongation, and myocardial injury. The most common toxicity is systolic dysfunction or cardiomyopathy, potentially leading to heart failure, which is most likely mediated through direct toxicity of cardiomyocytes (Albini et al., 2010; Eschenhagen et al., 2011; Force and Kolaja, 2011; Raschi and De Ponti, 2012; Ewer and Ewer, 2015).

Trastuzumab, an inhibitor of the HER2 receptor tyrosine kinase (Slamon et al., 2001; Piccart-Gebhart et al., 2005; Romond et al., 2005; Force et al., 2007) was both the first monoclonal antibody TKI given FDA approval (in 1998) and the first TKI reported to cause cardiotoxicity (Wu et al., 2016). Since the reports of trastuzumab-induced toxicity, several additional targeted cancer therapeutics have been classified as cardiotoxic, observations that have contributed to the emergence of a new research field, *cardio-oncology* (Albini et al., 2010; Bellinger et al., 2015).

Previous studies have shown that TKI-related cardiotoxicity, as seen with trastuzumab, is mostly due to the targeting of pathways that are shared between malignancies and cardiovascular cells (De Keulenaer et al., 2010; Bellinger et al., 2015). Investigations of these adverse events revealed that many of the tyrosine kinases targeted by TKIs serve critical roles in survival and maintenance of cardiomyocytes, leading to unintended *on-target* toxicity. At the same time, many TKIs inhibit multiple kinases simultaneously, which can cause *off-target* toxicity (Chen et al., 2008; Force and Kerkelä, 2008; Force and Kolaja, 2011).

Despite the risk of cardiotoxicity, TKIs are still one of the highly effective and favored cancer therapeutics on the market (Eschenhagen et al., 2011; Force and Kolaja, 2011). The success of drugs such as trastuzumab and imatinib, a small molecule inhibitor used to treat chronic myeloid leukemia (CML), has inspired the development of additional TKIs. As of April, 2015, 25 small molecule TKIs have entered the market (Shah and Morganroth, 2015), with many more under development (Bellinger et al., 2015). Given the booming research in the development of TKIs, it would be beneficial to develop a systematic strategy to: (1) evaluate and predict how new TKIs will affect signaling networks in cardiomyocytes; and (2) identify interventions that can reverse and/or mitigate any associated cardiotoxicity. These questions are well-suited to be addressed using a quantitative systems pharmacology (QSP) approach that combines large-scale measurements with mechanism-based mathematical modeling. The diversity of TKI targets and the complexity of cellular mechanisms responsible for cardiotoxicity mean that two drugs with similar targets may operate through different mechanisms, and the effects of two TKIs with different targets may converge on a common pathway. Untangling this type of complexity generally requires computational approaches that are based on biological mechanisms. Therefore, our aims in this Perspective are to review the progress that systems approaches have made in predicting TKI-induced cardiotoxicity and to offer suggestions for how mathematical modeling can be applied to elucidate mechanisms and predict potential adverse events caused by new drugs.

TYROSINE KINASE SIGNALING IN CANCER AND STRATEGIES UNDERLYING TKIs

The canonical roles of tyrosine kinases are found in mitogenesis and related processes such as differentiation, metabolism, and migration. Constitutive activation of tyrosine kinase (TK) signaling, via either gain-of-function (GOF) mutations or overexpression due to gene amplification, is found in about 70% of malignancies (Blume-Jensen and Hunter, 2001; Chen et al., 2008). Well-understood examples include overexpression of ERBB2 in HER2$^+$ breast cancer (Force et al., 2007) and the constitutively active oncogenic fusion protein BCR-ABL, which can cause CML (Force et al., 2007; Chen et al., 2008; Force and Kolaja, 2011). This dependency of tumor formation and proliferation on TK signaling led to the rise of TKIs as promising anti-cancer therapeutics.

Currently, there are two chemical classes of TKIs: (1) humanized monoclonal antibodies (mAbs) and (2) small molecule inhibitors (Force et al., 2007; Chen et al., 2008; Force and Kolaja, 2011). Small molecule TKIs can be further subcategorized based on whether they compete with ATP for the binding pocket or interact with other regions of the protein (Force and Kolaja, 2011). Additionally, TKIs are often identified by the intended target(s) or the target specificity (Force et al., 2007; Bellinger et al., 2015; Gharwan and Groninger, 2015). The most common target groups that are used to classify TKIs include EGFR/ERBB2 inhibitors, VEGFR inhibitors, ABL inhibitors, and multi-targeted drugs that are designed to inhibit at least two different target groups such as VEGFR and ABL (see **Table 1** for descriptions of the important cellular signaling proteins mentioned in the manuscript). **Figure 1A** shows the currently-approved TKIs, grouped by the published targets, and indicates how these classifications frequently overlap.

REPORTED SERIOUS CARDIAC SIDE EFFECTS OF TKIs

The initial discovery of TKI-induced cardiotoxicity was made during the groundbreaking clinical trials of trastuzumab, the first such drug to be marketed (Seidman et al., 2002; De Keulenaer et al., 2010). However, estimated cardiotoxicities of 3–7% with trastuzumab alone and 25% when the drug was administered with an anthracycline (Slamon et al., 2001) were only determined during a *post hoc* analysis. Similar retrospective analyses have been performed to estimate that sunitinib causes left ventricular dysfunction with an incidence of 4–11% (Yeh and Bickford, 2009; Lenneman and Sawyer, 2016) and the VEGFR inhibitor bevacizumab induces either cardiomyopathy or heart failure in 1.5–3% of patients (Yeh and Bickford, 2009). These examples demonstrate the difficulties associated with identifying cardiotoxicity during drug development. Because clinical trials are primarily focused on evaluating efficacy, they often lack appropriate safety screening measures to identify side effects (Force et al., 2007).

Overall, of the 30 TKIs currently marketed for use in the United States, 26 list serious cardiac side effects as a "black box warning" in their prescription information (FDA and CDER, 2012; Boehringer Ingelheim International GmbH, 2014; Gharwan and Groninger, 2015). The cardiac related black box warnings of TKIs can be categorized into: cardiomyopathy, arrhythmia, myocardial infarction,

TABLE 1 | Biological signaling components potentially relevant to toxicity.

Common name	Full name	Description
EGF	Epidermal growth factor	Extracellular peptide that signals through autocrine and paracrine mechanisms
Neuregulin1	N/A	Extracellular peptide that signals through autocrine and paracrine mechanisms
ERBB2/HER2	Human epidermal growth factor receptor 2	EGFR family receptor tyrosine kinase
ERBB1/EGFR	Receptor for EGF	EGFR family receptor tyrosine kinase
VEGF	Vascular endothelial-derived growth factor	Extracellular peptide that signals through autocrine and paracrine mechanisms
VEGFR	Receptor for VEGF	Receptor tyrosine kinase
PDGF	Platelet-derived growth factor	Extracellular peptide that signals through autocrine and paracrine mechanisms
PDGFR	Receptor for PDGF	Receptor tyrosine kinase
ABL1	Abelson murine leukemia viral oncogene homolog 1	cytoplasmic tyrosine kinase
BCR-ABL	Fusion protein of ABL1 and Breakpoint cluster region protein (BCR)	cytoplasmic fusion tyrosine kinase
Raf-1/c-Raf	N/A	cytoplasmic serine/threonine kinase
ERK	Extracellular signal-related kinase	cytoplasmic serine/threonine kinase
JNK	c-Jun N-terminal kinase	cytoplasmic serine/threonine kinase
PI3K	Phosphatidylinositide 3-kinase	cytoplasmic lipid kinase
Akt/PKB	Also known as Protein Kinase B	cytoplasmic serine/threonine kinase
Src/c-Src	N/A	cytoplasmic tyrosine kinase
AMPK	AMP-activated protein kinase	cytoplasmic serine/threonine kinase

hypertension, and pericardial effusion, based on the specific potential adverse events listed in the package insert. In **Figure 1B**, which indicates both the adverse events and the target class for each TKI, we observe no obvious association between the intended primary target, and the reported cardiac risks.

MECHANISMS UNDERLYING CARDIOTOXICITY CAUSED BY TKIs

The initial discovery of TKI-induced cardiotoxicity was met with surprise due to the fact that cardiomyocytes are non-dividing and terminally differentiated (Force et al., 2007). Since TKs were mostly known for their role in proliferation and their association with cancer, these kinases were not expected to have any essential role in cardiomyocytes, and toxicity in heart was not anticipated (Chen et al., 2008; Bellinger et al., 2015). The discovery of TKI-induced cardiotoxicity, therefore, became a driving force for uncovering the roles of tyrosine kinases in heart. The research spurred by these adverse events has allowed us to appreciate that many of the pathways responsible for proliferation in malignant cells also play important roles in cardiomyocytes in: (1) survival signaling; (2) mitochondrial and sarcoplasmic reticulum (SR) homeostasis; and (3) electrical and contractile function.

Survival Signaling

The role of tyrosine kinases in cardiomyocyte survival signaling was first discovered through the on-target cardiotoxicity caused by trastuzumab. Before the cardiotoxicity reports, expression of trastuzumab's target, ERBB2, was reported to be low in cardiomyocytes, and this receptor's role was unknown (Bellinger et al., 2015). However, subsequent studies have discovered that ERBB2 plays an important role in maintaining cardiomyocyte health, evidenced by the spontaneous dilated cardiomyopathy that results from ERBB2 knockout (Crone et al., 2002; De Keulenaer et al., 2010). More specifically, ERBB2 in cardiomyocytes has been shown to serve as a co-receptor in a critical cardiomyocyte survival pathway initiated by neuregulin-1 (Mellor et al., 2011; Bellinger et al., 2015). Neuregulin-1, a paracrine factor secreted by cardiac endothelial cells, activates mitogenic pathways through ERBB2 heterodimer formation with other members of the EGFR family, ERBB3 or ERBB4 (Chen et al., 2008; De Keulenaer et al., 2010).

Similarly, another EGFR family member, ERBB1, has also been implicated in cardioprotection and myocyte survival (Mellor et al., 2011; Bellinger et al., 2015), including cardiomyocyte defenses against the deleterious consequences caused by excessive β-adrenergic receptor stimulation (Chen et al., 2008). This role was based on the finding that an ERBB1 inhibitor, erlotinib, exacerbates isoproterenol-induced myocardial injury (Chen et al., 2008). Erlotinib is associated with cardiotoxicity, including cardiac arrhythmia and myocardial infarction (Gharwan and Groninger, 2015). One of the downstream pathways common to signaling through ERBB1 and ERBB2 is the lipid kinase PI3K, which in turn activates the protein kinase Akt. The PI3K-Akt axis is critical in survival signaling, and dysregulation of this pathway has been shown to induce ischemic heart disease, hypertrophy, and heart failure (Reichelt et al., 2017).

Raf-1, which belongs to the Raf family of serine/threonine kinases, is another important component of pro-survival signaling that has been linked to both inherited heart disease (Dhandapany et al., 2014), and TKI-induced cardiotoxicity. Specifically, Raf-1 has been identified as a critical component of cardiotoxicity caused by sorafenib (Force et al., 2007; Chen et al., 2008), a multi-target TKI used to treat renal and liver cancers. The inhibition of Raf-1 by sorafenib is thought to block survival

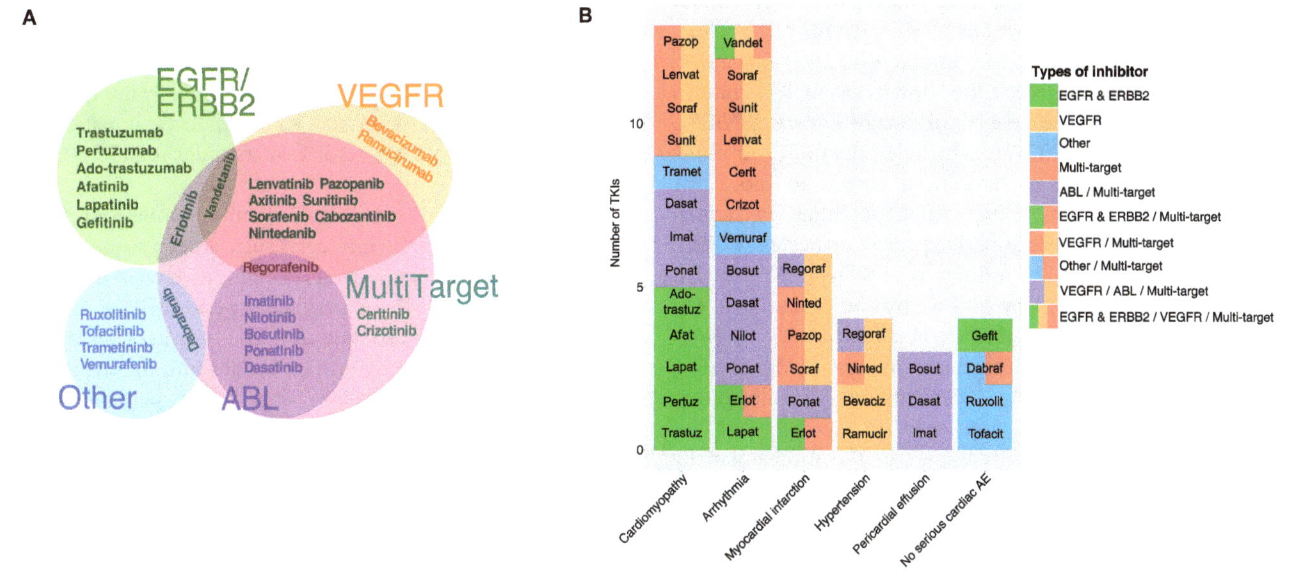

FIGURE 1 | TKI targets and associated adverse events. **(A)** Euler diagram of tyrosine kinase inhibitors grouped based on the primary intended target(s). The three major primary targets are EGFR/ERBB2 (8 TKIs), VEGFR (11 TKIs), and ABL (6 TKIs). The category "Other" comprises five relatively newer TKIs with primary targets in different categories, such as vemurafenib (B-Raf). Out of 30 approved TKIs, 18 were identified as having intended targets in more than one category. **(B)** Black box warnings associated with tyrosine kinase inhibitors are indicated, with closely-related toxicities grouped to ease visualization. *Cardiomyopathy* category includes: "cardiac dysfunction," "congestive heart failure," "left ventricular dysfunction," and "cardiomyopathy." *Arrhythmia* includes: "prolonged QT interval," "cardiac bradyarrhythmia," and "cardiac arrhythmia." *Pericardial effusion* includes both "pericardial/pleural effusion," and "cardiac tamponade." Four approved drugs have no cardiac associated boxed warning (i.e., no serious cardiac adverse events listed in the drug's package insert).

signaling through the protein kinase ERK, and concurrently to disinhibit pro-apoptotic kinases. This dual action of pro-survival signaling inhibition and apoptotic signaling activation can culminate in cell death (Force et al., 2007).

Sarcoplasmic Reticulum and Mitochondrial Homeostasis

In addition to pro-survival signaling, TKs are known to be closely linked to processes that maintain the health and function of cardiomyocytes through mitochondrial and SR homeostasis (Force and Kolaja, 2011). Mitochondria are responsible for matching the cellular supply of ATP with the energetic demand whereas the SR functions to both modulate the quantity of Ca^{2+} released with each heartbeat and to control the processing of many critical proteins.

When TKI-induced toxicity involves mitochondrial or SR function, the processes seem to be closely linked. Specifically, mitochondrial dysfunction resulting from TKI treatment can lead to membrane permeabilization and the release of reactive oxidative species to the cytoplasm. This oxidative stress can in turn lead to SR dysfunction through both altered Ca^{2+} release and the activation of signaling pathways that may ultimately lead to apoptosis (Groenendyk et al., 2010).

Cardiotoxicity caused by imatinib, a multi-targeted ABL inhibitor, has been proposed to follow this precise mechanism (Kerkelä et al., 2006; Force et al., 2007; Mellor et al., 2011). The on-target effect of imatinib has been linked to the disturbance of SR homeostasis via inhibition of an ABL isoform that is localized in the SR. This can eventually initiate apoptosis through JNK activation. Consistent with this hypothesis, postmortem histological examinations of patients treated with imatinib have revealed dilated SR structures, and experiments in isolated cardiomyocytes shown that imatinib can induce mitochondrial membrane potential collapse (Kerkelä et al., 2006).

Another example of interference with SR and mitochondrial homeostasis is cardiotoxicity caused by the multi-kinase inhibitor sunitinib. Sunitinib has been reported to cause ATP depletion in cardiomyocytes through an off-target effect involving AMP-activated protein kinase, or AMPK (Force et al., 2007). The unintentional inhibition of AMPK is thought to activate energy-consuming processes, including protein translation and lipid biosynthesis, which can deplete ATP. Given the tremendous energetic demands of the contracting cardiomyocyte, the improper activation of ATP-consuming processes can be highly toxic (Dyck and Lopaschuk, 2006; Zhang et al., 2008).

Excitation and Contraction

TKI-induced cardiotoxicity can also manifest itself as altered excitation or contraction of cardiac myocytes. These detrimental effects can occur through: (1) direct or indirect modulation of cardiac ionic currents, resulting in pro-arrhythmic electrical activity (Chen et al., 2008; Ghatalia et al., 2015); or (2) structural remodeling that leads to altered myocyte contraction.

TKIs can induce electrophysiological abnormalities directly, via block of ion channels, or indirectly, by altered intracellular signaling that leads to a decrease in K^+ currents. Because K^+

currents repolarize the cell membrane during action potentials, either direct or indirect reductions of K^+ currents can prolong electrocardiographic QT intervals and increase arrhythmia risk. TKIs that are known to block the most relevant K^+ channel ($K_V11.1$), encoded by the gene traditionally known as *hERG* (subsequently renamed *KCNH2*), include crizotinib, sunitinib, and nilotinib. These drugs have been shown to block the channel *in vitro* and to prolong action potentials in human induced pluripotent stem cell-derived cardiomyocytes (hiPSC-CMs) (Doherty et al., 2013). Indirect reductions in K^+ current may possibly be mediated by Src, a tyrosine kinase that can augment current carried by $K_V11.1$ (Schlichter et al., 2014). Thus, dasatinib and bosutinib, which are dual inhibitors of ABL and Src, can potentially cause reduced K^+ current and QT prolongation (Xu et al., 2009; Gharwan and Groninger, 2015).

Src may also be an important part of the mechanism by which TKIs can induce cellular structural remodeling and impaired contraction. In cardiomyocytes, Src is important for both the organization of sarcomeres and the formation of focal adhesions that connect adjacent cells (Kuramochi et al., 2006). In mice, genetic studies have shown that spontaneous cardiac chamber dilation and disorganization of myofibrils can result from knocking out any of several enzymes in the Src pathway (Peng et al., 2006). Thus, TKIs that inhibit Src may disrupt cardiac contraction by interfering with Src's role in maintaining myocyte structure.

COMPLEXITIES OF TKI-INDUCED CARDIOTOXICITY AND THE NEED FOR A SYSTEMS APPROACH

From survival and homeostasis to contractile function, tyrosine kinases perform a wide variety of important roles in the health and function of cardiomyocytes. Although considerable progress has been made to decipher the roles of individual TKs, the breadth of the different mechanisms involved makes it difficult to draw general conclusions about TKI-induced cardiotoxicity. Moreover, even when some mechanistic details have been uncovered, our understanding is primarily qualitative, and biological mechanisms cannot usually be connected to factors such as dosing and the physiological characteristics of individual patients. Given the past success of TKIs as cancer therapeutics and the drive to develop additional TKIs, it would be beneficial to develop a systematic strategy to: (1) evaluate the potential cardiotoxicity of new TKIs; (2) predict the mostly likely mechanisms involved; and (3) suggest strategies for mitigating and/or reversing toxicity. Systems approaches that perform large-scale measurements and quantitatively compare responses to multiple drugs are likely to be extremely useful for understanding the common and distinct features of cardiotoxicity caused by diverse TKIs.

A common approach in systems-level pharmacology studies is to utilize a cell based, high-throughput drug screening assay. Although cardiovascular pharmacology has traditionally not been well-suited for high throughput studies, the development of hiPSC-CMs has expanded the possibilities. For instance, a recent study described the development of a comprehensive assay that evaluated cellular effects of TKIs in hiPSC-CMs (Sharma et al., 2017). Using hiPSC lines from 13 individuals, the investigators examined how 21 FDA-approved small molecule TKIs affected cell viability, contractility, and gene expression. By integrating the results with literature-reported TKI serum levels in patients, the authors developed a novel cardiac safety index for TKIs (Sharma et al., 2017).

Although this study represents a significant milestone in that it integrates cutting edge technologies such as deep sequencing and high-throughput imaging, room for improvement nonetheless remains. Specifically, the experiments performed in this study represent snapshots of cell state after TKI treatment, and the data can therefore provide only limited insight into the dynamics of toxicity development. Moreover, experiments performed using individual drugs cannot predict how either a second drug or a circulating hormone (e.g., adrenaline, angiotensin) might either exacerbate or protect against cardiotoxicity. Although it is of course possible to expand the assay to treat cells with drug pairs and/or add relevant physiological stimuli, it is not clear *a priori* which additional perturbations might be informative or relevant. Finally, even when unambiguous results are seen in cellular high-throughput assays, the mechanistic details often remain hidden. It would therefore be helpful to couple such high-throughput measurements with integrative computational analyses that can potentially overcome these limitations.

MECHANISTIC MATHEMATICAL MODELING TO IMPROVE TOXICITY TESTING

One way to address the aforementioned limitations is to use mathematical models that mechanistically describe biological dynamics. When the processes simulated by these models overlap with toxicity mechanisms, the simulations can be used to generate testable predictions, to guide experimental studies, and ultimately to make decisions about new drugs based on a quantitative understanding of benefits and risks. In this context, models that describe biological mechanisms through differential equations are frequently referred to as QSP models (Leil and Bertz, 2014; Gadkar et al., 2016). Although precise definitions remain a matter of debate, QSP models are generally distinguished from both purely empirical, statistical approaches such as computing a risk score for a drug based on a series of measurements (Kramer et al., 2013; Mistry et al., 2015), and pharmacokinetic models that can predict the effects of dosing on cardiotoxicity (van Hasselt et al., 2012) but generally offer only limited mechanistic insight. Although QSP models have been exploited to understand cardiotoxicity caused by anthracyclines (de Oliveira et al., 2016), the application of QSP to TKI-induced cardiotoxicity is still in its early stages. Given the recent development of QSP modeling, it is instructive to consider examples in which mechanistic models have been successfully applied to the study of adverse events, in particular drug-induced liver injury (DILI) (Huang et al., 2013; Shoda et al., 2014; Yang et al., 2015), and drug-induced arrhythmias (Moreno et al., 2011; Sarkar and Sobie, 2011; Britton et al., 2013; Cummins et al., 2014; Grandi and Maleckar, 2016; Yang et al., 2016). Specifically, we emphasize how mechanistic models can be integrated with large *in vitro* data sets, as these studies may provide an important blueprint for future research on cardiotoxicity caused by kinase inhibitors.

An example of the success of QSP models for toxicity applications can be found in the development of DILIsym®, a mathematical model and software package used for predicting DILI. DILIsym® comprises multiple sub-models describing relevant biological processes involved in hepatotoxicity such as drug distribution in the liver, bile acid homeostasis, reactive metabolite generation and disposition, oxidative stress, immune responses, and the hepatocyte life cycle (Woodhead et al., 2017). The value of this approach was recently demonstrated in studies that examined differences in hepatotoxicity between acetaminophen and its less toxic isomer 3′-hydroxyacetnilide. Although the former drug can cause toxicity across many species, the latter has been shown to cause DILI in humans and rats, but not in mice. Using the mechanistic DILIsym® model, a testable hypothesis was generated in which the amount of reactive metabolite produced from each isomer was identified as an important contributor to the observed species differences, and this prediction was confirmed experimentally in a later study (Kyriakides et al., 2016). In addition to the consortium that has developed the DILIsym® package, other groups have gained important insight into DILI through mathematical modeling (Smith et al., 2016; Blais et al., 2017; Thiel et al., 2017).

To understand and predict drug-induced arrhythmias, e.g., Torsades de Pointes (TdP), the Comprehensive *in vitro* Proarrhythmia Assay (CiPA) initiative is highly relevant. This effort, part of the FDA's Critical Path Initiative, aims to improve the accuracy and cost effectiveness of screening for TdP risk. Whereas current *in vitro* methods for predicting TdP risk focus almost exclusively on block of $K_V11.1$ (i.e., the *hERG* channel), an approach that is often inadequate, CiPA intends to both assess how drugs block multiple ion channels and to combine these measurements with recordings in hiPSC-CMs and mechanistic simulations (Sager et al., 2014; Fermini et al., 2016). A couple of recently-published studies highlight the value that is gained by utilizing QSP models. Lancaster and Sobie, for example, used models of human ventricular myocytes to simulate physiological changes caused by 67 unique drugs, some that are known to cause TdP, and others that are apparently safe. In addition to providing a classification model that was superior to $K_V11.1$ block alone, the simulations provided testable predictions about the most informative assays to perform in cellular experiments and the specific ion transport pathways that, when affected by a drug, may contribute to TdP risk (Lancaster and Sobie, 2016). More recently, Li et al. showed that incorporating the kinetics of $K_V11.1$ block into simulations provides superior identification of TdP risk than simply considering steady-state block measurements (i.e., an IC_{50}-value), and the study suggested an experimental protocol for measuring drug block kinetics (Li et al., 2017).

The examples of both DILI and drug-induced TdP demonstrate the value that can be added when mechanistic modeling is used to address toxicity. The simulations can uncover the reasons for counterintuitive results, such as drugs that block $K_V11.1$ but are nonetheless safe (Kramer et al., 2013; Lancaster and Sobie, 2016; Li et al., 2017), or drugs that only cause hepatotoxicity in some species (Kyriakides et al., 2016; Smith et al., 2016; Blais et al., 2017; Thiel et al., 2017; Woodhead et al., 2017). The simulations can also suggest the prioritization of experiments that are most likely to provide additional insight.

INITIAL EFFORTS TO USE QSP APPROACHES TO UNDERSTAND TKI-INDUCED CARDIOTOXICITY

TKI-induced cardiotoxicity is a problem that seems well-suited to a QSP approach because tyrosine kinase signaling encompasses large, complex networks with numerous feedback loops, and understanding how a drug alters TK cascades is therefore extremely complicated. Although mechanistic modeling to predict TKI-induced cardiotoxicity is much less well-developed than for DILI or TdP, efforts that may yield breakthroughs in the next few years are currently underway.

As noted above, an important recent study by Sharma et al. (2017) derived a "toxicity index" by examining effects of TKIs in hiPSC-CMs through several assays. Although the large-scale nature of this study justifies the "systems" label, and the toxicity index is a quantitative risk score, it's important to emphasize that QSP modeling, which can provide mechanistic insight and actionable predictions, is complementary to a high-throughput, data-driven strategy such as that used in this study (Sharma et al., 2017).

Another notable recent effort is a study by Shin et al. (2014). These investigators combined experimental measurements with simulations to uncover mechanisms by which high and sustained doses of the β-adrenergic receptor agonist isoproterenol could increase myocyte susceptibility to apoptosis (Shin et al., 2014). This study is an important example of how simulations often generate novel experimentally-testable predictions, and the work can potentially be extended to examine TKI-induced toxicity.

To fill current gaps in knowledge and obtain new mechanistic insight, the Drug Toxicity Signature Generation (DToxS) Center at Mount Sinai has initiated a large-scale project to advance cellular assays and computational approaches that can improve our understanding of TKI-induced cardiotoxicity. One aspect of this project involves employing QSP models that describe biological processes potentially involved in this cardiotoxicity. We outline here an approach by which whole transcriptome expression assays can be integrated with mechanistic models to classify drugs and generate novel, experimentally-testable predictions.

For this part of the analysis, the project has designed a standard experimental protocol (DtoxS—Drug Toxicity Signature Generation Center—SOP, https://martip03.u.hpc.mssm.edu/sop.php) that captures early effects of drugs, as reflected in gene expression changes. The experiments treat cultured cardiomyocyte-derived cells with potentially cardiotoxic TKIs as well as drugs from different classes that are presumably safe. After 48 h, mRNA is harvested, and sequencing is performed to quantify drug-induced changes in gene expression (compared with vehicle-treated controls). Data are released at the DToxS website and can be freely-downloaded (DtoxS—Drug Toxicity Signature Generation Center—Data

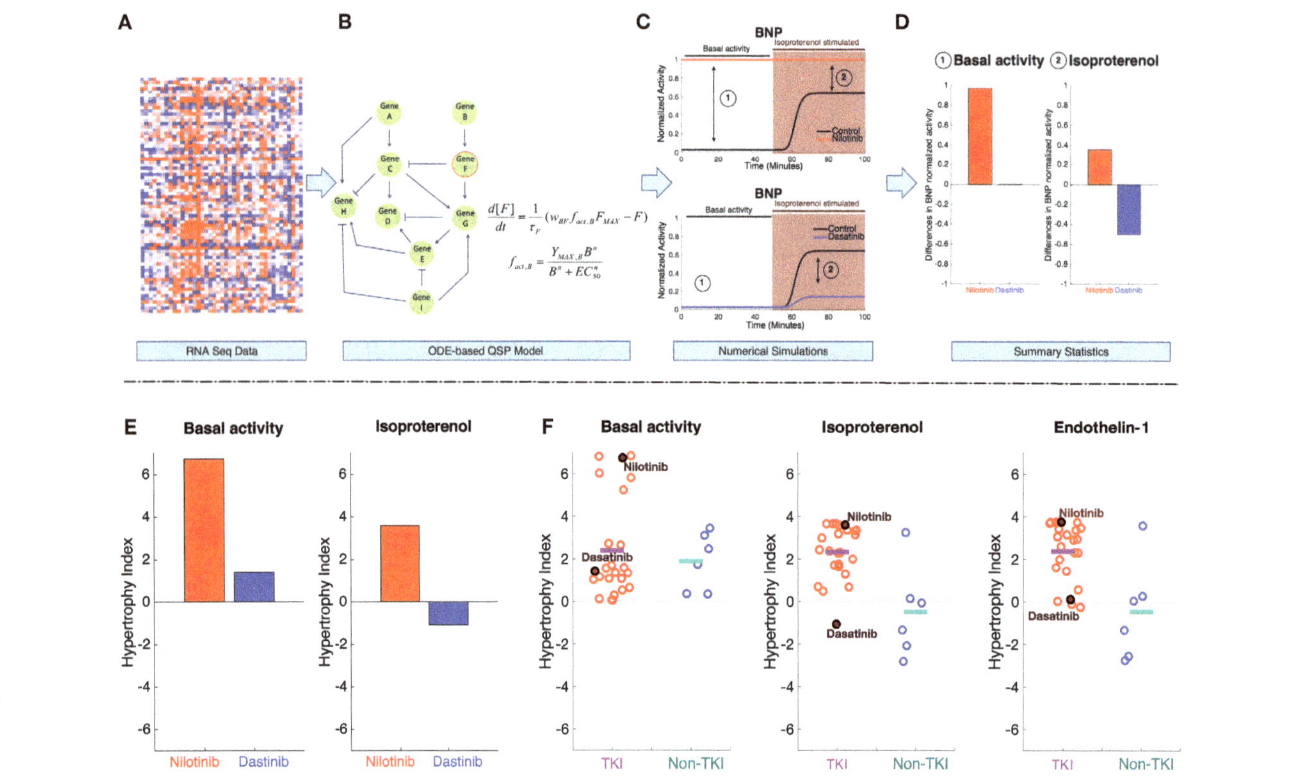

FIGURE 2 | Computational pipeline for integrating gene expression data with QSP models to enable understanding of TKI-induced cardiotoxicity. The pipeline starts with **(A)** mRNAseq data generated from drug treated cells. Using the mRNAseq data, parameters in the QSP model are altered to reflect changes in cell state after 48 h of drug treatment. Specifically, parameters describing maximal activity of model species are scaled based on the changes in gene expression (drug-treated vs. untreated cells). **(B)** The QSP model (Ryall et al., 2012) is composed of ordinary differential equations (ODEs) that describe activation and inactivation of cellular signaling dynamics. Simulations are performed to predict how drug-induced changes in gene expression will influence both basal signaling activity and how cells respond to stimuli. For instance, example simulation results in **(C)** show BNP activity, before, and after stimulation with isoproterenol (a β-adrenergic receptor agonist), in both untreated cells, and cells that have been exposed to two different TKIs for 48 h. These time course simulations predict drug-specific changes, such as an increase in BNP signaling after nilotinib treatment (top) compared with a decrease after dasatinib treatment (bottom). From these time courses, summary statistics **(D)** are collected from steady-state levels of BNP under two conditions (① basal activity and ② stimulus). **(E)** Using this pipeline, steady state changes in seven model outputs were computed and summed to generate a metric that we termed the "hypertrophy index." This provides a summary statistic of the overall hypertrophic risk of a drug under different conditions (e.g., basal activity, left, and isoproterenol stimulation, right). **(F)** Hypertrophy indices computed, under three different conditions, from data obtained in a single cell line after treatment with 24 TKIs, and six non-TKIs (control drugs that are presumed to not cause cardiotoxicity). Each circle represents an individual drug, the line indicates the mean value for each group under basal activity (left), isoproterenol stimulation (middle), and endothelin-1 stimulation (right).

& Resources, https://martip03.u.hpc.mssm.edu/data.php). The pipeline for integrating these released data with mechanistic mathematical models is shown in **Figure 2**, top. Changes in mRNA levels in drug treated cells (**Figure 2A**) can be translated into parameter alterations in models that describe processes potentially relevant to the toxicity (**Figure 2B**), and simulations are then performed with these models. This workflow assumes that before overt toxicity is induced, drugs can alter the cellular state in relatively subtle ways. Mechanistic simulations may then allow one to predict how this drug-induced altered cellular state influences the response to various physiological stimuli.

For example, results shown here are obtained with a QSP model that describes signaling events relevant to cardiac hypertrophy through a system of 106 ordinary differential equations, each one describing activity of a signaling component (Ryall et al., 2012). This model was chosen for initial simulations because the progression to heart failure due to pathological remodeling often includes a transient induction of hypertrophy. In addition, many known TKI targets (e.g., ERBB2, Raf-1) and critical nodes in cardiac survival signaling (e.g., PI3K, Akt, and ERK) are included. Using this model, simulations were performed to predict how drug-induced network alterations affected 7 hypertrophy biomarkers (the model's "outputs"), under conditions meant to simulate a variety of physiological or pharmacological stimuli (e.g., stretch, angiotensin, EGF, phenylephrine). For instance, time courses in **Figure 2C** show simulated normalized levels of Brain Natriuretic Peptide (BNP) under six conditions: before and after isoproterenol stimulation, and in three groups of cells: untreated (control), nilotinib-treated, and dasatinib-treated. BNP is an appropriate output to consider because it is both measured in patients with hypertrophy and heart failure and has been shown to be relevant for drug-induced cardiotoxicity (Nousiainen et al., 2002; Sandri et al., 2005; Skovgaard et al., 2014).

These example simulation results, summarized in **Figure 2D**, suggest that nilotinib leads to increases in BNP, both before and after isoproterenol, whereas dasatinib may reduce the upregulation of BNP that isoproterenol normally causes. The *hypertrophy index*, a summary statistic, condenses results by summing drug-induced changes across seven biomarkers in response to different stimuli applied in the model. The hypertrophy index confirms the impression from the simulated time courses, namely a pro-hypertrophic response to nilotinib contrasted with a slight anti-hypertrophic response to dasatinib (**Figure 2E**).

By simulating responses to stimuli, using gene expression changes induced by all drugs, patterns begin to emerge. Specifically, in myocytes that are not exposed to a physiological stimulus, TKIs and non-TKIs cause similar changes in hypertrophy biomarkers (**Figure 2F**). However, simulations predict that when TKI-treated myocytes are also exposed to isoproterenol or endothelin-1, agonists that are used experimentally to induce hypertrophy (Ichikawa et al., 1996; Yamazaki et al., 1996; Shohet et al., 2004; Ryall et al., 2012), the pro-hypertrophic response is exaggerated compared with non-TKI-treated cells.

These preliminary simulation results indicate the potential strengths of combining large scale measurements with mechanism-based mathematical models. First the simulations do not simply describe existing data—they can predict how drug-treated cells will respond to an additional stimulus that has not yet been applied experimentally. These predictions can be subsequently tested. Second, the simulation approach does not merely generate qualitative predictions; because the quantitative models predict that some drugs and/or stimuli may cause large effects whereas others cause only minor effects, this provides a means to prioritize experimental tests and use resources efficiently. Third, when clear differences are observed, for instance between individual drugs or between drug classes, the simulations predict the mechanisms responsible for the differences.

FUTURE DIRECTIONS

Although the preliminary simulation results shown here are encouraging, they also hint at the future research that must be performed to fully realize the potential of this approach. First, although the simulations predict how drug-induced changes in gene expression may influence both baseline signaling and cellular responses to stimuli, they do not describe direct inhibition of kinase activity by drugs, which is of course the more traditional and straightforward method for simulating drug effects. We excluded these effects from initial simulations because many TKI targets are not included in the model, but future work will expand the model by systematically adding drug targets based on published protein-protein interaction databases (Warde-Farley et al., 2010) and large-scale kinase inhibition assays (Anastassiadis et al., 2011; Davis et al., 2011). For such work, a promising way to expand the model will be to use large-scale, data-driven network identification algorithms (Thiagarajan et al., 2017) that can provide an unbiased approach for identifying potential off-targets.

A second important extension of the work will be to simulate additional biological processes potentially involved in cardiotoxicity. For instance, cell death via apoptosis, which may be important in the development of toxicity caused by some TKIs, has been described mathematically by many previous models (Schleich and Lavrik, 2013; Shin et al., 2014). Once these are tuned to reflect apoptotic signaling in cardiac myocytes, the models can be integrated with the experimental gene expression data to generate novel predictions. Similarly, models describing mitochondrial function, including the production of reactive oxygen species (Aon and Cortassa, 2012; Bazil et al., 2016; Wacquier et al., 2016), and the coupling of electrical excitation, and contractile function (Rice et al., 2008; Tewari et al., 2016), are also likely to be relevant. Finally, once a number of QSP models, describing additional processes, have been added, further secondary analyses can be performed. These include sensitivity analysis to identify the most important nodes in each model (Sobie, 2009), systematic simulations to potential targets for toxicity mitigation or reversal, and effects of combination therapy.

CONCLUSIONS

Here, we have discussed contemporary challenges in understanding TKI-induced cardiotoxicity and have illustrated how a QSP approach can be used to address unresolved questions and improve understanding. Previous successes of QSP in illuminating and predicting other forms of drug toxicity, including hepatotoxicity and drug-induced arrhythmia, demonstrate its potential utility for other drug toxicities. The initial results presented here show how mechanistic models can be integrated with "omics" measurements such as mRNA-seq, generating simulations that can suggest underlying mechanisms and help in prioritizing costly experiments. In the coming years, future work along these lines can be used to develop strategies to mitigate or reverse TKI-induced cardiotoxicity, thereby contributing to the development of therapeutic regimens that are both effective and safe.

AUTHOR CONTRIBUTIONS

JVS and BC performed an extensive literature review and analysis of published clinical and experimental data. JVS performed simulations and analysis. JVS and ES wrote the initial draft of the manuscript. BC, JvH, MB, and JJS provided critical feedback and editorial suggestions.

ACKNOWLEDGMENTS

This work was supported as a part of the National Institutes of Health (NIH) Common Fund's Library of Integrated Network-Based Cellular Signatures (LINCS) program through grants U54 HG008098 and U54 HL127624. Additional support has been provided by NIH grants and R01 HL137100 (to JJS) and U01 HL136297 (to ES), and National Science Foundation grant 1252854 to JJS.

REFERENCES

Albini, A., Pennesi, G., Donatelli, F., Cammarota, R., De Flora, S., and Noonan, D. M. (2010). Cardiotoxicity of anticancer drugs: the need for cardio-oncology and cardio-oncological prevention. *J. Natl. Cancer Inst.* 102, 14–25. doi: 10.1093/jnci/djp440

Anastassiadis, T., Deacon, S. W., Devarajan, K., Ma, H., and Peterson, J. R. (2011). Comprehensive assay of kinase catalytic activity reveals features of kinase inhibitor selectivity. *Nat. Biotechnol.* 29, 1039–1045. doi: 10.1038/nbt.2017

Aon, M. A., and Cortassa, S. (2012). Mitochondrial network energetics in the heart. *Wiley Interdiscip. Rev. Syst. Biol. Med.* 4, 599–613. doi: 10.1002/wsbm.1188

Bazil, J. N., Beard, D. A., and Vinnakota, K. C. (2016). Catalytic coupling of oxidative phosphorylation, atp demand, and reactive oxygen species generation. *Biophys. J.* 110, 962–971. doi: 10.1016/j.bpj.2015.09.036

Bellinger, A. M., Arteaga, C. L., Force, T., Humphreys, B. D., Demetri, G. D., Druker, B. J., et al. (2015). Cardio-oncology. *Circulation* 132, 2248–2258. doi: 10.1161/CIRCULATIONAHA.115.010484

Blais, E. M., Rawls, K. D., Dougherty, B. V., Li, Z. I., Kolling, G. L., Ye, P., et al. (2017). Reconciled rat and human metabolic networks for comparative toxicogenomics and biomarker predictions. *Nat. Commun.* 8:14250. doi: 10.1038/ncomms14250

Blume-Jensen, P., and Hunter, T. (2001). Oncogenic kinase signalling. *Nature* 411, 355–365. doi: 10.1038/35077225

Boehringer Ingelheim International GmbH (2014). *Ofev (Nintedanib) [Package Insert]*. 1–18. Available online at: https://www.accessdata.fda.gov/drugsatfda_docs/label/2014/205832s000lbl.pdf (Accessed June 26, 2017).

Britton, O. J., Bueno-Orovio, A., Van Ammel, K., Lu, H. R., Towart, R., Gallacher, D. J., et al. (2013). Experimentally calibrated population of models predicts and explains intersubject variability in cardiac cellular electrophysiology. *Proc. Natl. Acad. Sci. U.S.A.* 110, E2098–E2105. doi: 10.1073/pnas.1304382110

Chen, M. H., Kerkel, R., and Force, T. (2008). Mechanisms of cardiac dysfunction associated with tyrosine kinase inhibitor cancer therapeutics. *Circulation* 118, 84–95. doi: 10.1161/CIRCULATIONAHA.108.776831

Crone, S. A., Zhao, Y.-Y., Fan, L., Gu, Y., Minamisawa, S., Liu, Y., et al. (2002). ErbB2 is essential in the prevention of dilated cardiomyopathy. *Nat. Med.* 8, 459–465. doi: 10.1038/nm0502-459

Cummins, M. A., Dalal, P. J., Bugana, M., Severi, S., and Sobie, E. A. (2014). Comprehensive analyses of ventricular myocyte models identify targets exhibiting favorable rate dependence. *PLoS Comput. Biol.* 10:e1003543. doi: 10.1371/journal.pcbi.1003543

Davis, M. I., Hunt, J. P., Herrgard, S., Ciceri, P., Wodicka, L. M., Pallares, G., et al. (2011). Comprehensive analysis of kinase inhibitor selectivity. *Nat. Biotechnol.* 29, 1046–1051. doi: 10.1038/nbt.1990

De Keulenaer, G. W., Doggen, K., and Lemmens, K. (2010). The vulnerability of the heart as a pluricellular paracrine organ: lessons from unexpected triggers of heart failure in targeted ErbB2 anticancer therapy. *Circ. Res.* 106, 35–46. doi: 10.1161/CIRCRESAHA.109.205906

de Oliveira, B. L., Niederer, S., Imlay, J., Chen, J., Winslow, R., and Hsu, C. (2016). A biophysical systems approach to identifying the pathways of acute and chronic doxorubicin mitochondrial cardiotoxicity. *PLoS Comput. Biol.* 12:e1005214. doi: 10.1371/journal.pcbi.1005214

Dhandapany, P. S., Razzaque, M. A., Muthusami, U., Kunnoth, S., Edwards, J. J., Mulero-Navarro, S., et al. (2014). RAF1 mutations in childhood-onset dilated cardiomyopathy. *Nat. Genet.* 46, 635–639. doi: 10.1038/ng.2963

Doherty, K. R., Wappel, R. L., Talbert, D. R., Trusk, P. B., Moran, D. M., Kramer, J. W., et al. (2013). Multi-parameter *in vitro* toxicity testing of crizotinib, sunitinib, erlotinib, and nilotinib in human cardiomyocytes. *Toxicol. Appl. Pharmacol.* 272, 245–255. doi: 10.1016/j.taap.2013.04.027

Dyck, J. R., and Lopaschuk, G. D. (2006). AMPK alterations in cardiac physiology and pathology: enemy or ally? *J. Physiol.* 574, 95–112. doi: 10.1113/jphysiol.2006.109389

Eschenhagen, T., Force, T., Ewer, M. S., de Keulenaer, G. W., Suter, T. M., Anker, S. D., et al. (2011). Cardiovascular side effects of cancer therapies: a position statement from the heart failure association of the European society of cardiology. *Eur. J. Heart Fail.* 13, 1–10. doi: 10.1093/eurjhf/hfq213

Ewer, M. S., and Ewer, S. M. (2015). Cardiotoxicity of anticancer treatments. *Nat. Rev. Cardiol.* 12, 547–558. doi: 10.1038/nrcardio.2015.65

FDA and CDER (2012). *Xeljanz (tofacitinib)* [package insert] (New York, NY; Pfizer Inc.), 1–33. Available online at: https://www.accessdata.fda.gov/drugsatfda_docs/label/2012/203214s000lbl.pdf (Accessed June 26, 2017).

Fermini, B., Hancox, J. C., Abi-Gerges, N., Bridgland-Taylor, M., Chaudhary, K. W., Colatsky, T., et al. (2016). A new perspective in the field of cardiac safety testing through the comprehensive *in vitro* proarrhythmia assay paradigm. *J. Biomol. Screen.* 21, 1–11. doi: 10.1177/1087057115594589

Force, T., and Kerkelä, R. (2008). Cardiotoxicity of the new cancer therapeutics - mechanisms of, and approaches to, the problem. *Drug Discov. Today* 13, 778–784. doi: 10.1016/j.drudis.2008.05.011

Force, T., and Kolaja, K. L. (2011). Cardiotoxicity of kinase inhibitors: the prediction and translation of preclinical models to clinical outcomes. *Nat. Rev. Drug Discov.* 10, 111–126. doi: 10.1038/nrd3252

Force, T., Krause, D. S., and Van Etten, R. A. (2007). Molecular mechanisms of cardiotoxicity of tyrosine kinase inhibition. *Nat. Rev. Cancer* 7, 332–344. doi: 10.1038/nrc2106

Gadkar, K., Kirouac, D., Parrott, N., and Ramanujan, S. (2016). Quantitative systems pharmacology: a promising approach for translational pharmacology. *Drug Discov. Today Technol.* 21–22, 57–65. doi: 10.1016/j.ddtec.2016.11.001

Gharwan, H., and Groninger, H. (2015). Kinase inhibitors and monoclonal antibodies in oncology: clinical implications. *Nat. Rev. Clin. Oncol.* 13, 209–227. doi: 10.1038/nrclinonc.2015.213

Ghatalia, P., Je, Y., Kaymakcalan, M. D., Sonpavde, G., and Choueiri, T. K. (2015). QTc interval prolongation with vascular endothelial growth factor receptor tyrosine kinase inhibitors. *Br. J. Cancer* 112, 296–305. doi: 10.1038/bjc.2014.564

Grandi, E., and Maleckar, M. M. (2016). Anti-arrhythmic strategies for atrial fibrillation. *Pharmacol. Ther.* 168, 126–142. doi: 10.1016/j.pharmthera.2016.09.012

Groenendyk, J., Sreenivasaiah, P. K., Kim, D. H., Agellon, L. B., and Michalak, M. (2010). Biology of endoplasmic reticulum stress in the heart. *Circ. Res.* 107, 1185–1197. doi: 10.1161/CIRCRESAHA.110.227033

Huang, S.-M., Abernethy, D. R., Wang, Y., Zhao, P., and Zineh, I. (2013). The utility of modeling and simulation in drug development and regulatory review. *J. Pharm. Sci.* 102, 2912–2923. doi: 10.1002/jps.23570

Ichikawa, K.-I., Hidai, C., Okuda, C., Kimata, S.-I., Matsuoka, R., Hosoda, S., et al. (1996). Endogenous endothelin-1 mediates cardiac hypertrophy and switching of myosin heavy chain gene expression in rat ventricular myocardium. *J. Am. Coll. Cardiol.* 27, 1286–1291. doi: 10.1016/0735-1097(95)00568-4

Kerkelä, R., Grazette, L., Yacobi, R., Iliescu, C., Patten, R., Beahm, C., et al. (2006). Cardiotoxicity of the cancer therapeutic agent imatinib mesylate. *Nat. Med.* 12, 908–916. doi: 10.1038/nm1446

Kramer, J., Obejero-Paz, C. A., Myatt, G., Kuryshev, Y. A., Bruening-Wright, A., Verducci, J. S., et al. (2013). MICE models: superior to the HERG model in predicting torsade de pointes. *Sci. Rep.* 3:2100. doi: 10.1038/srep02100

Kuramochi, Y., Guo, X., and Sawyer, D. B. (2006). Neuregulin activates erbB2-dependent src/FAK signaling and cytoskeletal remodeling in isolated adult rat cardiac myocytes. *J. Mol. Cell. Cardiol.* 41, 228–235. doi: 10.1016/j.yjmcc.2006.04.007

Kyriakides, M., Maitre, L., Stamper, B. D., Mohar, I., Kavanagh, T. J., Foster, J., et al. (2016). Comparative metabonomic analysis of hepatotoxicity induced by acetaminophen and its less toxic meta-isomer. *Arch. Toxicol.* 90, 3073–3085. doi: 10.1007/s00204-015-1655-x

Lancaster, M. C., and Sobie, E. (2016). Improved prediction of drug-induced torsades de pointes through simulations of dynamics and machine learning algorithms. *Clin. Pharmacol. Ther.* 100, 371–379. doi: 10.1002/cpt.367

Leil, T. A., and Bertz, R. (2014). Quantitative Systems pharmacology can reduce attrition and improve productivity in pharmaceutical research and development. *Front. Pharmacol.* 5:247. doi: 10.3389/fphar.2014.00247

Lenneman, C. G., and Sawyer, D. B. (2016). Cardio-oncology. *Circ. Res.* 118, 1008–1020. doi: 10.1161/CIRCRESAHA.115.303633

Li, Z., Dutta, S., Sheng, J., Tran, P. N., Wu, W., Chang, K., et al. (2017). Improving the *in silico* assessment of proarrhythmia risk by combining hERG (human ether-à-go-go-related gene) channel–drug binding kinetics and multichannel pharmacology. *Circ. Arrhythmia Electrophysiol.* 10:e004628. doi: 10.1161/CIRCEP.116.004628

Mellor, H. R., Bell, A. R., Valentin, J.-P., and Roberts, R. R. A. (2011). REVIEW cardiotoxicity associated with targeting kinase pathways in cancer. *Toxicol. Sci.* 120, 14–32. doi: 10.1093/toxsci/kfq378

Mistry, H. B., Davies, M. R., and Di Veroli, G. Y. (2015). A new classifier-based strategy for *in-silico* ion-channel cardiac drug safety assessment. *Front. Pharmacol.* 6:59. doi: 10.3389/fphar.2015.00059

Moreno, J. D., Zhu, Z. I., Yang, P.-C., Bankston, J. R., Jeng, M.-T., Kang, C., et al. (2011). A computational model to predict the effects of class I anti-arrhythmic drugs on ventricular rhythms. *Sci. Transl. Med.* 3:98ra83. doi: 10.1126/scitranslmed.3002588

Nousiainen, T., Vanninen, E., Jantunen, E., Puustinen, J., Remes, J., Rantala, A., et al. (2002). Natriuretic peptides during the development of doxorubicin-induced left ventricular diastolic dysfunction. *J. Intern. Med.* 251, 228–234. doi: 10.1046/j.1365-2796.2002.00951.x

Peng, X., Kraus, M. S., Wei, H., Shen, T.-L., Pariaut, R., Alcaraz, A., et al. (2006). Inactivation of focal adhesion kinase in cardiomyocytes promotes eccentric cardiac hypertrophy and fibrosis in mice. *J. Clin. Invest.* 116, 217–227. doi: 10.1172/JCI24497

Piccart-Gebhart, M. J., Procter, M., Leyland-Jones, B., Goldhirsch, A., Untch, M., Smith, I., et al. (2005). Trastuzumab after adjuvant chemotherapy in HER2-positive breast cancer. *N. Engl. J. Med.* 353, 1659–1672. doi: 10.1056/NEJMoa052306

Raschi, E., and De Ponti, F. (2012). Cardiovascular toxicity of anticancer-targeted therapy: emerging issues in the era of cardio-oncology. *Intern. Emerg. Med.* 7, 113–131. doi: 10.1007/s11739-011-0744-y

Reichelt, M. E., O'Brien, S., Thomas, W. G., and Headrick, J. P. (2017). Transactivation of the epidermal growth factor receptor in responses to myocardial stress and cardioprotection. *Int. J. Biochem. Cell Biol.* 83, 97–110. doi: 10.1016/j.biocel.2016.12.014

Rice, J. J., Wang, F., Bers, D. M., and de Tombe, P. P. (2008). Approximate model of cooperative activation and crossbridge cycling in cardiac muscle using ordinary differential equations. *Biophys. J.* 95, 2368–2390. doi: 10.1529/biophysj.107.119487

Romond, E. H., Perez, E. A., Bryant, J., Suman, V. J., Geyer, C. E. Jr., Davidson, N. E., et al. (2005). Trastuzumab plus adjuvant chemotherapy for operable HER2-positive breast cancer. *N. Engl. J. Med.* 353, 1673–1684. doi: 10.1056/NEJMoa052122

Ryall, K. A., Holland, D. O., Delaney, K. A., Kraeutler, M. J., Parker, A. J., and Saucerman, J. J. (2012). Network reconstruction and systems analysis of cardiac myocyte hypertrophy signaling. *J. Biol. Chem.* 287, 42259–42268. doi: 10.1074/jbc.M112.382937

Sager, P. T., Gintant, G., Turner, J. R., Pettit, S., and Stockbridge, N. (2014). Rechanneling the cardiac proarrhythmia safety paradigm: a meeting report from the cardiac safety research consortium. *Am. Heart J.* 167, 292–300. doi: 10.1016/j.ahj.2013.11.004

Sandri, M. T., Salvatici, M., Cardinale, D., Zorzino, L., Passerini, R., Lentati, P., et al. (2005). N-Terminal Pro-B-type natriuretic peptide after high-dose chemotherapy: a marker predictive of cardiac dysfunction? *Clin. Chem.* 51, 1405–1410. doi: 10.1373/clinchem.2005.050153

Sarkar, A. X., and Sobie, E. A. (2011). Quantification of repolarization reserve to understand interpatient variability in the response to proarrhythmic drugs: a computational analysis. *Heart Rhythm* 8, 1749–1755. doi: 10.1016/j.hrthm.2011.05.023

Schleich, K., and Lavrik, I. N. (2013). Mathematical modeling of apoptosis. *Cell Commun. Signal.* 11, 44. doi: 10.1186/1478-811X-11-44

Schlichter, L. C., Jiang, J., Wang, J., Newell, E. W., Tsui, F. W. L., and Lam, D. (2014). Regulation of hERG and hEAG channels by Src and by SHP-1 tyrosine phosphatase via an ITIM Region in the cyclic nucleotide binding domain. *PLoS ONE* 9:e90024. doi: 10.1371/journal.pone.0090024

Seidman, A., Hudis, C., Pierri, M. K., Shak, S., Paton, V., Ashby, M., et al. (2002). Cardiac dysfunction in the trastuzumab clinical trials experience. *J. Clin. Oncol.* 20, 1215–1221. doi: 10.1200/JCO.2002.20.5.1215

Shah, R. R., and Morganroth, J. (2015). Update on cardiovascular safety of tyrosine kinase inhibitors: with a special focus on QT interval, left ventricular dysfunction and overall risk/benefit. *Drug Saf.* 38, 693–710. doi: 10.1007/s40264-015-0300-1

Sharma, A., Burridge, P. W., McKeithan, W. L., Serrano, R., Shukla, P., Sayed, N., et al. (2017). High-throughput screening of tyrosine kinase inhibitor cardiotoxicity with human induced pluripotent stem cells. *Sci. Transl. Med.* 9:eaaf2584. doi: 10.1126/scitranslmed.aaf2584

Shin, S.-Y., Kim, T., Lee, H.-S., Kang, J. H., Lee, J. Y., Cho, K.-H., et al. (2014). The switching role of β-adrenergic receptor signalling in cell survival or death decision of cardiomyocytes. *Nat. Commun.* 5:5777. doi: 10.1038/ncomms6777

Shoda, L. K. M., Woodhead, J. L., Siler, S. Q., Watkins, P. B., and Howell, B. A. (2014). Linking physiology to toxicity using DILIsym®, a mechanistic mathematical model of drug-induced liver injury. *Biopharm. Drug Dispos.* 35, 33–49. doi: 10.1002/bdd.1878

Shohet, R. V., Kisanuki, Y. Y., Zhao, X.-S., Siddiquee, Z., Franco, F., and Yanagisawa, M. (2004). Mice with cardiomyocyte-specific disruption of the endothelin-1 gene are resistant to hyperthyroid cardiac hypertrophy. *Proc. Natl. Acad. Sci. U.S.A.* 101, 2088–2093. doi: 10.1073/pnas.0307159101

Skovgaard, D., Hasbak, P., and Kjaer, A. (2014). BNP predicts chemotherapy-related cardiotoxicity and death: comparison with gated equilibrium radionuclide ventriculography. *PLoS ONE* 9:e96736. doi: 10.1371/journal.pone.0096736

Slamon, D. J., Leyland-Jones, B., Shak, S., Fuchs, H., Paton, V., Bajamonde, A., et al. (2001). Use of chemotherapy plus a monoclonal antibody against HER2 for metastatic breast cancer that overexpresses HER2. *N. Engl. J. Med.* 344, 783–792. doi: 10.1056/NEJM200103153441101

Smith, A. K., Petersen, B. K., Ropella, G. E. P., Kennedy, R. C., Kaplowitz, N., Ookhtens, M., et al. (2016). Competing mechanistic hypotheses of acetaminophen-induced hepatotoxicity challenged by virtual experiments. *PLoS Comput. Biol.* 12:e1005253. doi: 10.1371/journal.pcbi.1005253

Sobie, E. A. (2009). Parameter sensitivity analysis in electrophysiological models using multivariable regression. *Biophys. J.* 96, 1264–1274. doi: 10.1016/j.bpj.2008.10.056

Tewari, S. G., Bugenhagen, S. M., Palmer, B. M., and Beard, D. A. (2016). Dynamics of cross-bridge cycling, ATP hydrolysis, force generation, and deformation in cardiac muscle. *J. Mol. Cell. Cardiol.* 96, 11–25. doi: 10.1016/j.yjmcc.2015.02.006

Thiagarajan, R., Alavi, A., Podichetty, J. T., Bazil, J. N., and Beard, D. A. (2017). The feasibility of genome-scale biological network inference using graphics processing units. *Algorithms Mol. Biol.* 12:8. doi: 10.1186/s13015-017-0100-5

Thiel, C., Cordes, H., Fabbri, L., Aschmann, H. E., Baier, V., Smit, I., et al. (2017). A comparative analysis of drug-induced hepatotoxicity in clinically relevant situations. *PLoS Comput. Biol.* 13:e1005280. doi: 10.1371/journal.pcbi.1005280

van Hasselt, J. G. C., Schellens, J. H. M., Mac Gillavry, M. R., Beijnen, J. H., and Huitema, A. D. R. (2012). Model-based evaluation and optimization of cardiac monitoring protocols for adjuvant treatment of breast cancer with trastuzumab. *Pharm. Res.* 29, 3499–3511. doi: 10.1007/s11095-012-0845-y

Wacquier, B., Combettes, L., Van Nhieu, G. T., Dupont, G., Zimmermann, B., Szabadkai, G., et al. (2016). Interplay between intracellular Ca^{2+} oscillations and Ca^{2+}-stimulated mitochondrial metabolism. *Sci. Rep.* 6:19316. doi: 10.1038/srep19316

Warde-Farley, D., Donaldson, S. L., Comes, O., Zuberi, K., Badrawi, R., Chao, P., et al. (2010). The GeneMANIA prediction server: biological network integration for gene prioritization and predicting gene function. *Nucleic Acids Res.* 38, W214–W220. doi: 10.1093/nar/gkq537

Woodhead, J. L., Watkins, P. B., Howell, B. A., Siler, S. Q., and Shoda, L. K. M. (2017). The role of quantitative systems pharmacology modeling in the prediction and explanation of idiosyncratic drug-induced liver injury. *Drug Metab. Pharmacokinet.* 32, 40–45. doi: 10.1016/j.dmpk.2016.11.008

Wu, P., Nielsen, T. E., and Clausen, M. H. (2016). Small-molecule kinase inhibitors: an analysis of FDA-approved drugs. *Drug Discov. Today* 21, 5–10. doi: 10.1016/j.drudis.2015.07.008

Xu, Z., Cang, S., Yang, T., and Liu, D. (2009). Cardiotoxicity of tyrosine kinase inhibitors in chronic myelogenous leukemia therapy. *Hematol. Rep.* 1:4. doi: 10.4081/hr.2009.e4

Yamazaki, T., Komuro, I., Kudoh, S., Zou, Y., Shiojima, I., Hiroi, Y., et al. (1996). Endothelin-1 is involved in mechanical stress-induced cardiomyocyte hypertrophy. *J. Biol. Chem.* 271, 3221–3228. doi: 10.1074/jbc.271.6.3221

Yang, P.-C., Moreno, J. D., Miyake, C. Y., Vaughn-Behrens, S. B., Jeng, M.-T., Grandi, E., et al. (2016). *In silico* prediction of drug therapy in catecholaminergic polymorphic ventricular tachycardia. *J. Physiol.* 594, 567–593. doi: 10.1113/JP271282

Yang, Y., Nadanaciva, S., Will, Y., Woodhead, J. L., Howell, B. A., Watkins, P. B., et al. (2015). MITOsym®: a mechanistic, mathematical model of hepatocellular respiration and bioenergetics. *Pharm. Res.* 32, 1975–1992. doi: 10.1007/s11095-014-1591-0

Yeh, E. T. H., and Bickford, C. L. (2009). Cardiovascular complications of cancer therapy. *J. Am. Coll. Cardiol.* 53, 2231–2247. doi: 10.1016/j.jacc.2009.02.050

Zhang, P., Hu, X., Xu, X., Fassett, J., Zhu, G., Viollet, B., et al. (2008). AMP activated protein kinase-alpha2 deficiency exacerbates pressure-overload-induced left ventricular hypertrophy and dysfunction in mice. *Hypertension* 52, 918–924. doi: 10.1161/HYPERTENSIONAHA.108.114702

11

In Vitro and In silico Risk Assessment in Acquired Long QT Syndrome: The Devil is in the Details

William Lee[1,2], *Monique J. Windley*[1,2], *Jamie I. Vandenberg*[1,2] *and Adam P. Hill*[1,2*]

[1] *Molecular Cardiology and Biophysics Division, Victor Chang Cardiac Research Institute, Darlinghurst, NSW, Australia,* [2] *St. Vincent's Clinical School, University of New South Wales, Sydney, NSW, Australia*

Correspondence:
Adam P. Hill
a.hill@victorchang.edu.au

Acquired long QT syndrome, mostly as a result of drug block of the Kv11. 1 potassium channel in the heart, is characterized by delayed cardiac myocyte repolarization, prolongation of the T interval on the ECG, syncope and sudden cardiac death due to the polymorphic ventricular arrhythmia Torsade de Pointes (TdP). In recent years, efforts are underway through the Comprehensive *in vitro* proarrhythmic assay (CiPA) initiative, to develop better tests for this drug induced arrhythmia based in part on *in silico* simulations of pharmacological disruption of repolarization. However, drug binding to Kv11.1 is more complex than a simple binary molecular reaction, meaning simple steady state measures of potency are poor surrogates for risk. As a result, there is a plethora of mechanistic detail describing the drug/Kv11.1 interaction—such as drug binding kinetics, state preference, temperature dependence and trapping—that needs to be considered when developing *in silico* models for risk prediction. In addition to this, other factors, such as multichannel pharmacological profile and the nature of the ventricular cell models used in simulations also need to be considered in the search for the optimum *in silico* approach. Here we consider how much of mechanistic detail needs to be included for *in silico* models to accurately predict risk and further, how much of this detail can be retrieved from protocols that are practical to implement in high throughout screens as part of next generation of preclinical *in silico* drug screening approaches?

Keywords: kv11.1, herg, acquired long QT syndrome, arrhythmia, pharmacology, CiPA, modeling

INTRODUCTION

In the past 20 years, a range of structurally unrelated drugs, including antihistamines, antibiotics and antipsychotics, have been withdrawn from the market due to adverse effects on cardiac repolarization - so called acquired long QT syndrome (aLQTS). aLQTS is characterized by prolongation and sometimes morphological deformation of QT segments on the 12-lead electrocardiogram (ECG), syncope and sudden cardiac death due to the polymorphic ventricular arrhythmia Torsade de Pointes (TdP). Theoretically, aLQTS can occur due to unwanted drug induced modulation of any of the ionic channels that contribute to cardiac repolarization either through direct modulation of channel conductance (Cavero et al., 2000; Perrin et al., 2008a) or up/down regulation of channel trafficking and expression on the cell membrane (Dennis et al., 2007; Ballou et al., 2015). In practice however, the overwhelming majority of these drugs cause aLQTS through blockade of the Kv11.1 potassium channel that carries the rapid component of the delayed rectifier current in the heart (I_{Kr}) (Perrin et al., 2008b).

As a result of the prevalence of these proarrhythmic side effects, regulatory guidelines have been put in place as part of preclinical drug development to ensure such dangerous compounds do not get to market. In their current form, these guidelines use simple steady-state measures of Kv11.1 inhibitory concentration and action potential prolongation to estimate arrhythmic risk (E14, 2005; S7B, 2005). However, while these steady-state measures of Kv11.1 block are very sensitive (no new proarrhythmic drugs have knowingly come to market since the inception of these guidelines), they are not specific. The link between Kv11.1 block, repolarization delay, and TdP is poorly understood meaning these measures are poor surrogates for actual risk of TdP. Given that not all drugs that block Kv11.1 are going to be proarrhythmic, this has likely resulted in an unnecessarily high attrition rate of drugs in development (Redfern et al., 2003; Sager et al., 2014).

To address this issue, the Comprehensive *in vitro* Proarrhythmia assay (CiPA) has been proposed as a new safety paradigm in understanding TdP and assessing proarrhythmia risk (Sager et al., 2014). CiPA has two primary objectives: (1) Detailed *in vitro* electrophysiological characterization of drug interaction with Kv11.1 (and other cardiac ion channels) and integration of this data into *in silico* models to predict proarrhythmia in simulations of the cardiac action potential and (2) Validation of *in silico* models using human induced pluripotent stem cell derived cardiac cardiomyocytes (Fermini et al., 2016). Central to the first of these objectives is our understanding of the mechanistic subtleties of how drugs interact with Kv11.1. There are several key factors that contribute to a drug's pharmacological profile and hence contribute to proarrhythmic risk, including the kinetics of drug binding and unbinding, gating-state preference and temperature dependence. These factors are not easily quantified by simple steady-state measures, yet can have significant effects on the measured potency of a drug as well as profound impact on the degree of repolarization delay and the emergence of proarrhythmic markers seen in *in silico* simulations. For example, **Figure 1** demonstrates an *in silico* simulation of 6,561 theoretical drugs that block Kv11.1 all at calculated IC_{50} doses and yet the simulated action potential prolongation is significantly varied. Furthermore, whilst Kv11.1 is the major repolarizing current in the cardiac action potential, there are multiple other currents that contribute to repolarization, a concept known as repolarization reserve (Roden, 1998). In this context, the evolution of drug induced TdP may involve block of multiple ion channel currents and a drug's affinity for a variety of targets may modify the proarrhythmic risk associated with its block of Kv11.1. Determination of the proarrhythmic risk profile of Kv11.1 blocking drugs is therefore a multifaceted problem that goes beyond simple measures of potency. As a result, using *in silico* means to predict the risk associated with individual drugs is a complex process for which the optimal implementation remains to be decided upon. In this article we will consider what level of mechanistic detail describing the interaction between drug and ion channel target needs to be included for *in silico* models to accurately predict risk and further, how much of this detail can be retrieved from protocols that are practical to

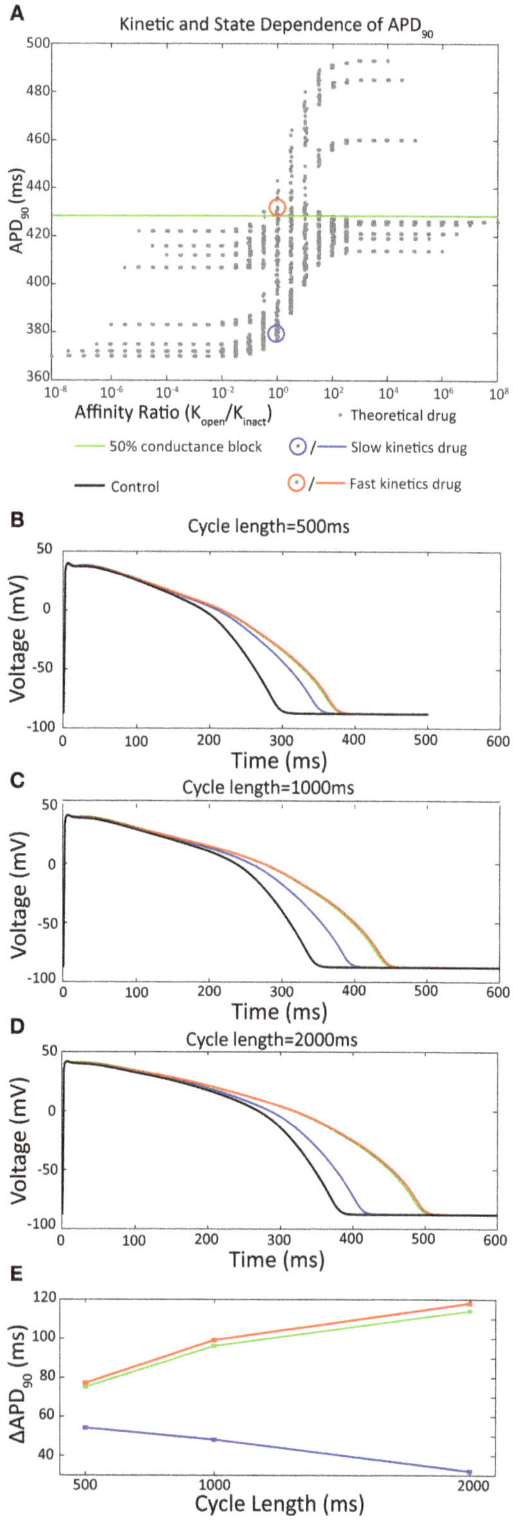

FIGURE 1 | (A) *In silico* analysis of APD_{90} with respect to the ratio of affinity for the open vs inactivated state, K_O /K_i. A family of theoretical drugs was constructed using permutations of the forward and reverse rates for binding to the open state of the channel (kf,open and kb,open respectively) and the inactivated state of the channel (kf,inact and kb,inact respectively) in the range *(Continued)*

FIGURE 1 | Continued
0.01–100 s-1 using half-logarithmic increments. An IC_{50} dose of each drug, calculated *in silico* using a simulated direct drug application of the drug at a holding potential of 0 mV, was applied to the O'Hara Rudy action potential at 1000 ms pacing cycle length. Drugs with higher affinity for the open state are shown on the right (K_O / K_i > 1) and drugs with higher affinity for the inactivated state are shown to the left (K_O / K_i < 1). The green line shows the APD_{90} for IK_r50 (a 50 % conductance block of I_{kr}) of 428 ms. *Adapted from* Lee et al. (2016). **(B–E)** Drug binding kinetics contribute to reverse rate dependence. **(B)** Action potentials simulated at 500 ms pacing interval in response to an IC_{50} dose of the drugs selected in **(A)**. Black line represents a control action potential with no drug applied. **(C)** Action potentials at 1,000 ms pacing interval. **(D)** Action potentials at 2,000 ms pacing interval. **(E)** Pacing cycle dependence of ΔAPD_{90}.

implement in high throughout screens as part of preclinical development?

COMPLEXITY OF THE KV11.1/DRUG INTERACTION

In many cases, a drug's interactions with its ion channel pharmacological target can be described as a simple bimolecular reaction according to the equation:

$$O \underset{k_b}{\overset{k_f[D]}{\rightleftharpoons}} OD \quad (1)$$

Where O represents the open ion channel, D is drug, and $k_f$and k_b are the rates of association and dissociation respectively. A dissociation constant (K_D), describing the affinity of binding can then be defined as the quotient of k_b from k_f:

$$K_D = \frac{k_b}{k_f} \quad (2)$$

In the scenario where this binding results in block of the ion channel current, the IC_{50}, the drug concentration at which 50% of channels are blocked, approximates the K_D. Whilst Kv11.1 interaction with drugs does not follow this simple rule (Windley et al., 2016), it nevertheless provides a useful framework for discussion of drug binding to Kv11.1. A detailed consideration of the factors that contribute to the complexity of block of these channels is presented in the following sections.

Drug Binding Kinetics

The inclusion of drug binding kinetics in *in silico* simulations has been demonstrated to significantly alter predictions of cardiac action potential prolongation (Di Veroli et al., 2014; Lee et al., 2016). Specifically, drugs of equivalent affinity for Kv11.1 demonstrate varying degrees of action potential prolongation (**Figures 1B–D**). In some experiments, up to 4-fold increased difference in prolongation can be observed when comparing equipotent drugs with fast kinetics (τ_{on} = 0.1 s) to those with slow kinetics (τ_{on} = 100 s) (Di Veroli et al., 2014), which is within the range of time constants for drug binding observed for known drugs (Windley et al., 2017). Moreover, this differential prolongation is accentuated at different pacing frequencies; fast drugs cause greater prolongation at lower pacing frequencies while the opposite is true for slow drugs. At a pacing cycle length of 1,000 ms this leads to a difference in prolongation of APD_{90} of 52 ms when these parameters are incorporated into *in silico* simulations (**Figure 1C**; Lee et al., 2016).

These rate dependent effects therefore contribute to one of the most commonly measured indicators of proarrhythmic propensity—reverse rate dependence (RRD)—where an inverse relationship exists between action potential prolongation and depolarization frequency (Hondeghem et al., 2001a,b). The implied mechanism of this is that drugs with different kinetics of binding reach different levels of steady state block as a function of the relative rates of drug binding, unbinding and cycle length. Specifically, for the drugs shown in **Figures 1B–D**, this manifests as a maximal 30% block of Kv11.1 achieved with application of slow drugs at an IC_{50} dose during 1 Hz pacing, compared to 50% block for fast drugs under the same conditions (Lee et al., 2016). While it is known that other factors including genetic background and environmental factors including adrenergic upregulation of I_{Ks} (Sanguinetti et al., 1991; Bosch et al., 2002; Bányász et al., 2009) contribute to RRD, it is clear that the kinetics of the drug/channel interaction are also central to this established measure of proarrhythmia.

Another characteristic of drug interaction with Kv11.1 that is at least partially underpinned by the kinetics of binding and unbinding is that of "trapping" (Carmeliet, 1992; Yang et al., 1995; Mitcheson et al., 2000b; Perry et al., 2004; Stork et al., 2007). For some drugs, this phenomenon is due to true drug trapping. In these cases the drug molecule remains within the channel pore, sterically prevented from diffusing out as a result of closing of the cytoplasmic gate when the channel deactivates (Mitcheson et al., 2000b; Stork et al., 2007). Other compounds however, are more likely to display "virtual trapping," where drug unbinding is significantly slower than the rate of channel deactivation (Perry et al., 2004). In these cases, depending on the voltage protocol used, the drug will appear to be "virtually trapped" if the interpulse time is insufficient for complete drug dissociation. (Lee et al., 2016; Windley et al., 2017). However, the extent to which the degree and type of trapping can be measured *in vitro* using simple voltage protocols is limited. For example, in the step depolarization protocol used by Windley et al. (2017) and Li et al. (2017), the degree of trapping is estimated with a fixed 15 s interpulse interval. The limitations of this approach are twofold. First, it is not possible to distinguish between true trapping and virtually trapped drugs. In practical terms, *in silico* simulation has demonstrated that true trapping results in significantly greater APD_{90} prolongation and greater pro-arrhythmic risk, Di Veroli et al. (2014) and therefore it is important to distinguish between the two. Second, any virtually trapped drug that dissociates quicker than 15 s will be described as non-trapped. Even if there was significant residual block evident at 5 or 10 s, the protocol cannot test this. In the context of cardiac cycle, where a typical diastolic interval might be on the order of 600 ms, this might be a significant shortcoming. Even so, Li et al. have shown that including an approximation of trapping and kinetics based on this protocol in their *in silico* models is useful in improving proarrhythmic prediction. For example, discrimination between drugs with low, medium and high risk of proarrhythmia using the metric ability of the "cqInward" (which represents the net inward current during the cardiac action potential) is incrementally improved when descriptions of trapping and kinetics are included in simulation as compared to simple IC_{50} measures of drug potency (Li et al., 2017; **Figure 2**). This is therefore clearly an important factor to consider, even if it is described with some degree of simplicity.

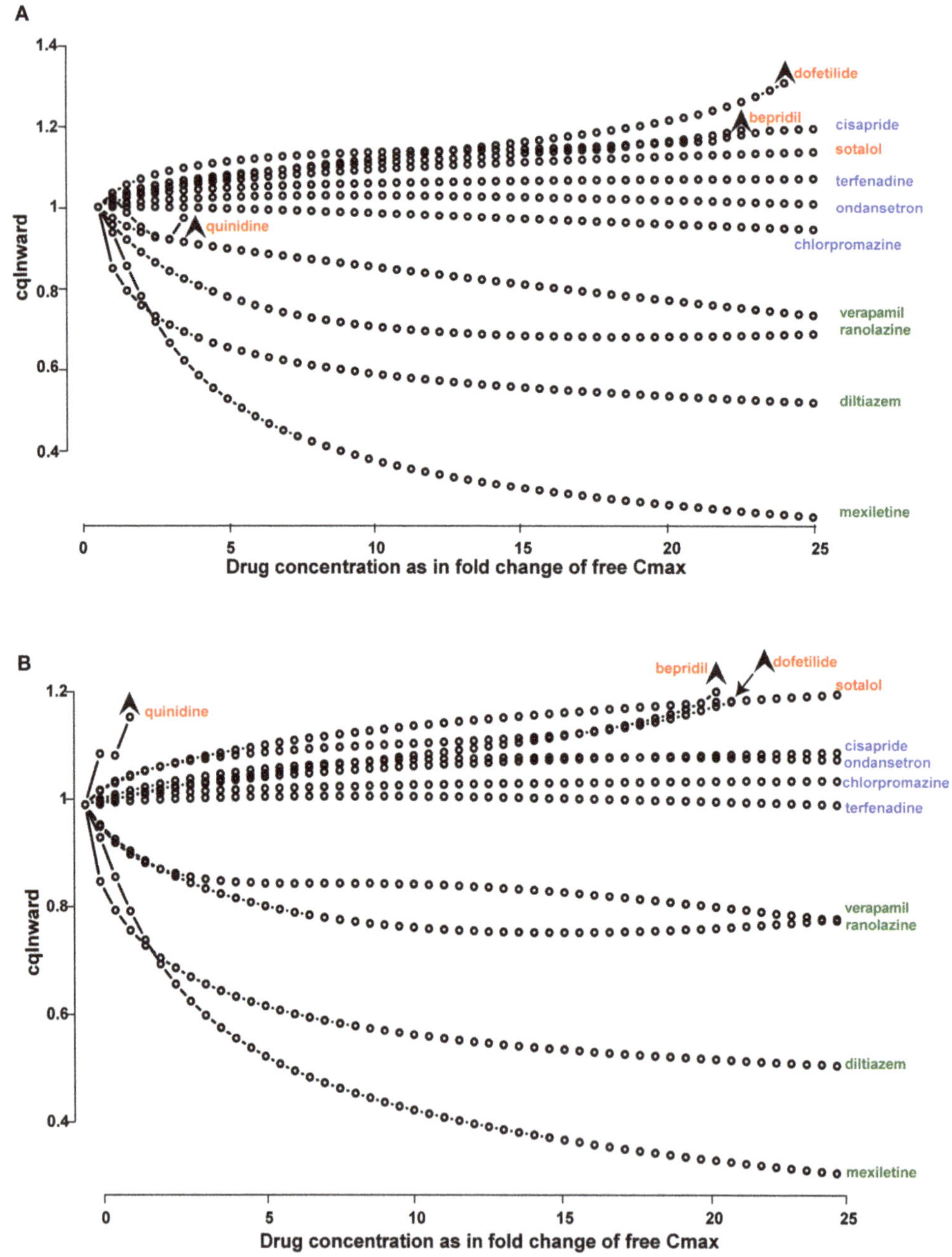

FIGURE 2 | Drug binding kinetics improves risk prediction. **(A,B)** Concentration-dependent cqInward for all CiPA (Comprehensive *in vitro* Proarrhythmia Assay) training compounds. (High risk drugs are labeled in red, intermediate risk in blue and low risk in green) x-axis is the ratio between the simulated concentration and free Cmax; y-axis is the cqInward metric. Stars indicate the threshold dose, which is the highest dose that did not elicit an early afterdepolarization (EAD). The metric cqInward is the net inward current for each drug and is calculated as (INaL_AUC_drug/INaL_AUC_control+ICaL_AUC_drug/ICaL_AUC_control)/2, where AUC is the integrated area under the curve of the late sodium (INaL) and L-type calcium (ICaL) current traces during steady-state action potential simulation with (_drug) or without (_control) drugs. **(A)** Simulations are performed using instantaneous block of Kv11.1 base on dose response curves. **(B)** Simulations are performed using a dynamic model of Kv11.1-drug binding with incremental improvement in arrhythmia risk stratification. Reproduced from Li et al. (2017).

In summary, the kinetics of binding and unbinding of drugs to Kv11.1 play an important role in accurate prediction of prolongation of repolarization and proarrhythmic propensity. The addition of greater complexity, such as variability in ionic channel densities/function seen in different layers of the ventricular myocardium (Saiz et al., 2011) or congenital LQTS mutants (Romero et al., 2014), will further compound these effects. Consequently, in pursuit of a robust and comprehensive risk prediction assay, detailed understanding of these baseline measures of drug binding kinetics are likely an important component for *in silico* risk prediction and inaccurate estimation will likely lead to compounding errors as we continue to build and refine prediction models.

State Dependent Binding

The vast majority of drugs which target Kv11.1 require channel opening in order to gain access to the receptor site within the inner cavity of the channel pore (Kiehn et al., 1996; Walker et al., 1999; Vandenberg et al., 2012). However, a drug's affinity can be relatively greater for either the open state (K_O) or inactivated state (K_I) resulting in a state preference in drug binding. To date, there are no studies that have been able to demonstrate drug binding in the closed state. Several studies have demonstrated that some, but not all, drugs with high affinity binding to Kv11.1 show preferential binding to the inactivated state (Suessbrich et al., 1997; Ficker et al., 1998; Numaguchi et al., 2000; Perrin et al., 2008a; Du et al., 2014). These studies show that Kv11.1 binding potency in certain high affinity drugs is reduced by using inactivation attenuated mutants, such as N588K or S631A (Perrin et al., 2008a; Du et al., 2014), or the inactivation deficient mutant S620T (Suessbrich et al., 1997; Ficker et al., 1998; Perrin et al., 2008a; Wu et al., 2015). The inference being that these drugs favor binding to the inactivated state, hence channel mutants which reduced inactivation are less likely to bind the drug in question.

However, it is important to note that it is not always the case that there is a direct correlation between the extent of inactivation and the affinity of drug binding, even for state-dependent blockers. Electrophysiological studies using concatenated Kv11.1 tetramers containing variable number of inactivation deficient subunits have demonstrated changes in drug binding affinity that occur independent of inactivation (Chen et al., 2002; Wu et al., 2015). The major molecular determinants for drug binding to Kv11.1 are two aromatic residues Y652 and F56 in the S6 helix (Mitcheson et al., 2000a; Chen et al., 2002; Wu et al., 2015). In addition to these two S6 aromatics, Thr623, Ser624, and Val625 at the base of the selectivity filter, and Phe557 on the S5 helix also contribute to drug binding at least for some drugs (Mitcheson et al., 2000a,b; Saxena et al., 2016). It is likely that conformational changes that accompany inactivation, but that are not strictly necessary for the open to inactivated state transition, alter the arrangement of these residues within the pore cavity to allow for additional close molecular interactions that result in preferential binding to the inactivated state (Durdagi et al., 2012). This is supported by evidence from molecular dynamics simulations, albeit those limited to using homology models of Kv11.1, which demonstrate these conformational changes (Durdagi et al., 2012).

Of course, there are also non-state dependent drugs whose potencies are not affected by inactivation deficient mutants. These drugs include: quinidine, erythromycin, perhexiline (Perrin et al., 2008a), and clozapine (Hill et al., 2014). Moreover, studies have suggested that some compounds may also have an open state preference with minimal binding to the inactivated state (Kamiya et al., 2001; Park et al., 2002; Su et al., 2004). However, the contention with these studies is that rather than using mutagenesis to manipulate state occupancy, they utilize complex non-standardized voltage protocols to demonstrate state preference since an open deficient Kv11.1 mutant is not useful due to an absence of current. It is likely that the recent advent of high resolution structures of Kv11.1 (Wang and MacKinnon, 2017) and the potential this presents to generate more structures of drugs interacting with inactivation deficient Kv11.1 channels, will allow more accurate molecular dynamic simulations to probe these questions around state-dependent drug binding in more detail.

How important then is the consideration of state dependent binding for *in silico* prediction of arrhythmic risk? The data in **Figures 3A,B** shows that an IC_{50} dose of two drugs with opposite state preferences differ in the degree of observed APD prolongation by 56 ms—clearly a significant amount in predicting their proarrhythmic potential. However, this relationship also needs to be considered through the prism of the limitation that the measured IC_{50} is itself influenced by the state preference and how this manifests as a function of the voltage protocol used to measure the potency. Current safety guidelines mandate equilibrium testing of drugs to estimate potency to estimate arrhythmic risk (S7B, 2005). However, measures of drug potency vary between voltage protocols for some drugs but not for others (Kirsch et al., 2004; Yao et al., 2005; Milnes et al., 2010). These differences, which can be an order of magnitude in disparity, are in part due to using voltage protocols which favor occupancy of either the open or inactivated state, so favoring drug binding to that state (Milnes et al., 2010). Therefore, how can one measure state preference for incorporation into *in silico* simulations? The processes of channel opening and inactivation occur over overlapping voltage ranges, so it is almost impossible to tease out the relative affinities for the two states from a single, relatively simple voltage protocol. One potential approach to this might be to examine multiple protocols, that each sample the state occupancy of open vs. inactive differently, and attempt to infer information about state preference from the differences in IC_{50}s measured using each. However, this is a relatively complex task that may not be amenable to high throughput screens.

Temperature Dependence

The temperature dependence of potency of Kv11.1 block is a phenomenon that has been described in the literature for many drugs (Guo et al., 2005; Yao et al., 2005; Alexandrou et al., 2006; Hill et al., 2007). For instance, Guo et al. (2005) and Alexandrou et al. (2006) demonstrate an increase in potency with respect to increasing temperature from 22 to 37°C for fluoroquinolone antibiotics (erythromycin and moxifloxacin respectively), although not to the same magnitude. In contrast, other drugs, including loratadine and bepridil, exhibit reduced

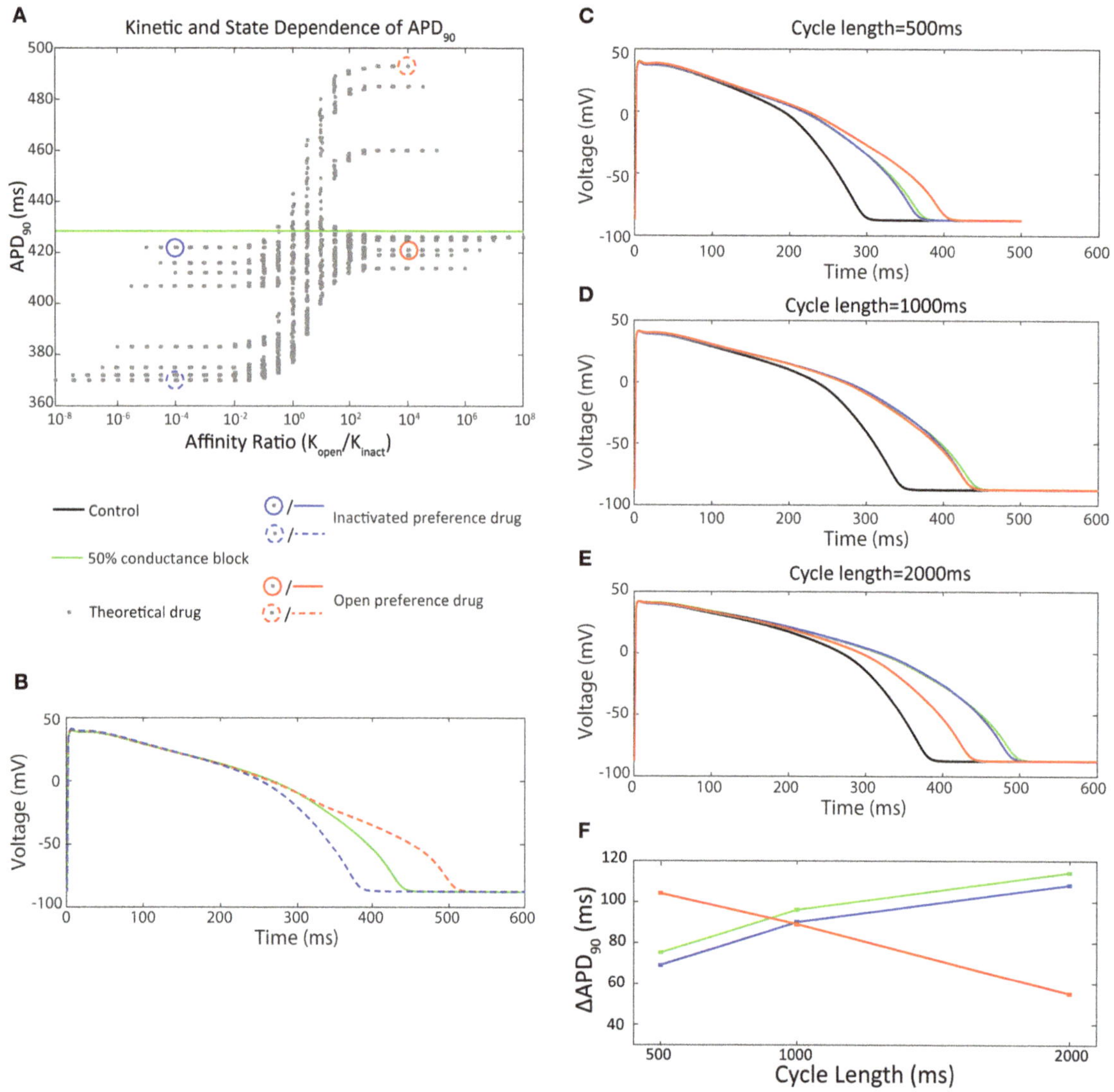

FIGURE 3 | Effect of state preference on cardiac action potential prolongation. **(A)** 2 drugs with equal but opposite ratio of affinity for the open vs. inactivated state were selected from the dataset in **(A)**. The inactivated state preference drug ($K_O/K_i = 10^{-4}$) is shown in blue-dash. The open state preference drug ($K_O/K_i = 10^4$) is shown in red-dash. **(B)** Ventricular action potentials corresponding to the two drugs in **(A)** in comparison to IK_r50. **(C–F)** Effect of pacing cycle length on cardiac action potential prolongation**.** 2 drugs with equal and opposite ratio of affinity for the open vs inactivated state and equal APD_{90} at a pacing cycle length of 1,000 ms were selected from **(A)**. The inactivated state preference drug ($K_O/K_i = 10^{-4}$) is shown in blue-solid. The open state preference drug ($K_O/K_i = 10^4$) is shown in red-solid. **(C)** Action potentials at 500 ms pacing interval. **(D)** Action potentials at 1,000 ms pacing interval. **(E)** Action potentials at 2,000 ms pacing interval. **(F)** Pacing cycle dependence of ΔAPD_{90}

potency at physiological temperatures (Kirsch et al., 2004). Larger scale studies have also established that a range of different drugs have a variable degree of Kv11.1 blockade when examined at ambient temperature compared to physiological temperatures (Kirsch et al., 2004; Yao et al., 2005). Moreover, differences in temperature sensitivity can be accentuated by different voltage protocols (Kirsch et al., 2004).

In relation to gathering data to constrain *in silico* models, this problem is further complicated by recent studies by Windley et al. (Windley et al., 2016), that revealed some mechanistic insights into the temperature dependence of drug binding to Kv11.1. Using a direct measurement of kinetics at 0 mV rather than a pulsed voltage protocol, Windley et al. demonstrated that for cisapride, increasing temperature from 22 to 37°C did not affect affinity of binding, but significantly altered kinetics. *In silico* the temperature dependence of binding and unbinding kinetics could not be described by a simple bi-molecular interaction, but required inclusion of an "encounter-complex"; a conducting intermediary state between unblocked and blocked channels states. This change in kinetics could also be used to potentially explain apparent differences in drug potency when using varying pulsed voltage protocols as discussed in the following section

For example: at 20 nM comparing 22–37°C, Windley et al. observed a 5.5-fold increase in cisapride binding rates to Kv11.1. Based on the analysis in Lee et al. (2016), this could account for a ~20 ms increase in drug-induced APD_{90} prolongation, despite no change in affinity. In addition to these effects of temperature on drug binding, the gating of the Kv11.1 channel itself is sensitive to temperature. Specifically, at 37°C there are increases in channel conductance, a hyperpolarizing shift in activation and a depolarizing shift in inactivation (Vandenberg et al., 2006), resulting in an overall increase in in open state that will also influence the measured potency of drugs that display state dependent binding (see Section State Dependent Binding).

The implications of these studies are that for some drugs, measures of potency and kinetics made at ambient temperatures may not be useful in constraining *in silico* models used to predict proarrhythmia at physiological temperatures (Windley et al., 2016). This is potentially a concern for large scale, high-throughput drug screening as many of the current generations of automated patch clamp platforms are limited to recording at ambient temperature (Fermini et al., 2016). However, efforts are currently underway, through the CiPA *in silico* Working Group and High Throughout stream to establish the practical importance and consequences of this issue.

MEASURING AND MODELING DRUG BINDING TO KV11.1

The complexity of Kv11.1-drug interactions therefore has clear implications for how the field should approach both measuring of these phenomena *in vitro*, as well as how we describe them using *in silico* models that can be used for risk prediction. Current guidelines stipulate the I_{Kr} current should be assayed but do not specify voltage protocols, or details, such as temperature or cellular expression systems. As a result there is a lack of standardization in how block of I_{Kr} current is measured (Fermini et al., 2016). Redfern et al. (2003) proposed a 30-fold safety margin between the measured IC_{50} of a drug and its maximum unbound plasma concentration (C_{max}) to distinguish between safe and unsafe drugs. However, many studies have shown variance in drug potency dependent as a function of temperature and voltage protocol (Kirsch et al., 2004; Yao et al., 2005; Milnes et al., 2010) and this safety margin becomes unreliable if a true IC_{50} value cannot be agreed upon. For example, the reported IC_{50} values for cisapride, span a 60-fold range (Potet et al., 2001; Rezazadeh et al., 2004). One approach therefore is to use *in silico* modeling to "fine-tune" *in vitro* experimental protocols to more closely mimic *in vivo* conditions (Ellinwood et al., 2017). However, even if a standardized protocol could be agreed upon, such as using a physiological cardiac action potential to reproduce the state transitions of Kv11.1 that are seen during the cardiac cycle, this would not take into account the impact of variations in heart rate or action potential prolongation which are paramount to the highly dynamic binding kinetics of the drug/Kv11.1 interaction. For example the data in **Figures 3C–F** shows two drugs with equal and opposite gating state preference. At 1,000 ms pacing cycle length the APD_{90} differs by 1 ms. However, at 500 ms pacing cycle length the open state preference drug prolongs the APD_{90} by 35 ms *more* than the inactivated state preference drug; while at 2,000 ms pacing cycle length the open state preference drug prolongs the APD_{90} by 53 ms *less* than the inactivated state preference drug. (**Figures 3C–F**) Moreover, these standardized conditions also lack the ability to predict variations in physiological conditions, such as hyper/hypo-kalaemia (Wang et al., 1997) or low pH (and the consequent changes in protonation of drug compounds) (Moreno et al., 2011; Wang et al., 2016), all of which are known to affect the state-dependence of drug binding. An alternative therefore, is to use non-physiological voltage protocols to accurately constrain *in silico* models of drug binding (Hill et al., 2014; Beattie et al., 2017) that can then be used *in silico* to evaluate a limitless range of physiological conditions.

This approach however brings with it a new set of challenges. There exists a wide variety of models of Kv11.1/drug interaction in the literature, each with different structures and each constrained by different *in vitro* datasets. Furthermore, they differ substantially in their ability to describe the key features of Kv11.1/drug binding dynamics discussed above, such as kinetics and state dependence (**Figures 4A,B**; Di Veroli et al., 2013; Hill et al., 2014), drug trapping (**Figure 4C**; Li et al., 2017) and temperature dependence (**Figure 4D**; Windley et al., 2016). While each of these models represents a good description of drug binding under certain conditions, they differ significantly in their predicted state occupancies over any given voltage protocol (**Figures 4Aii,Cii**), so will result in a difference in state-dependent drug binding. As yet, no Markov model provides a universal solution that we can be sure would be useful for prediction of proarrhythmic risk. As a result, further complexity may need to be added, or the existing models constrained with new *in vitro* data, to improve the model's predictive accuracy (Fermini et al., 2016). The issue of what is the optimum approach to measuring and modeling drug binding to Kv11.1 is therefore an open question and the optimum balance between how much and what type of data is required to constrain *in silico* models and what is practical to do in the context of high throughput data acquisition is yet to be determined.

MULTICHANNEL PHARMACOLOGY

The final piece of the puzzle that needs to be considered in developing ventricular cell simulations for *in silico* risk prediction is the role of multichannel pharmacology, and how this contributes to characteristics of the cellular action potential. Whilst Kv11.1 blockade is certainly critical to understanding aLQTS and drug induced TdP, it is not the sole determinant of arrhythmogenesis since drugs that block Kv11.1 can often also block other cardiac ion channels (Bril et al., 1996; Aiba et al., 2005; Wu et al., 2008; Vicente et al., 2015) to suppress or promote arrhythmogenesis (Fermini et al., 2016). An evaluation of the potency of a panel of 30 drugs against the seven major currents that contribute to repolarization demonstrated that the primary pharmacological targets that determine proarrhythmia were I_{Kr} (Kv11.1), I_{CaL} (Cav 1.2), and I_{NaL} (Nav1.5-late). Furthermore,

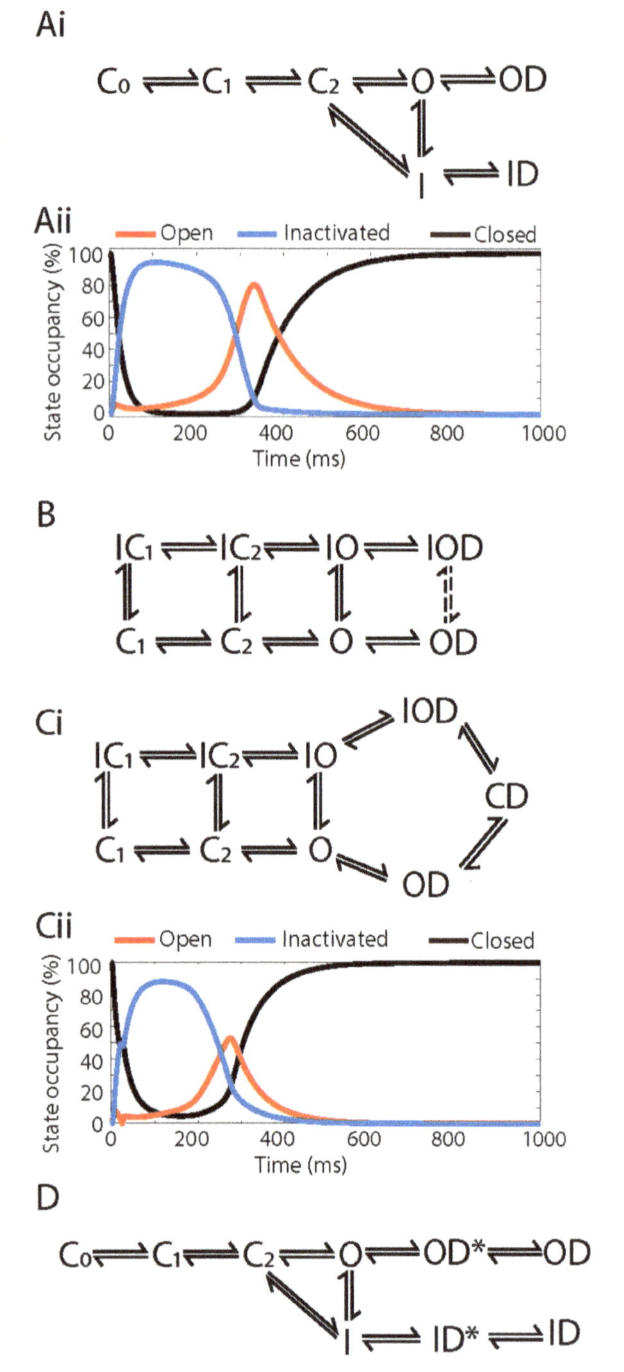

FIGURE 4 | Example Markov models of drug binding to Kv11.1. **(Ai)** Kinetic and gating-state dependent model *adapted from* Lee et al. (2016). **(Aii)** State occupancies of the combined closed (C-black), open (O-red) and inactivated (I-blue) states using the Markov model in **(Ai)**, simulated in an O'Hara Rudy action potential at 1 Hz. **(B)** Kinetic and gating-state dependent model *adapted from* Di Veroli et al. (2013). **(Ci)** Drug trapping model *adapted from* Li et al. (2017). **(Cii)** State occupancies of the combined closed (C-black), open (O-red) and inactivated (I-blue) states using the Markov model in **(Ci)**, simulated in an O'Hara Rudy action potential at 1 Hz. **(D)** Temperature dependent model *adapted from* Windley et al. (2016). C_0, C_1, C_2, Closed states; IC_1, IC_2, Inactivated-closed states; I, IO, Inactivated states; O, Open state; ID, IOD, Drug bound-inactivated states; OD, Drug bound-open state; CD, Drug trapped state.

drugs with high TdP risk tended toward unopposed Kv11.1 block, while drugs with low TdP risk had similar or higher potency for the inward currents (I_{CaL} and I_{NaL}) in conjunction with Kv11.1 block (Crumb et al., 2016). These multichannel pharmacological profiles are reflected in the morphology of the AP waveform (and hence the surface ECG). The AP waveform is formed through summed contribution of all the individual ionic currents in the cardiac myocytes. As a result, varied drug block of different ionic currents will result in a spectrum of AP morphologies and durations, which is idiosyncratic to individual drugs that manifests *in vivo* as differences in QT duration as well as T wave morphology (**Figures 5Ci–Cii**; Vicente et al., 2015). Critically for *in silico* risk prediction, this "AP morphology signature" is in turn linked to the drug's pro-arrhythmic potential and potentially can be used to predict TdP.

In this regard, drug induced morphological changes in the cardiac AP have been shown to correlate with risk of TdP (Hondeghem et al., 2001a). Specifically, this study suggested the presence of AP "triangulation" (slow repolarization, without a distinct plateau or rapid repolarization phase) was a marker of risk of drug induced TdP. Several single drug studies exemplify this point and support the link with multichannel pharmacology. Drugs that block Kv11.1 without significant inward current block, such as Sotalol (Milberg et al., 2004) and dofetilide (Osadchii, 2012; **Figure 5Aii**), produce AP triangulation in addition to prolongation, (**Figure 5Bii**) and are considered high TdP risk drugs. Conversely, Verapamil, a potent blocker of Cav1.2 as well as Kv11.1 (**Figure 5Ai**), does not manifest in triangulation or prolongation of the AP (**Figure 5Bi**) and is considered a low TdP-risk drug (Aiba et al., 2005). Similarly, other drugs with multichannel pharmacological profiles, such as ranolazine (Jia et al., 2011) and tolterodine (Martin et al., 2006) demonstrate dose dependent AP prolongation without AP triangulation and are also considered low risk. It is clear therefore, that multichannel pharmacology, and its manifestation in morphology of the AP, is an important detail that must be considered for risk prediction.

In silico modeling again provides an ideal solution to integrating pharmacological data from multiple cardiac ion channels. Indeed, recent studies by Li et al. (2017) and Dutta et al. (2017) have shown the value of this approach and demonstrated that incorporating Cav1.2 and Nav1.5-late block into action potential simulations improves arrhythmia risk prediction (Yang et al., 2016; Li et al., 2017). However, in a similar vein to that discussed above for models of the Kv11.1/drug interaction, there are several models of the ventricular cardiac action potential that have been proposed in the literature including the ten Tusscher 2006 (TT06) (Ten Tusscher and Panfilov, 2006), Grandi-Bers 2010 (GB10) (Grandi et al., 2010), and O'hara Rudy 2011 (ORD11) models (O'Hara et al., 2011). Population based studies using these cell models have allowed interrogation of how the variation in repolarization reserve that occurs as a result of differential expression of ion channels between individuals can influence predicted drug effects as well as develop our understanding of multichannel pharmacology (Sobie, 2009; Lancaster and Sobie, 2016). However, each of the models is considerably different in relation to the conductance levels of

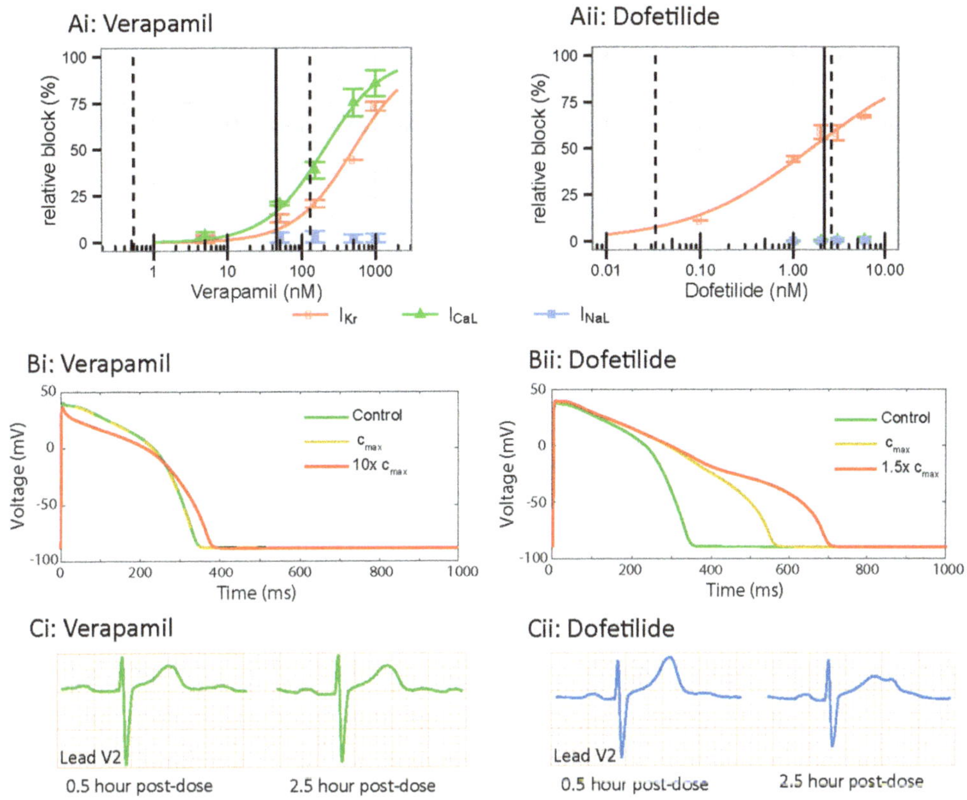

FIGURE 5 | *In vitro, in silico* and *in vivo* comparison of multi-channel pharmacology. **(A)** *In vitro* drug block of Kv11.1 (I_{Kr}-red), Cav1.2 (I_{CaL}-green) and Nav1.5-Late (I_{NaL}-blue) for (i) verapamil and (ii) dofetilide. Adapted from Vicente et al. (2015). **(B)** *In silico* cardiac action potential prolongation and morphology based on *in vitro* data from Vicente et al. (2015), simulated using the O'Hara Rudy ventricular action potential. Control is shown in green, C_{max} dose in yellow and super-C_{max} dose in red. Verapamil demonstrates less action potential prolongation and triangulation compared to Dofetilide. **(C)** *In vivo* ECG data demonstrating lead V2 in a patient at 0.5 and 2.5 h post injection of 120 mg verapamil or 500 ug dofetilide. Verapamil demonstrates no change in prolongation or T-wave morphology while Dofetilide shows marked changes in prolongation and T-wave notching between the 2 time points. Reproduced from Vicente et al. (2015).

individual cardiac ion channels. As a result, predictions around APD prolongation and emergence of proarrhythmic markers that each of the models make in response to drug block are significantly different (Mirams et al., 2014) and do not reproduce *in vivo* data (Britton et al., 2017). For example, Mann et al showed that 50% inhibition of Kv11.1 caused 113, 22, and 34 ms prolongation of APD_{90} for ORD11, TT06 and GB10 respectively (Mann et al., 2016). This issue is being considered by the field and recent efforts have focused on refining cell models by rescaling their ionic conductances using either patient data from subjects with various subtypes of the long QT syndrome (Mann et al., 2016) or published drug data (Britton et al., 2013; Dutta et al., 2016). Even so, significant disparity still exists between the "optimized" versions of the cell models, meaning the differences in predicted risk that result from using different models are likely to outweigh, or at least match, the differences associated with descriptions of the drug/channel interaction. It may also prove to be true that similar mechanistic descriptors that are becoming routine for drug binding to Kv11.1, such as kinetics and state dependence, also need to be incorporated for other cardiac ion channels for optimum risk prediction. However, the benefit of this relative to the cost of acquiring the data may preclude such an approach. What is clear, is that each of these facets of *in silico* risk prediction—the Markov descriptions of drug/channel interaction *as well as* the model of the ventricular cell in which they are incorporated, should each be considered as a priority for the field.

CONCLUSION

Understanding the intricacies of the Kv11.1/drug interaction and optimizing our approaches to measuring and modeling these characteristics is critical to developing better preclinical *in silico* risk prediction. In doing this it is important to remember that all models are simplifications. Therefore, the challenge is to determine how much information needs to be included to make them useful rather than how much information is needed to make them accurate for every drug scenario, which would potentially necessitate the collection of very large amounts of data that may be redundant for many drugs. Given the potential significance of factors, such as drug binding kinetics, temperature dependence, state dependence and multichannel pharmacology discussed above, it seems clear that these factors need to be included at some level in models of drug binding. The major challenge faced by the field in the short term is determining what level of detail is necessary, and balancing this against the practicalities of data acquisition in high throughout screens.

AUTHOR CONTRIBUTIONS

WL, MW, JV, and AH all contributed to planning, writing and editing of the manuscript and figures contained herein.

FUNDING

WL is supported by a National Heart Foundation of Australia Health Professional Scholarship (101552). AH is supported by an Australian National Health and Medical Research Council project grant (1088214). JV is supported by an Australian National Health and Medical Research Council Fellowship (1019693).

ACKNOWLEDGMENTS

Special thanks to Dr. Melissa Mangala and Dr. Matthew Perry for intellectual input in the editing of this manuscript; and to Dr. Jose Vicente and Dr. Zhihua Li for providing data for figures.

REFERENCES

Aiba, T., Shimizu, W., Inagaki, M., Noda, T., Miyoshi, S., Ding, W. G., et al. (2005). Cellular and ionic mechanism for drug-induced long QT syndrome and effectiveness of verapamil. *J. Am. Coll. Cardiol.* 45, 300–307. doi: 10.1016/j.jacc.2004.09.069

Alexandrou, A. J., Duncan, R. S., Sullivan, A., Hancox, J. C., Leishman, D. J., Witchel, H. J., et al. (2006). Mechanism of hERG K^+ channel blockade by the fluoroquinolone antibiotic moxifloxacin. *Br. J. Pharmacol.* 147, 905–916. doi: 10.1038/sj.bjp.0706678

Ballou, L. M., Lin, R. Z., and Cohen, I. S. (2015). Control of cardiac repolarization by phosphoinositide 3-kinase signaling to ion channels *Circ. Res.* 116, 127–137. doi: 10.1161/CIRCRESAHA.116.303975

Bányász, T., Horváth, B., Virág, L., Bárándi, L., Szentandrássy, N., Harmati, G., et al. (2009). Reverse rate dependency is an intrinsic property of canine cardiac preparations. *Cardiovasc. Res.* 84, 237–244. doi: 10.1093/cvr/cvp213

Beattie, K. A., Hill, A. P., Bardenet, R., Cui, Y., Vandenberg, J. I., Gavaghan, D . J., et al. (2017). Sinusoidal voltage protocols for rapid characterization of ion channel kinetics. *bioRxiv.* doi: 10.1101/100677

Bosch, R. F., Schneck, A. C., Kiehn, J., Zhang, W., Hambrock, A., Eigenberger, B. W., et al. (2002). beta3-adrenergic regulation of an ion channel in the heart-inhibition of the slow delayed rectifier potassium current I(Ks) in guinea pig ventricular myocytes. *Cardiovasc. Res.* 56, 393–403. doi: 10.1016/S0008-6363(02)00601-6

Bril, A., Gout, B., Bonhomme, M., Landais, L., Faivre, J. F., Linee, P., et al. (1996). Combined potassium and calcium channel blocking activities as a basis for antiarrhythmic efficacy with low proarrhythmic risk: experimental profile of BRL-32872. *J. Pharmacol. Exp. Ther.* 276, 637–646.

Britton, O. J., Abi-Gerges, N., Page, G., Ghetti, A., Miller, P. E., and Rodriguez, B. (2017). Quantitative comparison of effects of dofetilide, sotalol, quinidine, and verapamil between human *ex vivo* trabeculae and *in silico* ventricular models incorporating inter-individual action potential variability. *Front. Physiol.* 8:597. doi: 10.3389/fphys.2017.00597

Britton, O. J., Bueno-Orovio, A., Van Ammel, K., Lu, H. R., Towart, R., Gallacher, D. J., et al. (2013). Experimentally calibrated population of models predicts and explains intersubject variability in cardiac cellular electrophysiology. *Proc. Natl. Acad. Sci. U.S.A.* 110, E2098–E2105. doi: 10.1073/pnas.1304382110

Carmeliet, E. (1992). Voltage- and time-dependent block of the delayed K^+ current in cardiac myocytes by dofetilide. *J. Pharmacol. Exp. Ther.* 262, 809–817.

Cavero, I., Mestre, M., Guillon, J. M., and Crumb, W. (2000). Drugs that prolong QT interval as an unwanted effect: assessing their likelihood of induction hazardous cardiac dysrhythmias. *Expert Opin. Pharmacother.* 1, 947–973. doi: 10.1517/14656566.1.5.947

Chen, J., Seebohm, G., and Sanguinetti, M. C. (2002). Position of aromatic residues in the S6 domain, not inactivation, dictates cisapride sensitivity of HERG and eag potassium channels. *Proc. Natl. Acad. Sci. U.S.A.* 99, 12461–12466. doi: 10.1073/pnas.192367299

Crumb, W. J. Jr., Vicente, J., Johannesen, L., and Strauss, D. G. (2016). An evaluation of 30 clinical drugs against the comprehensive *in vitro* proarrhythmia assay (CiPA) proposed ion channel panel. *J. Pharmacol. Toxicol. Methods* 81, 251–262. doi: 10.1016/j.vascn.2016.03.009

Dennis, A., Wang, L., Wan, X., and Ficker, E. (2007). hERG channel trafficking: novel targets in drug-induced long QT syndrome. *Biochem. Soc. Trans.* 35, 1060–1063. doi: 10.1042/BST0351060

Di Veroli, G. Y., Davies, M. R., Zhang, H., Abi-Gerges, N., and Boyett, M. R. (2013). High-throughput screening of drug-binding dynamics to HERG improves early drug safety assessment. *Am. J. Physiol. Heart Circ. Physiol.* 304, H104–H117. doi: 10.1152/ajpheart.00511.2012

Di Veroli, G., Davies, M. R., Zhang, H., Abi-Gerges, N., and Boyett, M. R. (2014). hERG inhibitors with similar potency but different binding kinetics do not pose the same proarrhythmic risk: implications for drug safety assessment. *J. Cardiovasc. Electrophysiol.* 25, 197–207. doi: 10.1111/jce.12289

Du, C., Zhang, Y., El Harchi, A., Dempsey, C. E., and Hancox, J. C. (2014). Ranolazine inhibition of hERG potassium channels: drug-pore interactions and reduced potency against inactivation mutants. *J. Mol. Cell Cardiol.* 74, 220–230. doi: 10.1016/j.yjmcc.2014.05.013

Durdagi, S., Deshpande, S., Duff, H. J., and Noskov, S. Y. (2012). Modeling of open, closed, and open-inactivated states of the hERG1 channel: structural mechanisms of the state-dependent drug binding. *J. Chem. Inf. Model.* 52, 2760–2774. doi: 10.1021/ci300353u

Dutta, S., Chang, K. C., Beattie, K. A., Sheng, J., Tran, P. N., Wu, W. W., et al. (2017). Optimization of an *in silico* cardiac cell model for proarrhythmia risk assessment. *Front. Physiol.* 8:616. doi: 10.3389/fphys.2017.00616

Dutta, S., Chang, K. C., Beattie, K. A., Sheng, J., Tran, P. N. and Wu, W. W. (2016). Optimization of an *in silico* cardiac cell model for proarrhythmia risk assessment. *Comput. Cardiol.* 43. doi: 10.22489/CinC.2016.253-483

E14, I. (2005). *Note for Guidance on the Clinical Evaluation of QT/QTc Interval Prolongation and Proarrhythmic Potential for Non-Antiarrhythmic Drugs.* International Council for Harmonisation.

Ellinwood, N., Dobrev, D., Morotti, S., and Grandi, E. (2017). Revealing kinetics and state-dependent binding properties of I_{Kur}-targeting drugs that maximize atrial fibrillation selectivity. *Chaos* 27:093918. doi: 10.1063/1.5000226

Fermini, B., Hancox, J. C., Abi-Gerges, N., Bridgland-Taylor, M., Chaudhary, K. W., Colatsky, T., et al. (2016). A new perspective in the field of cardiac safety testing through the comprehensive *in vitro* proarrhythmia assay paradigm. *J. Biomol. Screen.* 21, 1–11. doi: 10.1177/1087057115594589

Ficker, E., Jarolimek, W., Kiehn, J., Baumann, A., and Brown, A. M. (1998). Molecular determinants of dofetilide block of HERG K^+ channels. *Circ. Res.* 82, 386–395. doi: 10.1161/01.RES.82.3.386

Grandi, E., Pasqualini, F. S., and Bers, D. M. (2010). A novel computational model of the human ventricular action potential and Ca transient. *J. Mol. Cell. Cardiol.* 48, 112–121. doi: 10.1016/j.yjmcc.2009.09.019

Guo, J., Zhan, S., Lees-Miller, J. P., Teng, G., and Duff, H. J. (2005). Exaggerated block of hERG (KCNH2) and prolongation of action potential duration by erythromycin at temperatures between 37 degrees C and 42 degrees C. *Heart Rhythm* 2, 860–866. doi: 10.1016/j.hrthm.2005.04.029

Hill, A. P., Perrin, M. J., Heide, J., Campbell, T. J., Mann, S. A., and Vandenberg, J. I. (2014). Kinetics of drug interaction with the Kv11.1 potassium channel. *Mol. Pharmacol.* 85, 769–776. doi: 10.1124/mol.114.091835

Hill, A. P., Sunde, M., Campbell, T. J., and Vandenberg, J. I. (2007). Mechanism of block of the hERG K^+ channel by the scorpion toxin CnErg1. *Biophys. J.* 92, 3915–3929. doi: 10.1529/biophysj.106.101956

Hondeghem, L. M., Carlsson, L., and Duker, G. (2001a). Instability and triangulation of the action potential predict serious proarrhythmia, but action potential duration prolongation is antiarrhythmic. *Circulation* 103, 2004–2013. doi: 10.1161/01.CIR.103.15.2004

Hondeghem, L. M., Dujardin, K., and De Clerck, F. (2001b). Phase 2 prolongation, in the absence of instability and triangulation, antagonizes class III proarrhythmia. *Cardiovasc. Res.* 50, 345–353. doi: 10.1016/S0008-6363(01)00259-0

Jia, S., Lian, J., Guo, D., Xue, X., Patel, C., Yang, L., et al. (2011). Modulation of the late sodium current by ATX-II and ranolazine affects the reverse use-dependence and proarrhythmic liability of IKr blockade. *Br. J. Pharmacol.* 164, 308–316. doi: 10.1111/j.1476-5381.2010.01181.x

Kamiya, K., Mitcheson, J. S., Yasui, K., Kodama, I., and Sanguinetti, M. C. (2001). Open channel block of HERG K^+ channels by vesnarinone. *Mol. Pharmacol.* 60, 244–253. doi: 10.1124/mol.60.2.244

Kiehn, J., Lacerda, A. E., Wible, B., and Brown, A. M. (1996). Molecular physiology and pharmacology of HERG. single-channel currents and block by dofetilide. *Circulation* 94, 2572–2579. doi: 10.1161/01.CIR.94.10.2572

Kirsch, G. E., Trepakova, E. S., Brimecombe, J. C., Sidach, S. S., Erickson, H. D., Kochan, M. C., et al. (2004). Variability in the measurement of hERG potassium channel inhibition: effects of temperature and stimulus pattern. *J. Pharmacol. Toxicol. Methods* 50, 93–101. doi: 10.1016/j.vascn.2004.06.003

Lancaster, M. C., and Sobie, E. A. (2016). Improved prediction of drug-induced torsades de pointes through simulations of dynamics and machine learning algorithms. *Clin. Pharmacol. Ther.* 100, 371–379. doi: 10.1002/cpt.367

Lee, W., Mann, S. A., Windley, M. J., Imtiaz, M. S., Vandenberg, J. I., and Hill, A. P. (2016). In silico assessment of kinetics and state dependent binding properties of drugs causing acquired LQTS. *Prog. Biophys. Mol. Biol.* 120, 89–99. doi: 10.1016/j.pbiomolbio.2015.12.005

Li, Z., Dutta, S., Sheng, J., Tran, P. N., Wu, W., Chang, K., et al. (2017). Improving the *in silico* assessment of proarrhythmia risk by combining hERG (Human Ether-a-go-go-Related Gene) channel-drug binding kinetics and multichannel pharmacology. *Circ. Arrhythm. Electrophysiol.* 10:e004628. doi: 10.1161/CIRCEP.116.004628

Mann, S. A., Imtiaz, M., Winbo, A., Rydberg, A., Perry, M. D., Couderc, J. P., et al. (2016). Convergence of models of human ventricular myocyte electrophysiology after global optimization to recapitulate clinical long QT phenotypes. *J. Mol. Cell. Cardiol.* 100, 25–34. doi: 10.1016/j.yjmcc.2016.09.011

Martin, R. L., Su, Z., Limberis, J. T., Palmatier, J. D., Cowart, M. D., Cox, B. F., et al. (2006). *In vitro* preclinical cardiac assessment of tolterodine and terodiline: multiple factors predict the clinical experience. *J. Cardiovasc. Pharmacol.* 48, 199–206. doi: 10.1097/01.fjc.0000246853.15926.d4

Milberg, P., Ramtin, S., Mönnig, G., Osada, N., Wasmer, K., Breithardt, G., et al. (2004). Comparison of the *in vitro* electrophysiologic and proarrhythmic effects of amiodarone and sotalol in a rabbit model of acute atrioventricular block. *J. Cardiovasc. Pharmacol.* 44, 278–286. doi: 10.1097/01.fjc.0000129581.81508.78

Milnes, J. T., Witchel, H. J., Leaney, J. L., Leishman, D. J., and Hancox, J. C. (2010). Investigating dynamic protocol-dependence of hERG potassium channel inhibition at 37 degrees C: cisapride vs dofetilide. *J. Pharmacol. Toxicol. Methods* 61, 178–191. doi: 10.1016/j.vascn.2010.02.007

Mirams, G. R., Davies, M. R., Brough, S. J., Bridgland-Taylor, M. H., Cui, Y., Gavaghan, D. J., et al. (2014). Prediction of thorough QT study results using action potential simulations based on ion channel screens. *J. Pharmacol. Toxicol. Methods* 70, 246–254. doi: 10.1016/j.vascn.2014.07.002

Mitcheson, J. S., Chen, J., Lin, M., Culberson, C., and Sanguinetti, M. C. (2000a). A structural basis for drug-induced long QT syndrome. *Proc. Natl. Acad. Sci. U.S.A.* 97, 12329–12333. doi: 10.1073/pnas.210244497

Mitcheson, J. S., Chen, J., and Sanguinetti, M. C. (2000b). Trapping of a methanesulfonanilide by closure of the HERG potassium channel activation gate. *J. Gen. Physiol.* 115, 229–240. doi: 10.1085/jgp.115.3.229

Moreno, J. D., Zhu, Z. I., Yang, P.-C., Bankston, J. R., Jeng, M.-T., Kang, C., et al. (2011). A Computational model to predict the effects of class I anti-arrhythmic drugs on ventricular rhythms. *Sci. Trans. Med.* 3, 98ra83–98ra83. doi: 10.1126/scitranslmed.3002588

Numaguchi, H., Mullins, F. M., Johnson, J. P. Jr., Johns, D. C., Po, S. S., Yang, I. C., et al. (2000). Probing the interaction between inactivation gating and Dd-sotalol block of HERG. *Circ. Res.* 87, 1012–1018. doi: 10.1161/01.RES.87.11.1012

O'Hara, T., Virág, L., Varró, A., and Rudy, Y. (2011). Simulation of the undiseased human cardiac ventricular action potential: model formulation and experimental validation. *PLoS Comput. Biol.* 7:e1002061. doi: 10.1371/journal.pcbi.1002061

Osadchii, O. E. (2012). Dofetilide promotes repolarization abnormalities in perfused Guinea-pig heart. *Cardiovasc. Drugs Ther.* 26, 489–500. doi: 10.1007/s10557-012-6405-1

Park, J. B., Choe, H., Lee, Y. K., Ha, K. C., Rhee, K. S., Ko, J. K., et al. (2002). Open channel block by KCB-328 [1-(2-amino-4-methanesulfonamidophenoxy)-2-[N-(3,4-dimethoxyphenethyl)-N-methylam ino]ethane hydrochloride] of the heterologously expressed human ether-a-go-go-related gene K^+ channels. *J. Pharmacol. Exp. Ther.* 302, 314–319. doi: 10.1124/jpet.302.1.314

Perrin, M. J., Kuchel, P. W., Campbell, T. J., and Vandenberg, J. I. (2008a). Drug binding to the inactivated state is necessary but not sufficient for high-affinity binding to human ether-a-go-go-related gene channels. *Mol. Pharmacol.* 74, 1443–1452. doi: 10.1124/mol.108.049056

Perrin, M. J., Subbiah, R. N., Vandenberg, J. I., and Hill, A. P. (2008b). Human ether-a-go-go related gene (hERG) K^+ channels: function and dysfunction. *Prog. Biophys. Mol. Biol.* 98, 137–148. doi: 10.1016/j.pbiomolbio.2008.10.006

Perry, M., de Groot, M. J., Helliwell, R., Leishman, D., Tristani-Firouzi, M., Sanguinetti, M. C., et al. (2004). Structural determinants of HERG channel block by clofilium and ibutilide. *Mol. Pharmacol.* 66, 240–249. doi: 10.1124/mol.104.000117

Potet, F., Bouyssou, T., Escande, D., and Baró, I. (2001). Gastrointestinal prokinetic drugs have different affinity for the human cardiac human ether-a-gogo K^+ channel. *J. Pharmacol. Exp. Ther.* 299, 1007–1012.

Redfern, W. S., Carlsson, L., Davis, A. S., Lynch, W. G., MacKenzie, I., Palethorpe, S., et al. (2003). Relationships between preclinical cardiac electrophysiology, clinical QT interval prolongation and torsade de pointes for a broad range of drugs: evidence for a provisional safety margin in drug development. *Cardiovasc. Res.* 58, 32–45. doi: 10.1016/S0008-6363(02)00846-5

Rezazadeh, S., Hesketh, J. C., and Fedida, D. (2004). Rb+ flux through hERG channels affects the potency of channel blocking drugs: correlation with data obtained using a high-throughput Rb+ efflux assay. *J. Biomol. Screen.* 9, 588–597. doi: 10.1177/1087057104264798

Roden, D. M. (1998). Taking the "idio" out of "idiosyncratic": predicting torsades de pointes. *Pacing Clin. Electrophysiol.* 21, 1029–1034. doi: 10.1111/j.1540-8159.1998.tb00148.x

Romero, L., Trenor, B., Yang, P. C., Saiz, J., and Clancy, C. E. (2014). In silico screening of the impact of hERG channel kinetic abnormalities on channel block and susceptibility to acquired long QT syndrome. *J. Mol. Cell. Cardiol.* 72, 126–137. doi: 10.1016/j.yjmcc.2014.02.018

S7B, I. (2005). *Note for Guidance on the Nonclinical Evaluation of the Potential for Delayed Ventricular Repolarization (QT Interval Prolongation) by Human Pharmaceuticals).* International Council for Harmonisation.

Sager, P. T., Gintant, G., Turner, J. R., Pettit, S., and Stockbridge, N. (2014). Rechanneling the cardiac proarrhythmia safety paradigm: a meeting report from the cardiac safety research consortium. *Am. Heart J.* 167, 292–300. doi: 10.1016/j.ahj.2013.11.004

Saiz, J., Gomis-Tena, J., Monserrat, M., Ferrero, J. M. Jr., Cardona, K., and Chorro, J. (2011). Effects of the antiarrhythmic drug dofetilide on transmural dispersion of repolarization in ventriculum. a computer modeling study. *IEEE Trans. Biomed. Eng.* 58, 43–53. doi: 10.1109/TBME.2010.2077292

Sanguinetti, M. C., Jurkiewicz, N. K., Scott, A., and Siegl, P. K. (1991). Isoproterenol antagonizes prolongation of refractory period by the class III antiarrhythmic agent E-4031 in guinea pig myocytes. mechanism of action. *Circ. Res.* 68, 77–84. doi: 10.1161/01.RES.68.1.77

Saxena, P., Zangerl-Plessl, E. M., Linder, T., Windisch, A., Hohaus, A., Timin, E., et al. (2016). New potential binding determinant for hERG channel inhibitors. *Sci. Rep.* 6:24182. doi: 10.1038/srep24182

Sobie, E. A. (2009). Parameter sensitivity analysis in electrophysiological models using multivariable regression. *Biophys. J.* 96, 1264–1274. doi: 10.1016/j.bpj.2008.10.056

Stork, D., Timin, E. N., Berjukow, S., Huber, C., Hohaus, A., Auer, M., et al. (2007). State dependent dissociation of HERG channel inhibitors. *Br. J. Pharmacol.* 151, 1368–1376. doi: 10.1038/sj.bjp.0707356

Su, Z., Martin, R., Cox, B. F., and Gintant, G. (2004). Mesoridazine: an open-channel blocker of human ether-a-go-go-related gene K^+ channel. *J. Mol. Cell. Cardiol.* 36, 151–160. doi: 10.1016/j.yjmcc.2003.10.017

Suessbrich, H., Schönherr, R., Heinemann, S. H., Lang, F., and Busch, A. E. (1997). Specific block of cloned Herg channels by clofilium and its tertiary analog LY97241. *FEBS Lett.* 414, 435–438. doi: 10.1016/S0014-5793(97)01030-2

Ten Tusscher, K. H., and Panfilov, A. V. (2006). Cell model for efficient simulation of wave propagation in human ventricular tissue under normal and pathological conditions. *Phys. Med. Biol.* 51, 6141–6156. doi: 10.1088/0031-9155/51/23/014

Vandenberg, J. I., Perry, M. D., Perrin, M. J., Mann, S. A., Ke, Y., and Hill, A. P. (2012). hERG K^+ channels: structure, function, and clinical significance. *Physiol. Rev.* 92, 1393–1478. doi: 10.1152/physrev.00036.2011

Vandenberg, J. I., Varghese, A., Lu, Y., Bursill, J. A., Mahaut-Smith, M. P., and Huang, C. L. (2006). Temperature dependence of human ether-a-go-go-related gene K+ currents. *Am. J. Physiol. Cell Physiol.* 291, C165–175. doi: 10.1152/ajpcell.00596.2005

Vicente, J., Johannesen, L., Mason, J. W., Crumb, W. J., Pueyo, E., Stockbridge, N., et al. (2015). Comprehensive T wave morphology assessment in a randomized clinical study of dofetilide, quinidine, ranolazine, and verapamil. *J. Am. Heart Assoc.* 4:e001615. doi: 10.1161/JAHA.114.001615

Walker, B. D., Singleton, C. B., Bursill, J. A., Wyse, K. R., Valenzuela, S. M., Qiu, M. R., et al. (1999). Inhibition of the human ether-a-go-go-related gene (HERG) potassium channel by cisapride: affinity for open and inactivated states. *Br. J. Pharmacol.* 128, 444–450. doi: 10.1038/sj.bjp.0702774

Wang, S., Liu, S., Morales, M. J., Strauss, H. C., and Rasmusson, R. L. (1997). A quantitative analysis of the activation and inactivation kinetics of HERG expressed in Xenopus oocytes. *J. Physiol.* 502, 45–60. doi: 10.1111/j.1469-7793.1997.045bl.x

Wang, W., and MacKinnon, R. (2017). Cryo-EM Structure of the open human ether-a-go-go-related K^+ channel hERG. *Cell* 169, 422.e10–430.e10. doi: 10.1016/j.cell.2017.03.048

Wang, Y., Guo, J., Perissinotti, L. L., Lees-Miller, J., Teng, G., Durdagi, S., et al. (2016). Role of the pH in state-dependent blockade of hERG Currents. *Sci. Rep.* 6:32536. doi: 10.1038/srep32536

Windley, M. J., Abi-Gerges, N., Fermini, B., Hancox, J. C., Vandenberg, J. I., and Hill, A. P. (2017). Measuring kinetics and potency of hERG block for CiPA. *J. Pharmacol. Toxicol. Methods* 87, 99–107. doi: 10.1016/j.vascn.2017.02.017

Windley, M. J., Mann, S. A., Vandenberg, J. I., and Hill, A. P. (2016). Temperature effects on kinetics of KV11.1 drug block have important consequences for *in silico* proarrhythmic risk prediction. *Mol. Pharmacol.* 90, 1–11. doi: 10.1124/mol.115.103127

Wu, L., Guo, D., Li, H., Hackett, J., Yan, G. X., Jiao, Z., et al. (2008). Role of late sodium current in modulating the proarrhythmic and antiarrhythmic effects of quinidine. *Heart Rhythm* 5, 1726–1734. doi: 10.1016/j.hrthm.2008.09.008

Wu, W., Gardner, A., and Sanguinetti, M. C. (2015). The Link between inactivation and high-affinity block of hERG1 channels. *Mol. Pharmacol.* 87, 1042–1050. doi: 10.1124/mol.115.098111

Yang, P. C., El-Bizri, N., Romero, L., Giles, W. R., Rajamani, S., Belardinelli, L., et al. (2016). A computational model predicts adjunctive pharmacotherapy for cardiac safety via selective inhibition of the late cardiac Na current. *J. Mol. Cell. Cardiol.* 99, 151–161. doi: 10.1016/j.yjmcc.2016.08.011

Yang, T., Snyders, D. J., and Roden, D. M. (1995). Ibutilide, a methanesulfonanilide antiarrhythmic, is a potent blocker of the rapidly activating delayed rectifier K^+ current (IKr) in AT-1 cells. concentration-, time-, voltage-, and use-dependent effects. *Circulation* 91, 1799–1806. doi: 10.1161/01.CIR.91.6.1799

Yao, J. A., Du, X., Lu, D., Baker, R. L., Daharsh, E., and Atterson, P. (2005). Estimation of potency of HERG channel blockers: impact of voltage protocol and temperature. *J. Pharmacol. Toxicol. Methods* 5, 146–153. doi: 10.1016/j.vascn.2005.04.008

12

Simultaneous Quantification of Spatially Discordant Alternans in Voltage and Intracellular Calcium in Langendorff-Perfused Rabbit Hearts and Inconsistencies with Models of Cardiac Action Potentials and Ca Transients

Ilija Uzelac[1†], Yanyan C. Ji[1†], Daniel Hornung[2], Johannes Schröder-Scheteling[2], Stefan Luther[2], Richard A. Gray[3], Elizabeth M. Cherry[4] and Flavio H. Fenton[1]*

[1] School of Physics, Georgia Institute of Technology, Atlanta, GA, United States, [2] Max Planck Institute for Dynamics and Self-Organization, Gottingen, Germany, [3] Center for Device and Radiological Health, Food and Drug Administration, Silver Spring, MD, United States, [4] School of Mathematical Sciences, Rochester Institute of Technology, Rochester, NY, United States

***Correspondence:**
Flavio H. Fenton
flavio.fenton@physics.gatech.edu

† These authors have contributed equally to this work.

Rationale: Discordant alternans, a phenomenon in which the action potential duration (APDs) and/or intracellular calcium transient durations (CaDs) in different spatial regions of cardiac tissue are out of phase, present a dynamical instability for complex spatial dispersion that can be associated with long-QT syndrome (LQTS) and the initiation of reentrant arrhythmias. Because the use of numerical simulations to investigate arrhythmic effects, such as acquired LQTS by drugs is beginning to be studied by the FDA, it is crucial to validate mathematical models that may be used during this process.

Objective: In this study, we characterized with high spatio-temporal resolution the development of discordant alternans patterns in transmembrane voltage (V_m) and intracellular calcium concentration ($[Ca_i]^{+2}$) as a function of pacing period in rabbit hearts. Then we compared the dynamics to that of the latest state-of-the-art model for ventricular action potentials and calcium transients to better understand the underlying mechanisms of discordant alternans and compared the experimental data to the mathematical models representing V_m and $[Ca_i]^{+2}$ dynamics.

Methods and Results: We performed simultaneous dual optical mapping imaging of V_m and $[Ca_i]^{+2}$ in Langendorff-perfused rabbit hearts with higher spatial resolutions compared with previous studies. The rabbit hearts developed discordant alternans through decreased pacing period protocols and we quantified the presence of multiple nodal points along the direction of wave propagation, both in APD and CaD, and compared these findings with results from theoretical models. In experiments, the nodal lines of CaD alternans have a steeper slope than those of APD alternans, but not as steep as predicted by numerical simulations in rabbit models. We further quantified several additional discrepancies between models and experiments.

Conclusions: Alternans in CaD have nodal lines that are about an order of magnitude steeper compared to those of APD alternans. Current action potential models lack the necessary coupling between voltage and calcium compared to experiments and fail to reproduce some key dynamics such as, voltage amplitude alternans, smooth development of calcium alternans in time, conduction velocity and the steepness of the nodal lines of APD and CaD.

Keywords: discordant alternans, calcium dynamics, voltage-calcium coupling, arrhythmia, optical mapping, long QT syndrome, cardiac cell modeling

INTRODUCTION

Long-QT syndrome (LQTS), characterized by abnormal prolongation of the QT interval (Schwartz et al., 1993), is a result of delayed repolarizations in the heart and can increase the risk of life-threatening arrhythmias, with a mortality rate of 20% within the first year after first detection and up to 50% in the next 10 years for untreated patients (Schwartz, 1985). The known dangers of LQTS have resulted in guidelines by the FDA concerning the design and testing of *any* new drug and in the interpretation and analysis of these drugs in clinical trials (Food and Drug Administration, 2005). In addition, many currently available medications can be very dangerous to some patients with heart problems, as they are known to further prolong QT intervals as shown in the compendium maintained by the Sudden Arrhythmia Death Syndromes Foundation (sads.org). LQTS is usually accompanied by T-wave alternans (Zareba et al., 1994) where the duration of the T wave can vary from one beat to the next (Jayakrishnan and Krishnakumar, 2006). This long-short alternation in duration and in some cases amplitude has been shown to arise from a period-doubling bifurcation (Nolasco and Dahlen, 1968; Guevara et al., 1984) originating at the cellular level (Pastore et al., 1999). In space, alternans can lead to complex spatiotemporal patterns along the epicardium and endocardium (Gizzi et al., 2013) and eventually to conduction block and fibrillation (Fenton et al., 2002; Choi et al., 2007).

During fast pacing, alternate patterns of action potential duration (APD) in space can be classified as concordant alternans (CA), in which all the tissue responds with a long APD on one beat and with a short APD on the following beat with the sequence repeating, or discordant alternans (DA), in which one section of tissue responds with a long APD and another with a short APD on the same beat followed by the reverse on the next beat. During DA, the regions of long and short APDs that alternate out-of-phase are separated by nodes, which are regions where the APDs have the same values for successive beats and hence do not alternate (Qu et al., 2000; Watanabe et al., 2001).

To date, two main mechanisms for the development of discordant alternans have been proposed, one driven by voltage and another by calcium (Saitoh et al., 1988, 1989). The first mechanism identified (Nolasco and Dahlen, 1968) was purely voltage-driven (Guevara et al., 1984); in space it is coupled through the dynamical interaction between the APD restitution curve and the conduction velocity (CV) restitution curve. When tissue is paced rapidly, diastolic intervals are shorter, causing slower CV near the stimulating site while CV increases downstream along wavefront propagation, causing a large spatial dispersion in the APD that can lead to DA (Qu et al., 2000; Watanabe et al., 2001).

The other mechanism, calcium-driven, is considered more complex, with DA caused by instabilities in $[Ca_i]^{+2}$ cycling that in turn impacts APD through $[Ca_i]^{+2}$–V_m coupling (Chudin et al., 1999; Sato et al., 2006). $[Ca_i]^{+2}$–V_m coupling depends on a dynamical balance between the influx through the L-type calcium current (I_{CaL}) and extrusion through the Na-Ca exchanger current (I_{NCX}) (Weiss et al., 2006). If the effect of I_{NCX} dominates, positive $[Ca_i]^{+2}$–V_m coupling will occur, where a large $[Ca_i]^{+2}$ causes prolonged APD by an enhanced calcium extrusion through I_{NCX}. Otherwise, when a large Ca transient reduces I_{CaL} through increased calcium-dependent inactivation, APD will be shortened (Edwards and Blatter, 2014). Ca instability is another multifactorial process. The key components are the fractional Ca release from the sarcoplasmic reticulum (SR), which refers to the relation between the Ca released from the SR and the SR calcium load, and the cytosolic Ca sequestration, which refers to the efficiency of Ca removal from the cytosol through the reuptake to the SR and the extrusion through the Na-Ca exchanger (Weiss et al., 2011). In general, factors increasing fractional Ca release promote Ca alternans and factors increasing Ca sequestration reduce alternans (Edwards and Blatter, 2014). Many studies have attributed cardiac alternans to disturbances of $[Ca_i]^{+2}$ signaling, with APD alternans considered a secondary consequence (Eisner et al., 2006; Clusin, 2008; Laurita and Rosenbaum, 2008; Myles et al., 2008; Kanaporis and Blatter, 2015).

Alternans was observed in cardiac tissue as early as 1872 (Traube, 1872), and some of the earliest mathematical models of cardiac action potentials were able to produce such phenomena (Noble, 1962; Beeler and Reuter, 1977). However, later generations of models often failed to produce alternans (DiFrancesco and Noble, 1985; Luo and Rudy, 1991, 1994; Faber and Rudy, 2000), with more detailed species-specific models for rabbit (Puglisi and Bers, 2001; Shannon et al., 2004), dog (Winslow et al., 1999) and human (Priebe and Beuckelmann, 1998; Iyer et al., 2004; ten Tusscher et al., 2004) ventricular action potentials among them. In time, other models have been specifically designed to account for alternans (Fox et al., 2002; Mahajan et al., 2008; O'Hara et al., 2011; Sato et al., 2013).

Recently the FDA's sponsored Cardiac Safety Research Consortium (Sager et al., 2014) proposed a new initiative, the Comprehensive *in-Vitro* Pro-arrhythmia Assay (CiPA), which specifies the use of mathematical models of cardiac action potentials in the aid of pro-arrhythmic drug risk assessments. Many recently developed ionic models are complex single-cell models with a large number of variables. There exists a large variability in dynamics between them as well as failures to reproduce key physiological features when they are tested in tissue (alternans, reentrant wave dynamics, dominant frequencies, etc.). The known differences between many cell and tissue models make it imperative to validate and verify models with experiments.

Toward this end, in this study, we performed dual optical-mapping recordings with high spatial and temporal resolution for $[Ca_i]^{+2}$–V_m during discordant alternans in Langendorff-perfused rabbit hearts to better quantify the alternans mechanism as it relates to LQTS. We then used the data for validation and verification of the Sato et al. voltage-calcium rabbit cell model (Sato et al., 2013).

MATERIALS AND METHODS

Heart Preparation

All experiments conform to the current Guide for Care and Use of Laboratory Animals published by the National Institutes of Health (NIH Publication No. 85–23, revised 1996), and approved by the Office of Research and Integrity Assurance at Georgia Tech. New Zealand white rabbits (2–3 kg, $n = 8$) were anesthetized with ketamine/xylazine/ace-promazine (17/9/0.9 mg/kg) and then injected with heparin (300 U/Kg). After 5 min, euthanasia was induced with 120 mg/kg pentobarbital. Hearts were then quickly removed via a left thoracotomy and perfused retrogradely via the aorta with cardioplegic solution (NaCl: 6.43 g/L, KCl: 1.19 g/L, $NaHCO_3$: 0.84 g/L, $MgCl{\cdot}6H_2O$: 3.25 g/L, $CaCl_2$: 0.13 g/L), gassed with 95% O_2 and 5% CO_2. Then the hearts were immersed in a chamber kept at $37.0 \pm 0.3°C$ and perfused with Tyrode's solution (NaCl: 7.24 g/L, KCl: 0.30 g/L, $NaHCO_3$: 2.02 g/L, $NaH_2PO_4{\cdot}H_2O$: 0.12 g/L, $MgCl{\cdot}6H_2O$: 0.14 g/L, dextrose: 0.99 g/L, $CaCl_2{\cdot}2H_2O$: 0.29 g/L) gassed with 95% O_2 and 5% CO_2 at a pressure of about 60 mmHg maintained by a peristaltic pump. Motion was suppressed by using blebbistatin at a concentration of 3–5 mM (dissolved in DMSO at the ratio of 5 mg/mL). For imaging, the heart was stained with the voltage-sensitive dye JPW-6003 (0.4 mg dissolved in 40 µL of pure ethanol) and intracellular calcium-sensitive dye Rhod-2 (1 mg dissolved in 1 mL of DMSO).

Optical Mapping

The optical system was previously described (Fenton et al., 2009; Ji et al., 2017). Briefly, six high-power LEDs were used for excitation (LED Engin, San Jose CA). Three LEDs were used for V_m imaging, coupled with OD4 650/20 nm excitation filters (Edmund Optics), and the other three were used for $[Ca_i]^{+2}$ imaging, coupled with OD4 550/20 nm excitation filters. The operations and the intensity of the LEDs were controlled by custom-designed apparatus. Series of fluorescent images corresponding to $[Ca_i]^{+2}$ and V_m dynamics were obtained using the time-multiplexing method with a single camera (Photometric Evolve 128 EMCCD), with which the switching of the different excitation LEDs was synchronized. Fluorescence images from the anterior view (partial RV and LV) were obtained at spatial resolution of 128 × 128 pixels (full frame) at 500 fps digitized with a 16-bit dynamic range A/D.

Stimulation Protocol

External bipolar stimuli (3–5 ms, strength twice diastolic threshold) were applied from the apex or the base using a downsweep pacing protocol with the pacing cycle length (PCL) starting from 400 ms. For each PCL, 150–200 stimuli were delivered to allow the system to reach steady state. The PCL was gradually shortened with decreasing steps once alternans started to appear until the occurrence of VF or wave block at any point along the wavefront propagation, usually between 150 and 130 ms. The programming sequence was coordinated with the internal camera trigger clock using an Arduino (Uno R3) so that each pacing stimulus was delivered at a known time point when the camera started to acquire a certain frame. This method allowed us to perform image stacking (Uzelac and Fenton, 2015) once steady state was reached and to detect APD and CaD variations with temporal resolution better than the 2 ms sampling rate of the camera. We found the ability to reach faster pacing rates without inducing fibrillation was highly correlated with uniform physiological temperature across the entire heart and with smaller PCL steps, especially when the PCL was less than 160 ms. To achieve stable and uniform temperature, the heart was submerged in heated Tyrode's solution and a thermometer calibrated to the precision of 0.01°C (Thermo-Fisher) was used for temperature measurement. In case of VF, the heart was defibrillated via low-energy anti-fibrillation pacing (Fenton et al., 2009) or with cardioplegia and was allowed to recover for 30 min before performing subsequent downsweep pacing for comparison.

Data Analysis

As part of the experimental data processing, stacking (ensemble averaging) was used to obtain a high S/N ratio to avoid filtering the $[Ca_i]^{+2}$–V_m signals (Uzelac and Fenton, 2015), which degraded both spatial and temporal resolutions. For each pixel, we recorded at least 150 cycles for one pacing period, then we stacked (summed) the signals for even and odd beats, excluding the first 10 cycles at the start of each PCL to allow the heart to reach the steady state.

Alternans in voltage were quantified by measuring the action potential duration (APD) and the alternans in calcium by measuring calcium transient duration (CaD). When calculating the APD and CaD, the voltage and calcium signals were first normalized between 0 and 1 for each pixel. Then the APD was calculated using a threshold of 0.5, and the CaD was calculated using a threshold of 0.4.

Numerical Simulations

The Sato et al. (2013) model for rabbit ventricular cells in space was used under conditions similar to those of the rabbit experiments. Briefly, each cardiac cell of a one-dimensional cable of tissue is modeled by 75 sarcomeres connected through the diffusion of cytosolic calcium (Cai) and network sarcoplasmic reticulum (NSR) calcium. The diffusion strengths are 8×10^{-9} cm^2/ms and 4×10^{-10} cm^2/ms, respectively. Voltage in the 75 sarcomeres within one cell is considered to be the same due to the fast diffusion inside a cell. Each sarcomere consists of four compartments: cytosol, submembrane, NSR and junctional SR (JSR). The calcium fluctuation is model by the Langevin equation with a noise term depending on the number of SERCA pumps.

One-dimensional tissue is modeled by the cable equation:

$$\frac{\partial V}{\partial t} = -\frac{I_{ion}}{C_m} + D_V \frac{\partial^2 V}{\partial x^2}, \quad (1)$$

where C_m is the membrane capacitance (1 $\mu F/cm^2$), D_v is the voltage diffusion coefficient (10^{-3} cm^2/ms), and I_{ion} is the total transmembrane current, which is the sum of all the ionic currents:

$$I_{ion}^i = I_{Na}^i + I_K^i + \sum\nolimits_{j=1}^{M} (I_{Ca}^{i,j} + I_{NaCa}^{i,j}) \quad (2)$$

Here I_{ion}^i is the ionic current (Sato et al., 2013). Index i is the cell index in the 1D cable and index j is the index for the jth sarcomere in the ith cell. M is the total number of sarcomeres in one cell (i.e., 75 in our simulations). The cable equation is integrated using an operator splitting approach with $\Delta x = 0.015$ cm and $\Delta t = 0.1$ ms. The diffusion of calcium between cells is considered negligible.

Three different pacing protocols were used for the 1D simulations, with each using a stimulus current applied to the first five cells for a duration of 2 ms. In the first pacing protocol, we started by pacing with PCL = 600 ms until steady state was reached, then decreased the PCL to 300 ms and paced until steady state was reached. In the second pacing protocol, we initially assigned to the whole cable the steady state variables for the leftmost cell for PCL = 600 ms, then we gradually decreased the PCL to 300, 295, 290, 285, 280, 270, and 260 ms. For PCLs longer than 300 ms, we used the third pacing protocol, in which we used the steady state of PCL = 300 ms from the second protocol as the initial condition. When calculating APD, −80 mV (about 80% repolarization) was used as the threshold. When calculating CaD, the threshold was set to be between 10 and 20% of the repolarization, adjusted among different pacing cycle lengths to make sure both even and odd beats can be captured.

RESULTS

[Ca]$_i$ Alternans Develops at Longer PCLs than APD Alternans

The spatiotemporal dynamics of voltage and calcium in cardiac tissue depends on the pacing period. **Figure 1A** shows snapshots of voltage (upper two rows) and calcium (lower two rows) in a rabbit ventricle for a series of PCLs from 350 to 140 ms when stimulation was applied at the base of the heart (black arrow). Each column shows consecutive even and odd images during steady state 120 ms after stimulus application; all frame over two successive beats at steady state are shown in Supplementary Movie 1. **Figure 1B** shows the same situation but when the stimulus is applied to the apex, and Supplementary Movie 2 shows all frames over two successive beats at steady state for this case. In all rabbit experiments, Ca alternans clearly developed at longer PCLs than voltage alternans. As the tissue was paced more rapidly, inhomogeneity emerged in both voltage and calcium patterns with calcium displaying more spatial heterogeneity compared to voltage. **Figures 2A,B** shows the voltage and calcium signals, respectively, over time for one pixel indicated by a marker in **Figure 1** for all PCLs. As the PCL decreases, alternans was detected first in calcium amplitude (250 ± 10 ms), then in calcium duration (220 ± 15 ms), and finally in APD (200 ± 15 ms). The shortest PCLs can barely generate an excitation in calcium for the short beats (last two panels in **Figure 2B**), and alternans is more pronounced in both duration and amplitude for the calcium signal.

Discordant Alternans Nodes Are More Pronounced in [Ca]$_i$ than in APD

Figure 3A shows the spatial dispersion of APD for successive beats at steady state. Several important features are worth noticing. At long PCLs (e.g., >250 ms), there is no difference between even and odd beats (no alternans), but there is an intrinsic smooth spatial dispersion of APDs in the range of 15 ms for each beat. As concordant alternans and then discordant alternans develop, the gradient of APD increases to around 30 ms as the PCL decreases. The distance between the locations of the longest and shortest APD decreases during DA, similar to what has been observed in canine hearts (Gizzi et al., 2013). During DA, the regions of long-short and short-long APD are separated by a collection of nodes (nodal lines) where the APD remains constant from beat to beat (shown as white lines in **Figure 3**), with more nodes forming as the PCL decreases. **Figure 3B** shows the CaD dispersion in tissue, similar to **Figure 3A**. However, during DA, the nodal lines are thicker and more pronounced compared to voltage nodal lines. **Figures 3C,D** shows plots similar to **Figures 3A,B** for the same preparation but with the pacing site located at the apex instead of the base. The progression from no alternans to CA and then to DA occurs at the same PCLs, but the spatial patterns are different. This difference of patterns depending on pacing site was observed in all 8 rabbit experiments as well as in previous studies using canine hearts (Gizzi et al., 2013).

Previous numerical studies of alternans (Qu et al., 2000; Watanabe et al., 2001; Fenton et al., 2002; Skardal et al., 2014) have used one-dimensional cables to quantify the spatial profiles of APDs, including the number of nodes present. In the same way, **Figure 4** displays the values of APD and CaD along a line across the heart's surface for two successive beats during alternans. As in **Figure 3**, it can be seen that there is no alternans for PCL >250 ms, then concordant alternans in voltage and calcium appears for PCLs between 200 and 180 ms. At 170 ms, there is CA in voltage but DA for calcium, and for PCL <170 ms DA is present for both voltage and calcium. We calculated in **Table 1** the steepness (slope) of the APD and CaD nodal lines for PCL between 160 and 146 ms corresponding to **Figures 4I–L** when the DA are most pronounced. Data was presented as mean ± s.d., averaged among the slopes at each node for even and odd

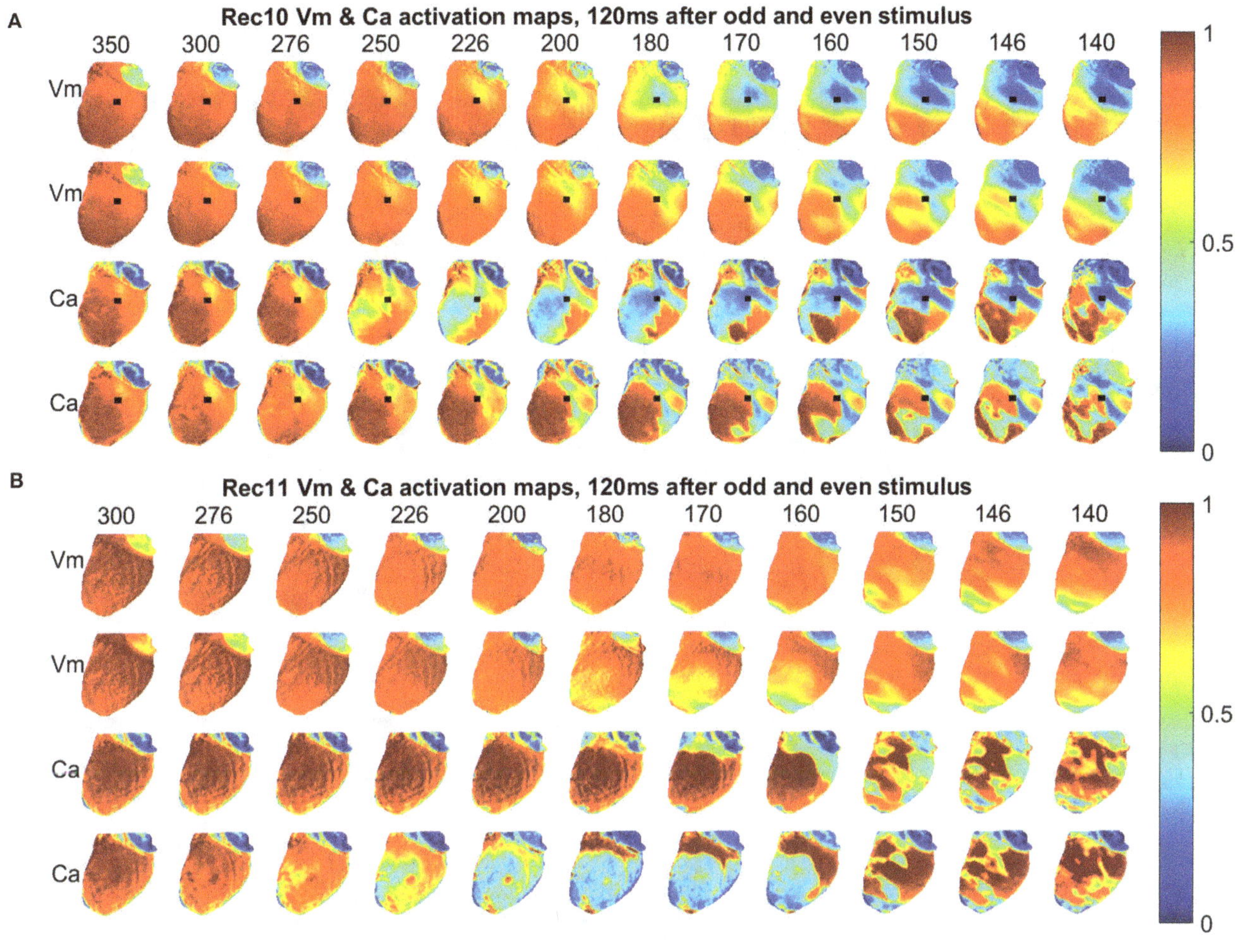

FIGURE 1 | Snapshots of normalized voltage (upper two rows) and intracellular Ca (lower two rows) 120 ms after stimulus application on consecutive beats for decreasing pacing cycle lengths (PCL) from 350 to 140 ms (left to right). Stimulus is applied at **(A)** the base and **(B)** the apex.

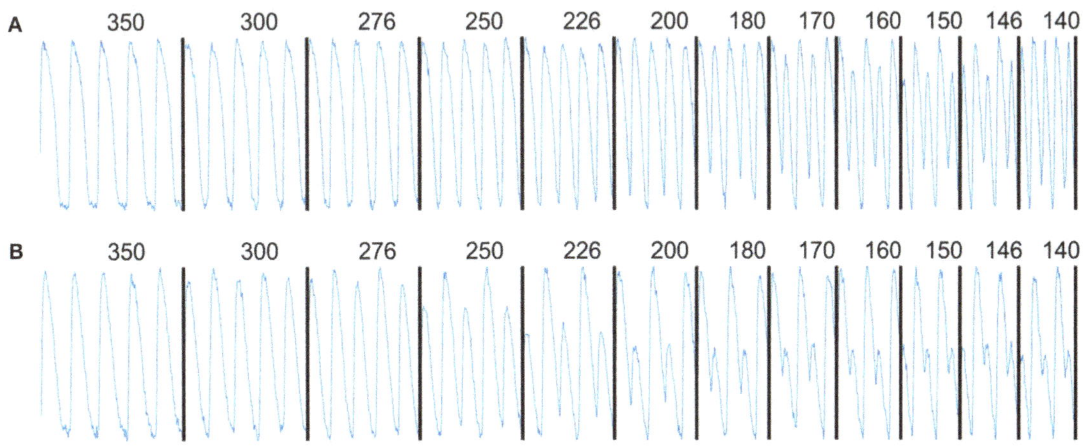

FIGURE 2 | Time traces of normalized voltage **(A)** and $[Ca]_i$ **(B)** signals from a single pixel marked in **Figure 1A** for the same PCLs.

beats for each pacing cycle length. It clearly shows that CaD nodal lines are about one order of magnitude steeper than APD nodal lines, indicating the diffusive connection among cells differs in voltage and calcium signals (Shiferaw and Karma, 2006; Gaeta et al., 2009), as the lack of diffusion in calcium leads to calcium profiles that are sharper in space compared to voltage.

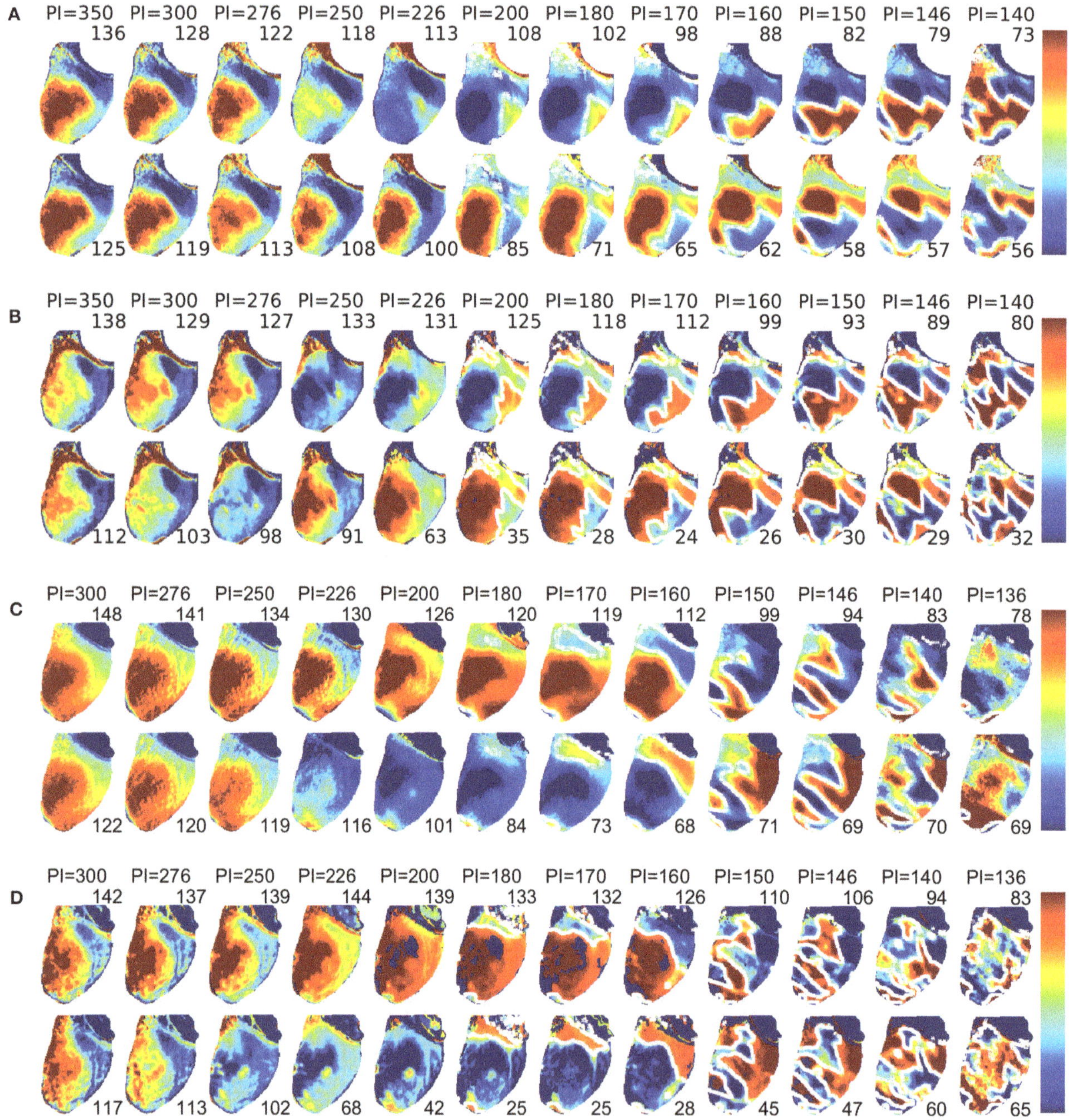

FIGURE 3 | (A) Spatial distribution in APD for even (top) and odd (bottom) beats at various PCLs with stimulation applied to the base. Numbers next to the maps indicate maximum and minimum values used in the color map in ms. Notice there is no alternans for PCL > 275 ms, concordant alternans for PCL between 250 and 225 ms, and discordant alternans for PCLs below 225 ms. Nodal lines are shown in white. **(B)** [Ca]i spatial distribution for even (top) and odd (bottom) beats as in **(A)** but transitions between discordant alternans phases are sharper and nodes are more pronounced. **(C,D)** Spatial distributions as in **(A,B)** but for pacing from the apex.

Experimental Alternans Features Smoother Spatial Profiles and Slower Alternans Amplitude Growth than Simulated Alternans

Simulation results using the Sato et al. model confirm that alternans appear as the PCL is decreased. However, the PCLs at which they appear are much longer compared to experiments. **Figures 5**, **6** show voltage and calcium alternans in a 1D cable 3 cm in length. **Figure 5** illustrates APD as a function of length in the left column for even and odd beats at PCLs of 400, 300, and 260 ms. The right column shows the voltage signal for the corresponding PCL for two cells, one near the left end and one near the right end of the cable, so that if it

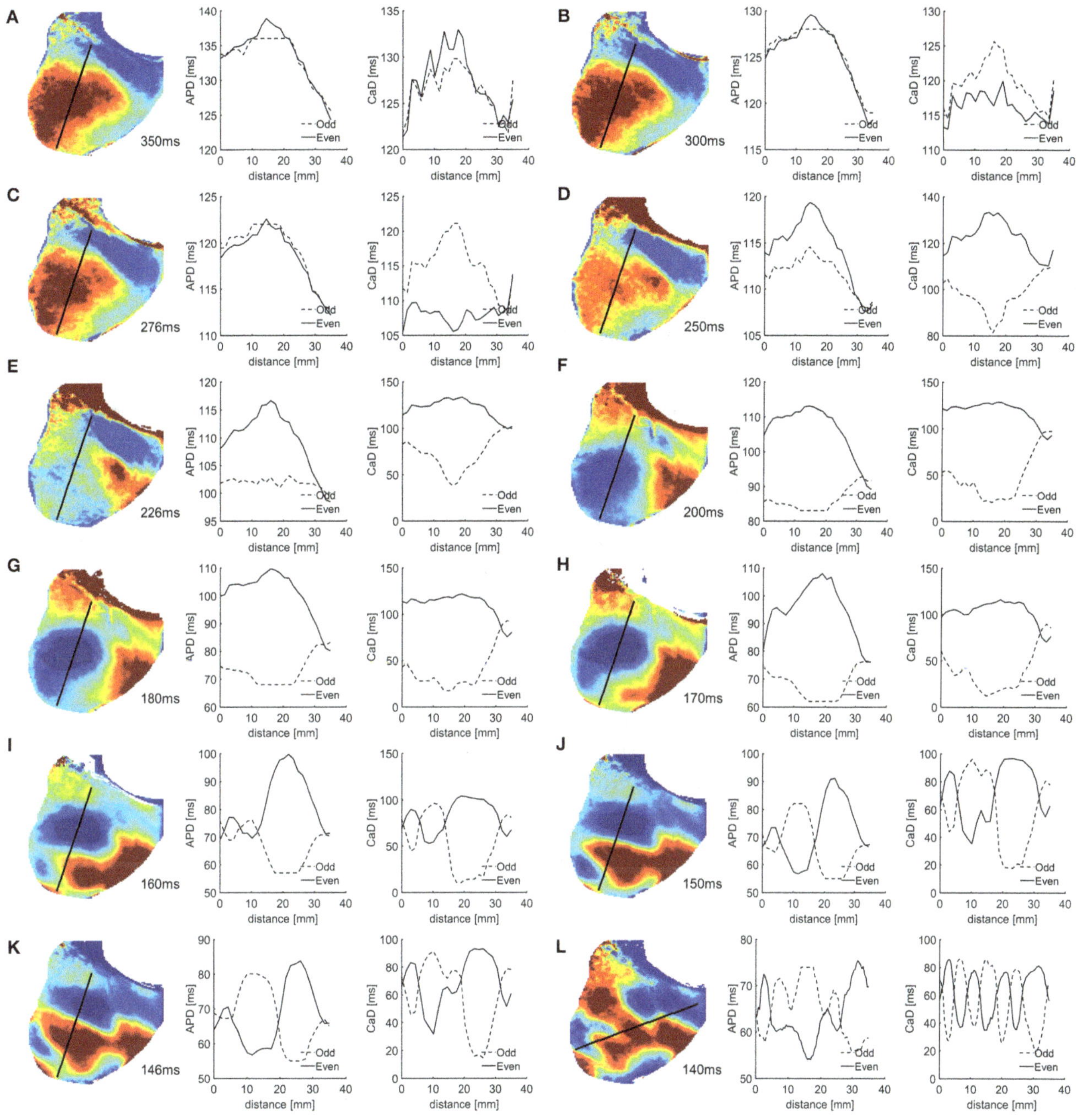

FIGURE 4 | APD contour and APD and $[Ca]_i$ alternans duration in ms for even and odd beats measured along a one-dimensional line shown in black for different PCLs as in **Figure 3**.

undergoes discordant alternans, the voltage signal of the two cells should be out of phase. **Figure 6** shows similar plots but for calcium. The left column indicates CaD over the cable for even and odd beats for the same PCLs as in **Figure 5**. The right column of **Figure 6** displays the calcium signal from two sarcomeres for corresponding PCLs, with the two sarcomeres chosen so that if there is discordant alternans in calcium, the two sarcomeres should be out of phase. Results for other PCLs (600, 500, 450, 350, 290, 280, and 270 ms) are presented in Supplementary Figure 1 for APD and Supplementary Figure 2 for CaD.

For large PCLs (>400 ms), there is no alternans in either voltage or calcium (Supplementary Figures 1A–C, 2A–C). When the PCL drops to 400 ms, concordant alternans appears (**Figures 5A**, **6A**). For PCLs 300 ms or below, discordant alternans occurs (**Figures 5C,D**, **6C,D** and Supplementary Figures 1E–G, 2E–G). In all these simulations, voltage and calcium alternans are "synchronized," such that if there is

TABLE 1 | Steepness of APD and CaD nodal lines.

	PCL = 160 ms	PCL = 150 ms	PCL = 146 ms	PCL = 140 ms
Steepness of APD nodal lines (ms/mm)	2.20 ± 0.87	3.11 ± 1.54	2.75 ± 1.51	1.12 ± 0.38
Steepness of CaD nodal lines (ms/mm)	12.1 ± 4.8	12.5 ± 3.7	9.94 ± 2.91	20.1 ± 5.6

no voltage alternans, there is no calcium alternans, and if there is discordant voltage alternans, there is discordant calcium alternans, with the exception of **Figures 5B, 6B**. In **Figures 5B, 6B**, where we used the second pacing protocol and the PCL is the same as **Figure 5C**, we obtained concordant voltage alternans, whereas the calcium alternans is discordant with multiple nodes. By using different initial conditions, it is possible to obtain completely different dynamics for the same PCL. The Sato et al. model is very sensitive to initial conditions due to the random fluctuation term in the SERCA pump, and in this respect, it is similar to experiments, where it has been shown that small changes in initial conditions can result in very different alternans patterns (Gizzi et al., 2013). In all the simulations presented in this paper, the random noise was generated using the same seed. We did not observe significant changes when we repeat the simulations with different seeds (data not shown).

One major difference between the experiments and the simulations is how sharp the calcium transition is between different alternans phases. In the experiments, both APD and CaD have relatively similar smooth transitions between the maximum and minimum values (**Figures 3**, **4**), with calcium showing only a slightly faster transition, whereas in simulations, CaD has a significantly sharper transition than APD (**Figures 5**, **6**). In addition, in experiments, as the PCL is decreased, CaD transitions from no alternans to concordant alternans and then to discordant alternans with the alternans amplitude increasing smoothly. In simulations, on the other hand, CaD changes drastically from no alternans to concordant alternans with an amplitude of 150 ms when the PCL decreases from 450 to 400 ms.

Figure 7 shows a bifurcation diagram for APD (left) and CaD (right) as a function of PCL calculated at one point from the numerical simulation of the 1D cable (top) and experimental data (bottom) where the alternans has the largest amplitude. As the PCL is decreased from 600 to 260 ms in the numerical simulations, the bifurcation appears simultaneously for both voltage and intracellular calcium just above a CL of 400 ms (PCL_c). The bifurcation amplitude for voltage grows at a rate of the square root away from the bifurcation point ($\Delta APD \sim (PCL - PCL_c)^{1/2}$) (Cherry and Fenton, 2008). The bifurcation amplitude in calcium experiences a sharp discontinuous jump (see Supplementary Figure 3 for the curve fitting). In contrast, the experimental bifurcations occur at much lower PCLs close to 250 ms, and the amplitude of alternans just beyond the bifurcation can be fit better into a linear function with a smoother growth than in the simulations.

DISCUSSION

Patients with LQTS have a higher risk of cardiac arrhythmias due to augmentation of the T-wave and increased spatial dispersion. For many years now, detection of LQTS and T-wave alternans in the ECG has been used as a quantitative tool for predicting dangerous spatial variations in dispersion, which are dynamically induced at the cellular level and can induce arrhythmias. Since 2005, the FDA has required that new drugs be tested for QT prolongation and development of T-wave alternans and recently an FDA-sponsored consortium proposed an initiative to use mathematical action potential models in the aid of drug risk assessment. If models are indeed to be used to investigate pro-arrhythmic and anti-arrhythmic effects of drugs, they first need to be validated against experimental data in normal conditions. The main goal of this study is to create an in tissue experimental data set of simultaneous voltage and calcium optical mapping recordings from Langendorff-perfused rabbit hearts at high temporal and spatial resolution and in particular during alternans for use in validating the dynamics from numerical simulations from the most recent model of rabbit ventricular action potentials (Sato et al., 2013).

We found that alternans in voltage and calcium develops similarly in both experiments and simulations as the pacing cycle length is decreased; however, the model developed alternans much sooner at longer periods close to 420 ms compared to 240 ± 10 ms in experiments. Likewise, the minimum period of stimulation before conduction block developed earlier at 260 ms in the model vs. 140 ± 5 ms in the experiments. Also, it is important to notice that in experiments, as in the models, the magnitude in variations of the APD were much smaller than the variations in CaD during alternans. However, the magnitudes in alternans duration were about twice as large in the model as in the experiments, with maximum values of 55 ms for APD and 150 ms for CaD in the model vs. 25 ± 4 and 65 ± 5 ms, respectively, for the experiments.

More crucial differences arise from the larger differences in how alternans develops. In experiments, alternans in voltage develops gradually, appearing to be more consistent with a border-collision bifurcation (Cherry and Fenton, 2007, 2008; Zhao et al., 2008), where small changes in duration grow slowly and mostly linearly, whereas in the model alternans grows much faster, as with a pitchfork bifurcation (Cherry and Fenton, 2008). Furthermore, the model does not yield action potential amplitude (APA) alternans as observed in the experiments when the tissue is paced at very short pacing cycle lengths (see Supplementary Figure 4 for the APA bifurcation map from experiment), an important additional pro-arrhythmic mechanism recently described by Myles et al. (2011); Chen et al. (2017). On the other hand, while intracellular calcium does display amplitude alternans in both experiments and simulations, in experiments amplitude alternans develops slowly, while in the model a large difference in amplitude appears as soon as alternans develops and persists with a similar amplitude for all periods where alternans is present, as shown in **Figure 6**.

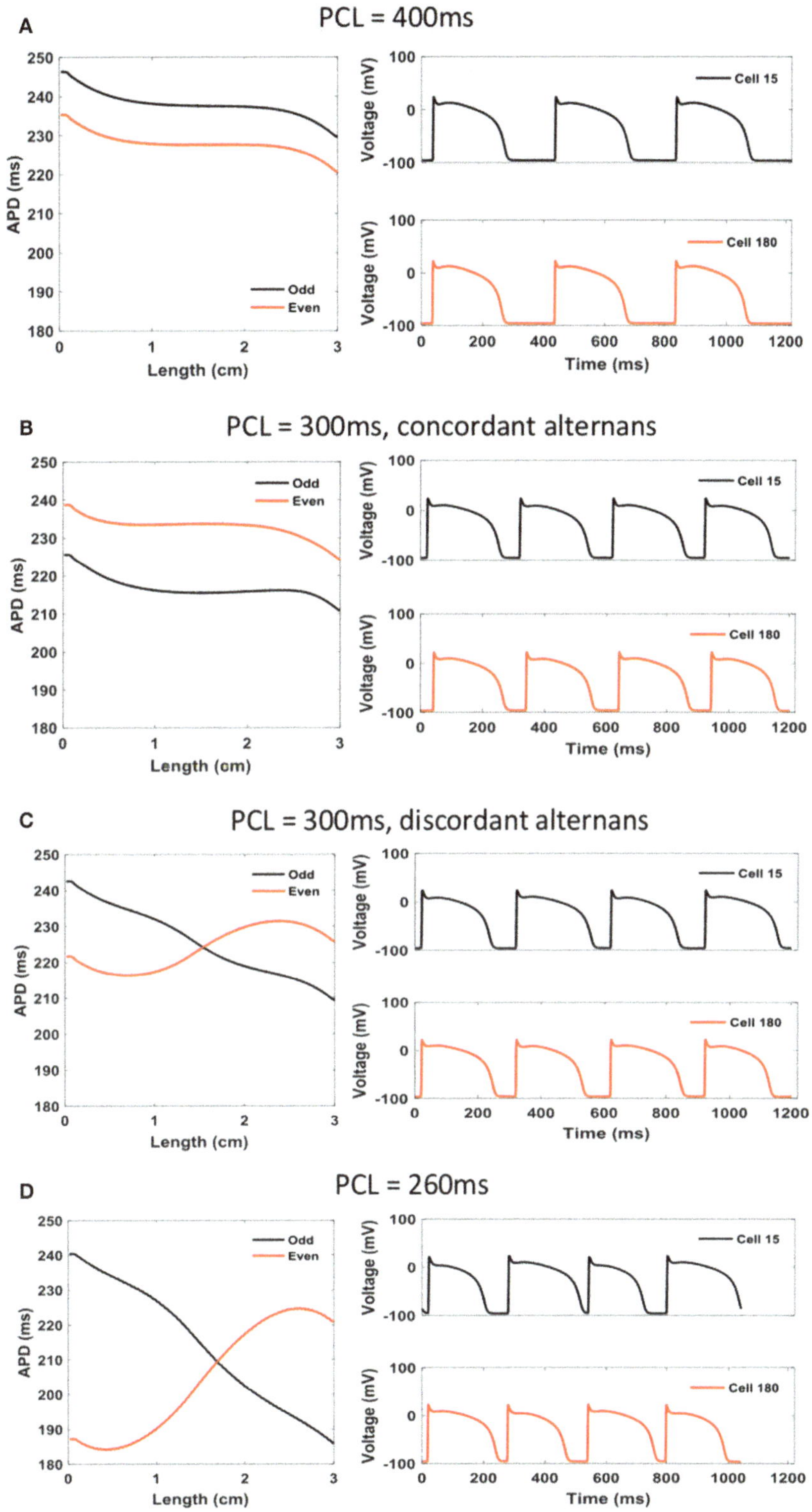

FIGURE 5 | Voltage alternans in a 1D cable ($L = 3$ cm, 200 cells) of the Sato et al. model for decreasing PCLs: **(A)** PCL = 400 ms, **(B)** PCL = 300 ms (concordant alternans), **(C)** PCL = 300 ms (discordant alternans), and **(D)** PCL = 260 ms (discordant alternans). Left: spatial profile of APD for odd (black) and even (red) beats. The amplitude of discordant alternans increases as PCL decreases. Right: voltage over time at two cells, one near the left end and the other near the right end of the cable.

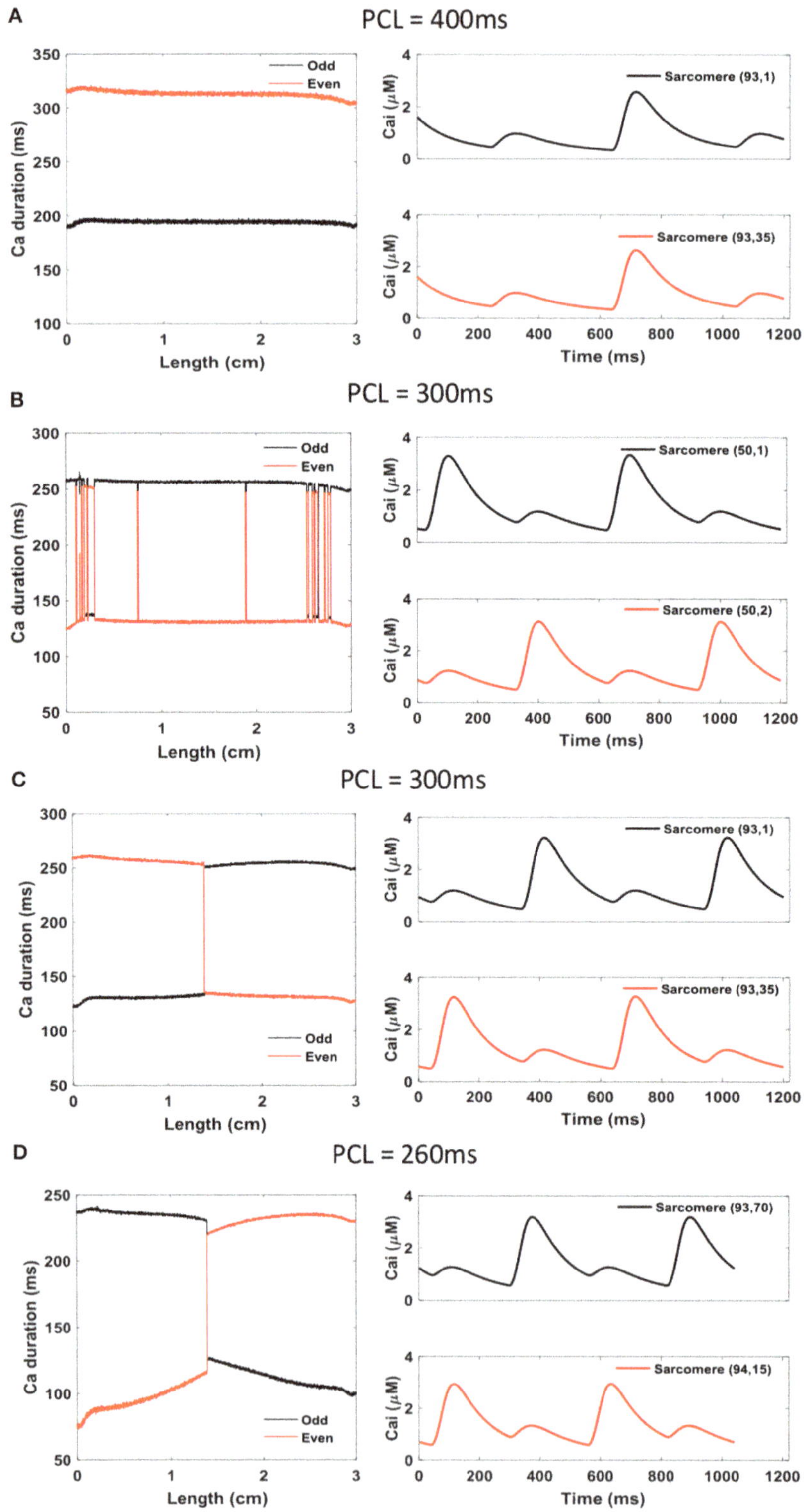

FIGURE 6 | Calcium alternans in a 1D cable ($L = 3$ cm, 200 cells, each cell consists of 75 sarcomeres). **(A)** PCL = 400 ms, **(B)** PCL = 300 ms, **(C)** PCL = 300 ms, and **(D)** PCL = 260 ms. Left: spatial profile of Ca duration for odd (black) and even (red) beats. Right: Ca over time at two sarcomeres that are around the CaD nodal point where they are completely out of phase when discordant alternans is present.

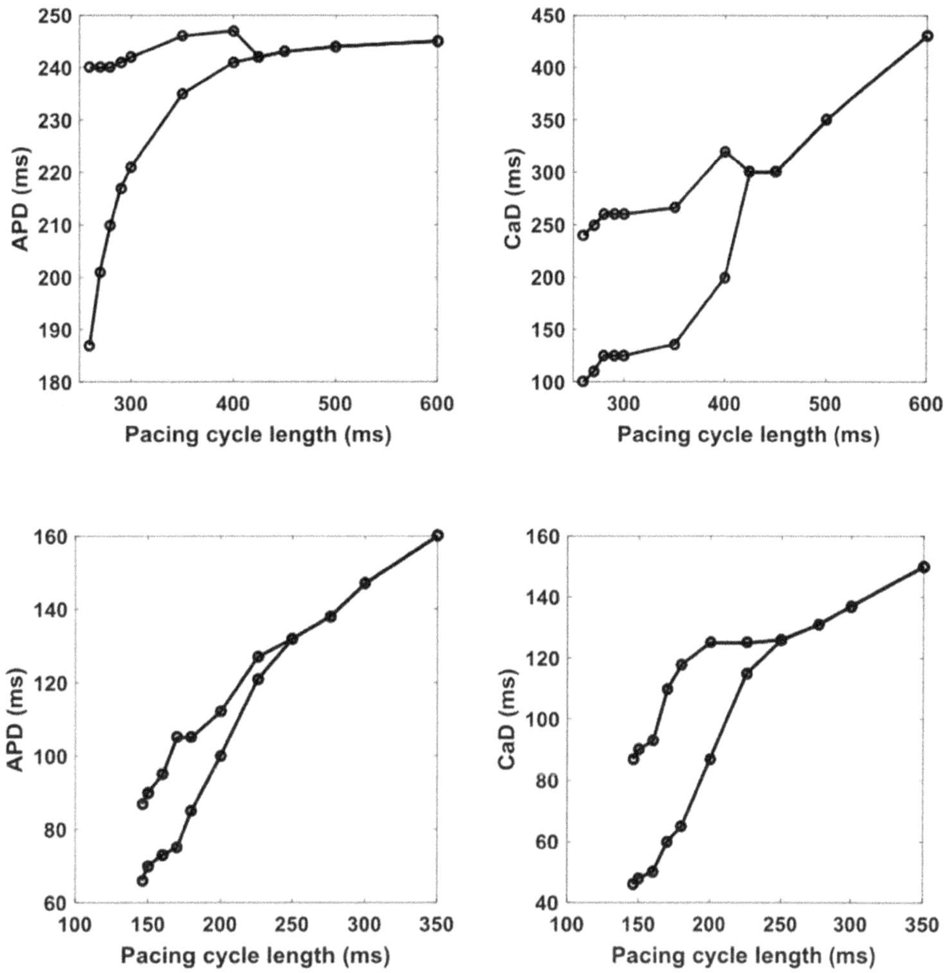

FIGURE 7 | Bifurcation plots of APD **(Left)** and CaD **(Right)** as a function of PCL for simulations (top) and experiments (bottom).

In regard to spatial distributions, in our experiments, we do not detect very sharp calcium duration transitions around nodal lines for most pacing cycle lengths; instead, we observe a smooth phase transition in both voltage and calcium, albeit with calcium appearing sharper, with more defined nodal lines than those in APD (**Figure 3** and **Table 1**). This is contrary to simulations where CaD alternans transition can happen within a cell. If the coupling between voltage and calcium is strong, calcium and voltage should have similar dynamics, i.e., the CaD alternans nodal line should follow that of the APD and vice versa. Therefore, we think the model, as it was published, lack necessary coupling between voltage and calcium. The resolution of our optical mapping is on the order of 200–250 microns; however, due to scattering (Bishop et al., 2007), the actual area may be smoothed to about a millimeter, which is still high enough to identify any possible sharp differences in heterogeneities between voltage and calcium. It is then possible that during pacing in tissue, calcium nodal lines still follow the smoother dynamics of voltage compared to when it is performed in single cell experiments (Gaeta et al., 2009).

Shortcomings of the Model

While the PCL at which alternans appears is much higher in the model than in the experiments by approximately 180 ms, this difference could be fixed with a simple re-scaling of some of the time constants of the model. Similarly, the difference between the minimum PCL for propagation (around 260 ms for the model compared to 140 ms for experiments) could also be fixed by modifications to the recovery and inactivation time constants of the sodium gating variables. Previous publication also showed that CaD alternans patterns can be smoothed by increasing voltage instability (and/or reducing Ca instability). However, there exist several other key physiological aspects that would require a more in-depth analysis and validation of the model's equations.

I. Type of bifurcation. The calcium dynamics should represent the fast nonlinear transition in the dynamical content of calcium in the sarcoplasmic reticulum (Díaz et al., 2004) that can result in a border-collision bifurcation with slow linear growth.

II. Development of alternans in calcium duration. In the model, as soon as alternans develops in calcium, its amplitude is almost at its maximum (**Figure 6**), whereas in the experiments, there is a very smooth transition in Ca alternans with decreasing cycle length (**Figure 2B**).
III. Development of alternans in amplitude. In the model, when alternans in the AP duration develops, at no point does alternans in AP amplitude appear (**Figure 5**). This is in contrast to experiments, where at very short cycle lengths alternans in amplitude is readily observed (**Figure 2A**). Recent experiments and theory predict that the presence of amplitude alternans is key in the development of reentrant arrhythmias (Myles et al., 2011; Chen et al., 2017).
IV. CV and nodal lines. In both simulations and experiments, concordant and discordant alternans appears in tissues of similar size of about 3 cm. The conduction velocities are very different between simulations having a maximum velocity at about 47 cm/s, vs. experiments at around 100 cm/s. Numerically, this means that if the model's diffusion coefficient was modified to fit the experimental CV values, it will result in tissues of more than twice the size needed experimentally to support discordant alternans.

Limitations

The mechanical and electrical behaviors of the heart are strongly coupled through calcium signaling. Very few mathematical models incorporate both aspects (Ji et al., 2015) even though there exists a strong bi-directional coupling between them. We did not study the effect of alternans on contraction or vice versa in either experiments or simulations and we did not study the effect of temperature on calcium and voltage alternans. It has been shown that mammalian hearts can largely increase the magnitude of alternans when temperature is lowered (Pastore et al., 1999; Fenton et al., 2013; Filippi et al., 2014).

DISCLOSURE

The mention of commercial products, their sources, or their use in connection with material reported herein is not to be construed as either an actual or implied endorsement of such products by the Department of Health and Human Services.

AUTHOR CONTRIBUTIONS

IU: experiment, data analysis and writing. YJ and EC: simulation and writing. DH, JS, SL, amd RG: experiment. FF: experiment, simulation and writing.

REFERENCES

Beeler, G. W., and Reuter, H. (1977). Reconstruction of the action potential of ventricular myocardial fibres. *J. Physiol.* 268, 177–210. doi: 10.1113/jphysiol.1977.sp011853

Bishop, M. J., Rodriguez, B., Qu, F., Efimov, I. R., Gavaghan, D. J., and Trayanova, N. A. (2007). The role of photon scattering in optical signal distortion during arrhythmia and defibrillation. *Biophys. J.* 93, 3714–3726. doi: 10.1529/biophysj.107.110981

Chen, D. D., Gray, R. A., Uzelac, I., Herndon, C., and Fenton, F. H. (2017). Mechanism for amplitude alternans in electrocardiograms and the initiation of spatiotemporal chaos. *Phys. Rev. Lett.* 118:168101. doi: 10.1103/PhysRevLett.118.168101

Cherry, E. M., and Fenton, F. H. (2007). A tale of two dogs: analyzing two models of canine ventricular electrophysiology. *Am. J. Physiol. Heart Circ. Physiol.* 292, H43–H55. doi: 10.1152/ajpheart.00955.2006

Cherry, E. M., and Fenton, F. H. (2008). Visualization of spiral and scroll waves in simulated and experimental cardiac tissue. *New J. Phys.* 1012:125016. doi: 10.1088/1367-2630/10/12/125016

Choi, B.-R., Jang, W., and Salama, G. (2007). Spatially discordant voltage alternans cause wavebreaks in ventricular fibrillation. *Heart Rhythm Off. J. Heart Rhythm Soc.* 4, 1057–1068. doi: 10.1016/j.hrthm.2007.03.037

Chudin, E., Goldhaber, J., Garfinkel, A., Weiss, J., and Kogan, B. (1999). Intracellular Ca2+ dynamics and the stability of ventricular Tachycardia. *Biophys. J.* 77, 2930–2941. doi: 10.1016/S0006-3495(99)77126-2

Clusin, W. T. (2008). Mechanisms of calcium transient and action potential alternans in cardiac cells and tissues. *Am. J. Physiol. Heart Circ. Physiol.* 294, H1–H10. doi: 10.1152/ajpheart.00802.2007

Díaz, M. E., O'Neill, S. C., and Eisner, D. A. (2004). Sarcoplasmic Reticulum calcium content fluctuation is the key to cardiac alternans. *Circ. Res.* 94, 650–656. doi: 10.1161/01.RES.0000119923.64774.72

DiFrancesco, D., and Noble, D. (1985). A model of cardiac electrical activity incorporating ionic pumps and concentration changes. *Philos. Trans. R. Soc. Lond. B Biol. Sci.* 307, 353–398. doi: 10.1098/rstb.1985.0001

Edwards, J. N., and Blatter, L. A. (2014). Cardiac alternans and intracellular calcium cycling. *Clin. Exp. Pharmacol. Physiol.* 41, 524–532. doi: 10.1111/1440-1681.12231

Eisner, D. A., Li, Y., and O'Neill, S. C. (2006). Alternans of intracellular calcium: mechanism and significance. *Heart Rhythm* 3, 743–745. doi: 10.1016/j.hrthm.2005.12.020

Faber, G. M., and Rudy, Y. (2000). Action potential and contractility changes in [Na(+)](i) overloaded cardiac myocytes: a simulation study. *Biophys. J.* 78, 2392–2404. doi: 10.1016/S0006-3495(00)76783-X

Fenton, F. H., Cherry, E. M., Hastings, H. M., and Evans, S. J. (2002). Multiple mechanisms of spiral wave breakup in a model of cardiac electrical activity. *Chaos Woodbury N* 12, 852–892. doi: 10.1063/1.1504242

Fenton, F. H., Gizzi, A., Cherubini, C., Pomella, N., and Filippi, S. (2013). Role of temperature on nonlinear cardiac dynamics. *Phys. Rev. E Stat. Nonlin. Soft Matter Phys.* 87:042717. doi: 10.1103/PhysRevE.87.042717

Fenton, F. H., Luther, S., Cherry, E. M., Otani, N. F., Krinsky, V., Pumir, A., et al. (2009). Termination of atrial fibrillation using pulsed low-energy far-field stimulation. *Circulation* 120, 467–476. doi: 10.1161/CIRCULATIONAHA.108.825091

Filippi, S., Gizzi, A., Cherubini, C., Luther, S., and Fenton, F. H. (2014). Mechanistic insights into hypothermic ventricular fibrillation: the role of temperature and tissue size. *Eur. Eur. Pacing Arrhythm. Card. Electrophysiol. J. Work. Groups Card. Pacing Arrhythm. Card. Cell. Electrophysiol. Eur. Soc. Cardiol.* 16, 424–434. doi: 10.1093/europace/euu031

Food and Drug Administration (2005). *Guidance for Industry E14 Clinical Evaluation of QT/QTc Interval Prolongation and Proarrhythmic Potential for Non-antiarrhythmic Drugs*. Silver Spring, MD: FDA.

Fox, J. J., McHarg, J. L., and Gilmour, R. F. (2002). Ionic mechanism of electrical alternans. *Am. J. Physiol. Heart Circ. Physiol.* 282, H516–H530. doi: 10.1152/ajpheart.00612.2001

Gaeta, S. A., Bub, G., Abbott, G. W., and Christini, D. J. (2009). Dynamical mechanism for subcellular alternans in cardiac myocytes. *Circ. Res.* 105, 335–342. doi: 10.1161/CIRCRESAHA.109.197590

Gizzi, A., Cherry, E., Gilmour, R. F. J., Luther, S., Filippi, S., and Fenton, F. H. (2013). Effects of pacing site and stimulation history on alternans dynamics and the development of complex spatiotemporal patterns in cardiac tissue. *Front. Physiol.* 4:71. doi: 10.3389/fphys.2013.00071

Guevara, M., Ward, G., and Glass, L. (1984). Electrical alternans and period doubling bifurcations. *IEEE Comp. Cardiol.* 562, 167–170.

Iyer, V., Mazhari, R., and Winslow, R. L. (2004). A computational model of the human left-ventricular epicardial myocyte. *Biophys. J.* 87, 1507–1525. doi: 10.1529/biophysj.104.043299

Jayakrishnan, M. P., and Krishnakumar, P. (2006). Macroscopic T wave alternans in long QT syndrome. *Indian J. Pediatr.* 73, 539–540. doi: 10.1007/BF02759905

Ji, Y. C., Gray, R. A., and Fenton, F. H. (2015). Implementation of contraction to electrophysiological ventricular myocyte models, and their quantitative characterization via post-extrasystolic potentiation. *PLoS ONE* 10:e0135699. doi: 10.1371/journal.pone.0135699

Ji, Y. C., Uzelac, I., Otani, N., Luther, S., Gilmour, R. F., Cherry, E. M., et al. (2017). Synchronization as a mechanism for low-energy anti-fibrillation pacing. *Heart Rhythm* 14, 1254–1262. doi: 10.1016/j.hrthm.2017.05.021

Kanaporis, G., and Blatter, L. A. (2015). The mechanisms of calcium cycling and action potential dynamics in cardiac alternans. *Circ. Res.* 116, 846–856. doi: 10.1161/CIRCRESAHA.116.305404

Laurita, K. R., and Rosenbaum, D. S. (2008). Cellular mechanisms of arrhythmogenic cardiac alternans. *Prog. Biophys. Mol. Biol.* 97, 332–347. doi: 10.1016/j.pbiomolbio.2008.02.014

Luo, C. H., and Rudy, Y. (1991). A model of the ventricular cardiac action potential. depolarization, repolarization, and their interaction. *Circ. Res.* 68, 1501–1526. doi: 10.1161/01.RES.68.6.1501

Luo, C. H., and Rudy, Y. (1994). A dynamic model of the cardiac ventricular action potential. I. simulations of ionic currents and concentration changes. *Circ. Res.* 74, 1071–1096. doi: 10.1161/01.RES.74.6.1071

Mahajan, A., Shiferaw, Y., Sato, D., Baher, A., Olcese, R., Xie, L. H., et al. (2008). A rabbit ventricular action potential model replicating cardiac dynamics at rapid heart rates. *Biophys. J.* 94, 392–410. doi: 10.1529/biophysj.106.98160

Myles, R. C., Burton, F. L., Cobbe, S. M., and Smith, G. L. (2008). The link between repolarisation alternans and ventricular arrhythmia: does the cellular phenomenon extend to the clinical problem? *J. Mol. Cell. Cardiol.* 45, 1–10. doi: 10.1016/j.yjmcc.2008.03.024

Myles, R. C., Burton, F. L., Cobbe, S. M., and Smith, G. L. (2011). Alternans of action potential duration and amplitude in rabbits with left ventricular dysfunction following myocardial infarction. *J. Mol. Cell. Cardiol.* 50, 510–521. doi: 10.1016/j.yjmcc.2010.11.019

Noble, D. (1962). A modification of the Hodgkin—Huxley equations applicable to Purkinje fibre action and pacemaker potentials. *J. Physiol.* 160, 317–352. doi: 10.1113/jphysiol.1962.sp006849

Nolasco, J. B., and Dahlen, R. W. (1968). A graphic method for the study of alternation in cardiac action potentials. *J. Appl. Physiol.* 25, 191–196.

O'Hara, T., Virág, L., Varró, A., and Rudy, Y. (2011). Simulation of the undiseased human cardiac ventricular action potential: model formulation and experimental validation. *PLoS Comput. Biol.* 7:e1002061. doi: 10.1371/journal.pcbi.1002061

Pastore, J. M., Girouard, S. D., Laurita, K. R., Akar, F. G., and Rosenbaum, D. S. (1999). Mechanism linking T-wave alternans to the genesis of cardiac fibrillation. *Circulation* 99, 1385–1394. doi: 10.1161/01.CIR.99.10.1385

Priebe, L., and Beuckelmann, D. J. (1998). Simulation study of cellular electric properties in heart failure. *Circ. Res.* 82, 1206–1223. doi: 10.1161/01.RES.82.11.1206

Puglisi, J. L., and Bers, D. M. (2001). LabHEART: an interactive computer model of rabbit ventricular myocyte ion channels and Ca transport. *Am. J. Physiol. Cell Physiol.* 281, C2049–2060.

Qu, Z., Garfinkel, A., Chen, P. S., and Weiss, J. N. (2000). Mechanisms of discordant alternans and induction of reentry in simulated cardiac tissue. *Circulation* 102, 1664–1670. doi: 10.1161/01.CIR.102.14.1664

Sager, P. T., Gintant, G., Turner, J. R., Pettit, S., and Stockbridge, N. (2014). Rechanneling the cardiac proarrhythmia safety paradigm: a meeting report from the cardiac safety research consortium. *Am. Heart J.* 167, 292–300. doi: 10.1016/j.ahj.2013.11.004

Saitoh, H., Bailey, J. C., and Surawicz, B. (1988). Alternans of action potential duration after abrupt shortening of cycle length: differences between dog Purkinje and ventricular muscle fibers. *Circ. Res.* 62, 1027–1040. doi: 10.1161/01.RES.62.5.1027

Saitoh, H., Bailey, J. C., and Surawicz, B. (1989). Action potential duration alternans in dog Purkinje and ventricular muscle fibers. further evidence in support of two different mechanisms. *Circulation* 80, 1421–1431. doi: 10.1161/01.CIR.80.5.1421

Sato, D., Bers, D. M., and Shiferaw, Y. (2013). Formation of spatially discordant alternans due to fluctuations and diffusion of calcium. *PLoS ONE* 8:e85365. doi: 10.1371/journal.pone.0085365

Sato, D., Shiferaw, Y., Garfinkel, A., Weiss, J. N., Qu, Z., and Karma, A. (2006). Spatially discordant alternans in cardiac tissue: role of calcium cycling. *Circ. Res.* 99, 520–527. doi: 10.1161/01.RES.0000240542.03986.e7

Schwartz, P. J. (1985). Idiopathic long QT syndrome: progress and questions. *Am. Heart J.* 109, 399–411. doi: 10.1016/0002-8703(85)90626-X

Schwartz, P. J., Moss, A. J., Vincent, G. M., and Crampton, R. S. (1993). Diagnostic criteria for the long QT syndrome. an update. *Circulation* 88, 782–784. doi: 10.1161/01.CIR.88.2.782

Shannon, T. R., Wang, F., Puglisi, J., Weber, C., and Bers, D. M. (2004). A mathematical treatment of integrated Ca dynamics within the ventricular myocyte. *Biophys. J.* 87, 3351–3371. doi: 10.1529/biophysj.104.047449

Shiferaw, Y., and Karma, A. (2006). Turing instability mediated by voltage and calcium diffusion in paced cardiac cells. *Proc. Natl. Acad. Sci. U.S.A.* 103, 5670–5675. doi: 10.1073/pnas.0511061103

Skardal, P. S., Karma, A., and Restrepo, J. G. (2014). Spatiotemporal Dynamics of calcium-driven cardiac alternans. *Phys. Rev. E Stat. Nonlin. Soft Matter Phys.* 89:052707. doi: 10.1103/PhysRevE.89.052707

ten Tusscher, K. H. W. J., Noble, D., Noble, P. J., and Panfilov, A. V. (2004). A model for human ventricular tissue. *Am. J. Physiol. Heart Circ. Physiol.* 286, H1573–H1589. doi: 10.1152/ajpheart.00794.2003

Traube, L. (1872). Ein fall von pulsus bigeminus nebst bemerkungen tiber die lebershwellungen bei klappenfehlern und uber acute leberatrophic. *Ber Klin Wschr* 9.

Uzelac, I., and Fenton, F. (2015). Robust framework for quantita tive analysis of optical mapping signals without filtering. *Comput. Cardiol.* 42, 461–464. doi: 10.1371/journal.pcbi.1005063

Watanabe, M. A., Fenton, F. H., Evans, S. J., Hastings, H. M., and Karma, A. (2001). Mechanisms for discordant alternans. *J. Cardiovasc. Electrophysiol.* 12, 196–206. doi: 10.1046/j.1540-8167.2001.00196.x

Weiss, J. N., Karma, A., Shiferaw, Y., Chen, P.-S., Garfinkel, A., and Qu, Z. (2006). From pulsus to pulseless: the saga of cardiac alternans. *Circ. Res.* 98, 1244–1253. doi: 10.1161/01.RES.0000224540.97431.f0

Weiss, J. N., Nivala, M., Garfinkel, A., and Qu, Z. (2011). Alternans and arrhythmias: from cell to heart. *Circ. Res.* 108, 98–112. doi: 10.1161/CIRCRESAHA.110.223586

Winslow, R. L., Rice, J., Jafri, S., Marbán, E., and O'Rourke, B. (1999). Mechanisms of altered excitation-contraction coupling in canine tachycardia-induced heart failure, II. *Circ. Res.* 84, 571–586. doi: 10.1161/01.RES.84.5.571

Zareba, W., Moss, A. J., le Cessie, S., and Hall, W. J. (1994). T wave alternans in idiopathic long QT syndrome. *J. Am. Coll. Cardiol.* 23, 1541–1546. doi: 10.1016/0735-1097(94)90653-X

Zhao, X., Schaeffer, D. G., Berger, C. M., Krassowska, W., and Gauthier, D. J. (2008). Cardiac alternans arising from an unfolded border-collision bifurcation. *J. Comput. Nonlin. Dyn.* 3:041004-041004-7. doi: 10.1115/1.296046

13

Composite Biomarkers Derived from Micro-Electrode Array Measurements and Computer Simulations Improve the Classification of Drug-Induced Channel Block

Eliott Tixier[1,2], *Fabien Raphel*[1,2], *Damiano Lombardi*[1,2] *and Jean-Frédéric Gerbeau*[1,2*]

[1] Inria Paris, Paris, France, [2] Sorbonne Universités, Université Pierre et Marie Curie—Paris 6, UMR 7598 LJLL, Paris, France

Correspondence:
Jean-Frédéric Gerbeau
jean-frederic.gerbeau@inria.fr

The Micro-Electrode Array (MEA) device enables high-throughput electrophysiology measurements that are less labor-intensive than patch-clamp based techniques. Combined with human-induced pluripotent stem cells cardiomyocytes (hiPSC-CM), it represents a new and promising paradigm for automated and accurate *in vitro* drug safety evaluation. In this article, the following question is addressed: which features of the MEA signals should be measured to better classify the effects of drugs? A framework for the classification of drugs using MEA measurements is proposed. The classification is based on the ion channels blockades induced by the drugs. It relies on an *in silico* electrophysiology model of the MEA, a feature selection algorithm and automatic classification tools. An *in silico* model of the MEA is developed and is used to generate synthetic measurements. An algorithm that extracts MEA measurements features designed to perform well in a classification context is described. These features are called composite biomarkers. A state-of-the-art machine learning program is used to carry out the classification of drugs using experimental MEA measurements. The experiments are carried out using five different drugs: mexiletine, flecainide, diltiazem, moxifloxacin, and dofetilide. We show that the composite biomarkers outperform the classical ones in different classification scenarios. We show that using both synthetic and experimental MEA measurements improves the robustness of the composite biomarkers and that the classification scores are increased.

Keywords: cardiac electrophysiology, numerical simulations, bidomain model, micro-electrode array, classification, drug safety evaluation

INTRODUCTION

One of the main goals of safety pharmacology studies is to anticipate how drugs affect cardiomyocytes. Among other adverse effects, it focuses on predicting arrhythmic behaviors which may lead to torsades de pointes (TdP). The most common risk factors under consideration are QT prolongation and hERG block. However these risk factors are now considered insufficient and the guidelines need to be improved (Fermini et al., 2016). For instance, an observed QT prolongation is not necessarily associated with TdP risk (Antzelevitch et al., 2004). Several advances in technology and computational modeling may favor the emergence of new methods for more efficient drug safety evaluation. On the hardware side, the Micro-Electrode Array (MEA) technology[1] (Meyer et al., 2004) enables high-throughput electrophysiology measurements that are less labor-intensive than patch-clamp based techniques. This device has been successfully used in large drug studies (Blinova et al., 2016). On the biological side, the use of human-induced pluripotent stem cells (hiPSC) has developed (Scott et al., 2013) and their recent large-scale production makes it a viable human model replacement. The combined use of the MEA technology and hiPSC cardiomyocytes (hiPSC-CM) represents a new and promising paradigm for automated and accurate *in vitro* drug safety evaluation (Clements and Thomas, 2014; Cavero et al., 2016). The CIPA initiative (Cavero et al., 2016; Fermini et al., 2016) promotes disruptive drug safety guidelines, in particular the use of hiPSC-CM and *in silico* modeling. In parallel of these technological breakthroughs, several efforts have been recently made toward promoting the use of computational tools in drug safety evaluation (Davies et al., 2016; Lancaster and Sobie, 2016). In this context, a framework for drug safety evaluation using *in silico* models and experimental measurements using a MEA device is hereby presented. The device considered in the present work is a six-well nine-electrode MEA but, as shown in Raphel et al. (2017), the approach is general enough to be extended to other types of MEA.

The framework aims at predicting the effect of a drug onto the cardiomyocytes ion channels activities from the knowledge of MEA experimental recordings. More precisely, the goal is to determine which ion channels are affected by a given drug. Note that the aim of the present study is not to predict the drugs propensities to induce cardiac arrhythmias but rather to identify which ion channel is primarily blocked. This represents a first step toward the use of the MEA-hiPSC-CM platform in arrhythmogenicity studies. Even though patch-clamp experiments are the gold standard to assess drug-induced channel block, it was shown in a recent study (Raphel et al., 2017) that it is possible to do so also using MEA field potential measurements. The approach is based on an *in silico* model of the MEA and the hiPSC-CM tissue, a feature selection algorithm and a classification model. The *in silico* model is based on a simple ionic model (Bueno-Orovio et al., 2008) for the cardiomyocytes electrical activity and on the bidomain equations (Tung, 1978) for the spatial propagation of the electrical potentials. The ionic model counts three different currents (fast inward, slow inward, slow outward), each being associated with an ionic species (respectively sodium, calcium, potassium). The activity of each current is controlled by a scaling parameter that is referred to as conductance in the following. In the present work, the drugs considered are assumed to affect one of those three currents. Thus, the inactivation of a current caused by a drug is modeled by a diminution of the corresponding conductance in the ionic model. The conductances and some other parameters of the model can be varied in order to replicate the variability observed in the experimental measurements. The *in silico* model is used to generate what is later referred to as synthetic MEA measurements. The experimental data set itself consists of MEA electrode recordings which come in the form of time series. Each recording is done in control conditions (no drug) and with different drug concentration levels. The experimental data is also labeled, meaning the affected ionic channels are known for each drug.

As explained above, the MEA measurements, whether synthetic or experimental, come in the form of time series. For classification purposes, it is more efficient to extract features from these time series. Some features, also called biomarkers, are already widely used in the community such as the field potential duration (Clements and Thomas, 2014) which may be associated with the QT segment in ECGs. These common features are referred to as classical biomarkers. We propose a way to automatically extract features from the MEA measurements that are designed to perform well in a classification context. First a set of biomarkers is built. The set is referred to as dictionary and each biomarker is referred to as an entry in the following. Then we define new features, referred to as composite biomarkers, as linear combinations of the dictionary entries. The weights of these linear combinations are found by solving a sparse optimization problem. The optimization procedure uses a data set which consists of experimental MEA measurements, simulated ones or a combination of both.

To predict the effects of drugs onto channel block, we propose to adopt a Machine Learning approach. Machine Learning is a family of statistical methods whose aim is to build predictive models given a (ideally large) data set. There exists a wide variety of such methods: neural networks (Kiranyaz et al., 2016), Support Vector Machine (Hua and Sun, 2001), decision trees (Arikawa et al., 1993), etc. All these methods have proved their performances in many different scenarios of regression and classification, in particular when applied to biological data. In the present work, we propose to use Support Vector Classification (SVC) (Boser et al., 1992) which derives from Support Vector Machine. This method seeks a hyperplane that separates the data samples with a maximum margin. The samples are then classified according to their position with respect to the separating hyperplane.

The paper is organized as follows. First, the methods are described. The *in silico* model is presented and the generation of synthetic data is explained. The algorithm that computes the composite biomarkers is described and the classification tools are presented. Second, the performance of the composite biomarkers and of the classification tools are studied in different drug classification scenarios. The composite biomarkers are compared to the classical ones using two different classification strategies. Finally, composite biomarkers computed with experimental data only and with a mixed set of experimental and synthetic data are compared.

[1]Systems, M. Microelectrode array (mea) manual. http://www.multichannelsystems.com/sites/multichannelsystems.com/files/documents/manuals/MEA_Manual.pdf.

METHODS

Equations

Bidomain Equations and Ionic Model

Let Ω be the domain representing a MEA's well. The thickness of the layer of cells being small compared to the size of the well, the problem is assumed to be two-dimensional. We denote by A_m, C_m the surface area of membrane per unit volume of tissue, the membrane capacitance, and the thickness of the cell layer, respectively. The intra and extra-cellular conductivity tensors σ_i and σ_e are assumed to be scalar. The parameters values are reported in **Table 1**. The propagation of the transmembrane potential V_m and the extracellular potential ϕ_e are modeled in Ω with the bidomain model (Tung, 1978):

$$\begin{cases} A_m C_m \dfrac{\partial V_m}{\partial t} + A_m I_{ion}(V_m, w) - \nabla \cdot (\sigma_i \nabla V_m) - \nabla \cdot (\sigma_i \nabla \phi_e) = A_m I_{app}, \\ -\nabla \cdot ((\sigma_i + \sigma_e) \nabla \phi_e) - \nabla \cdot (\sigma_i \nabla V_m) = \frac{1}{z_{thick}} \sum_{e_k} \dfrac{I_{el}^k}{|e_k|} \chi_{e_k}. \end{cases} \quad (1)$$

In the second equation, I_{el}^k is the electric current which goes through the electrode located at e_k, $|e_k|$ is the electrode surface and χ_{e_k} is the characteristic function of e_k (which takes the value 1 on the electrode and 0 elsewhere). An imperfect model for the electrode is used to compute I_{el}^k and described in the Supplementary Material. The activation is assumed to be triggered by a current I_{app} that is applied in an arbitrary region of the well with a cycle length of 1,200 ms. The locations of the stimulations are randomized to model the uncertainties of the spontaneous stimulus locations in *in vitro* measurements. This is further explained in the Heterogeneity modeling subsection. The computational domain Ω corresponds to one well of the MEA device as shown in **Figure 1**. Let $\boldsymbol{n}$ be the outward normal to the boundary of the domain Ω. Equations (1) are completed with the following boundary conditions: $\sigma_i \nabla \phi_i \cdot \boldsymbol{n} = 0$ (where $\phi_i = V_m + \phi_e$), and either $\phi_e = 0$ on the region connected to the ground or $\sigma_e \nabla \phi_e \cdot \boldsymbol{n} = 0$ elsewhere. The ground location is indicated in **Figure 1**.

The transmembrane ionic current I_{ion} is described with the Minimal Ventricular (MV) model (Bueno-Orovio et al., 2008) which includes three currents: fast inward (fi), slow inward (si) and outward (so) currents. The reader is referred to the original publication for more details. Schematically, I_{ion} depends on V_m and on gating variables $\mathbf{w} = (w_j)_{1 \le j \le 3}$, solution of a system of three non-linear ordinary differential equations. A conductance coefficient g_s, with $s = fi, si$ or so, controls the activity of the idealized channels associated with each of three currents of the model.

The partial differential equations are discretized in space by means of P1 finite elements, and in time by using backward differentiation formula (BDF) schemes with adaptive time steps and order provided by Sundials' CVODE library (Hindmarsh et al., 2005). The quantity of interest is the extra-cellular potential, also referred to as field potential (FP). It is a function of time and recorded at the electrodes locations.

TABLE 1 | Bidomain model parameters.

A_m	C_m	σ_i	σ_e	z_{thick}
200 cm^{-1}	1 $\mu F.cm^{-2}$	5 $mS.cm^{-1}$	5 $mS.cm^{-1}$	10 μm

Synthetic measurements

In the present work, the computational model is used to generate synthetic MEA measurements. The main idea is to enrich the experimental data set with *in silico* measurements to make the classification more robust, in particular by exploring regions of the parametric space that are not covered by the experience. For a given set of conductances, the model is evaluated and the electrodes FPs are recorded. The conductances are chosen as to represent meaningful scenarios, as explained later in the Results section. To mimic experimental measurements, a zero-mean Gaussian noise of standard deviation 10 μV is added to the FPs (see **Figure 2**). A heterogeneity model of some ionic parameters is also considered to replicate the variability exhibited by the experimental measurements. This model is described later in this section. The stimulation location is also varied to model the uncertainty of the spontaneous stimulus location in the experiments. **Figure 3** shows examples of synthetic recordings generated using the aforementioned *in silico* model. The FPs are simulated for three different scenarios. The scenarios consist in simulating the effects of sodium, calcium and potassium antagonist drugs, in each case with five different concentrations. In Supplementary Figure 1 a simulated FP recorded on an electrode is shown with the simulated action potential recorded on the same electrode.

Steady-state regime

Because the initial conditions of the ionic model do not correspond to those of a steady-state regime, several beats may need to be simulated before reaching a regime where there is negligible beat-to-beat variations. A numerical experiment was carried out to determine when this regime is reached. **Figure 4** shows superimposed consecutive simulated FPs and the normalized beat-to-beat variations in the FP. When considering noisy synthetic measurements as described above, the steady-state is assumed to be reached when the beat-to-beat variations are comparable to variations induced by noise only. The beat-to-beat variability observed after this beat may be imputed to the coarseness of the mesh, the time discretization errors and the fluctuations of the ionic model itself. In the present work, the steady-state is assumed to be reached at the second beat. Therefore, the simulations are run for two cardiac cycles and the second beat is recorded to be used as a synthetic measurement.

Drug Modeling

We chose to model the action of drugs on the ion channels by the conductance-block formulation of the pore block model (Bottino et al., 2006; Mirams et al., 2011; Zemzemi et al., 2013). This simple approach, which relies on a small number of parameters, was shown in Abbate et al. (2017) to be able to reproduce the expected effects of several drugs on MEA signals. The conductance of a

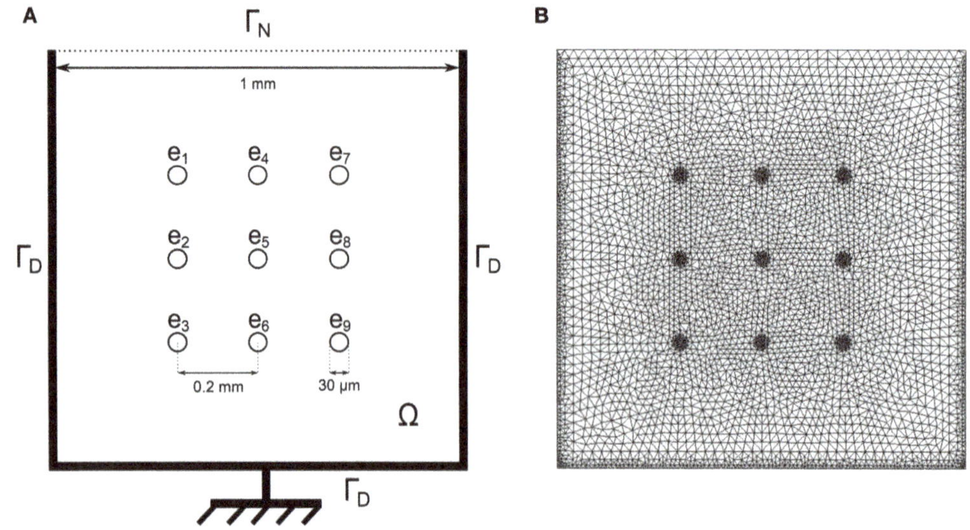

FIGURE 1 | (A) Schematic of one well of the nine-electrode MEA device. The bidomain equations are solved in the domain Ω with homogeneous Neumann boundary conditions on Γ_N: $\nabla\phi_e \cdot \vec{n} = 0$ and homogeneous Dirichlet boundary conditions on Γ_D: $\phi_e = 0$ where the ground is located. **(B)** Corresponding finite element mesh.

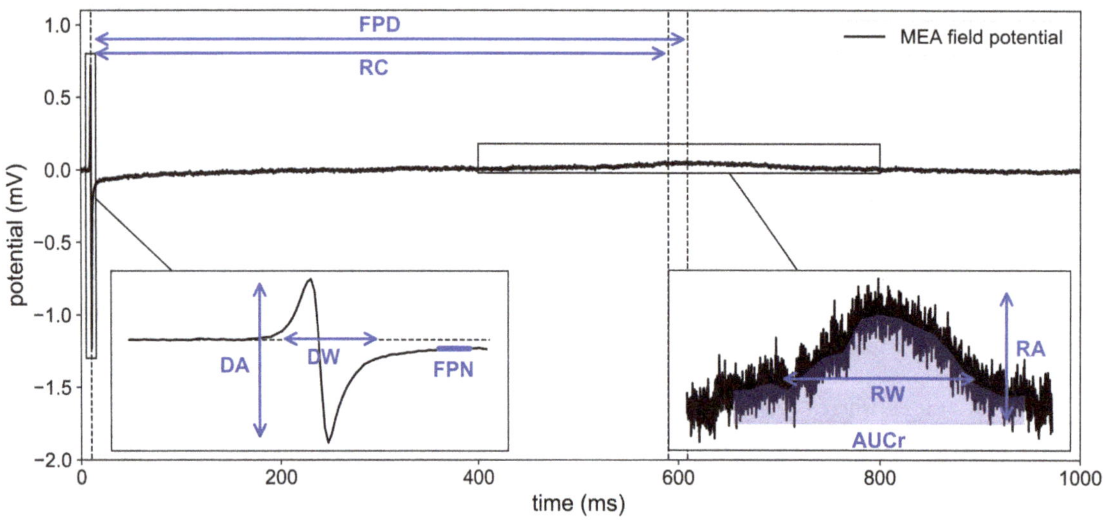

FIGURE 2 | Experimental recording of MEA field potential. Eight biomarkers are extracted from the time series: DA, depolarization amplitude; DW, depolarization width; RA, repolarization amplitude; FPD, field potential duration; AUCr, area under repolarization curve; RC, repolarizarion center; RW, repolarization width; FPN, field potential notch.

given channel s is given by:

$$g_s = g_{control,s}\left[1 + \left(\frac{[D]}{\mathrm{IC}_{50}}\right)^n\right]^{-1}, \quad (2)$$

where $g_{control,s}$ is the drug-free maximal conductance, $[D]$ is the drug concentration, IC_{50} is the value of the drug concentration at which the peak current is reduced of 50%, n is the Hill coefficient. In this work, n will be assumed to be equal to 1.

Heterogeneity Modeling

A typical experimental MEA FP measurement exhibits both a depolarization spike and a repolarization wave (see **Figure 2**). Using the computational model described above, the repolarization wave is usually too small compared to what is observed in experiments. As noted in Abbate et al. (2017), the repolarization wave provided by this model is larger when the domain includes cells with different APDs. In Abbate et al. (2017), the cell heterogeneity was defined on a checkerboard arbitrarily chosen in the MEA's well. We propose here a different approach, based on a probabilistic description of the

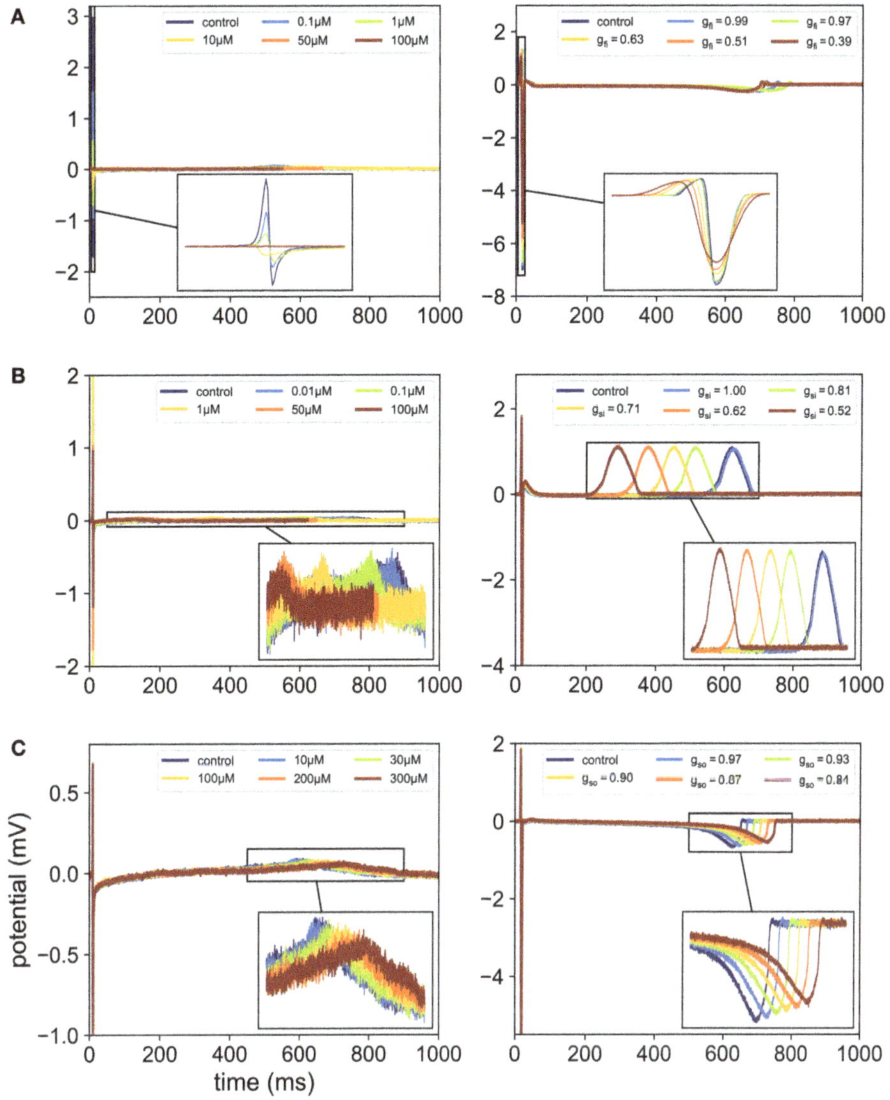

FIGURE 3 | Comparison between *in vitro* and *in silico* MEA FP recordings. In each case, the FPs are recorded in control conditions and for five different drug concentrations. For the *in silico* measurements, the drugs effects are modeled using Equation (2), which amounts to reducing g_{fi}, g_{si} or g_{so} depending on the ion channel affected by the drug. **(A)** Effect of flecainide (sodium antagonist drug) on experimental recordings (left) and effect of a virtual sodium antagonist drug on simulated MEA FPs (right). **(B)** Effect of diltiazem (assumed to be mainly calcium antagonist in this study) on experimental recordings (left) and effect of a virtual calcium antagonist drug on simulated MEA FPs (right). **(C)** Effect of moxifloxacin (potassium antagonist drug) on experimental recordings (left) and effect of a virtual potassium antagonist drug on simulated MEA FPs (right).

heterogeneity. The tissue is supposed to be a continuous mixture of two cell types: A and B. We make the assumption that the transition between these two types can be described by a single space dependent parameter $c(x, y)$ as follows:

$$\mathbf{p}(x,y) = (1 - c(x,y))\mathbf{p}^{(A)} + c(x,y)\mathbf{p}^{(B)}, \tag{3}$$

where c is a random process with values in $[0, 1]$ and $\mathbf{p}^{(A)}$ (resp. $\mathbf{p}^{(B)}$) the set of 19 parameters of the MV model corresponding to cell type A (resp. B). The values of $\mathbf{p}^{(A)}$ and $\mathbf{p}^{(B)}$ are given in Supplementary Table 1. The APs corresponding to different realizations of c are shown in **Figure 5**. We make the hypothesis that the spatial variations of c are structured by a normal correlation function f_c:

$$f_c\left[\begin{pmatrix}x\\y\end{pmatrix}, \begin{pmatrix}x'\\y'\end{pmatrix}\right] = \exp\left[-\frac{(x-x')^2 + (y-y')^2}{2l_c^2}\right], \tag{4}$$

where l_c is the correlation length, set to $l_c = 0.25$ mm in the present work. To discretize the random process c, we compute the correlation matrix on the finite element mesh used for the discretization of the bidomain equations. The correlation matrix

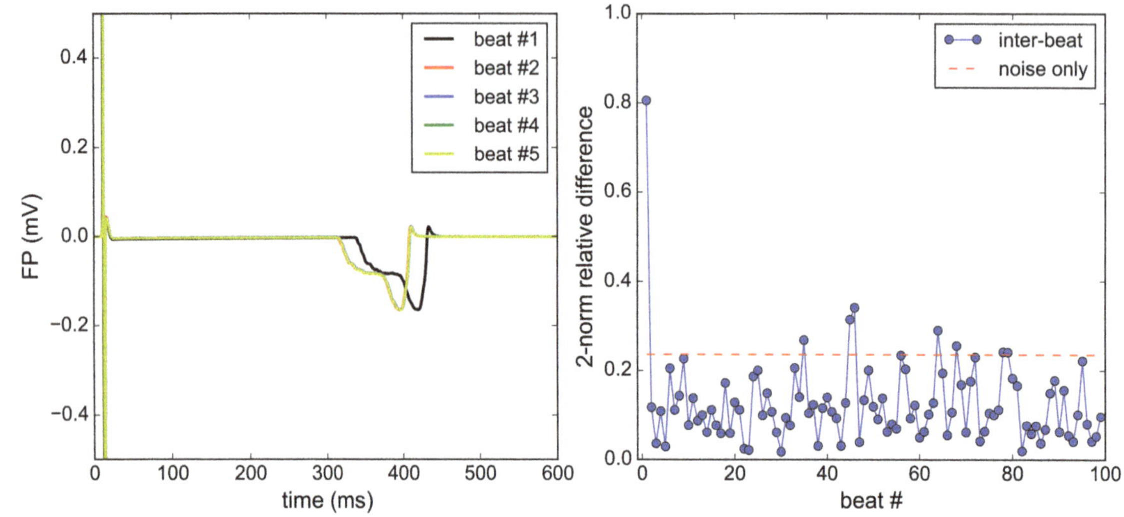

FIGURE 4 | Steady-state analysis: the Bidomain equations are solved for 100 consecutive beats. Qualitatively, a satisfactory steady state is reached at the second beat **(left)**. The beat-to-beat relative difference of the FP is monitored (right) and is to be compared to the relative difference between two identical solutions, each polluted by an independent noise **(right)**.

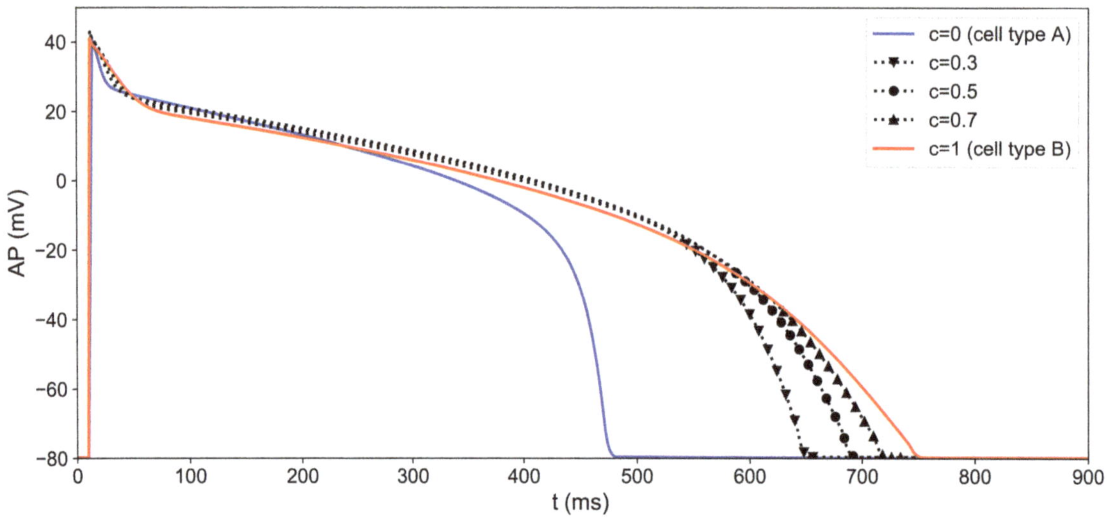

FIGURE 5 | Heterogeneity modeling: different APs obtained by simulating the MV model with different values of the heterogeneity parameter *c*. The heterogeneity parameter is a function of space and its pattern differs from one well to another (see **Figure 6**).

$\mathbf{C} = [C_{i,j}] \in \mathbb{R}^{N_{\text{mesh}} \times N_{\text{mesh}}}$ reads:

$$C_{i,j} = f_c\left[\begin{pmatrix}\hat{x}_i\\ \hat{y}_i\end{pmatrix}, \begin{pmatrix}\hat{x}_j\\ \hat{y}_j\end{pmatrix}\right], \tag{5}$$

where N_{mesh} is the total number of mesh nodes and $(\hat{x}_i, \hat{y}_i)$ are the coordinates of the ith node. The eigenpairs of $\mathbf{C}$ are denoted by (λ_i, Φ_i), and ordered by decreasing order of the eigenvalues λ_i. By a convenient abuse of notation, we denote by $(\hat{x}, \hat{y}) \rightarrow \Phi_i(\hat{x}, \hat{y})$ the function of the finite element space associated with the eigenmode Φ_i. Finally, the discretized heterogeneity field is approximated by the following truncated expansion:

$$c(\hat{x}, \hat{y}, \boldsymbol{\xi}) = \sum_{i=1}^{n_c} \xi_i \Phi_i(\hat{x}, \hat{y}) \tag{6}$$

where $\boldsymbol{\xi} = (\xi_i)_{i=1...n_c}$ is a random vector and n_c a truncation index chosen so that the truncation explains at least 99% of the variance. In other words, n_c is the smallest index n such that the following criterion is verified:

$$\frac{\sum_{i=1}^{n} \lambda_i}{\sum_{i=1}^{N_{\text{mesh}}} \lambda_i} > 0.99\,. \tag{7}$$

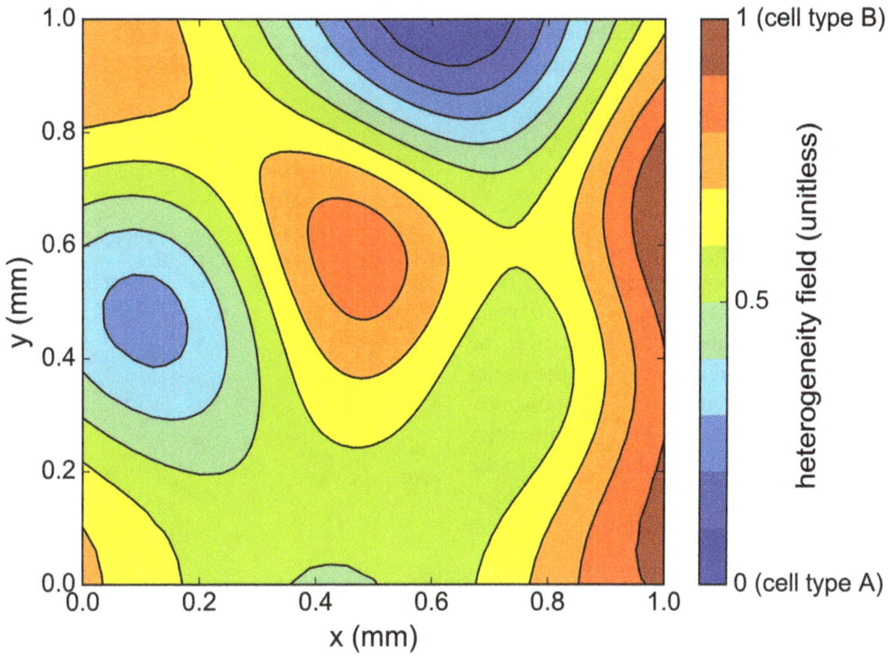

FIGURE 6 | One sample of cell heterogeneity field $c(x, y)$ generated using the correlation matrix method. As c ranges from 0 to 1, the cell action potential varies from that of cell type "A" to cell type "B" (see **Figure 5**).

In our case, the choice of l_c and the domain geometry yields $n_c = 14$. Heterogeneity fields can now be generated simply by sampling the random variable ξ. In the present work, $N_h = 128$ heterogeneity fields were generated by sampling ξ from an uncorrelated uniform distribution over $[-1, 1]^{n_c}$, and each sample is rescaled to range between 0 and 1. An example of heterogeneity field is presented in **Figure 6**.

The observed variations in the experimental MEA FP recordings are also attributable to fluctuations in the stimulation location. In practice, the hiPSC-CM are not electrically stimulated: a stimulus arises spontaneously in the medium, probably due to the presence of pacemaker cells. The location of the spontaneous stimulation is not known to the experimentalist. We make the assumption that the location is random and therefore model it with a random uniform law over the square $[0.15, 0.85]^2$ where $\Omega = [0, 1]^2$ is the complete domain.

To conclude, in a given experimental setting, we know neither the stimulation position nor the cell distribution inside the well and we would like the classification method to be robust with respect to all these unknown, random elements. This is why, when generating synthetic MEA FPs using our *in silico* model, we introduce two sources of uncertainty: the heterogeneous CM field and the stimulation location.

Biomarkers

Biomarkers may be defined as quantities extracted from a signal that convey information about hidden quantities of interest. In our case, the biomarkers are features extracted from the MEA FP which would ideally provide information about the conductances of interest: g_{fi}, g_{so}, g_{si}. In this section, we present different choices of biomarkers to be used in a classification context.

"Classical" Biomarkers

The MEA FP can be split into two regions of interest: the depolarization and the repolarization. The depolarization observed at one electrode corresponds to the local depolarization of the cardiomyocytes. The depolarization amplitude (DA, referred to as spike amplitude in Clements and Thomas, 2014) may be qualitatively linked to the AP upstroke velocity. This biomarker is commonly associated with the activity of the fast sodium channel (g_{fi} for the MV model). The repolarization amplitude (RA) may be qualitatively linked to some extent to the AP repolarization slope and to a bigger extent to spatial heterogeneities in AP durations. Once the depolarization and repolarization have been detected, it is possible to measure the FP duration (FPD), simply as the difference between the repolarization and depolarization times. The FPD is a commonly used biomarker (Navarrete et al., 2013; Clements and Thomas, 2014) which may be seen as a surrogate for APD in patch clamp experiments and QT interval in electrocardiograms. Both biomarkers RA and FPD are associated with the activity of the potassium and calcium currents (g_{so} and g_{si} in the MV model). As explained above, each (real or numerical) experiment is performed both in drug-block conditions and in control condition. Because of the significant variability of measurements in MEA, it is important to consider the variations observed in the FP in drug block conditions with respect to the control conditions to isolate the effect of the drug from other sources of variability: tissue variability, stimulation protocol, etc. Therefore, as proposed in Raphel et al. (2017), the features of interest are the biomarkers in drug block condition divided by the biomarkers in control conditions. For instance, the depolarization amplitude is actually the following ratio:

$$\mathrm{DA}_{\mathrm{ratio}} = \frac{\mathrm{DA}_{\mathrm{drug}}}{\mathrm{DA}_{\mathrm{control}}} \tag{8}$$

For the sake of clarity in the notation, the subscript "ratio" is omitted in the following and any biomarker actually refers to a ratio with the control value. For each MEA measurement, the FP is recorded at each of the nine electrodes. Again, the important variability in the measurements motivates the use of robust features. Since the behavior of the FP may greatly vary from one electrode to another, the median of the biomarkers over all electrodes is in practice a good choice of features. In the following, the set of biomarkers $\{\tilde{\mathrm{DA}}, \tilde{\mathrm{RA}}, \tilde{\mathrm{FPD}}\}$ is referred to as the classical biomarkers, where the $\tilde{}$ operator denotes the median over all nine electrodes.

Composite Biomarkers

The rationale behind the choice of biomarkers described above is only qualitative and oftentimes does not represent the best set of features in a classification context. Here, we adopt a more automatic strategy to select the best set of biomarkers for a given experimental scenario. First, the set of features to be extracted from a given FP is enriched with other features.

It is indeed possible to extract additional quantities from the FP other than DA, RA, and FPD. We propose to compute also, for each electrode of the MEA, the following features: the area under curve of the repolarization wave (AUCr), the repolarization center (RC), the repolarization width (RW), the FP notch (FPN), and the depolarization width (DW). The details on how to compute these additional biomarkers are described in Appendix A (Supplementary Material) and illustrated in **Figure 2**. Ratios of these quantities are also added to the dictionary of features: RA/DA, DA/RA, RA/FPD, FPD/RA, DA/FPD, FPD/DA, RA/RW, RW/RA. Each feature is actually a ratio with its control counterpart as described in Equation (8). To include the information of all nine electrodes, the median (denoted by the $\tilde{}$ operator), mean (denoted by the <> operator) and maximum values (denoted by a max subscript) over the electrodes are retained in the dictionary. We finally add the conduction velocity (CV) which is not an electrode-wise quantity but defined using all nine electrodes signals as explained in Appendix A (Supplementary Material). This amounts to a total of $N_b = 41$ features reported in **Table 2**. The extended set of features is referred to as the dictionary or the biomarkers dictionary. Each biomarker is referred to as an entry, denoted by b_j, $1 \leq j \leq N_b$, in the following.

Before going into further details about the numerical methods, let us now explain the purpose of the composite biomarkers. The purpose of the method is to associate each conductance g_{fi}, g_{si}, g_{so} with a composite biomarker that is maximally correlated with it and minimally correlated with the others. For instance, the composite biomarker, denoted by y_1, associated with g_{fi} is maximally correlated with g_{fi} while being minimally correlated with g_{si} and g_{so}. The main idea is that by observing y_1 we have good information about the hidden variations of g_{fi} which is not tampered by simultaneous variations of g_{si} or g_{so}. The composite biomarkers are defined as weighted linear combinations of the dictionary entries. We also require that the weights are sparse, meaning there are a lot of zero weights. This makes the composite biomarkers more easily interpretable. Indeed, they can be seen as a combination of only a small subset of the dictionary entries, ideally including the classical biomarkers as seen in **Figure 7**.

TABLE 2 | Indices of the biomarkers dictionary entries.

Index (median)	Index (mean)	Index (max)	Entry
0	8		DA
1	9		RA
2	10		FPD
3	11		$\mathrm{AUC_r}$
4	12		RC
5	13		RW
6	14		FPN
7	15		DW
16	24	32	RA/DA
17	25	33	DA/RA
18	26	34	RA/FPD
19	27	35	FPD/RA
20	28	36	DA/FPD
21	29	37	FPD/DA
22	30	38	RA/RW
23	31	39	RW/RA
	40		CV

The weights of such a combination are solution of an optimization problem. First, let us introduce some notation. We denote by y_1 (resp. y_2, y_3) the composite biomarker (to be determined) associated with g_{fi} (resp. g_{si}, g_{so}). From now on, the conductances (g_{fi}, g_{si}, g_{so}) are denoted by $\boldsymbol{\theta} = (\theta_1, \theta_2, \theta_3)$. Each dictionary entry is considered as a function of $\boldsymbol{\theta}$. The composite biomarkers are sought as a linear combination of the dictionary entries:

$$y_h(\boldsymbol{\theta}) = \sum_{j=1}^{N_b} w_j^{(h)} b_j(\boldsymbol{\theta}), \quad 1 \leq h \leq 3, \tag{9}$$

where the weights $\boldsymbol{w}^{(h)} = (w_j^{(h)}) \in \mathbb{R}^{N_b}$ are the unknowns of the problem. These weights are sought so that $y_h(\boldsymbol{\theta})$ is maximally correlated with θ_h and minimally correlated with $\theta_k, \forall k \neq h$. This may be stated as follows:

$$\forall h \in \{1, \ldots, 3\}, \quad \begin{cases} \max\limits_{y_h} \quad \mathrm{cov}\left(y_h(\boldsymbol{\theta}), \theta_h\right) & (10a) \\ \min\limits_{y_h} \quad \left|\mathrm{cov}\left(y_h(\boldsymbol{\theta}), \theta_k\right)\right|, \quad \forall k \neq h & (10b) \\ \text{s.t.} \quad \mathrm{var}\left(y_h(\boldsymbol{\theta})\right) = 1 & (10c) \end{cases}$$

where $\mathrm{cov}(\cdot,\cdot)$ and $\mathrm{var}(\cdot)$ are respectively the covariance and variance operators. In the following, we assume that each

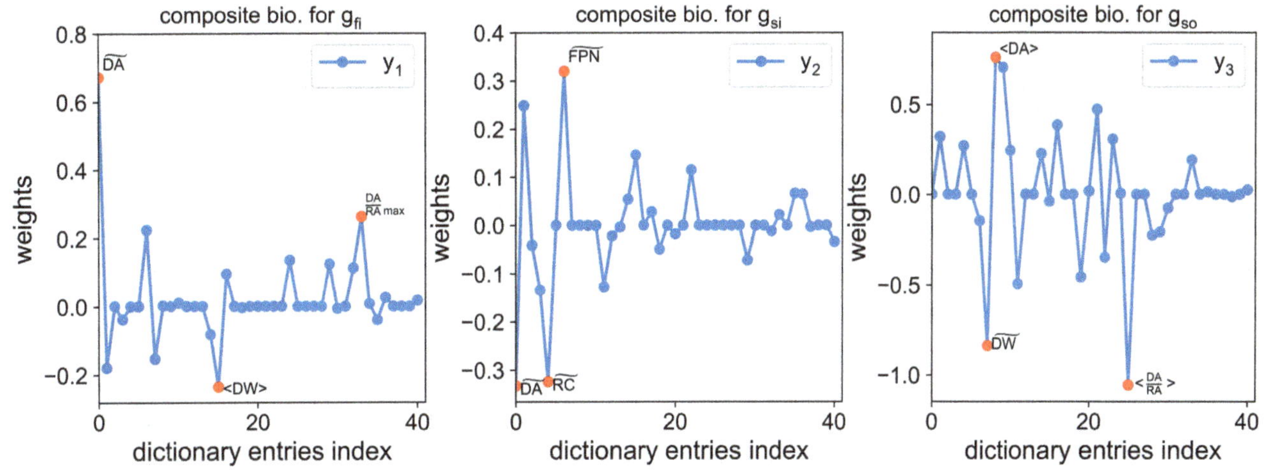

FIGURE 7 | Example of composite biomarkers weights. The three highest weights (in absolute value) are highlighted by a red dot for each composite biomarker. Note that some classical biomarkers are selected by the method: $\tilde{DA}$ for g_{fi}, $\tilde{RC}$ (closely related to the FPD) for g_{si} and RA in the ratio (DA/RA) for g_{so}.

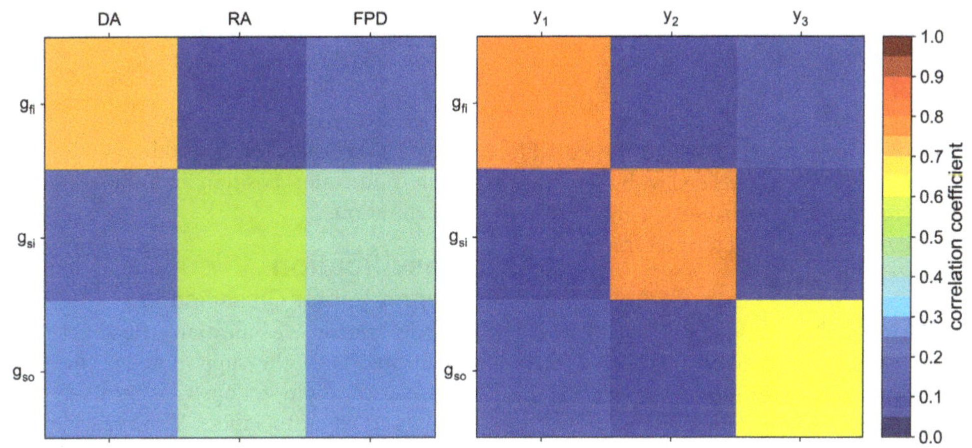

FIGURE 8 | Correlation matrix of the conductances of interest with the "classical" biomarkers **(Left)** and with the composite biomarkers **(Right)**.

component of $\boldsymbol{\theta}$ is a zero-mean unit-variance random variable. This is achieved in practice by a simple rescaling of the conductances samples. We also adopt the following notation:

$$\tilde{b}_j(\boldsymbol{\theta}) = b_j(\boldsymbol{\theta}) - \mathbb{E}\left[b_j(\boldsymbol{\theta})\right], \tag{11}$$

where $\mathbb{E}\left[\cdot\right]$ is the expectation operator. The problem may now be recast into an optimization problem where the cost function to be minimized reads:

$$\mathcal{J}(\boldsymbol{w}^{(h)}) = \mathcal{J}_C(\boldsymbol{w}^{(h)}) + \mathcal{J}_N(\boldsymbol{w}^{(h)}) + \mathcal{J}_P(\boldsymbol{w}^{(h)}), \tag{12}$$

where

$$\mathcal{J}_C(\boldsymbol{w}^{(h)}) = \frac{1}{2}\|\mathbf{C}\boldsymbol{w}^{(h)} - \mathbf{e}^{(h)}\|^2 \text{ where } C_{kj} := \mathbb{E}(\theta_k\tilde{b}_j),\ e_k^{(h)} := \delta_{kh}, \tag{13a}$$

$$\mathcal{J}_N(\boldsymbol{w}^{(h)}) = \frac{\xi}{2}\left(\boldsymbol{w}^{(h)T}\mathbf{G}\boldsymbol{w}^{(h)} - 1\right)^2 \text{ where } G_{ij} := \mathbb{E}(\tilde{b}_i\tilde{b}_j), \tag{13b}$$

$$\mathcal{J}_P(\boldsymbol{w}^{(h)}) = \frac{\lambda_h}{N_b}\|\boldsymbol{w}^{(h)}\|_1. \tag{13c}$$

Let us now explain each term of Equation (13). $\mathcal{J}_C(\boldsymbol{w}^{(h)})$ corresponds to Equations (10a,b). It measures the discrepancy to the ideal situation where $\text{cov}\left(y_h(\boldsymbol{\theta}), \theta_h\right) = 1$ and $\text{cov}\left(y_h(\boldsymbol{\theta}), \theta_k\right) = 0, \forall k \neq h$.

$\mathcal{J}_N(\boldsymbol{w}^{(h)})$ is a relaxation of the constraint in Equation (10c). ξ is a regularization parameter that is set to 1 in practice.

$\mathcal{J}_P(\boldsymbol{w}^{(h)})$ is a regularization term by penalization of the 1-norm of $\boldsymbol{w}^{(h)}$, where λ_h, $1 \leq h \leq 3$, are regularization parameters. ℓ_1 penalized cost functions tend to promote sparse solutions (Tibshirani, 1996). Sparse solutions for $\boldsymbol{w}^{(h)}$ are interesting in that they offer a more interpretable decomposition onto the dictionary entries (since most weights are zero) than what an ℓ_2 penalization would yield.

We now discretize the problem by considering N samples of the parameters $\boldsymbol{\theta}$ drawn over a parameter space $\Theta \subset \mathbb{R}^3$. The expectation operator is approximated using a quasi-Monte-Carlo quadrature rule and the cost function in Equation (12) is minimized using a Nesterov accelerated gradient descent (O'Donoghue and Candes, 2015). The Monte-Carlo samples may come from synthetic or experimental measurements. For synthetic measurements, the conductances are known, but this is not the case for experimental measurements. In that case, an approximation of these conductances is computed using Equation (2). Note that the solution weights depend strongly on the choice of samples used for the Monte-Carlo approximations.

An example of the obtained weights is shown in **Figure 7**. Interestingly, the classical biomarkers are still among the most weighted features. The correlation between the conductances of interest and the composite biomarkers is compared to the correlation with the classical biomarkers in **Figure 8**. The correlation between two quantities u and v is defined as follows:

$$\mathrm{cor}(u, v) = \frac{\mathrm{cov}(u, v)}{\sqrt{\mathrm{var}(u)\mathrm{var}(v)}}. \qquad (14)$$

As expected, each composite biomarker is well correlated with its associated conductance whereas uncorrelated with the others. This is not the case for the classical biomarkers. The results in the next section show that such a choice of features improves the classification performance.

Experimental Data Set

The MEA considered in the present work is a 6-well MEA with nine electrodes per well. Its geometry as well as the corresponding finite element mesh is shown in **Figure 1**. The MEA measurements come in the form of FP recordings corresponding to the different electrodes of the different wells of the MEA. These recordings come in the form of time series where several cardiac cycles, or beats, are recorded. The time resolution of the MEA recordings is 10 kHz. We extracted several beats on each electrode from each well of the MEA. Data were provided by Janssen Pharmaceutica NV using MC_Rack (Multi Channel Systems GmbH) and post-processed by NOTOCORD Systems (NOTOCORD-FPS 3.0 software). The hiPSC-CM used in this study are a commercially available line of cells (iCell Cardiomyocytes) and were provided by the CDI (Cellular Dynamics International) company.

After thawing, the hiPSC-CM were precultivated for 7 days before being plated on the MEA. Then the cells were cultivated again from 6 to 7 days. Prior to the experiments, the cells rested for 15 min inside the MEA. The recordings come in series of 2 min each and a wash-in period of 5 min was allocated before changing compound concentrations. Up to two different hiPSC-CM cultures were used and each experiment was repeated from 5 to 12 times.

As explained earlier the recordings were made in control conditions (no drug) and with different drugs at different concentrations levels. **Figure 3** shows examples of experimental recordings in control conditions and with five different concentrations of flecainide, diltiazem and moxifloxacin. The drugs used for the present study are summarized in **Table 3**. The corresponding concentrations are presented in **Table 4**. The IC_{50} values that were used in the study are also reported and are in the range of those reported in Crumb et al. (2016). Note that the diltiazem was recorded in two different wells (A and B) since it was the only calcium-antagonist drug in the experimental data that were made available to the authors. The experimental process consists in adding five times a compound at increasing concentrations in a given well. Thus, including the control condition record, we finally obtain field potentials for six contexts in each well. Equation (2) was used to obtain an approximation of the conductances values associated with the experimental measurements which are needed for the composite biomarkers calculations. The Hill coefficients and IC_{50} values are given in the Supplementary Material of Kramer et al. (2013) and Mirams et al. (2011). Concerning the dictionary of features, a few adjustments need to be made in some cases. Indeed, it appears that at some high concentration levels of mexiletine, there is simply no action potential (because the sodium channels are too blocked) and therefore the field potential is a flat line. To take this into account, the values of dictionary entries are set to the ones at the last concentration where an action potential was observed. In addition, all features where DA is in the numerator position in a ratio are set to zero for this concentration.

Classification

Support Vector Classification

Support vector classification (Boser et al., 1992) (SVC) is an adaptation of the support vector machine (SVM) method in a classification setting. Classification generally consists in attributing labels to inputs. The available data set, comprising both inputs and labels, is generally split into a training set used to build the classifier and a validation set to test the classifier. The inputs are often multidimensional and in our case

TABLE 3 | Repartition of the available (experimental and synthetic) data set.

Drug name	Blocked ionic channel	Associated conductance	ID	SVC class label	# Experiments
Mexiletine	Sodium	g_{fi}	0	0	160
Flecainide	Sodium	g_{fi}	1	0	120
Diltiazem A	Calcium	g_{si}	2	1	160
Diltiazem B	Calcium	g_{si}	3	1	160
Moxifloxacin	Potassium	g_{so}	4	2	120
Dofetilide	Potassium	g_{so}	5	2	160
Synth. A	Sodium	g_{fi}	6	0	155
Synth. B	Calcium	g_{si}	7	1	155
Synth. C	Potassium	g_{so}	8	2	155

The ID is used in the data set splitting (see ***Table 5****). The SVC class label corresponds to the associated blocked channel conductance.*

TABLE 4 | Summary of the drugs information constituting the experimental measurement set.

Concentration index	Mexiletine	Flecainide	Diltiazem	Moxifloxacin	Dofetilide
1	0.01 μM	0.1 μM	0.01 μM	10.0 μM	0.1 nM
2	0.1 μM	1.0 μM	0.1 μM	30.0 μM	1.0 nM
3	1.0 μM	10.0 μM	1.0 μM	100.0 μM	10.0 nM
4	10.0 μM	50.0 μM	5.0 μM	200.0 μM	50.0 nM
5	50.0 μM	100.0 μM	10.0 μM	300.0 μM	100.0 nM
Main channel blocked	Sodium	Sodium	Calcium	Potassium	Potassium
IC_{50}	43.0 μM	6.2 μM	0.75(or 0.45) μM	86.2 μM	30.0(or 5.0) nM

Five concentrations were studied for each drug. The IC_{50} values are reported as well as the main channel blocked by each drug (in the scope of the single channel block assumption).

correspond to the biomarkers, whether classical or composite. The labels are integers that represent the classes to which the inputs are assigned. These classes are mutually exclusive, meaning one sample can only belong to a single class. SVC belongs to the so-called supervised methods since the labels are known, at least for the training set. The main idea behind SVC is to maximize the margin between the inputs and the decision boundary (Boser et al., 1992). In the linear case, the decision boundary is a hyperplane of the input space. In general, however, this is not sufficient to properly separate the samples according to their classes. A common way to obtain more complex boundary decisions is to use a so-called "kernel trick" (Schölkopf and Smola, 2002) which is based on a mapping from the input space to a higher-dimensional space where the existence of a separating hyperplane is more likely. In the present case, the labels are "sodium antagonist," "calcium antagonist," and "potassium antagonist," respectively associated with labels 0, 1, and 2. Among various possible choices of kernels, a Gaussian kernel is employed in this work.

We used a Python implementation of SVC through the Scikit-learn (Pedregosa et al., 2011) machine learning library which itself uses the LIBSVM library (Chang and Lin, 2011). For a given training set, a so-called classifier is built. The classifier is then called to predict the labels of the validation set samples. The predictions are finally compared to the true labels. There exist several metrics to quantify the prediction quality. Two different metrics are considered here: the Cohen's kappa and the receiver operating characteristic area under curve (AUC). The Cohen's kappa is a single scalar designed to measure the performance of multi-class classifiers. Its value ranges from −1 (worst possible classifier) to 1 (perfect classifier), 0 corresponding to a coin-flip classifier. The AUC is defined for each class and measures how a classifier performs with respect to a given class. Its value ranges from 0 (worst) to 1 (best), 0.5 being a coin-flip. Because the classification is repeated several times with different data set splittings, the classification metrics are summarized using their means and standard deviations. The "averaged AUC" corresponds to the average of all AUCs (one AUC per class).

Both metrics are described in detail in the Supplementary Material. We now present two different strategies to employ SVC in the context of drug classification.

3-vs.-3 classification

Since there are three distinct classes in the experimental set, those three classes need to be included in the training set, preferably in equal proportions. The strategy of 3-vs.-3 (3v3) classification consists in dividing the experimental set into a training set and validation set that both include samples from the three classes. Each class is divided into two sub-classes. This is naturally done for the sodium and potassium antagonist classes since they are each comprised of data from two different drugs. For the calcium antagonist class, the diltiazem data is artificially split into two drugs "diltiazem A" and "diltiazem B" (see **Table 3**). Each subclass is associated with an identification number (ID) from 0 to 5. Therefore, there are 8 possible choices for the training and validation set combinations as summarized in **Table 5**.

One-vs.-all classification

The One-vs.-All (OvA) classification strategy consists in training one classifier for each class. For each class *j*, the training set labels are modified to take the value 1 for samples in class *j* and 0 otherwise and a classifier is trained on this relabeled training set. In other words, the classifier for class *j* is only trained to recognize whether or not a sample belongs to class *j*. For the validation step, the classifiers do not predict a class label but a probability for a given sample to be in their respective class. Each sample of the validation step goes through each of the three classifiers and the predicted class corresponds to the classifier returning the highest probability. The splitting between training and validation sets is done in the same way as in the 3-vs.-3 classification strategy.

RESULTS

Comparison between Classical and Composite Biomarkers

Here the performance of the composite biomarkers in a classification context is compared to that of the classical biomarkers for two different classification strategies. The data set is composed of 880 experiments, each counting one control measurement and 5 measurements at different drug concentration levels. For each experiment, the conductances values and FP features are computed as explained in the Methods section and the labels are defined according to **Table 3**. The classification results are summarized in the following and more detailed results may be found in Supplementary Tables 3, 4.

TABLE 5 | Different possible splittings of the experimental data set.

Splitting index	0	1	2	3	4	5	6	7
Training set IDs	{0, 2, 4}	{0, 2, 5}	{0, 3, 4}	{0, 3, 5}	{1, 2, 4}	{1, 2, 5}	{1, 3, 4}	{1, 3, 5}
Validation set IDs	{1, 3, 5}	{1, 3, 4}	{1, 2, 5}	{1, 2, 4}	{0, 3, 5}	{0, 3, 4}	{0, 2, 5}	{0, 2, 4}

The statistical significance of the potential improvements in the classification scores attributable to the use of composite biomarkers is studied using an analysis of variance (ANOVA) with a significance level of 0.05.

3v3 Classification

The performance of the composite biomarkers compared to the classical ones is evaluated using the 3v3 classification strategy. The classification procedure is carried out for each different splitting of the data set as summarized in **Table 5**. First, the classification inputs are the 3 classical biomarkers for each drug concentration level:

$$\left\{\tilde{DA}_{c1}, \tilde{RA}_{c1}, \tilde{FPD}_{c1}, \ldots, \tilde{DA}_{c5}, \tilde{RA}_{c5}, \tilde{FPD}_{c5}\right\}, \quad (15)$$

where c_k is the k-th concentration level. Then, the classification inputs are the composite biomarkers for each concentration, computed as explained in the Methods section using the classification training set as samples for the Monte-Carlo approximations. The inputs now read:

$$\left\{y_{1,c1}, y_{2,c1}, y_{3,c_1}, \ldots, y_{1,c5}, y_{2,c5}, y_{3,c_5}\right\}. \quad (16)$$

In both cases, the inputs are therefore of dimension 15. Note that for each splitting of the data set, new weights for the composite biomarkers are computed. The classification procedure is carried out in both cases and the results are summarized in **Table 6**. Regardless of the chosen classification score, the results are significantly better using the composite biomarkers as inputs.

OvA Classification

The same procedure as in the 3v3 case is applied to the OvA strategy. The classification procedure is carried out with both classical and composite biomarkers as inputs and the results are summarized in **Table 7**. The prediction of slow outward current block is significantly improved using the composite biomarkers as inputs. Furthermore, the results are overall better when using the OvA approach rather than the 3v3 one.

In the next section, the addition of synthetic measurements in the computation of the composite biomarkers is investigated. To test whether potential improvements are due to the nature of the added data and not to the increase in the size of the data set, the classification framework was applied to a smaller data set of 440 experiments (i.e., half of the previous data set) for which the results are reported in Supplementary Tables 5, 6. The conclusions of this additional study being similar, this suggests that the classification results are weakly impacted by the size of the data set.

TABLE 6 | Comparison between classical and composite biomarkers with the 3v3 classification strategy.

Score	Classical biomarkers		Composite biomarkers	
	Mean	Std.	Mean	Std.
Cohen's kappa	0.27	0.16	$0.56^{+,*}$	0.25
g_{fi} AUC	0.74	0.15	$0.90^{+,*}$	0.09
g_{si} AUC	0.98	0.01	$1.00^{+,*}$	0.00
g_{so} AUC	0.69	0.04	$0.84^{+,*}$	0.04
Averaged AUC	0.80	–	0.92	–

*Variation (+increase, −decrease) in the classification scores attributable to the composite biomarkers. ANOVA study: *significant at the 0.05 probability level.*

TABLE 7 | Comparison between classical and composite biomarkers. Classification scores in the one-vs.-all scenario.

Score	Classical biomarkers		Composite biomarkers	
	Mean	Std.	Mean	Std.
Cohen's kappa	0.44	0.24	$0.54^{+,\dagger}$	0.24
g_{fi} AUC	0.83	0.10	$0.74^{-,\dagger}$	0.24
g_{si} AUC	0.89	0.10	$0.94^{+,\dagger}$	0.07
g_{so} AUC	0.77	0.13	$0.92^{+,*}$	0.08
Averaged AUC	0.83	–	0.87	–

*Variation (+increase, −decrease) in the classification scores attributable to the composite biomarkers. ANOVA study: *significant at the 0.05 probability level, †non-significant at the 0.05 probability level.*

Using Combined Experimental and Synthetic Measurements for the Composite Biomarkers Computation

Having established that composite biomarkers outperform classical ones in two different classification scenarios, we now investigate the addition of synthetic measurements for the computation of the composite biomarkers weights. To enrich the set of experimental samples used to compute the composite biomarkers, a set of synthetic measurements is built. First, conductances samples are chosen to mimic the effect of drugs as shown in **Figure 9**. Depending on the most affected conductance, these samples are associated with a synthetic sodium (resp. calcium and potassium) antagonist drug called "synth A" (resp. B and C). 775 samples per drug are chosen which amounts to 155 experiments per drug. and their repartition is summarized in **Table 3**. This approximately corresponds to a 50/50% split between experimental and synthetic measurements. For each conductance sample, the computational model described in the

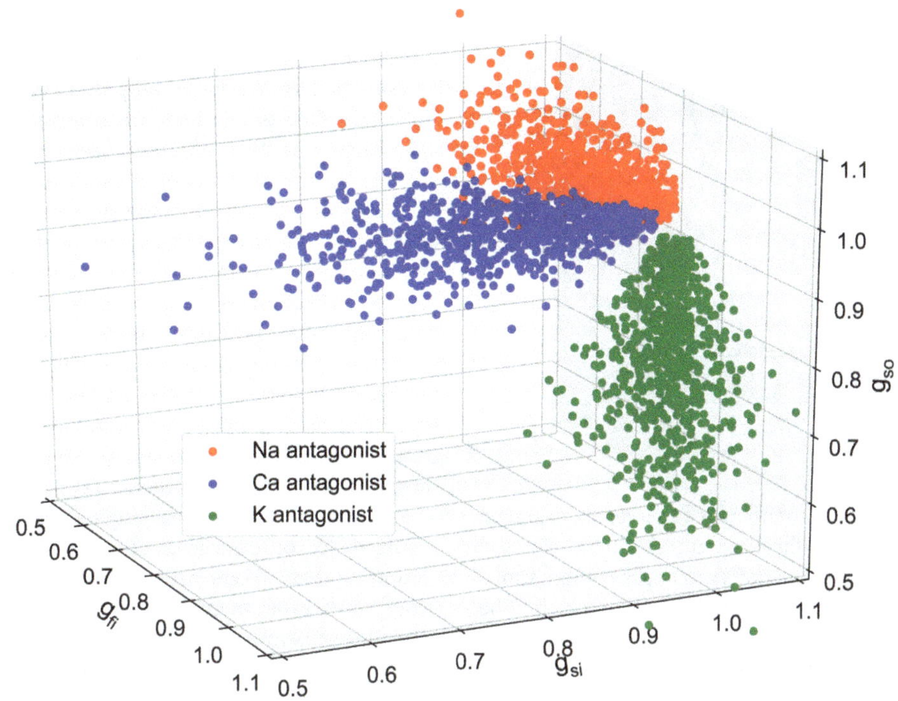

FIGURE 9 | Plot of the 2,325 *in silico* conductances samples. Three populations of 155 virtual drugs were generated according to their ion channel targets: sodium antagonist drugs (red), calcium antagonist (blue) and potassium antagonist (green). For each drug, 5 different concentrations are considered which correspond to 5 different set of conductances. These conductances are then used as inputs to generate *in silico* MEA measurements using the bidomain equations.

Methods section is evaluated and the dictionary entries are computed from the simulated FPs. For each experiment, the computational model is also evaluated in control conditions, i.e., with $g_{fi} = g_{si} = g_{so} = 1$ in order to compute the ratios as defined in Equation (8). The *in silico* measurements are incorporated in the experimental set to create an augmented set. This augmented set is then used to compute the composite biomarkers weights. The same data set splitting procedure as described before is carried out. Note that the synthetic measurements are only used for the composite biomarkers computation and are included neither in the training set nor in the validation set. Again, two classification strategies are explored.

Classification Results

The classification is carried out using both 3v3 and OvA approaches. The results are summarized in **Tables 8**, **9** and reported in detail in Supplementary Tables 4, 7. The statistical significance of the modifications in the classification scores standard deviations attributable to the use of synthetic data is assessed using the *F*-test with a significance level of 0.05.

In the 3v3 case, the Cohen's kappa standard deviation is significantly decreased when using the mixed set of experiments and synthetic data. In the OvA case, the standard deviation of the g_{si} AUC is significantly decreased while that of the g_{so} AUC is increased.

TABLE 8 | Comparison between composite biomarkers computed from experiments only and combined experiments and synthetic measurements.

	Experiments only		Experiments + synthetic	
Score	Mean	Std.	Mean	Std.
Cohen's kappa	0.56	0.25	0.59	$0.10^{-,*}$
g_{fi} AUC	0.90	0.09	0.89	$0.06^{-,\dagger}$
g_{si} AUC	1.00	0.00	1.00	$0.00^{=}$
g_{so} AUC	0.84	0.04	0.85	$0.06^{+,\dagger}$
Averaged AUC	0.92	–	0.91	–

3v3 classification strategy.
Variation ($^{+}$increase, $^{-}$decrease) in the classification scores standard deviations attributable to the use of numerical simulations in the composite biomarkers computation.
*F-test of variances: *significant at the 0.05 probability level, †non-significant at the 0.05 probability level, $^{=}$no variation.*

DISCUSSION

In this study, a framework for an automatic classification of drugs from MEA measurements has been presented. The framework relies on an *in silico* model of a MEA device, on a feature selection algorithm and on state-of-the-art machine learning tools. The *in silico* model is a PDE model (the bidomain equations) coupled with an ionic model that describes the transmembrane current of the cardiomyocytes. The ionic model is a phenomenological model consisting of a set of coupled non-linear ODEs. The feature selection algorithm proposes a way to compute a so-called

TABLE 9 | Comparison between composite biomarkers computed from experiments only and combined experiments and synthetic measurements.

	Experiments only		Experiments + synthetic	
Score	Mean	Std.	Mean	Std.
Cohen's kappa	0.54	0.24	0.63	$0.19^{-,\dagger}$
g_{fi} AUC	0.74	0.24	0.81	$0.14^{-,\dagger}$
g_{si} AUC	0.94	0.07	0.99	$0.01^{-,*}$
g_{so} AUC	0.92	0.08	0.81	$0.17^{+,*}$
averaged AUC	0.87	–	0.87	–

OvA classification strategy.
*Variation (+ increase, − decrease) in the classification scores standard deviations attributable to the use of numerical simulations in the composite biomarkers computation. F-test of variances: * significant at the 0.05 probability level, † non-significant at the 0.05 probability level.*

composite biomarker for each conductance of interest, designed to perform better in a classification context than classical biomarkers. The composite biomarkers are linear combinations of the entries of a dictionary of features which is given. The calculation of the weights involves Monte-Carlo approximations which use experimental or synthetic (or both) conductances and FP samples. It has been applied to drug classification problems using experimental MEA recordings. The classification was carried out using the Scikit-Learn Python library (Pedregosa et al., 2011) which includes several classification tools. In the present work a Support Vector Classification was used. The data used for the classification consist in FP features extracted from experimental measurements and their associated labels corresponding to the type of drug that is considered.

The purpose of the present work is twofold. First, it intends to establish that the classically used biomarkers may be improved, at least in a classification context, by using composite biomarkers instead. Second, it intends to show that the classification performance may benefit from the addition of synthetic measurements in the calculation of the composite biomarkers. More generally, the authors intend to show that numerical simulations are useful to cardiac electrophysiology in general, beyond the sole scope of drug classification.

First, a comparison between classical and composite biomarkers was carried out. The comparison consists in classifying drugs from experimental measurements using two different strategies: 3v3 and OvA. For each strategy, the classification is performed using classical or composite biomarkers as inputs. As expected, the classification results in both cases are improved when using the composite biomarkers. The latter were indeed designed to be maximally correlated to their associated conductance and minimally correlated to the others. As a consequence, they are more revealing of the underlying conductances than the classical biomarkers. In the 3v3 case, all classification scores significantly increase when using composite biomarkers instead of classical ones. In the OvA case, the improvement is less clear, mainly because most variations in the classification scores are not statistically significant. Nevertheless, the improvement is significant for the g_{so} AUC and overall the OvA strategy yields better classification results than the 3v3 strategy.

Second, the use of combined experimental and synthetic measurements to compute composite biomarkers is investigated. The composite biomarkers are computed using Monte-Carlo approximations that require conductances and FP features samples. In the previous case, these samples are experimental. The idea is to improve the robustness of the composite biomarkers by incorporating synthetic measurements which better span the parameters (i.e., conductances) space. This approach is meant to compensate the scarcity of experimental data and more generally the fact that the experiments do not cover every possible drug block scenario. The *in silico* measurements allow for a more thorough exploration of the parameter space. Conductances samples were drawn and the computational model was evaluated to generate noisy FPs. From these FPs, the entries of the dictionary of features were computed. The composite biomarkers weights are then computed using a mixed set of experimental and synthetic samples. These composite biomarkers are compared to the ones computed using only experimental data. The same two classification strategies as before are used to compare both approaches. In the 3v3 case, the standard deviation of the Cohen's kappa is significantly decreased, which suggests that this approach makes the classification more robust, at least when considering this metric. The variations of the other classification scores are not statistically significant. In the OvA case, the Cohen's kappa seems to increase in average while its standard deviation decreases. This finding must however be mitigated by the fact that it is not statistically significant. As for the AUC scores, the same observation can be made concerning the g_{fi} AUC. The standard deviation of the g_{si} AUC is significantly decreased but the standard deviation of the g_{so} AUC is increased. Overall, the use of mixed experimental and synthetic measurements seems to improve the classification and make it more robust even though the statistical significance of the results is not conclusive. The use of a larger experimental data set could help assessing the statistical significance of the previous findings.

The use of FP features in a classification context is now discussed. In classification problems, and in machine learning in general, a large number of inputs tend to provoke an over-fitting of the model. This means that the classifier tends to have satisfactory training scores but generalizes poorly on a validation test. This is in part solved by the regularization used but the number of inputs still remains important. When dealing with experimentally recorded FPs, the different signals are often not perfectly synchronized, making timestep-wise comparisons meaningless. Furthermore, an important variability of the signal amplitudes is observed in practice, making even perfectly synchronized signals difficult to compare. Using features extracted from the FP that are do not depend on time shifts and amplitude variations are therefore more robust in a classification context.

Limitations

The limitations of the proposed approach are now discussed. First we discuss the heterogeneity modeling. In the present work, we make the assumption that the hiPSC-CM medium is a continuous mixture of two cell types ("A" and "B") based on a ventricular endocardium cell model, modified to match the action potential duration of the experimental recordings. The actual nature of the hiPSC-CM types is still quite unknown, to the authors knowledge, even though some studies suggest it is a mixture of atrial, ventricular and pacemaker cells (Matsa et al., 2011). Even if the medium can be well characterized in a particular setting, it varies greatly from one cell line to another. In the present work, we propose a general method to generate heterogeneous media and for the sake of simplicity we restricted our study to a continuous mixture of two cell types. The approach is easily generalizable to more realistic heterogeneities, including for instance atrial, ventricular and pacemaker cells. Second, the conductances values associated with the experimental measurements are not known and are therefore approximated using Equation (2). This approximation is, however, subject to several sources of uncertainty such as the IC_{50} whose value for a given drug may vary according to the source considered (Mirams et al., 2011; Kramer et al., 2013). The uncertainties also come from the Hill's equation which is an imperfect model. Knowing the exact values for the conductances is, however, not critical since those values are only needed to derive the composite biomarkers and are not directly used during the classification procedure. Furthermore, the drugs studied in the present work are assumed to be single channel blockers. In reality, some drugs (e.g., diltiazem) are known to target more than one ion channel. In fact, it can be considered that any drug affects every ion channel with different IC_{50} values. In the present work, we make the strong assumption of single channel blocking as a first step toward a finer description of the drugs effects. This assumption is also motivated by the simplicity of the considered ionic model which only counts three different currents. Note also that mexiletine primarily blocks the late sodium channel current and not the fast one. In the MV model, there is no distinction between these two currents.

Another limitation comes from the computational model used in the present work. The sources of error are multiple: space and time discretizations, conductivities errors, modeling errors, etc. These errors are not critical either since the computational model is only used to compute the composite biomarkers weights. This study shows that, despite the modeling errors, adding synthetic measurements simulated by the computational model leads to a better and more robust classification. In the present study, we based our *in silico* modeling on the MV ionic model. It is a very simplistic model which is not able to reproduce complex behaviors such as early after depolarizations for instance. Furthermore, the hiPSC-CM are spontaneously excitable cells in our case while the MV model is not sophisticated enough to reproduce such a behavior. For this reason, it is not suited to the study of drug arrhythmogenicity. However, in the scope of the present work, we have established that it is suited to the characterization of drug-induced channel block, at least for a coarse description of it. Furthermore, it was also established in Raphel et al. (2017) that it is possible to identify which of the three main currents is affected by a drug using the MV model. Other limitations come from the classification strategies. Both classification strategies are non-exhaustive in that they do not explore every possible way of splitting the data set. Furthermore, the classification metrics used to compare the different approaches are not flawless. In some cases comparing AUCs for instance is not the best way to compare classifiers (Adams and Hand, 2000). Other metrics exist, such as the mean squared error, but were not investigated in this work. Finally, the composite biomarkers derived in the present work are not optimal in the sense that their correlation with their associated conductances is not equal to one, as seen in **Figure 8**.

The limitations of the study also arise from the MEA measurements themselves. Variations of the repolarization wave morphology and the depolarization amplitude from one experiment to another constitute a technical challenge when one tries to extract meaningful information from the measurements. In the present study, we propose to model the heterogeneities of the experimental settings (CM cell types and stimulation location) to account for the observed variability in the data. Furthermore, considering ratios of biomarkers with their control counterparts makes the approach more robust and less dependent on fluctuations from one experiment to another.

Perspectives

We now discuss some perspectives that could lead to interesting future works. Other classification methods than SVC exist, such as neural networks or random forests for instance. It would be interesting to assess whether the findings of this work are still valid when considering other classification tools. It would also be interesting to evaluate which classification tool generally performs best in the present drug classification context. Other perspectives concern the composite biomarkers computed using a mixed set of synthetic and experimental measurements. In the present work, the mixed set is roughly composed of half synthetic and half experimental measurements. However, other proportions could be investigated and an optimal proportion with respect to the classification score could be found. In the present work, only sodium, potassium and calcium antagonists drugs are considered but other types of drugs exist. Drugs that affect other ionic channels or even simultaneously several of them could be investigated. In parallel, more sophisticated ionic models including more current types would need to be used to model these new drugs. This would, of course, come at the expense or more computationally intensive simulations. Another interesting perspective would be to train the classifiers with only synthetic measurements instead of experimental ones. This would be very useful when experimental data are insufficient or even not available. The classifiers could also be trained with a mixed set of synthetic and experimental data just like it is done in this work for the computation of composite biomarkers. Finally, as explained earlier, the point of the present work is not the direct assessment of drugs arrhythmogeneicity but rather the identification of the main channel block induced by the drugs. This is, in the author's opinions, a necessary first step toward a better understanding of MEA measurements and *in fine* its use in drug safety evaluation. Considering a larger set of drugs and more realistic ionic models in order to perform drugs classification based on their arrhythmogenicity (or TdP risk) will be the purpose of future works.

AUTHOR CONTRIBUTIONS

All authors listed have made substantial, direct and intellectual contribution to the work, and approved it for publication.

FUNDING

ET was funded by a doctoral grant from the French Ministry of Research and Higher Education. FR was funded by Instem. This work was partially supported by the Agency for Interaction in Mathematics with Business and Society (AMIES).

ACKNOWLEDGMENTS

We would like to thank Janssen Pharmaceutica NV for providing us with the raw experimental data and Philippe Zitoun for many fruitful discussions.

REFERENCES

Abbate, E., Boulakia, M., Coudière, Y., Gerbeau, J.-F., Zitoun, P., and Zemzemi, N. (2017). *In silico* assessment of the effects of various compounds in MEA/hiPSC-CM assays: modelling and numerical simulations. *J. Pharm. Toxicol. Methods* 89, 59–72. doi: 10.1016/j.vascn.2017.10.005

Adams, N. M., and Hand, D. J. (2000). Improving the practice of classifier performance assessment. *Neural Comput.* 12, 305–311. doi: 10.1162/089976600300015808

Antzelevitch, C., Belardinelli, L., Zygmunt, A. C., Burashnikov, A., Di Diego, J. M., Fish, J. M., et al. (2004). Electrophysiological effects of ranolazine, a novel antianginal agent with antiarrhythmic properties. *Circulation* 110, 904–910. doi: 10.1161/01.CIR.0000139333.83620.5D

Arikawa, S., Miyano, S., Shinohara, A., Kuhara, S., Mukouchi, Y., and Shinohara, T. (1993). A machine discovery from amino acid sequences by decision trees over regular patterns. *New Gen. Comput.* 11, 361–375. doi: 10.1007/BF03037183

Blinova, K., Stohlman, J., Vicente, J., Chan, D., Johannesen, L., Hortigon-Vinagre, M. P., et al. (2016). Comprehensive translational assessment of human-induced pluripotent stem cell derived cardiomyocytes for evaluating drug-induced arrhythmias. *Toxicol. Sci.* 155, 234–247. doi: 10.1093/toxsci/kfw200

Boser, B. E., Guyon, I. M., and Vapnik, V. N. (1992). "A training algorithm for optimal margin classifiers," in *Proceedings of the Fifth Annual Workshop on Computational Learning Theory* (Pittsburgh: ACM), 144–152.

Bottino, D., Penland, R. C., Stamps, A., Traebert, M., Dumotier, B., Georgieva, A., et al. (2006). Preclinical cardiac safety assessment of pharmaceutical compounds using an integrated systems-based computer model of the heart. *Prog. Biophys. Mol. Biol.* 90, 414–443. doi: 10.1016/j.pbiomolbio.2005.06.006

Bueno-Orovio, A., Cherry, E. M., and Fenton, F. H. (2008). Minimal model for human ventricular action potentials in tissue. *J. Theor. Biol.* 253, 544–560. doi: 10.1016/j.jtbi.2008.03.029

Cavero, I., Guillon, J.-M., Ballet, V., Clements, M., Gerbeau, J.-F., and Holzgrefe, H. (2016). Comprehensive *in vitro* proarrhythmia assay (CIPA): pending issues for successful validation and implementation. *J. Pharm. Toxicol. Methods* 81, 21–36. doi: 10.1016/j.vascn.2016.05.012

Chang, C.-C., and Lin, C.-J. (2011). Libsvm: a library for support vector machines. *ACM Trans. Intell. Syst. Technol.* 2:27. doi: 10.1145/1961189.1961199

Clements, M., and Thomas, N. (2014). High-throughput multi-parameter profiling of electrophysiological drug effects in human embryonic stem cell derived cardiomyocytes using multi-electrode arrays. *Toxicol. Sci.* 140, 445–461. doi: 10.1093/toxsci/kfu084

Crumb, W. J., Vicente, J., Johannesen, L., and Strauss, D. G. (2016). An evaluation of 30 clinical drugs against the comprehensive *in vitro* proarrhythmia assay (CIPA) proposed ion channel panel. *J. Pharmacol. Toxicol. Methods* 81, 251–262. doi: 10.1016/j.vascn.2016.03.009

Davies, M. R., Wang, K., Mirams, G. R., Caruso, A., Noble, D., Walz, A., et al. (2016). Recent developments in using mechanistic cardiac modelling for drug safety evaluation. *Drug Discov. Today* 21, 924–938. doi: 10.1016/j.drudis.2016.02.003

Fermini, B., Hancox, J. C., Abi-Gerges, N., Bridgland-Taylor, M., Chaudhary, K. W., Colatsky, T., et al. (2016). A new perspective in the field of cardiac safety testing through the comprehensive *in vitro* proarrhythmia assay paradigm. *J. Biomol. Screen.* 21, 1–11. doi: 10.1177/1087057115594589

Hindmarsh, A. C., Brown, P. N., Grant, K. E., Lee, S. L., Serban, R., Shumaker, D. E., et al. (2005). Sundials: suite of nonlinear and differential/algebraic equation solvers. *ACM Trans. Math. Softw.* 31, 363–396. doi: 10.1145/1089014.1089020

Hua, S., and Sun, Z. (2001). A novel method of protein secondary structure prediction with high segment overlap measure: support vector machine approach. *J. Mol. Biol.* 308, 397–407. doi: 10.1006/jmbi.2001.4580

Kiranyaz, S., Ince, T., and Gabbouj, M. (2016). Real-time patient-specific ecg classification by 1-d convolutional neural networks. *IEEE Trans. Biomed. Eng.* 63, 664–675. doi: 10.1109/TBME.2015.2468589

Kramer, J., Obejero-Paz, C. A., Myatt, G., Kuryshev, Y. A., Bruening-Wright, A., Verducci, J. S., et al. (2013). Mice models: superior to the HERG model in predicting torsade de pointes. *Sci. Rep.* 3:2100. doi: 10.1038/srep02100

Lancaster, M. C., and Sobie, E. (2016). Improved prediction of drug-induced torsades de pointes through simulations of dynamics and machine learning algorithms. *Clin. Pharmacol. Therapeut.* 100, 371–379. doi: 10.1002/cpt.367

Matsa, E., Rajamohan, D., Dick, E., Young, L., Mellor, I., Staniforth, A., et al. (2011). Drug evaluation in cardiomyocytes derived from human induced pluripotent stem cells carrying a long QT syndrome type 2 mutation. *Eur. Heart J.* 32, 952–962. doi: 10.1093/eurheartj/ehr073

Meyer, T., Boven, K.-H., Günther, E., and Fejtl, M. (2004). Micro-electrode arrays in cardiac safety pharmacology. *Drug Safety* 27, 763–772. doi: 10.2165/00002018-200427110-00002

Mirams, G., Cui, Y., Sher, A., Fink, M., Cooper, J., Heath, B., et al. (2011). Simulation of multiple ion channel block provides improved early prediction of compounds clinical torsadogenic risk. *Cardiovasc. Res.* 91, 53–61. doi: 10.1093/cvr/cvr044

Navarrete, E. G., Liang, P., Lan, F., Sanchez-Freire, V., Simmons, C., Gong, T., et al. (2013). Screening drug-induced arrhythmia using human induced pluripotent stem cell–derived cardiomyocytes and low-impedance microelectrode arrays. *Circulation* 128(11 Suppl. 1), S3–S13. doi: 10.1161/CIRCULATIONAHA.112.000570

O'Donoghue, B., and Candes, E. (2015). Adaptive restart for accelerated gradient schemes. *Found. Comput. Math.* 15, 715–732. doi: 10.1007/s10208-013-9150-3

Pedregosa, F., Varoquaux, G., Gramfort, A., Michel, V., Thirion, B., Grisel, O., et al. (2011). Scikit-learn: machine learning in Python. *J. Mach. Learn. Res.* 12, 2825–2830.

Raphel, F., Boulakia, M., Zemzemi, N., Coudière, Y., Guillon, J.-M., Zitoun, P., et al. (2017). Identification of ion currents components generating field potential recorded in MEA from hiPSC-CM. *IEEE Trans. Biomed. Eng.* doi: 10.1109/TBME.2017.2748798

Schölkopf, B., and Smola, A. J. (2002). *Learning with Kernels: Support Vector Machines, Regularization, Optimization, and Beyond.* (Cambridge, MA: MIT Press).

Scott, C. W., Peters, M. F., and Dragan, Y. P. (2013). Human induced pluripotent stem cells and their use in drug discovery for toxicity testing. *Toxicol. Lett.* 219, 49–58. doi: 10.1016/j.toxlet.2013.02.020

Tibshirani, R. (1996). Regression shrinkage and selection via the lasso. *J. R. Stat. Soc. Ser. B (Methodol.).* 58, 267–288.

Tung, L. (1978). *A Bi-domain Model for Describing Ischemic Myocardial D-C Potentials.* Ph.D. thesis, MIT. Available online at: https://hdl.handle.net/1721.1/16177

Zemzemi, N., Bernabeu, M., Saiz, J., Cooper, J., Pathmanathan, P., Mirams, G., et al. (2013). Computational assessment of drug-induced effects on the electrocardiogram: from ion channel to body surface potentials. *Brit. J. Pharmacol.* 168, 718–733. doi: 10.1111/j.1476-5381.2012.02200.x

14

Global Optimization of Ventricular Myocyte Model to Multi-Variable Objective Improves Predictions of Drug-Induced Torsades de Pointes

*Trine Krogh-Madsen[1,2,3], Anna F. Jacobson[3], Francis A. Ortega[4] and David J. Christini[1,2,3]**

[1] Greenberg Division of Cardiology, Department of Medicine, Weill Cornell Medicine, New York, NY, United States, [2] Institute for Computational Biomedicine, Weill Cornell Medicine, New York, NY, United States, [3] Cardiovascular Research Institute, Weill Cornell Medicine, New York, NY, United States, [4] Physiology, Biophysics and Systems Biology Graduate Program, Weill Cornell Graduate School, New York, NY, United States

***Correspondence:**
David J. Christini
dchristi@med.cornell.edu

In silico cardiac myocyte models present powerful tools for drug safety testing and for predicting phenotypical consequences of ion channel mutations, but their accuracy is sometimes limited. For example, several models describing human ventricular electrophysiology perform poorly when simulating effects of long QT mutations. Model optimization represents one way of obtaining models with stronger predictive power. Using a recent human ventricular myocyte model, we demonstrate that model optimization to clinical long QT data, in conjunction with physiologically-based bounds on intracellular calcium and sodium concentrations, better constrains model parameters. To determine if the model optimized to congenital long QT data better predicts risk of drug-induced long QT arrhythmogenesis, in particular Torsades de Pointes risk, we tested the optimized model against a database of known arrhythmogenic and non-arrhythmogenic ion channel blockers. When doing so, the optimized model provided an improved risk assessment. In particular, we demonstrate an elimination of false-positive outcomes generated by the baseline model, in which simulations of non-torsadogenic drugs, in particular verapamil, predict action potential prolongation. Our results underscore the importance of currents beyond those directly impacted by a drug block in determining torsadogenic risk. Our study also highlights the need for rich data in cardiac myocyte model optimization and substantiates such optimization as a method to generate models with higher accuracy of predictions of drug-induced cardiotoxicity.

Keywords: cardiac modeling, model optimization, safety pharmacology, long QT, *in silico* drug trial, cardiotoxicity

1. INTRODUCTION

Mathematical models of cardiac electrophysiology are at the cusp of usage in a variety of clinical and pre-clinical applications, including safety pharmacology (Mirams et al., 2012; Zhang et al., 2016). In particular, mathematical modeling forms a central component in the Comprehensive *in Vitro* Proarrhythmia Assay (CiPA) initiative, a proposed strategy for progressing drug safety testing (Sager et al., 2014; Colatsky et al., 2016; Fermini et al., 2016; Gintant et al., 2016).

In terms of cardiotoxicity, drug safety testing aims to avoid Torsades de Pointes (TdP), a life-threatening ventricular tachycardia. Indeed, occurrences of drug-induced TdP in patients have lead to regulatory bans and market withdrawals of several drugs (Mirams et al., 2011). TdP risk is associated with prolongation of the QT interval on the electrocardiogram, in particular due to block of the hERG channel, which carries the rapid delayed rectifier current (I_{Kr}; Sanguinetti et al., 1995; Straus et al., 2005; Hoffmann and Warner, 2006). However, multiple other currents and dynamics are of importance to torsadogenesis, and including measured effects of drugs on multiple channels, rather than just hERG, into TdP risk stratification improves risk prediction (Kramer et al., 2013; Mistry et al., 2015). Mechanistically, TdP initiation is linked to early afterdepolarizations (EADs) at the cellular level. Triggering of these EADs may depend directly on multiple different ionic currents, including the L-type calcium current (I_{CaL}) and the late sodium current (I_{NaL}) (Lankipalli et al., 2005; Hale et al., 2008), and may also depend on intracellular calcium and sodium dynamics (Terentyev et al., 2014; Kim et al., 2015; Xie et al., 2015; Krogh-Madsen and Christini, 2017), implying that the levels of the ionic transporters that control these concentrations (e.g., the sodium-calcium exchanger and the sodium-potassium pump) are important for torsadogenesis. Indeed, recent *in silico* work have pointed to the magnitudes of these two transporters as having large impact on TdP risk (Lancaster and Sobie, 2016).

Despite the proposed usage of mathematical models in safety pharmacology, even recent and sophisticated models of human ventricular myocyte electrophysiology perform poorly when simulating each of the most typical congenital long QT (LQT) syndromes (Mann et al., 2016). This naturally raises concerns about the ability of these *in silico* models to predict drug-induced LQT and TdP. However, using a global optimization strategy, *in silico* models can optimized to reproduce repolarization delays consistent with those seen clinically in the congenital LQT patient datasets, providing optimism for clinically-related model usage (Mann et al., 2016). A concern remains, however, as to whether these *in silico* models, optimized in terms of action potential properties, replicate dynamics of intracellular ionic concentrations well enough to reliably predict TdP risk. For example, when optimizing a model in terms of its electrical activity only, it can be difficult to correctly identify parameters that mainly control ionic concentrations (Groenendaal et al., 2015). Indeed, previous modeling studies have shown how identical-looking action potentials, modeled using different combinations of model parameters, can have differing calcium transients (Sarkar and Sobie, 2010).

To investigate this possible limitation, we therefore carried out a multi-variable optimization, using both clinical congenital LQT data and constraints on the concentrations on intracellular Ca^{2+} and intracellular Na^+ ($[Ca^{2+}]_i$ and $[Na^+]_i$). We then asked whether optimized models that better represent the congenital LQT syndromes might allow for more accurate and more reliable modeling of acquired LQT and TdP risk. To this end, we simulated 86 cases of multi-channel drug block with known TdP risk level (Lancaster and Sobie, 2016) and found that the model optimized in terms of both action potential and $[Ca^{2+}]_i$, and $[Na^+]_i$ data, better predicts TdP risk.

2. METHODS

2.1. Cell Model and Drug Simulations

Simulations were performed using the O'Hara-Rudy (ORd; O'Hara et al., 2011) human ventricular ionic model as the baseline model, as this is the model proposed to be used in the CiPA initiative (Colatsky et al., 2016; Fermini et al., 2016). We used endocardial myocyte parameter settings except where otherwise noted (**Figure 4A**). We used a 1 Hz pacing rate and corresponding steady-state initial conditions (O'Hara et al., 2011). For each perturbation to the model (simulating drug block or LQT syndromes and parameter changes during the optimization; detailed below), the model was simulated for 500 beats prior to collecting data. We quantified action potential duration to 90% (APD_{90}) or 50% (APD_{50}) repolarization, as indicated. Calcium transients were characterized by diastolic level (the minimum $[Ca^{2+}]_i$ attained within an action potential cycle cycle) and systolic concentration (the peak $[Ca^{2+}]_i$ reached during an action potential). The $[Na^+]_i$ varies little within a single action potential and was measured as the maximum value.

For our drug simulations, we used the datasets of Kramer et al. (2013) and Mirams et al. (2011) as curated by Lancaster and Sobie (2016) with an associated yes/no risk of torsadogenesis. For each drug, the dataset gives its estimated effective free therapeutic plasma concentration (EFTPC), along with IC_{50} values for block of the channels generating I_{Kr}, I_{CaL}, and the fast sodium current (I_{Na}). Drug effect on each channel type was modeled as a conductance block based on a Hill equation with a coefficient of 1:

$$G_{x,drug} = G_x \left(1 + \frac{\text{EFTPC}}{\text{IC}_{50,x}}\right)^{-1}, \quad (1)$$

where $G_{x,drug}$ is the maximal conductance of channel x in the presence of the drug. The dataset contains 86 entries, with some duplicate drugs modeled differently by the two original sources. There are therefore 68 different compounds in the set, covering a variety of intended clinical use, including anti-arrhythmics, anti-histamines, antipsychotics, hypertension/angina drugs, and others.

2.2. Drug Classification

To classify model output generated by these drug simulations we used a Support Vector Machine (SVM; Ben-Hur et al., 2008). We used linear decision boundaries separating two categories of data: TdP risk and no TdP risk. These decision boundaries were computed as the solution to a minimization of an error (E) calculated as the sum of squared distances between the location of miscategorized points and the boundary. Because the two variables used in the classification (APD_{50} and diastolic $[Ca^{2+}]_i$) have very different absolute values, we normalized them to baseline (i.e., no drug) values.

In general, the minimum value of E will take on different values when using different cell models to simulate drug effects, indicating that the separation of data points by category is better for some models than others. Therefore, to compare goodness of the classification between models and also to determine sensitivity of the decision boundaries, we calculate regions for which E remains below a threshold value (E*), which we set to twice the value of the lowest value of E found among the four tested models.

2.3. Model Optimization

We optimized the baseline ORd model based on clinical data from LQT patients, following a similar strategy as Mann et al. (2016) and using their QT interval data for control patients and patients with one of the three most prevalent congenital LQT syndromes: LQT1, LQT2, or LQT3. The QT interval data from LQT1 and LQT2 patients came from a patient cohort with heterozygote nonsense mutations only, as that can be mimicked in the model by decreasing the conductances of I_{Ks} and I_{Kr} by 50%, respectively. The LQT3 cohort data is more heterogenous and the subtype was simulated by increasing the conductance of I_{NaL} by a factor that was allowed to vary as part of the optimization process. The amount of QT interval prolongation in these patient groups was 12.2% for LQT1, 16.6% for LQT2, and 16.2% for LQT3. Mapping the delayed repolarization measured clinically as QT interval prolongation directly to APD_{90} prolongation in the cell model, the objective data set was 267.97 ms (control), 301.14 ms (LQT1), 312.20 ms (LQT2), and 311.55 (LQT3).

In its simplest setup, the optimization was designed to minimize a sum-of-squares error from the APD_{90} objective when subjecting the model to control conditions and each of the LQT subtypes 1, 2, and 3. We refer to this as the "APD_{LQT}" optimization. In other optimizations, we included $[Ca^{2+}]_i$ and $[Na^+]_i$ information in the objective to improve the optimization outcome. This "multi-variable" optimization was done by adding a hefty error (200 ms squared) if $[Ca^{2+}]_i$ and $[Na^+]_i$ fell outside a certain range during the control condition. We used a range of 0.05–0.15 μM for diastolic $[Ca^{2+}]_i$, 0.3–0.7 μM for systolic $[Ca^{2+}]_i$, and 7–10 mM for $[Na^+]_i$ based on measurements in human ventricular myocytes and recent modeling work (Beuckelmann et al., 1992; Piacentino et al., 2003; Grandi et al., 2010).

For the optimization method, we used a genetic algorithm (GA), which is a global optimization method that has been successful in optimizing cardiac ionic models to experimental and simulated data (Syed et al., 2005; Bot et al., 2012; Kaur et al., 2014; Groenendaal et al., 2015). We used a population size of 200 individual model instantiations and ran each GA for 50 generations. All other settings specific to the GA (detailing selection, crossover, mutation, and elitism) were defined as detailed previously (Bot et al., 2012). Because of the stochasticity inherent to the GA, each optimization was run ten times. We used the run resulting in the lowest error as the optimized model.

The parameters to be determined in the optimization process are scaling factors for the currents I_{Kr}, I_{CaL}, I_{NaL}, the slow delayed rectifier current (I_{Ks}), the sodium-calcium exchange current (I_{NCX}), the sodium-potassium pump current (I_{NaK}), and the extent of I_{NaL} increase with simulated LQT3. All scaling parameters were allowed to vary from 0.1% to 10-fold their values in the baseline model.

Note that for ease and consistency we will refer to current scaling factors as scaling of maximal conductances (and use G_{Kr}, G_{CaL}, G_{NaL}, G_{Ks}, G_{NCX}, and G_{NaK} for the currents defined above), although some currents are technically scaled by a permeability or a maximal charge carried.

3. RESULTS

3.1. Sensitivity of APD, $[Ca^{2+}]_i$, and $[Na^+]_i$ in Baseline Model

To help guide our optimization procedure, we first did a sensitivity analysis to the major conductances as parameters with low sensitivity are problematic to determine in an optimization.

In the baseline ORd model, the action potential duration of the ORd model is highly sensitive to changes in I_{Kr} (**Figure 1A**). For example, when decreasing G_{Kr} by 50% to simulate LQT2, the response is a prolongation of APD_{90} by 117 ms (44%), substantially larger than the QT interval prolongation of 68 ms (16.6%) seen in LQT2 patients with heterozygote nonsense mutations (Mann et al., 2016). The APD has an intermediate sensitivity on G_{CaL}, but shows little sensitivity to variations in G_{Ks} and G_{NaL}, the currents associated with LQT1 and LQT3, respectively. For example, reducing G_{Ks} by 50% to mimic LQT1, gives a modest 8-ms (3%) APD_{90} prolongation, much shorter than the 51 ms (12%) QT interval prolongation seen clinically (Mann et al., 2016).

As expected, the calcium transient has a very different parameter sensitivity dependence. It depends strongly on the conductances of I_{CaL} and I_{NCX}, with a 50% increase in G_{CaL} or a 50% reduction of G_{NCX} increasing systolic $[Ca^{2+}]_i$ by almost 0.2 μM (**Figure 1B**). The calcium dynamics also has a significant dependence on G_{NaK}, which only controls $[Ca^{2+}]_i$ indirectly via $[Na^+]_i$ changes that regulate I_{NCX}. Indeed, $[Na^+]_i$ depends sensitively on G_{NaK}, with a 50% reduction in G_{NaK} resulting in a 1.7 mM increase in $[Na^+]_i$ (**Figure 1C**). Variations in the remaining key conductances have little influence on $[Na^+]_i$ levels.

These results are consistent with those presented previously for ±10 and ±20% parameter variations in the ORd model (O'Hara et al., 2011).

3.2. Model Optimization

As it is difficult to estimate parameters to which an output is not sensitive, the above analysis suggests that if optimizing the baseline ORd model to APD data only, it will be problematic to estimate many of the conductance parameters. Including repolarization delay data from LQT types 1, 2, and 3 as additional information to the objective may help determine the scaling of G_{Ks}, G_{Kr}, and G_{NaL}. Further, pinpointing these parameters may narrow down other conductances that correlate with these more directly determined parameters (Groenendaal et al., 2015). The sensitivity analysis also indicates that inclusion of calcium transient data to the optimization objective should help determine G_{NCX} and G_{NaK} scaling, and that incorporation of $[Na^+]_i$ may further help determination of G_{NaK} scaling.

We therefore optimized the baseline ORd model to both clinical QT interval data from LQT patients and $[Ca^{2+}]_i$ and $[Na^+]_i$ as detailed in section 2.3. The model optimized to this multi-variable objective produces APD_{90} values that are within 3% of their target values (**Figure 2**). The optimized parameter

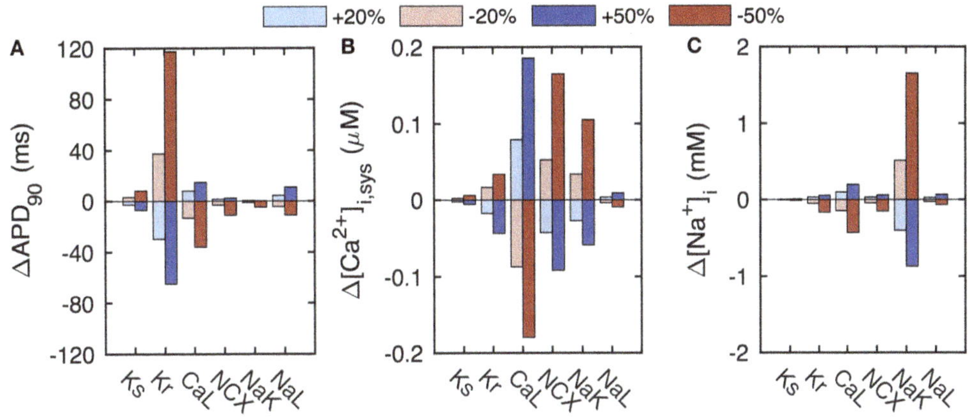

FIGURE 1 | Sensitivity of baseline ORd model to select conductances. **(A)** The APD of the baseline model has a strong sensitivity to the conductance of I_{Kr}. **(B)** The calcium transient (quantified here as systolic $[Ca^{2+}]_i$) depends sensitively on G_{CaL}, G_{NCX}, and G_{NaK}. **(C)** The level of $[Na^+]_i$ depends mainly on G_{NaK}. Conductances were varied by ±20% (light blue/red) and ±50% (dark blue/red) of baseline values.

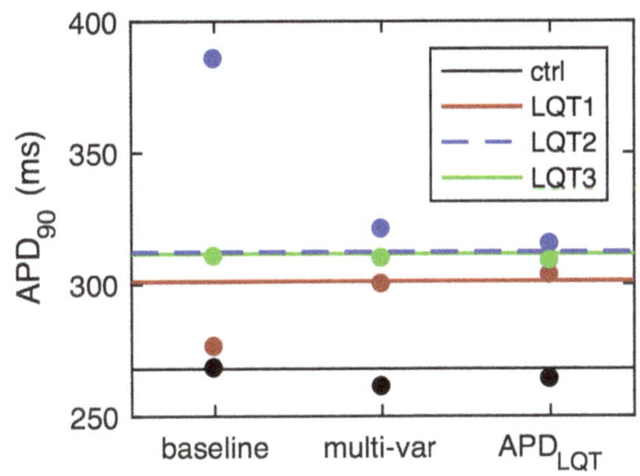

FIGURE 2 | APD values of optimized models. Horizontal lines give control APD_{90} (black) as well as APD_{90} surrogates for QT interval prolongation in LQT patients (colored). These APD values form the optimization objective in the simplest case ("APD_{LQT}"). For the multi-variable optimization ("multi-var"), the objective also include constraints on $[Ca^{2+}]_i$ and $[Na^+]_i$. Dots give APD_{90} values under control simulations (black) and during LQT simulations (LQT1, red; LQT2, blue; LQT3, green). The overestimation of the LQT2 response and the underestimation of the LQT1 response in the baseline ORd model are eliminated in the optimized models. Relative APD_{90} prolongation in the baseline model is 3.0, 43.8, and 15.8%, for LQT1, LQT2, and LQT3, respectively. For the multi-variable optimized model, relative APD_{90} prolongation is 14.9, 22.9, and 18.6% for LQT1-3, while for the APD_{LQT}-optimized model the corresponding values are 14.5, 19.4, and 17.0%. The target QT interval values are 12.2, 16.6, and 16.2%.

scaling factors are given in **Table 1**. The optimized model has a much increased G_{Ks}, resulting in a larger response to the simulated LQT1 condition, matching the target data (**Figure 2**).

Optimizing the baseline model to APD values only (i.e., omitting the $[Ca^{2+}]_i$ and $[Na^+]_i$ constraints) results in slightly better matching of the objective (**Figure 2**; errors with 2%). Optimized parameter values are very different, with large increases in scaling of G_{CaL} and G_{NaK} in addition to the enhanced G_{Ks} scaling (**Table 1**).

TABLE 1 | Scaling factors for optimized models.

Objective	Ks	Kr	CaL	NCX	NaK	NaL	NaL_{LQT3}
Multi-variable	8.09	1.17	3.57	3.05	1.91	1.70	4.17
APD_{LQT}	9.71	1.42	9.59	1.75	7.40	4.86	2.28

The optimization gave estimated parameters for scaling of the currents I_{Ks}, I_{Kr}, I_{CaL}, I_{NCX}, I_{NaK}, and I_{NaL}, and for the increase of I_{NaL} during simulated LQT3. Optimizing to APD values only (APD_{LQT}) resulted in a very different parameter set compared to the multi-variable optimization that include of $[Ca^{2+}]_i$ and $[Na^+]_i$ constraints. In particular, it resulted in much increased scalings for I_{CaL} and I_{NaK}.

Despite the diversity in parameter scalings among the baseline and the optimized models, the action potential morphology is quite similar across these differently parameterized models (**Figure 3A**). We also include for comparison the action potential generated by Mann et al. in an optimization to clinical LQT data under both baseline and β-adrenergic conditions ("$APD_{LQT\pm\beta Adr}$" optimization, Mann et al., 2016). The main difference among the action potential waveforms is a depolarization of phase 2 of the action potential, the amount of which correlates with the upscaling of G_{CaL} from the baseline model (about 2–4 in the multivariable and $APD_{LQT\pm\beta Adr}$ models, and almost 10 in the APD_{LQT} model).

However, calcium transients and $[Na^+]_i$ levels are vastly different across models (**Figures 3B,C**). When including $[Ca^{2+}]_i$ and $[Na^+]_i$ constraints in the optimization, the optimized calcium transient and $[Na^+]_i$ level are very close to those of the baseline model, despite the allowed ranges being relatively large (0.05–0.15 μM for diastolic $[Ca^{2+}]_i$, 0.3–0.7 μM for systolic $[Ca^{2+}]_i$, and 7–10 mM for $[Na^+]_i$). In our optimizations, when optimizing to APD only, the calcium transient is significantly enhanced. This is consistent with the much boosted G_{CaL} and the decreased G_{NCX} scaling (relative to the multi-variable optimization) both of which favor a larger calcium transient. In addition, the G_{NaK} scaling is much increased when optimizing to APD only, consistent with the lower $[Na^+]_i$. For the

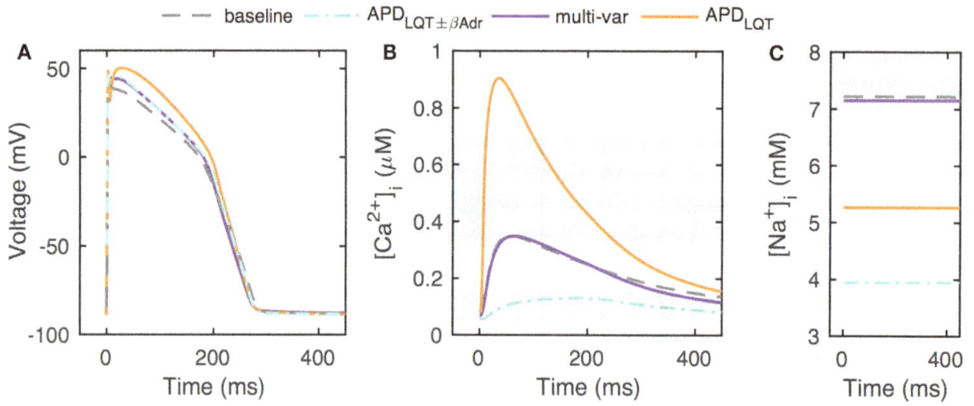

FIGURE 3 | Action potentials, calcium transients, and $[Na^+]_i$ in optimized models. **(A)** Optimized models have similar action potentials under control conditions, but the different parameter sets underlying the different solutions give rise to some waveform variation. **(B)** Despite having comparable action potentials, models optimized without constraints on $[Ca^{2+}]_i$ and $[Na^+]_i$ can have widely different calcium transients. Shaded areas give constraints on minimum and maximum $[Ca^{2+}]_i$ (0.05–0.15 and 0.3–0.7μM, respectively). **(C)** Without constraints on $[Ca^{2+}]_i$ and $[Na^+]_i$, optimization can result in models with very low $[Na^+]_i$ levels. Shaded area indicate constraint on $[Na^+]_i$ (7–10mM). "APD$_{LQT\pm\beta Adr}$" designates the original optimization to clinical LQT data under normal and β-adrenergic stimulation conditions by Mann et al. (2016).

$APD_{LQT\pm\beta Adr}$ optimized model (Mann et al., 2016), both G_{NCX} and G_{NaK} were much increased relative to baseline (scaling of 2.95 and 9.12, respectively), resulting in a small-amplitude calcium transient and a low $[Na^+]_i$.

3.3. TdP Prediction

To test how well the optimized models predict TdP risk, we used a dataset consisting of drugs blocking I_{Kr}, I_{CaL}, and I_{Na} to varying degrees, and their associated risk of torsadogenesis (TdP positive or TdP negative; Lancaster and Sobie, 2016). As demonstrated previously, while many of the drugs in this dataset that carry a TdP risk do prolong APD, some drug simulations predict an increased APD for TdP negative drugs (**Figure 4A**, Lancaster and Sobie, 2016). In particular, in the baseline model, simulations of three non-torsadogenic drugs results in action potential prolongation of 15–25 ms (one of these is noted by a black dot in **Figure 4A**). As demonstrated by Lancaster and Sobie, simulations of those three drugs also led to a decreased diastolic $[Ca^{2+}]_i$, which was not seen in the TdP positive drugs. Therefore, including diastolic $[Ca^{2+}]_i$ as a second metric (APD_{50} being the first) by which to classify the drugs, allows for a correct TdP risk categorization of these three otherwise false positives (**Figure 4A**, Lancaster and Sobie, 2016). Indeed, using APD_{50} and diastolic $[Ca^{2+}]_i$ in combination correctly classifies drugs in the dataset with high specificity and sensitivity (**Figure 4A**, Lancaster and Sobie, 2016).

For the $APD_{LQT\pm\beta Adr}$ optimized model (Mann et al., 2016), qualitatively similar results are observed (**Figure 4B**). The particular values of diastolic $[Ca^{2+}]_i$ over which TdP positive drugs are separated from TdP negative drugs are shifted, reflecting baseline differences. The same three TdP negative compounds that resulted in APD prolongation in the baseline model, give increased APD_{50} in this optimized model as well.

When simulating drug application in the multi-variable optimized model, predictions are improved (**Figure 4C**). In particular, none of the TdP negative drugs result in APD_{50} prolongation beyond 5 ms, implying that APD_{50} prolongation in itself is a strong predictor of torsadogenic risk in this model. In addition, many of the TdP negative compounds result in more substantial reductions in APD_{50} and/or diastolic $[Ca^{2+}]_i$ compared to the baseline and the $APD_{LQT\pm\beta Adr}$ optimized models. There is therefore an increased flexibility to the positioning of the decision boundary separating the TdP positive from the TdP negative drugs (dashed lines in **Figure 4C** mark off area within which the categorization error remains less than the threshold value, E*).

For the APD_{LQT} optimized model, the classification is less successful (**Figure 4D**). The same three TdP negative drugs that resulted in false positive APD prolongation in the baseline and in the $APD_{LQT\pm\beta Adr}$ optimized model do so here. Further, simulation of several TdP positive drugs result in decreased diastolic $[Ca^{2+}]_i$ without much change in APD and therefore form false negatives in this categorization. The presence of these false positives and negatives pose a challenge to the classification and prevents the categorization error from getting below the threshold value regardless of the location of the decision boundary.

What are the ionic mechanisms underlying the improvement in predictive ability by the multi-var model? The simulated drugs that give the false positive APD prolongations for the baseline and APD-optimized models are piperacillin and verapamil (note that two independent measurements for verapamil are included in the dataset). These drugs block both I_{CaL} and I_{Kr}. We investigated the ionics of verapamil (black dots in **Figure 4**) in more detail, as verapamil is a well-known example of an I_{Kr}-blocking agent that does not prolong the QT-interval and is not torsadogenic (Redfern et al., 2003).

A simulation of verapamil application in the baseline model is shown in **Figure 5A**. Drug-induced reductions in outward I_{Kr} and inward I_{CaL} are seen to be of similar amplitude and

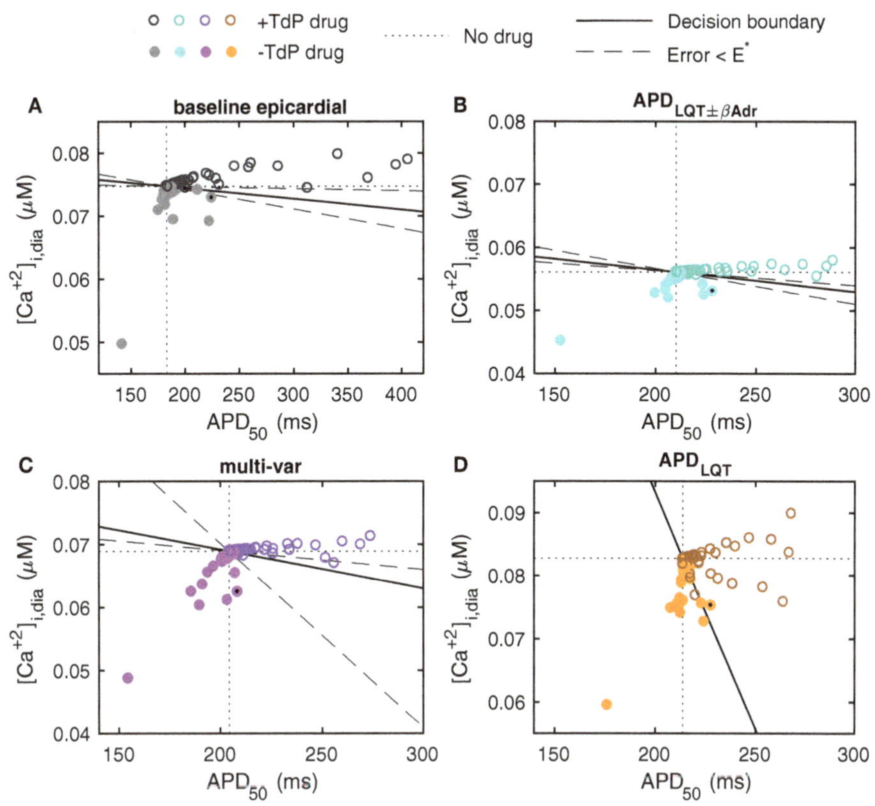

FIGURE 4 | Prediction of TdP risk from model simulations. **(A)** Baseline ORd model with epicardial myocyte parameter settings (the epicardial configuration is shown here as it was determined to give the best classification in Lancaster and Sobie, 2016. Using the endocardial baseline model yields very similar results). **(B)** $APD_{LQT\pm\beta Adr}$ optimized model. **(C)** Multi-variable optimized model. **(D)** APD_{LQT} optimized model. Dotted lines indicate no-drug control values of APD_{50} and diastolic $[Ca^{2+}]_i$. Colors for the different models correspond to the color scheme in **Figure 3**. Solid lines give decision boundaries between torsadogenic (open circles) and non-torsadogenic drugs (filled circles). Dashed lines demarcate regions within which the categorization error remains below a threshold value (E*). Using the multi-variable optimized model, all drugs that prolong APD_{50} by more than 5 ms are known TdP risk drugs. Verapamil (marked by black dot) is an example of a TdP negative drug that significantly prolongs the AP in the baseline and APD-optimized models but not in the multi-variable optimized model.

balance each other during the first 200 ms of the action potential. When I_{CaL} inactivates at this time, the loss of outward I_{Kr} is largely unopposed, leading to a decreased rate of repolarization and APD prolongation. In the multi-variable optimized model, the non-drug action potential is generated through a near-balance between a much increased I_{CaL} and a larger I_{NCX} providing inward current against the outward currents I_{Kr} and I_{Ks}, with I_{Ks} now being of similar size as I_{Kr} (**Figure 5B**). When simulating verapamil application in the multi-var optimized model, there is a loss of inward current by the direct effect of I_{CaL} conductance block and because of a reduction of I_{NCX} due to the decreased calcium transient. As both I_{CaL} and I_{NCX} are increased in the multi-variable optimized model relative to the baseline model, the loss of inward current with verapamil application is amplified, preventing repolarization delays. Further, the increased I_{Ks} in the multi-var model helps maintain repolarization under verapamil application. Thus, factors beyond the scaling of the directly blocked currents I_{Kr} and I_{CaL} contribute to the drug-induced response.

4. DISCUSSION

We investigated optimization of conductance parameters in a human ventricular myocyte model to match clinical data from LQT patients using constraints on the concentrations of intracellular calcium and sodium ions. Without these constraints, parameter optimization can lead to models with unphysiological calcium transient and $[Na^+]_i$. To test the hypothesis that the optimization would allow the model to make improved predictions of drug-induced arrhythmogenesis, we investigated the ability of the model to determine TdP risk in a large set of known drugs. We found that using the optimized model improves TdP prediction in two complementary manners. First, simulations of three TdP negative drugs that result in APD prolongation using the baseline model result in no or minimal APD prolongation when using the optimized model. Second, when using both diastolic $[Ca^{2+}]_i$ and APD_{50} for the model-based drug classification, the optimized model gives an improved separation between the TdP positive and negative drugs, measured as an increased flexibility in the positioning of the

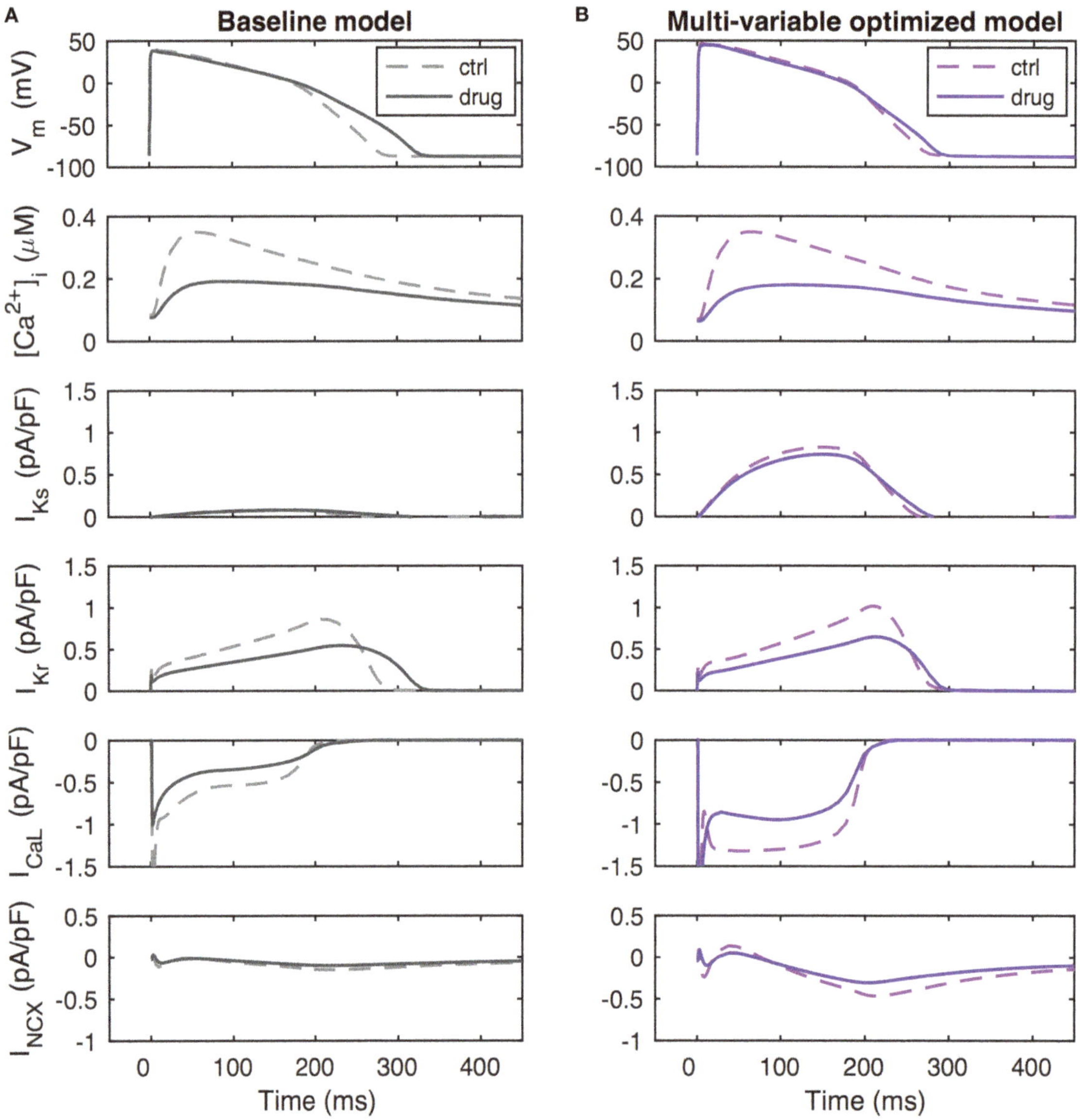

FIGURE 5 | Ionic mechanisms of repolarization dynamics during verapamil application. **(A)** Baseline model. **(B)** Multi-variable optimized model. Verapamil (simulated as a scaling of G_{CaL} by 0.64, a scaling of G_{Kr} by 0.55, and a scaling of G_{Na} by 0.998) decrease I_{Kr} by similar amounts in the baseline and in the multi-variable optimized models. However, due to the up-regulated I_{CaL} and I_{NCX} in the optimized model, it sustains a larger loss of inward current than the baseline model. Further, the increased I_{Ks} in this model provides a repolarization reserve. Together, these effects lead to a maintained APD_{50} value and an only slightly increased value of APD_{90}.

decision boundary. Based on these findings, our main conclusion is that intracellular ionic concentrations are important for safety pharmacology modeling.

4.1. *In Silico* TdP Prediction

Other studies have investigated ionic-model-based TdP prediction using different approaches. It is clear from these studies that a range of strategies can be applied to improve TdP prediction. First, there is improvement to the baseline model, which in itself can involve a number of approaches. One is to optimize a model to clinical LQT data, as done here or previously (Mann et al., 2016). Conceptually, fitting a cellular model to clinical ECG data rather than to experimental cellular-level data may appear counter-intuitive, but it makes sense given that the model is used to predict an organ-level, rather than a cellular-level, arrhythmia risk. Another model optimization approach is to tune the model to experimental data obtained with ion channel blockers. Such data can be additional to the data used originally to build the baseline model, as in the example of a canine model that upon optimization delivered improved prediction of test drug data (Davies et al., 2012). In another article in this Research Topic, Dutta et al. (2017) used drug data presented in the original ORd model paper to reparameterize the ORd model. This optimization was done in conjunction with another model improvement strategy: re-casting the I_{Kr} description as a Markov model with state- and voltage-dependent drug block (Li et al., 2017). An alternative strategy to optimizing a model is to generate a population of models to represent inter-individual and/or inter-cell variability, potentially recapitulating variability in drug response across a heterogeneous population (Lancaster and Sobie, 2016; Britton et al., 2017). Another contribution to this Research Topic demonstrates that such population models predict TdP risk better than using a single baseline model (Passini et al., 2017). Population models may also be used to gain mechanistic insights into arrhythmogenesis. For example, Passini et al. determined that different sub-populations of models had different propensities to repolarization abnormalities, with low conductances for the outward currents I_{Kr} and I_{NaK} and increased levels of I_{CaL} and I_{NCX} making models more prone to repolarization abnormalities, emphasizing that currents other than I_{Kr} are important in this aspect.

Second, TdP prediction may be improved by selection of better risk measures. While repolarization delay (APD or QT interval prolongation) has high sensitivity to TdP positive drugs, its specificity is more limited, with some drugs prolonging QT interval, yet carrying only low TdP risk (e.g., amiodarone; Sager et al., 2014). Measures that may be useful in risk stratification include diastolic $[Ca^{2+}]_i$ (Lancaster and Sobie, 2016) as employed here. While this measure was selected, in combination with APD_{50}, from a range of action potential and calcium transient biomarkers through a machine learning process, there is a mechanistic basis as to why $[Ca^{2+}]_i$ levels may be associated with TdP risk, as abnormal intracellular calcium dynamics and spontaneous calcium release is associated with EAD formation, a cellular-level trigger of TdP (Lancaster and Sobie, 2016; Němec et al., 2016). Another risk measure proposed from *in silico* work is the net charge carried during the action potential by six major ionic currents (Dutta et al., 2017; Li et al., 2017). This measure may also be mechanistically linked to TdP arrhythmogenesis, as it is indicative of robustness against EAD generation under a G_{Kr}-reduction challenge (Dutta et al., 2017). Use of repolarization abnormality occurrence (i.e., EADs or incomplete repolarization) in simulations as a metric for TdP risk may also present a viable stratification pathway (Passini et al., 2017). Given the direct link to arrhythmogenesis, this seems like a promising risk marker, but a possible limitation lies in its use of highly elevated drug concentrations to trigger the repolarization abnormalities, which may lead to an overestimation of the number of false negatives. Use of this metric rather than APD prolongation improves TdP prediction in a population of models, but not in the baseline ORd model (Passini et al., 2017).

In summary, it is clear that *in silico* cell models can be improved to better predict TdP risk and that measures beyond APD prolongation are helpful to this end, but it also apparent that significant uncertainties remain as to how to best carry out the modeling and the arrhythmia risk prediction.

4.2. Kr/Ks Balance

Our optimization resulted in significant rescaling of many parameters, in particular G_{Ks}, which was increased approximately eight-fold. This is comparable to the scaling of 5.75 found in Mann et al. (2016). In the baseline ORd model, I_{Ks} is relatively small under control conditions, its peak value during an action potential being roughly 10 times smaller than peak I_{Kr}. Significant upscaling of this current is therefore necessary to recapitulate the clinical LQT1 phenotype showing substantial QT interval prolongation with loss of I_{Ks}. Likewise, the Grandi-Bers model, another recent human ventricular myocyte model (Grandi et al., 2010) that has little reliance on I_{Ks} under control conditions, requires sizeable upscaling of G_{Ks} (about 25-fold) to reproduce the LQT1 clinical data (Mann et al., 2016). In contrast, the ten Tusscher-Panfilov human ventricular myocyte model (ten Tusscher and Panfilov, 2006) which has similarly sized I_{Ks} and I_{Kr}, requires increased G_{Kr} (2.65-fold) and decreased G_{Ks} (0.41-fold) to reproduce the clinical LQT dataset (Mann et al., 2016).

These substantial increases in G_{Ks} required for the ORd and the Grandi-Bers models to reproduce the clinical LQT data are at odds with the I_{Ks} ranges recorded experimentally. Factors that may contribute to this disagreement include: (1) Differences between levels of β-adrenergic-dependent kinases and phosphorylation which regulate I_{Ks} and exacerbate LQT1 (Wu et al., 2016); (2) Transmural or other intra-heart heterogeneity with some regions having especially delayed repolarization; (3) Methodological experimental limitations with I_{Ks} rundown and/or damage of the I_{Ks} channel due to enzymatic digestion—however, the recordings that formed the basis of G_{Ks} in the ORd model were done in small tissue preparations using microelectrodes for the express purpose of mitigating these complications (O'Hara et al., 2011).

The I_{Ks} conductance was also increased (by 87%) in the recent optimization of the ORd model with the Markov I_{Kr} formulation to the original O'Hara et al. data (Dutta et al., 2017). While this approximately doubled I_{Ks} at baseline, I_{Ks} remained much smaller than I_{Kr} (by about five-fold) and would not be expected to be able to reproduce the LQT1 phenotype. Because the particular balance between I_{Kr} and I_{Ks} can be important for action potential stability and EAD generation (Devenyi et al., 2017), one may expect a model with large G_{Ks} to behave differently from a model with smaller G_{Ks} model in terms of arrhythmogenesis. Because the reasons for the discrepancy between the experimental and the clinical I_{Ks} data are not known, it will likely be useful to the field to have both a model with large G_{Ks}, replicating the clinical LQT data, and a model with smaller G_{Ks}, replicating the experimental data.

The mismatch between the experimental and the clinically-based estimations of G_{Ks} also raises broader questions regarding how to best handle inconsistent data in model development. Our approach here has been to use data of perceived highest relevance to the particular type of predictions made, i.e., to use clinically-based parameter estimations to predict clinical arrhythmia risk. This approach is in line with the general strategy of using data specific to a particular system (e.g., a cell or a patient) to generate a model specific to that system. However, the best way forward may be to couple rigorously uncertainty in model parameters to uncertainty in model predictions using uncertainty quantification tools (Johnstone et al., 2016).

4.3. Effect of Verapamil on Action Potential Duration

The balance between different currents is also important for determining a model's response to simulated drug block. The anti-hypertension and anti-angina drug verapamil blocks I_{CaL} and I_{Kr}, does not prolong the QT interval, and does not prolong APD in recordings from human trabeculae (Redfern et al., 2003; Britton et al., 2017). However, different human *in silico* models give different responses to simulated verapamil application. The Grandi-Bers and the ten Tusscher-Panfilov models predict action potential shortening in response to verapamil (Mirams et al., 2011, 2012). In variations of the ORd model, verapamil almost always prolongs the APD, but the response varies depending on drug concentration, on how block is modeled, and on whether a Markov model is used for I_{Kr} (Britton et al., 2017; Dutta et al., 2017; Passini et al., 2017).

One hypothesis as to why verapamil does not prolong APD is that its block of I_{Kr} is compensated for by block of I_{CaL}. Using our multi-var optimized model, we show here that in addition to the block of I_{CaL}, a secondary reduction in I_{NCX} (due to the decreased calcium transient) is important in offsetting the I_{Kr} block by verapamil. The size of the I_{Ks} current is also important in determining APD under I_{Kr} block conditions as I_{Ks} provides a repolarization reserve. However, I_{Ks} level in itself is not predictive of APD shortening with verapamil since in the APD_{LQT} optimized model, which has a much increased repolarization reserve in I_{Ks}, verapamil leads to APD prolongation.

4.4. Limitations

There are several limitations to our modeling and optimization approach. We allowed large ranges of the scaling (0.1% to 10-fold) of the parameters to be estimated in the optimization. Consequentially, the conductance scalings may be unphysiologically large, with, e.g., G_{Ks} becoming larger than estimated experimentally. However, we are explicitly not attempting to make the best model of a single cell or small tissue, but, rather, a model capable of making clinically relevant predictions. We did not include the clinical data from control and LQT types 1, 2, and 3 patients during β-adrenergic stimulation (Mann et al., 2016) in the optimization objective as preliminary optimizations with this addition resulted in adrenergically stimulated action potentials having unsmooth repolarization profiles, characterized by slow late repolarization. Due to experimental difficulties in determining absolute values of $[Ca^{2+}]_i$ and $[Na^+]_i$, we based the allowed ranges of these mainly on modeling work, particularly the ORd and the Grandi-Bers models. While experimental measurements of $[Ca^{2+}]_i$ in human ventricular myocytes are consistent with the simulated values (Beuckelmann et al., 1992; Piacentino et al., 2003), reported measurements of $[Na^+]_i$ are much higher ($\sim$20 mM), but may be overestimated (Pieske et al., 2002; Grandi et al., 2010). While the inclusion of bounds on $[Ca^{2+}]_i$ and $[Na^+]_i$ provided additional information to constrain conductance parameters, it is likely that inclusion of more data into the objective would help constrain parameters further. Such data could include more repolarization markers, further calcium transient features, and drug block data.

We modeled the drug application using a simple conductance block, although some drugs are known to block in a state-dependent manner (Mirams et al., 2011; Di Veroli et al., 2014; Britton et al., 2017; Dutta et al., 2017). However, use of this simpler approach allowed us to simulate a larger drug data set. We used a single model for the drug simulations. It might be valuable in future work to generate a population of models around the optimized model to potentially improve predictions and to give insights into ionic mechanisms underlying population heterogeneity in drug responses.

AUTHOR CONTRIBUTIONS

TK-M: Designed study, carried out simulations, and analyzed data; AFJ and FAO: Implemented the optimization software. All authors contributed to critical revision of the manuscript.

REFERENCES

Ben-Hur, A., Ong, C. S., Sonnenburg, S., Schölkopf, B., and Rätsch, G. (2008). Support vector machines and kernels for computational biology. *PLoS Comput. Biol.* 4:e1000173. doi: 10.1371/journal.pcbi.1000173

Beuckelmann, D. J., Näbauer, M., and Erdmann, E. (1992). Intracellular calcium handling in isolated ventricular myocytes from patients with terminal heart failure. *Circulation* 85, 1046–1055.

Bot, C. T., Kherlopian, A. R., Ortega, F. A., Christini, D. J., and Krogh-Madsen, T. (2012). Rapid genetic algorithm optimization of a mouse computational model: benefits for anthropomorphization of neonatal mouse cardiomyocytes. *Front. Physiol.* 3:421. doi: 10.3389/fphys.2012.00421

Britton, O. J., Abi-Gerges, N., Page, G., Ghetti, A., Miller, P. E., and Rodriguez, B. (2017). Quantitative comparison of effects of dofetilide, sotalol, quinidine, and verapamil between human *ex vivo* trabeculae and *in silico* ventricular models incorporating inter-individual action potential variability. *Front. Physiol.* 8:597. doi: 10.3389/fphys.2017.00597

Colatsky, T., Fermini, B., Gintant, G., Pierson, J. B., Sager, P., Sekino, Y., et al. (2016). The Comprehensive *in Vitro* Proarrhythmia Assay (CiPA) initiative - Update on progress. *J. Pharmacol. Toxicol. Methods.* 81, 15–20. doi: 10.1016/j.vascn.2016.06.002

Davies, M. R., Mistry, H. B., Hussein, L., Pollard, C. E., Valentin, J. P., Swinton, J., et al. (2012). An *in silico* canine cardiac midmyocardial action potential duration model as a tool for early drug safety assessment. *Am. J. Physiol. Heart Circ. Physiol.* 302, H1466–H1480. doi: 10.1152/ajpheart.00808.2011

Devenyi, R. A., Ortega, F. A., Groenendaal, W., Krogh-Madsen, T., Christini, D. J., and Sobie, E. A. (2017). Differential roles of two delayed rectifier potassium currents in regulation of ventricular action potential duration and arrhythmia susceptibility. *J. Physiol.* 595, 2301–2317. doi: 10.1113/JP273191

Di Veroli, G. Y., Davies, M. R., Zhang, H., Abi-Gerges, N., and Boyett, M. R. (2014). hERG inhibitors with similar potency but different binding kinetics do not pose the same proarrhythmic risk: implications for drug safety assessment. *J. Cardiovasc. Electrophysiol.* 25, 197–207. doi: 10.1111/jce.12289

Dutta, S., Chang, K. C., Beattie, K. A., Sheng, J., Tran, P. N., Wu, W. W., et al. (2017). Optimization of an *in silico* cardiac cell model for proarrhythmia risk assessment. *Front. Physiol.* 8:616. doi: 10.3389/fphys.2017.00616

Fermini, B., Hancox, J. C., Abi-Gerges, N., Bridgland-Taylor, M., Chaudhary, K. W., Colatsky, T., et al. (2016). A new perspective in the field of cardiac safety testing through the Comprehensive *In Vitro* Proarrhythmia Assay paradigm. *J. Biomol. Screen.* 21, 1–11. doi: 10.1177/1087057115594589

Gintant, G., Sager, P. T., and Stockbridge, N. (2016). Evolution of strategies to improve preclinical cardiac safety testing. *Nat. Rev. Drug. Discov.* 15, 457–471. doi: 10.1038/nrd.2015.34

Grandi, E., Pasqualini, F. S., and Bers, D. M. (2010). A novel computational model of the human ventricular action potential and Ca transient. *J. Mol. Cell. Cardiol.* 48, 112–121. doi: 10.1016/j.yjmcc.2009.09.019

Groenendaal, W., Ortega, F. A., Kherlopian, A. R., Zygmunt, A. C., Krogh-Madsen, T., and Christini, D. J. (2015). Cell-specific cardiac electrophysiology models. *PLoS Comput. Biol.* 11:e1004242. doi: 10.1371/journal.pcbi.1004242

Hale, S. L., Shryock, J. C., Belardinelli, L., Sweeney, M., and Kloner, R. A. (2008). Late sodium current inhibition as a new cardioprotective approach. *J. Mol. Cell. Cardiol.* 44, 954–967. doi: 10.1016/j.yjmcc.2008.03.019

Hoffmann, P., and Warner, B. (2006). Are hERG channel inhibition and QT interval prolongation all there is in drug-induced torsadogenesis? A review of emerging trends. *J. Pharmacol. Toxicol. Methods* 53, 87–105. doi: 10.1016/j.vascn.2005.07.003

Johnstone, R. H., Chang, E. T. Y., Bardenet, R., de Boer, T. P., Gavaghan, D. J., Pathmanathan, P., et al. (2016). Uncertainty and variability in models of the cardiac action potential: Can we build trustworthy models? *J. Mol. Cell. Cardiol.* 96, 49–62. doi: 10.1016/j.yjmcc.2015.11.018

Kaur, J., Nygren, A., and Vigmond, E. J. (2014). Fitting membrane resistance along with action potential shape in cardiac myocytes improves convergence: application of a multi-objective parallel genetic algorithm. *PLoS ONE* 9:e107984. doi: 10.1371/journal.pone.0107984

Kim, J. J., Němec, J., Li, Q., and Salama, G. (2015). Synchronous systolic subcellular Ca^{2+}-elevations underlie ventricular arrhythmia in drug-induced long QT type 2. *Circ. Arrhythm. Electrophysiol.* 8, 703–712. doi: 10.1161/CIRCEP.114.002214

Kramer, J., Obejero-Paz, C. A., Myatt, G., Kuryshev, Y. A., Bruening-Wright, A., Verducci, J. S., et al. (2013). MICE models: superior to the HERG model in predicting Torsade de Pointes. *Sci. Rep.* 3:2100. doi: 10.1038/srep02100

Krogh-Madsen, T., and Christini, D. J. (2017). Slow $[Na^+]_i$ dynamics impacts arrhythmogenesis and spiral wave reentry in cardiac myocyte ionic model. *Chaos* 27, 93907–93912. doi: 10.1063/1.4999475

Lancaster, M. C., and Sobie, E. A. (2016). Improved prediction of drug-induced Torsades de Pointes through simulations of dynamics and machine learning algorithms. *Clin. Pharmacol. Ther.* 100, 371–379. doi: 10.1002/cpt.367

Lankipalli, R. S., Zhu, T., Guo, D., and Yan, G.-X. (2005). Mechanisms underlying arrhythmogenesis in long QT syndrome. *J. Electrocardiol.* 38(4 Suppl.), 69–73. doi: 10.1016/j.jelectrocard.2005.06.008

Li, Z., Dutta, S., Sheng, J., Tran, P. N., Wu, W., Chang, K., et al. (2017). Improving the *in silico* assessment of proarrhythmia risk by combining hERG (Human Ether-à-go-go-Related Gene) channel-drug binding iinetics and multichannel pharmacology. *Circ. Arrhythm. Electrophysiol.* 10:e004628. doi: 10.1161/CIRCEP.116.004628

Mann, S. A., Imtiaz, M., Winbo, A., Rydberg, A., Perry, M. D., Couderc, J.-P., et al. (2016). Convergence of models of human ventricular myocyte electrophysiology after global optimization to recapitulate clinical long QT phenotypes. *J. Mol. Cell. Cardiol.* 100, 25–34. doi: 10.1016/j.yjmcc.2016.09.011

Mirams, G. R., Cui, Y., Sher, A., Fink, M., Cooper, J., Heath, B. M., et al. (2011). Simulation of multiple ion channel block provides improved early prediction of compounds' clinical torsadogenic risk. *Cardiovasc. Res.* 91, 53–61. doi: 10.1093/cvr/cvr044

Mirams, G. R., Davies, M. R. M., Cui, Y. Y., Kohl, P. P., and Noble, D. D. (2012). Application of cardiac electrophysiology simulations to pro-arrhythmic safety testing. *Br. J. Pharmacol.* 167, 932–945. doi: 10.1111/j.1476-5381.2012.02020.x

Mistry, H. B., Davies, M. R., and Di Veroli, G. Y. (2015). A new classifier-based strategy for *in-silico* ion-channel cardiac drug safety assessment. *Front. Pharmacol.* 6:59. doi: 10.3389/fphar.2015.00059

Němec, J., Kim, J. J., and Salama, G. (2016). The link between abnormal calcium handling and electrical instability in acquired long QT syndrome - Does calcium precipitate arrhythmic storms? *Prog. Biophys. Mol. Biol.* 120, 210–221. doi: 10.1016/j.pbiomolbio.2015.11.00

O'Hara, T., Virág, L., Varró, A., and Rudy, Y. (2011). Simulation of the undiseased human cardiac ventricular action potential: model formulation and experimental validation. *PLoS Comput. Biol.* 7:e1002061. doi: 10.1371/journal.pcbi.1002061

Passini, E., Britton, O. J., Lu, H. R., Rohrbacher, J., Hermans, A. N., Gallacher, D. J., et al. (2017). Human *in silico* drug trials demonstrate higher accuracy than animal models in predicting clinical pro-arrhythmic cardiotoxicity. *Front. Physiol.* 8:668. doi: 10.3389/fphys.2017.00668

Piacentino, V., Weber, C. R., Chen, X., Weisser-Thomas, J., Margulies, K. B., Bers, D. M., et al. (2003). Cellular basis of abnormal calcium transients of failing human ventricular myocytes. *Circ. Res.* 92, 651–658. doi: 10.1161/01.RES.0000062469.83985.9B

Pieske, B., Maier, L. S., Piacentino, V., Weisser, J., Hasenfuss, G., and Houser, S. (2002). Rate dependence of $[Na^+]_i$ and contractility in nonfailing and failing human myocardium. *Circulation* 106, 447–453.

Redfern, W. S., Carlsson, L., Davis, A. S., Lynch, W. G., MacKenzie, I., Palethorpe, S., et al. (2003). Relationships between preclinical cardiac electrophysiology, clinical QT interval prolongation and torsade de pointes for a broad range of drugs: evidence for a provisional safety margin in drug development. *Cardiovasc. Res.* 58, 32–45.

Sager, P. T., Gintant, G., Turner, J. R., Pettit, S., and Stockbridge, N. (2014). Rechanneling the cardiac proarrhythmia safety paradigm: a meeting report from the Cardiac Safety Research Consortium. *Am. Heart J.* 167, 292–300. doi: 10.1016/j.ahj.2013.11.004

Sanguinetti, M. C., Jiang, C., Curran, M. E., and Keating, M. T. (1995). A mechanistic link between an inherited and an acquired cardiac arrhythmia: HERG encodes the IKr potassium channel. *Cell* 81, 299–307.

Sarkar, A. X., and Sobie, E. A. (2010). Regression analysis for constraining free parameters in electrophysiological models of cardiac cells. *PLoS Comput. Biol.* 6:e1000914. doi: 10.1371/journal.pcbi.1000914

Straus, S. M. J. M., Sturkenboom, M. C. J. M., Bleumink, G. S., Dieleman, J. P., van der Lei, J., de Graeff, P. A., et al. (2005). Non-cardiac QTc-prolonging drugs and the risk of sudden cardiac death. *Eur. Heart J.* 26, 2007–2012. doi: 10.1093/eurheartj/ehi312

Syed, Z., Vigmond, E., Nattel, S., and Leon, L. J. (2005). Atrial cell action potential parameter fitting using genetic algorithms. *Med. Biol. Eng. Comput.* 43, 561–571.

ten Tusscher, K. H. W. J., and Panfilov, A. V. (2006). Alternans and spiral breakup in a human ventricular tissue model. *Am. J. Physiol. Heart Circ. Physiol.* 291, H1088–H100. doi: 10.1152/ajpheart.00109.2006

Terentyev, D., Rees, C. M., Li, W., Cooper, L. L., Jindal, H. K., Peng, X., et al. (2014). Hyperphosphorylation of RyRs underlies triggered activity in transgenic rabbit model of LQT2 syndrome. *Circ. Res.* 115, 919–928. doi: 10.1161/CIRCRESAHA.115.305146

Wu, J., Ding, W.-G., and Horie, M. (2016). Molecular pathogenesis of long QT syndrome type 1. *J. Arrhythm.* 32, 381–388. doi: 10.1016/j.joa.2015.12.006

Xie, Y., Liao, Z., Grandi, E., Shiferaw, Y., and Bers, D. M. (2015). Slow $[Na]_i$ changes and positive feedback between membrane potential and $[Ca]_i$ underlie intermittent early afterdepolarizations and arrhythmias. *Circ. Arrhythm. Electrophysiol.* 8, 1472–1480. doi: 10.1161/CIRCEP.115.003085

Zhang, Y., Barocas, V. H., Berceli, S. A., Clancy, C. E., Eckmann, D. M., Garbey, M., et al. (2016). Multi-scale modeling of the cardiovascular system: Disease development, progression, and clinical intervention. *Ann. Biomed. Eng.* 44, 2642–2660. doi: 10.1007/s10439-016-1628-0

15

Trigger vs. Substrate: Multi-Dimensional Modulation of QT-Prolongation Associated Arrhythmic Dynamics by a hERG Channel Activator

Michael A. Colman [1], Erick A. Perez Alday [2], Arun V. Holden [1] and Alan P. Benson [1]*

[1] *School of Biomedical Sciences and Multidisciplinary Cardiovascular Research Centre, University of Leeds, Leeds, United Kingdom,* [2] *Division of Cardiovascular Medicine, Oregon Health and Science University, Portland, OR, United States*

Correspondence:
Michael A. Colman
m.a.colman@leeds.ac.uk

Background: Prolongation of the QT interval of the electrocardiogram (ECG), underlain by prolongation of the action potential duration (APD) at the cellular level, is linked to increased vulnerability to cardiac arrhythmia. Pharmacological management of arrhythmia associated with QT prolongation is typically achieved through attempting to restore APD to control ranges, reversing the enhanced vulnerability to Ca^{2+}-dependent afterdepolarisations (arrhythmia triggers) and increased transmural dispersion of repolarisation (arrhythmia substrate) associated with APD prolongation. However, such pharmacological modulation has been demonstrated to have limited effectiveness. Understanding the integrative functional impact of pharmacological modulation requires simultaneous investigation of both the trigger and substrate.

Methods: We implemented a multi-scale (cell and tissue) *in silico* approach using a model of the human ventricular action potential, integrated with a model of stochastic 3D spatiotemporal Ca^{2+} dynamics, and parameter modification to mimic prolonged QT conditions. We used these models to examine the efficacy of the hERG activator MC-II-157c in restoring APD to control ranges, examined its effects on arrhythmia triggers and substrates, and the interaction of these arrhythmia triggers and substrates.

Results: QT prolongation conditions promoted the development of spontaneous release events underlying afterdepolarisations during rapid pacing. MC-II-157c applied to prolonged QT conditions shortened the APD, inhibited the development of afterdepolarisations and reduced the probability of afterdepolarisations manifesting as triggered activity in single cells. In tissue, QT prolongation resulted in an increased transmural dispersion of repolarisation, which manifested as an increased vulnerable window for uni-directional conduction block. In some cases, MC-II-157c further increased the vulnerable window through its effects on I_{Na}. The combination of stochastic release event modulation and transmural dispersion of repolarisation modulation by MC-II-157c resulted in an integrative behavior wherein the arrhythmia trigger is reduced but the arrhythmia substrate is increased, leading to variable and non-linear overall vulnerability to arrhythmia.

Conclusion: The relative balance of reduced trigger and increased substrate underlies a multi-dimensional role of MC-II-157c in modulation of cardiac arrhythmia vulnerability associated with prolonged QT interval.

Keywords: QT interval, action potential duration, arrhythmia trigger, arrhythmia substrate, hERG activators, computational modeling

INTRODUCTION

Conditions in which the QT interval of the electrocardiogram (ECG) is prolonged, such as heart failure (Hart, 1994) and inherited or acquired long QT syndromes (LQTS) (Schwartz et al., 2012), are associated with an increased risk of ventricular arrhythmias (Tomaselli and Zipes, 2004; Moss and Kass, 2005). The prolonged QT interval reflects prolongation of the ventricular cellular action potential duration (APD), which can result in arrhythmias through an increase in cell-level arrhythmia triggers and/or modification of tissue-level arrhythmia substrates (Kalin et al., 2010; Benson et al., 2011a; Tse, 2016).

Cell-level triggers arise because delayed ventricular repolarisation modifies membrane and subcellular Ca^{2+} handling (Clusin, 2003; Němec et al., 2016), leading to either re-activation of the L-type Ca^{2+} current and early afterdepolarisations (Lankipalli et al., 2005), or Ca^{2+} overload of the sarcoplasmic reticulum (SR), causing spontaneous SR Ca^{2+} release events and delayed-afterdepolarisations through activation of the forward-mode Na^+-Ca^{2+} exchange current (I_{NaCa}), which in turn can result in triggered activity if the delayed afterdepolarisation is of sufficient magnitude (Janse, 2004). Cardiomyocytes typically exhibit a threshold dependence of the occurrence of spontaneous release events as a function of SR Ca^{2+} load, wherein the probability of a spontaneous release event rapidly rises from 0 to 1 within a critical region of SR Ca^{2+} (Venetucci et al., 2007; Campos et al., 2015). Although originating at the cell level, triggers need to be coordinated at the tissue level in order to develop into arrhythmias: a critical compact region of tissue simultaneously exhibiting triggered behavior is required to initiate propagation of the trigger (Noble, 1972; Clayton et al., 2011; Bezekci et al., 2015; Campos et al., 2015).

An increase in the tissue-level substrates for arrhythmias (that is, the necessary conditions for triggered activity to propagate and develop into arrhythmias) arise because APD prolongation is rarely homogenous in and between the different regions of the ventricles (e.g., transmurally, or from base to apex) (Antzelevitch, 2005; Glukhov et al., 2010). This heterogeneous APD prolongation increases the spatial dispersion of repolarisation, potentially leading to regions of recovered (i.e., excitable) tissue partially bordered by still refractory (i.e., unexcitable) tissue. A propagating trigger event occurring in such a location can be partially blocked by the refractory tissue, leading to re-entrant arrhythmias (Pandit and Jalife, 2013). The spatiotemporal region where such partial conduction block could occur is termed the "vulnerable window" (VW) (Starmer et al., 1993; Shaw and Rudy, 1995; Benson et al., 2008, 2011a). It follows that heterogeneous APD prolongation increases not only the spatial dispersion of repolarisation, but also the VW, i.e., the arrhythmia substrate.

The interaction of triggers and substrates determines the initiation of arrhythmia: an arrhythmia cannot be initiated without both a suitably-sized and -timed trigger and the necessary substrate to allow that trigger to propagate in a re-entrant manner (Kalin et al., 2010). Arrhythmias, therefore, are not cellular events, but tissue-level events.

Management of arrhythmias associated with QT prolongation can be achieved by attempting to restore the ventricular APD to control ranges (Nachimuthu et al., 2012), thus reversing the increases in arrhythmogenic triggers and substrates associated with APD prolongation. One such strategy is the use of human ether-a-go-go-related-gene channel (hERG) activators that enhance the repolarising rapid delayed rectifier K^+ current (I_{Kr}), thus reducing the APD (Grunnet et al., 2008; Wu and Sanguinetti, 2016). However, many anti-arrhythmic drugs have pro-arrhythmic effects (Kumar and Zimetbaum, 2013); such drugs can shorten the action potential and the QT interval (reducing arrhythmias associated with a prolonged QT interval), but they may have additional and unintended effects that increase (rather than reduce) the propensity for arrhythmias under certain conditions. For example, we have shown in a previous experimental and computational study that the hERG activator NS1643, one of the most effective and best characterized hERG activators (Hansen et al., 2006), successfully restores APD toward healthy durations and reduces arrhythmia triggers, but is associated with an increase in the VW, i.e., the substrate for arrhythmias, due to effects on the post-repolarisation refractory period (Peitersen et al., 2008). Furthermore, while low concentrations of NS1643 activates I_{Kr} and shortens APD, it has been shown that higher concentrations of NS1643 blocks (rather than activates) I_{Kr} (Bilet and Bauer, 2012).

The potentially pro-arrhythmic effects of hERG activators, such as NS1643 has prompted the search for novel hERG activators that do not display these effects. One recently-identified compound is MC-II-157c, an NS1643 analog. MC-II-157c activates I_{Kr} at low concentrations and, unlike NS1643, it continues to activate I_{Kr} at high concentrations; it may also block the sodium current (I_{Na}) (Guo et al., 2014). However, it remains unknown how the I_{Kr} activation and I_{Na} block seen with this new compound affect arrhythmia triggers and substrates, and importantly, how these (increased or decreased) triggers and substrates interact to induce arrhythmias (if at all).

Computational models provide powerful research tools to understand the intricacies of arrhythmia trigger and substrate interaction, as they allow us to modify parameters under precisely controlled conditions and quantify the resultant tissue-level arrhythmic behavior, and can predict how these arrhythmias will manifest in a clinical setting (e.g., changes to the ECG). We therefore used a computational approach to quantify the interaction of pharmacologically-modified arrhythmia trigger and substrate, using the novel hERG activator MC-II-157c as an example.

We wanted to quantify the modified triggers and substrate that result from MC-II-157c ion channel actions. To this end, we use detailed single cell and tissue level models to study the effect of QT prolongation and its modulation by MC-II-157c on: (i) APD heterogeneity in isolated cells; (ii) SR Ca^{2+} loading and subsequent spontaneous SR Ca^{2+} release events; (iii) the probability of spontaneous SR Ca^{2+} release manifesting as triggered action potentials in single cell and ectopic activity in tissue; and (iv) the vulnerability to the initiation of re-entrant like conduction patterns.

METHODS

We implemented a multi-scale *in silico* approach to study the interactions between arrhythmia trigger and substrate in conditions associated with prolonged QT intervals, and their modulation by the hERG activator MC-II-157c.

Isolated Cell Models – Intracellular Ca^{2+} Handling

In order to simulate triggered and ectopic activity underlain by spontaneous Ca^{2+} release events, a spatial model of intracellular Ca^{2+} handling which explicitly accounts for stochastic state transitions and spatial coupling is required. We therefore implemented an efficient, idealized reduction of a previously developed and validated general model of spatio-temporal Ca^{2+} handling with realistic structure (Colman et al., 2017), using a similar approach implemented by other groups (e.g., Restrepo et al., 2008). Briefly, 15 × 20 × 65 spatially-discrete individual calcium release units (CRUs) were modeled throughout the geometry of the cell (**Figure 1**). Each CRU comprises of five compartments with associated Ca^{2+} concentrations: the intracellular spaces of the dyadic cleft space ($[Ca^{2+}]_{ds}$), subspace ($[Ca^{2+}]_{SS}$) and bulk-cytosolic space ($[Ca^{2+}]_i$), and the network and junctional SR ($[Ca^{2+}]_{nSR}$, ($[Ca^{2+}]_{jSR}$). The bulk cytosol, subspace and network SR are diffusively coupled to neighboring CRUs; the dyadic cleft space and junctional SR are not spatially coupled to neighbors. The fundamental model equations describing this system are:

$$\frac{d[Ca^{2+}]_i}{dt} = \beta\left(\mathbf{D}\nabla^2[Ca^{2+}]_i + \varphi_i + (\nu_{SS}/\nu_i)J_{SS}\right)$$

$$\frac{d[Ca^{2+}]_{SS}}{dt} = \mathbf{D}\nabla^2[Ca^{2+}]_{SS} + \varphi_{SS} - J_{SS} + (\nu_{ds}/\nu_{SS})J_{ds}$$

$$\frac{d[Ca^{2+}]_{nSR}}{dt} = \beta_{nSR}\left(\mathbf{D}\nabla^2[Ca^{2+}]_{nSR} + \varphi_{nSR} - (\nu_{jSR}/\nu_{nSR})J_{jSR}\right)$$

$$\frac{d[Ca^{2+}]_{ds}}{dt} = \varphi_{ds} - J_{ds}$$

$$\frac{d[Ca^{2+}]_{jSR}}{dt} = \varphi_{jSR} - J_{jSR}$$

where transfer between compartments is given by:

$$J_{SS} = \left([Ca^{2+}]_{SS} - [Ca^{2+}]_i\right)\tau_{SS}^{-1}$$

$$J_{ds} = \left([Ca^{2+}]_{ds} - [Ca^{2+}]_{SS}\right)\tau_{ds}^{-1}$$

$$J_{jSR} = \left([Ca^{2+}]_{jSR} - [Ca^{2+}]_{nSR}\right)\tau_{jSR}^{-1}$$

where ν_x is the volume of compartment x, β_x is an instantaneous buffering term, and φ_x is the reaction term. Stochastic dynamics are modeled for the RyRs and LTCCs, which are part of the dyadic cleft space reaction term. All parameters and reaction terms are given in the Supplementary Material.

Isolated Cell Models - Action Potential Model

Ion currents were described by a simplified version of the O'Hara-Rudy dynamic (ORd) human ventricular cell model (O'Hara et al., 2011), wherein the major currents only (I_{Na}, I_{Kr}, I_{Ks}, I_{K1}, I_{to}, I_{NaK}) were included, without the further details of phosphorylation included in the original study; Ca^{2+} currents (I_{CaL}, I_{NaCa}, I_{Cap}, I_{Cab}) are described by the Ca^{2+} handling model. These simplifications were implemented to improve computational efficiency and for integration with the general stochastic Ca^{2+} handling model described above. The model provides specific formulations to describe the heterogeneity in ionic currents of the transmural cell types (endocardial, midmyocardial, and epicardial) found in the left ventricular free wall of the human heart (see O'Hara et al., 2011) for details.

This integrated stochastic framework captures spontaneous Ca^{2+} release events that could lead to triggered activity (see details in Simulating Spontaneous Release Events in Tissue Models below). Default model action potentials and cytosolic Ca^{2+} transients, for the three transmural cell types of the simplified ORd model with stochastic Ca^{2+} handling, are shown in **Figure 1B**. The updated cell model exhibits action potential and Ca^{2+} transient properties similar to the original cell model and within the range of experimental data presented in the original study (O'Hara et al., 2011): APD = 272–360 ms and intracellular Ca^{2+} transient magnitude of ~0.6 μM for the three cell-types during control pacing; note that the present study does not consider heterogeneity in the intracellular Ca^{2+} handling system and thus the Ca^{2+} transient is more homogeneous between the cell types than in the original study (see Limitations). The model is therefore considered suitable for the mechanistic study undertaken.

Prolonged QT and Pharmacological Modulation

We were interested in general cases of QT prolongation rather than modeling the kinetics of very specific conditions, while still making our results broadly applicable to clinical conditions, such as LQTS. We therefore simulated QT interval prolongation (i.e., prolongation of the ventricular APD) in one of three ways: (i) downregulation of the slow delayed rectifier K^+ current (I_{Ks}) maximal conductance by 50%, similar to LQTS1, which we term "prolonged QT variant a" (PQTa) in the remainder of the manuscript; (ii) downregulation of I_{Kr} maximal conductance by

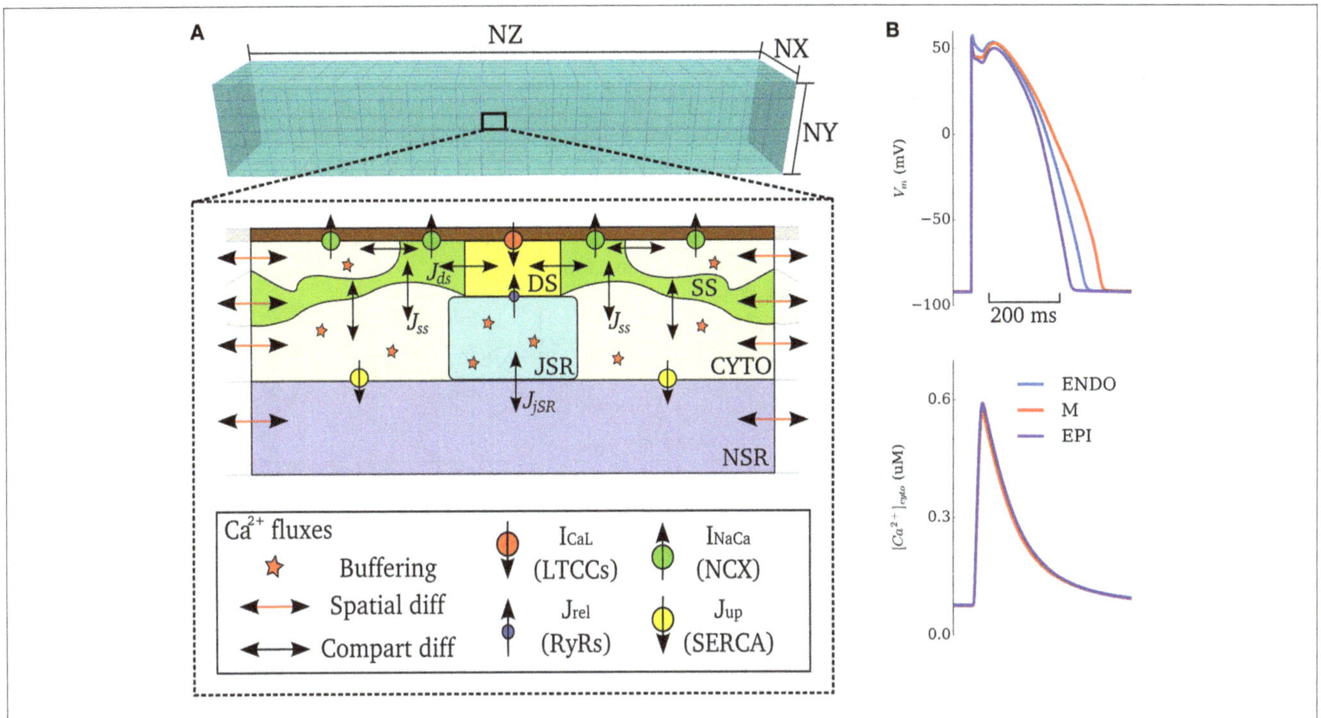

FIGURE 1 | Model schematic. **(A)** Schematic structure of the spatio-temporal Ca^{2+} handling model with the compartments comprising a single CRU, and coupling between compartments, illustrated. DS, dyadic cleft space; SS, subspace; CTYO, bulk intracellular space; JSR, junctional SR; NSR, network SR. NX, 15; NY, 20; NZ, 65. **(B)** Action potentials (upper) and Ca^{2+} transients (lower) during control pacing (BCL = 1, 000 ms) for the three cell types (ENDO, Endocardium; M, Midmyocardium; EPI, Epicardium).

50% (PQTb), similar to LQTS2; and (iii) upregulation of $I_{Ca,L}$ maximal conductance by 50% (PQTc), similar to LQT8 (Bohnen et al., 2017).

Effects of 10 μM of the hERG activator MC-II-157c on I_{Kr} were modeled by modifying the I_{Kr} formulation according to experimental data (Guo et al., 2014): maximal conductance was decreased by 12%, activation was shifted by −14 mV and inactivation by +14 mV, and deactivation kinetics were slowed 3.3-fold (note that, although the maximal conductance of I_{Kr} is reduced by MC-II-157c, its kinetic effects enhance the activity of the current; see The hERG Activator MC-II-157c Partially or Fully Reverses APD Prolongation Heterogeneously). Effects of MC-II-157c on blocking I_{Na} (which are not as well characterized as its effects on I_{Kr}; Guo et al., 2014) were simulated by reducing the maximal conductance of I_{Na} by 0, 40, and 80%.

Tissue Models

We used a 20 mm 1D virtual tissue strand (Kléber and Rudy, 2004) for quantifying transmural propagation and vulnerability, with equal spatial distributions of endocardial, midmyocardial and epicardial cells. A 20 × 40 mm 2D tissue sheet (Clayton et al., 2011) was used for simulations examining propagation of triggered activity, with equal distributions of endocardial, midmyocardial and epicardial tissue in the x direction. For examining intramural propagation and ectopic activity in 3D, we used an anatomically detailed 3D ventricular wedge model, obtained by diffusion tensor MRI, and used equal proportions of endocardial, midmyocardial and epicardial tissue in the transmural direction (see Benson et al., 2007, 2011b; Walton et al., 2013 for details).

All tissues were isotropic, i.e., conduction velocity was set to be equal in all directions: We used an electrical diffusion coefficient of $D = 0.048\ mm^2ms^{-1}$, to give a conduction time along the 1D strand (i.e., a transmural activation time) of 40 ms (cf. Glukhov et al., 2010), and a plane wave conduction velocity of 0.5 $m.s^{-1}$ in all tissues. The body surface potential was computed by placing the ventricular wedge model in a human torso mesh; the forward problem was solved by a boundary element method, as has been described in previous studies (Perez Alday et al., 2015, 2016, 2017). ECGs were derived from the body surface potential by selecting elements of the torso mesh which correspond to the ECG electrodes.

Simulating Spontaneous Release Events in Tissue Models

Performing tissue level simulations using the fully detailed spatial Ca^{2+} handling model to describe individual cells is computationally intractable due to the large number of equations that need to be solved in such situations. Furthermore, the focus of this study was not to dissect the mechanisms of spontaneous Ca^{2+} release in single cell, but rather to understand the considerations determining the manifestation of sub-cellular Ca^{2+} release as triggered action potentials and propagating electrical excitation in the presence of prolonged APD and its pharmacological modulation.

We therefore implemented a "non-spatial" simplification of the Ca^{2+} handling model (described in Isolated Cell Models–Intracellular Ca^{2+} Handling, above) for use in tissue-level simulations, to capture spontaneous Ca^{2+} release events at significantly reduced computational cost and with complete controllability. The non-spatial model consists of a single CRU (with RyR and LTCC dynamics solved deterministically) with additional analytical functions which describe the RyR waveform associated with whole-cell spontaneous release events, derived from analysis of the fully detailed spatial cell model, similar to the approach used in Campos et al. (2015) and Colman et al. (2015). For a simple transient-spike morphology (**Figure 2**) this function has the form:

$$N_{RyR\_O} = \frac{N_{RyR\_peak}}{\left(1+e^{-(t-(t_i+0.5t_{up}))/(0.1689t_{up}+0.00255)}\right)\left(1+e^{-(t-(t_i+t_{up}+0.5t_{decay}))/(0.1689t_{decay}+0.00255)}\right)}$$

where t_i is the initiation time of the spontaneous release and t_{up}, t_{decay} and N_{RyR_peak} describe the shape of the waveform and are all determined from the *duration* (**Figures 2**, **3** and described below). The function for the plateau-like waveform (corresponding to durations longer than 250 ms) is derived from the same parameters (note the peak time, t_p, is t_i+t_{up}):

$$N_{RyR\_O} = \frac{N_{RyR\_plateau}}{\left(1+e^{-(t-(t_i+17.5))/5.946}\right)\left(1+e^{(t-(t_f-17.5))/5.946}\right)} + \frac{N_{RyR\_peak}-N_{RyR\_plateau}}{\left(1+e^{-(t-(t_p-17.5))/5.946}\right)\left(1+e^{(t-(t_p+17.5))/5.946}\right)}$$

Thus, the waveform is completely described by the *initiation time* and the *duration*. The stochastic nature of spontaneous Ca^{2+} release is captured by randomly selecting these parameters from functions describing their physiological distributions. The distributions describing initiation time of whole-cell spontaneous release events in the spatial cell model are typically skewed (**Figure 3Aa**) and well approximated by two sigmoidal functions, split around the cumulative probability of 0.25 (corresponding to a specific initiation time, t_{i_sep}; **Figure 3Ab**). The initiation time can therefore be determined by passing a random number into the inverse of the two sigmoidal functions:

$$t_i = \begin{cases} -k_{F1}\ln\left(\frac{0.5}{rand}-1\right)+t_{i_{sep}}, & rand < 0.25 \\ -k_{F2}\ln\left(\frac{1.5}{rand+0.5}-1\right)+t_{i_{sep}}, & rand \geq 0.25 \end{cases}$$

where the gradient parameters of the two sigmoidal functions (k_{F1}, k_{F2}) and the t_i at the cumulative probability of 0.25, t_{i_sep}, completely control the resulting distribution. The duration, D, of the RyR waveform can be determined from distributions in an analogous manner:

$$D = \begin{cases} k_{1\_MD}\ln\left[1/\left(rand-1\right)\right]+MD, & rand < 0.5 \\ k_{2\_MD}\ln\left[1/\left(rand-1\right)\right]+MD, & rand \geq 0.5 \end{cases}$$

where MD refers to the median and k_{1_MD} and k_{2_MD} are functions of the median (in conditions where longer waveforms are observed, the variability in waveform duration between simulations is larger; **Figure 3Ba–c**):

$$k_{1\_MD} = 0.1366MD - 7.98$$
$$k_{2\_MD} = 0.12MD - 3.265$$

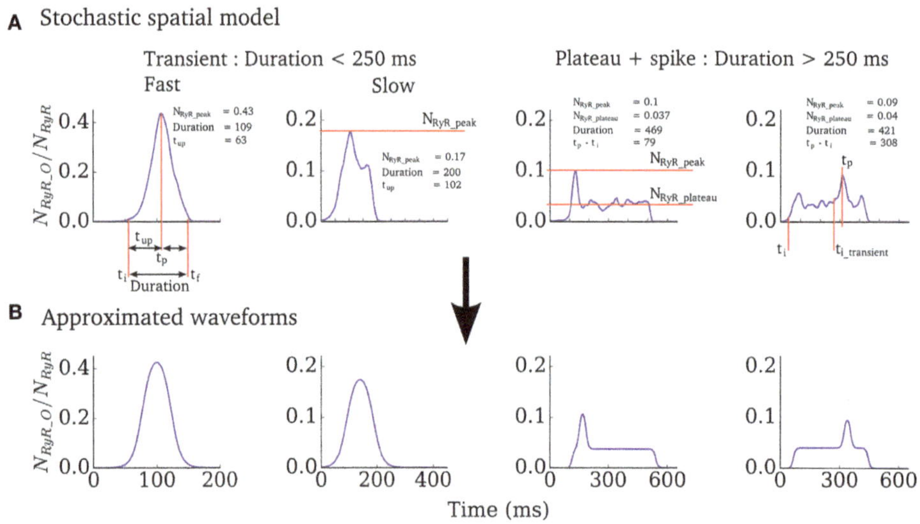

FIGURE 2 | Spontaneous excitation RyR waveforms and parameters. **(A)** Four examples of RyR waveforms associated with whole-cell spontaneous release events in the spatial cell model. Parameters describing the shape of the waveform are labeled. **(B)** Analytical waveforms approximating those in **(A)** using the input parameters listed.

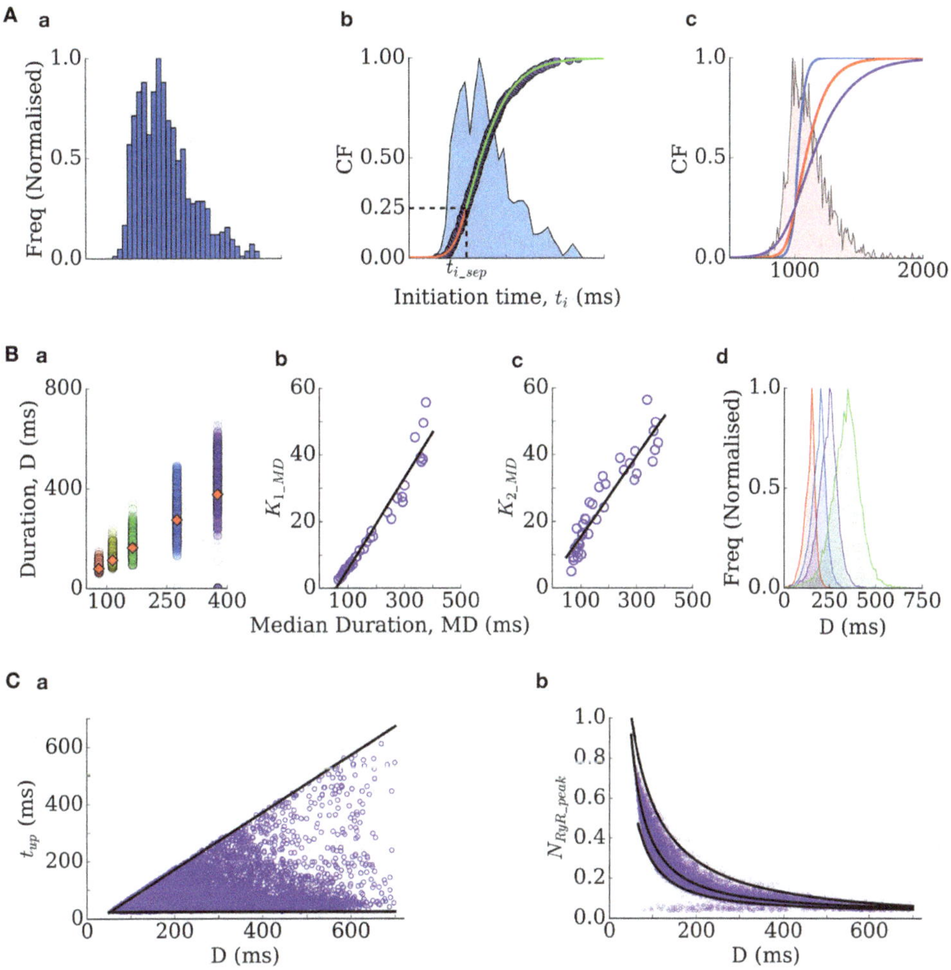

FIGURE 3 | Derivation of the RyR waveform parameters. **(A)** Initiation time distributions: **(a)** is an example distribution produced by the spatial cell model; **(b)** is the cumulative frequency of the distribution (purple dots) and two sigmoidal functions (red and green lines) which approximate it–the distribution itself is shown for reference (blue shading); **(c)** cumulative frequencies of the three distributions used in this study (t_i distribution widths of 350 ms–blue; 550 ms–red; 1,000 ms–purple), with the histogram corresponding to the red distribution shown for reference. **(B)** Duration distributions: **(a)** scatter-plot of the durations associated with multiple simulations under different conditions (colors), plotted against the median of each distribution, which is also shown as the red diamonds for reference; **(b,c)** correlation of the gradient parameters of sigmoidal functions describing the distribution either side of the median with the median value; **(d)** four duration distributions used in the present study (Median Duration = 150 ms–red; 200 ms–blue; 250 ms–purple; 300 ms–green). **(C)** Other parameters correlate with the duration–time to peak (t_{up}, **a**) and the waveform peak (N_{RyR_peak}, **b**).

Thus, the distribution is entirely described by the median. Finally, t_{up} and N_{RyR_peak} can be determined from the given duration (**Figure 3C**):

$$t_{up} = 24 + rand(D - 52)$$

$$N_{RyR\_peak} = \begin{cases} MRYR - rand(159.59(D^{-1.327} - D^{-1.4})), \; rand < 0.5 \\ MRYR - (1 - rand)(159.59\left((D+30)^{-1.15} + D^{-1.327}\right) + 0.08), \; rand \geq 0.5 \end{cases}$$

Where $MRYR$ refers to the median and is given by:

$$MRYR = 159.59D^{-1.327} + 0.028$$

And if duration > 250 ms, it is also necessary to compute $N_{RyR\_plateau}$:

$$N_{RyR\_plateau} = 31.09(0.01D)^{-7.39} + (rand - 0.5)(-5 \times 10^{-4}D\_0.0275) + 0.34$$

These formulations therefore allow complete control over spontaneous release dynamics through just four parameters (k_{F1}, k_{F2}, t_{i_sep}, median duration). We fix t_{i_sep} in simulations such that only the width of the initiation time distribution (k_{F1}, k_{F2}) and the median of the duration distribution are varied: t_i distribution widths of 350, 550, and 1,000 ms (**Figure 3Ac**) were used in tissue simulations; duration medians of 150, 200, 250, 300, and 350 ms (**Figure 3Bd**) were used in single-cell and tissue simulations. Derivation of these equations from the fully detailed spatial cell model ensures self-consistency and physiological validity of the resulting waveforms.

Computational Aspects

Models were coded in C/C++ and run on a Linux desktop machine, or using the University of Leeds ARC2 High Performance Computing facilities. Equations for isolated cell models were solved using a forward Euler method with a time step of $\Delta t = 0.05$ ms; ion channel gating equations were solved using the Rush-Larsen scheme (Rush and Larsen, 1978). For tissue models, the monodomain equation was solved using a Forward Time Centred Space method: Space steps of $\Delta x = 0.2$ mm were used in the 1D strand, $\Delta x = \Delta y = 0.2$ mm in the 2D tissue, and $\Delta x = \Delta y = 0.425$ mm and $\Delta z = 0.5$ mm in the 3D wedge model (as defined by the diffusion tensor MRI dataset). Parallelisation was implemented with OpenMP. Cell APD was measured from the time the membrane potential crossed −80 mV during the upstroke of the action potential, to when the membrane potential crossed back over −80 mV during the repolarisation phase.

RESULTS

The hERG Activator MC-II-157c Partially or Fully Reverses APD Prolongation Heterogeneously

The single cell model was paced at a cycle length of 1,000 ms for 100 beats under control (WT), PQT and PQT + MC-II-157c conditions to evaluate the efficacy of MC-II-157c on reversing PQT induced APD prolongation (**Figure 4**). **Figure 4A** shows effects on AP morphology of the PQTa, PQTb, and PQTc conditions in endocardial, midmyocardial, and epicardial cells, with WT action potentials shown as a reference. The PQTb condition (downregulation of I_{Kr}) has the largest effect on prolonging APD (from 360 to 649 ms in midmyocardial cells, an increase of 80%), due to the larger I_{Kr} conductance in human cells relative to I_{Ks} conductance, and its primary role in AP repolarisation. All three PQT conditions increase the transmural difference in APD (the difference between the longest and shortest APDs in the three cell types), from 88 ms in WT to 97, 279 and 122 ms with PQTa, PQTb, and PQTc, respectively.

Figure 4B shows how the hERG activator MC-II-157c reduces APD back towards control levels in all cell types and with all PQT conditions. The drug reduced APD back to control levels in PQTa (downregulation of I_{Ks}) due to the minimal effect this condition has on initially prolonging APD, but the largest decrease was seen with PQTb in midmyocardial cells, where APD was reduced from 649 to 540 ms, a reduction of 17% (**Figure 4C**). It should be noted, however, that MC-II-157c has transmurally heterogeneous effects; that is, the degree of APD reduction seen in the three different cell types is not identical, with the drug under PQTb conditions (for example) giving a 5% decrease in endocardial cells, 17% in midmyocardial cells and 4% in epicardial cells. Consequently, the maximal transmural difference in APD in PQTb reduces from 279 ms with the PQT condition alone to 184 ms with PQTb plus MC-II-157c, but does not reduce transmural difference in APD back down to WT levels (184 vs. 88 ms).

ECGs were computed for the different conditions using the 3D ventricular wedge model under normal pacing (BCL = 1,000 ms). QT-prolongation was observed for all three remodeling types (**Figure 4C**), with PQTb exhibiting the longest QT-interval, congruent with single cell results (QT = 310 ms in WT compared to 326, 418, and 329 ms in PQTa-c, respectively). MC-II-157c resulted in a delay in the QRS peak as well as earlier absolute repolarisation time and consequent shortening of the QT interval (QT = 309 ms, 403 and 310 ms in PQTa-c + MC-II-157c; **Figure 4C**); in PQTa and PQTc, MC-II-157c fully reverses QT prolongation.

The mechanism by which MC-II-157c shortens APD, despire reducing the maximal conductance of I_{Kr}, is illustrated in **Figure 5**: the shifts in the activation and inactivation curves and the slowing of deactivation kinetics result in an increased current during both voltage clamp and AP clamp experiments. These results are generally congruent with the original study of Guo et al. (2014), although the current traces do differ in morphology and extent of effect of MC-II-157c (see Limitations).

MC-II-157c has PQT-Type Dependent Effectiveness in Reversing SR Loading and Spontaneous Release Events

The vulnerability to the emergence of whole-cell spontaneous Ca^{2+} release events (such as intracellular Ca^{2+} waves, **Figure 6A**) is primarily controlled by the dynamics of the intracellular Ca^{2+} handling system and the SR Ca^{2+} load, wherein cells typically exhibit an SR load threshold above which the probability of spontaneous release events significantly increases (Wagner et al., 2015). The focus of this study is not on the mechanisms of spontaneous Ca^{2+} release, and therefore investigation of Ca^{2+} handling remodeling is beyond its scope. However, APD prolongation associated with PQT, and its subsequent reversal by MC-II-157c, may influence SR loading and consequently the vulnerability to the emergence of whole-cell spontaneous Ca^{2+} release.

An SR-loading protocol was used to analyse this behavior, by pacing the spatial cell model at a rapid rate (cycle length of 400 ms). The maximal flux rate of intracellular uptake was increased, simulating the effect of sympathetic stimulation, in order to promote SR loading. An increase by a factor of two was chosen as this loaded the SR-Ca^{2+} in the WT model to just above the spontaneous release threshold; the most suitable region to reveal the consequence of APD modulation on spontaneous activity.

The time series of SR-Ca^{2+} in WT and the PQTc condition in isolated epicardial cells illustrates the effect on SR-Ca^{2+} loading under rapid pacing and highlights that APD prolongation associated with PQT can promote loading (**Figure 6B**). The peak of the SR Ca^{2+} concentration during this time provides a measure of SR Ca^{2+} loading; these data are shown in **Figure 6C** for WT and all PQT conditions with and without MC-II-157c. The PQTa condition (downregulation of I_{Ks}) does not promote

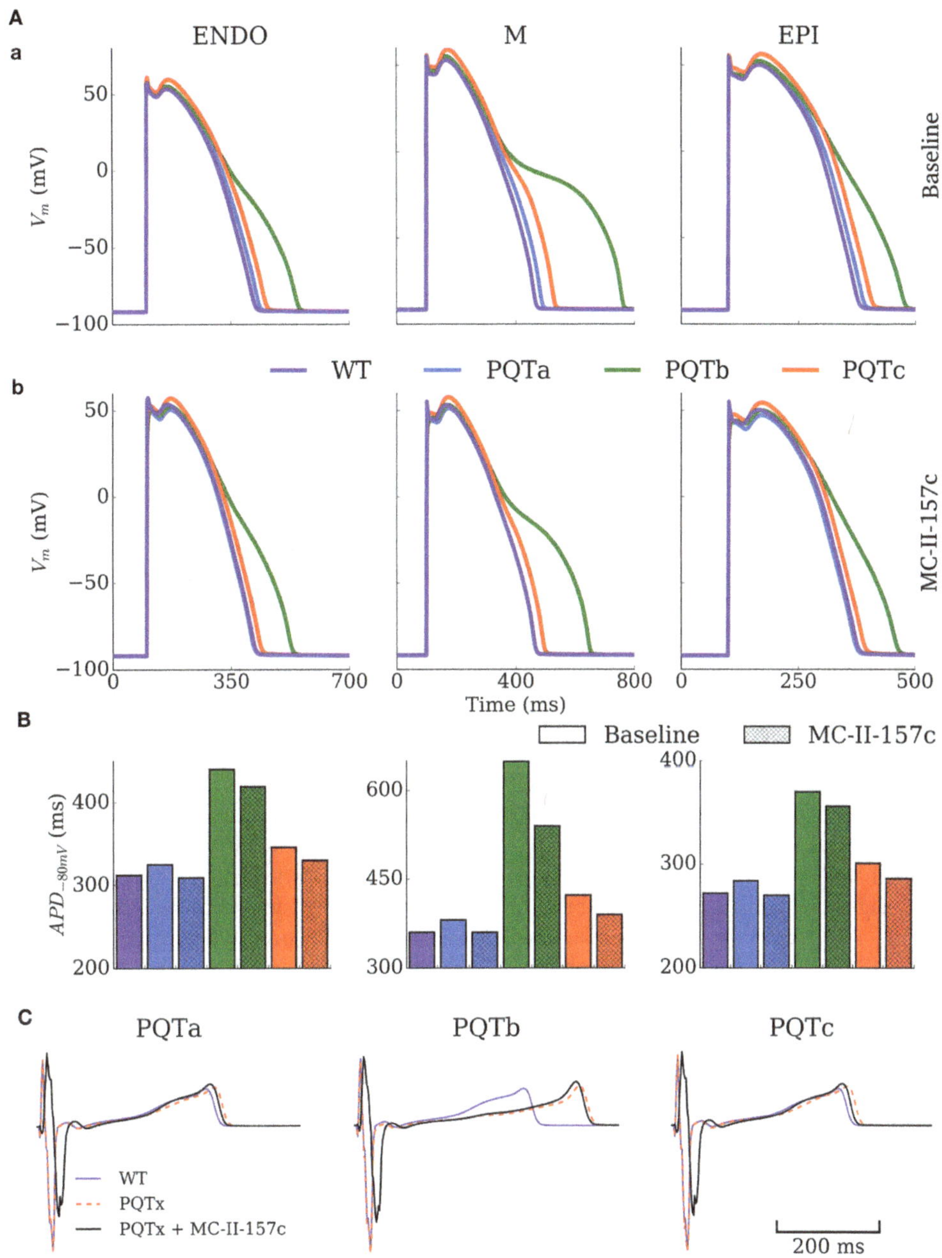

FIGURE 4 | Action potential and ECG morphology and duration in PQT and MC-II-157c. **(A)** Action potentials for the three cell types (ENDO, left; M, middle; EPI, right) under baseline (upper) and MC-II-157c (lower) conditions in control (WT, purple) and PQTa-c conditions (blue, green, red) in the spatial cell model. **(B)** Action potential duration at −80 mV for the same conditions in **(A)**. The colors in the key apply to both panels **(A,B)**. **(C)** Computed ECGs for the three conditions (dotted red line) and with the application of MC-II-157c (black line), relative to the WT (purple line). MC-II-157c was modeled as I_{Kr} modification + 40% I_{Na} block. Any impact of I_{Na} block on the upstroke velocity is not clear at this scale.

SR loading compared to WT (peak SR Ca^{2+} load of 1.07 mM in WT and 1.06 mM in PQTa), but the PQTb (downregulation of I_{Kr}) and PQTc (upregulation of $I_{Ca,L}$) conditions do (peak SR Ca^{2+} load of 1.106 and 1.13 mM, respectively), with PQTc having the largest effect due to the increase in the transmembrane Ca^{2+} current in this condition. MC-II-157c reverses SR Ca^{2+} loading in PQTb, reducing peak SR Ca^{2+} load at periodic steady-state to 1.05 mM, which is below WT levels. However, the drug has only a very small effect in PQTc (down to 1.108 mM) due to the minimal effect MC-II-157c has on APD in this condition, and the subsequently small change in the time course of $I_{Ca,L}$.

These relatively small changes in SR-Ca^{2+} can manifest as significant differences in the vulnerability to spontaneous Ca^{2+} release due to the non-linear threshold dependence on SR

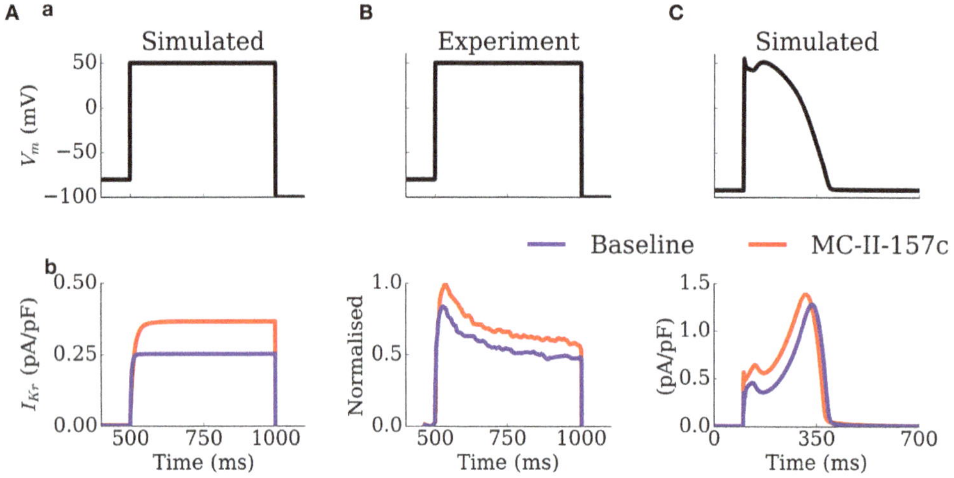

FIGURE 5 | Activity of I_{Kr} during voltage and AP clamp conditions under the application of MC-II-157c. I_{Kr} traces **(b)** elicited by a voltage step protocol **(a)** in simulation **(A)** and experiments of Guo et al. (2014); **(B)** and elicited by a simulated AP clamp **(C)**, for baseline (purple) and MC-II-157c (red) conditions. In **(B)**, the current traces have been normalized to the peak of the control current. Conditions in **(A)** were matched to those experimentally—the intracellular and extracellular concentrations of potassium were set to 120 and 5.4 mM, respectively.

Ca^{2+} concentration (**Figures 6D,E**). The probability of whole-cell spontaneous release events and the probability distributions describing the initiation time can be computed from a large set of simulations ($N = 1{,}000$ per condition). Example distributions are shown in **Figure 6E** for the WT and PQTc with and without MC-II-157c, highlighting that even the small change in SR Ca^{2+} as a result of MC-II-157c significantly reduces the probability of spontaneous release (~50% in PQTc with MC-II-157c compared to 98% in PQTc alone) as well as widening the distribution (although not fully reversed to WT). Due to the choice of loading parameters giving the WT close to threshold, no spontaneous release occurs for either PQTa or PQTb under the application of MC-II-157c as in these conditions threshold SR Ca^{2+} is not reached.

MC-II-157c Is Effective in Inhibiting DADs Turning into Triggered Activity

The effect of MC-II-157c on the probability of DADs manifesting as full triggered action potentials was investigated using the simplified, non-spatial model such that spontaneous release waveforms could be directly controlled. The initiation time was set to 1,000 ms and behavior of the cell models for WT, PQT and PQT + MC-II-157c was compared over multiple simulations ($N = 1{,}000$ per condition) for four different RyR waveform duration distributions (see details in Simulating Spontaneous Release Events in Tissue Models; the distribution determines the values of duration which can be selected from a random number input and thus the actual value of the duration will vary randomly within the 1,000 simulations according to the given distribution).

Examples of 100 simulations for WT and PQTb, with and without MC-II-157c, are shown in **Figure 7A**. In PQTb, more DADs turn into triggered activity compared to in WT (top two panels), while simulated application of MC-II-157c reduces the occurances of triggered activity (bottom two panels). These data are summarized for all conditions and two duration distributions (median 300 and 350 ms, see Simulating Spontaneous Release Events in Tissue Models) in **Figure 7B**, wherein the degree of block of I_{Na} associated with MC-II-157c is varied (0, 40, and 80% block). In all cases, the I_{Kr} modification reduces the probability of triggered activity (defined as the number of simulations in which triggered activity occurred as a proportion of the total), but the role of I_{Na} is less clear; blocking I_{Na} is important, but the degree of I_{Na} block has different effects depending on the condition. The mechanism of the drug's action is shown in **Figure 7C**: principally, an increase in repolarising I_{Kr} acts during the DAD to keep the cell's membrane potential below the threshold for triggered activity; reduced I_{Na} also pays a role (although not as great as that of I_{Kr}) in the drug's mechanism of action as it reduces excitability of the cell, again reducing the ease with which the cell's membrane potential can reach threshold.

MC-II-157c Reduces Vulnerability to Ectopic Activity in Tissue

The vulnerability to the development of ectopic activity (i.e., propagation of triggered activity in all directions through the tissue) was assessed in a 2D homogeneous sheet to provide a medium for the synchronization of independent stochastic release events. Ten simulations were performed for each condition (WT and PQT variants ± MC-II-157c for the combinations of t_i and duration median distributions; Epicardial cell model) wherein the tissue model was paced to steady state and then left quiescent for two simulation seconds within which time the spontaneous release occurs.

The occurrence of ectopic activity exhibits a largely "all-or-nothing" response, where most conditions lead to either 0 or 100% of simulations resulting in a premature excitation

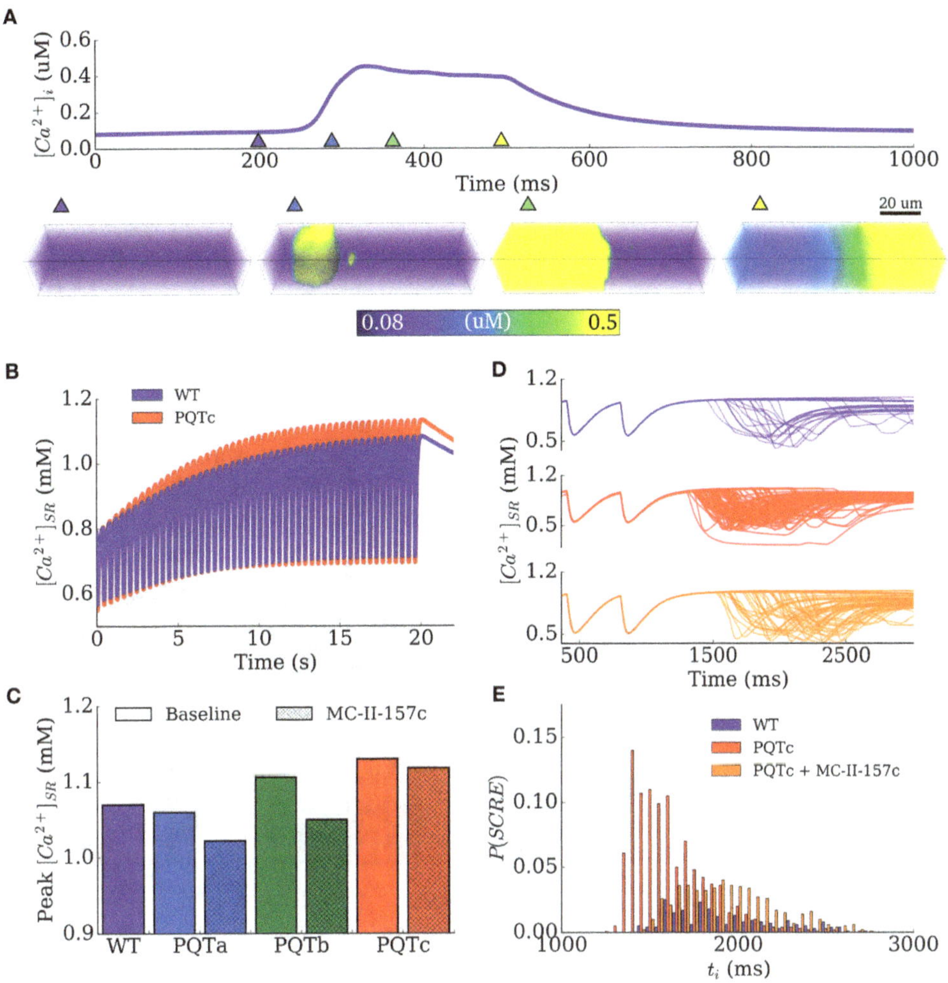

FIGURE 6 | SR Ca^{2+} loading and spontaneous Ca^{2+} release events. **(A)** Example of a whole-cell spontaneous Ca^{2+} release event (Ca^{2+}-wave), using the spatial model of stochastic intracellular Ca^{2+} handling, showing the Ca^{2+} transient (upper) and snapshots of Ca^{2+} concentration in the 3D cell volume (lower). The triangular makers in the upper panel indicate the timings of the snapshots in the lower panel. **(B)** Time-series of SR-Ca^{2+} during the SR-loading protocol, shown for control (WT, purple) and PQTc (red). **(C)** Peak SR-Ca^{2+} during the loading protocol for all conditions. **(D)** Examples of spontaneous release resulting from SR-loading for control (WT, purple), PQTc (red) and PQTc + MC-II-157c (orange). 100 simulations of each conditions are shown to indicate variation in spontaneous release. **(E)** Distributions of initiation time of spontaneous release events, corresponding to the same conditions shown in **(D)**. The time is relative to the start of the simulation (3 beats, initial conditions of dynamic steady state) to align with **(D)**. MC-II-157c was modeled as I_{Kr} modification + 40% I_{Na} block.

(**Table 1**). Ectopic activity was promoted by narrow distributions of initiation time (i.e., tight synchronization) and short RyR waveforms (i.e., large spontaneous Ca^{2+} transients), and conversely inhibited by wide distributions of initiation time (i.e., lose synchronization) and long RyR waveforms (i.e., small spontaneous Ca^{2+} transients). For example, no ectopic activity was observed for any condition with t_i distribution widths of 1,000 ms or duration medians of 300 ms or longer, whereas a t_i distribution width of 350 ms combined with median durations of 150 or 200 ms resulted in ectopic activity occurring in 100% of simulations (**Table 1**).

PQT variants were more susceptible to the development of ectopic activity in tissue than WT, congruent with the single-cell results (See MC-II-157c Is Effective in Inhibiting DADs Turning into Triggered Activity). Similarly in-line with single-cell results, MC-II-157c can inhibit ectopic activity (**Table 1**): for example, it reduces or entirely inhibits the occurrence of premature excitation in four conditions: PQTa with t_i width of 550 ms and duration median 150 ms; PQTc with t_i width of 550 ms and duration median 200 ms; PQTc with t_i width of 550 ms and duration median 150 ms; and PQTc with t_i width of 350 ms and duration median 250 ms. The effect of I_{Na} block is also congruent with single cell results: it contributes to the inhibition of ectopic activity, but to a smaller extent than I_{Kr} modification.

Figure 8A shows an example of synchronized triggered activity initiating in a region of the 2D tissue (shown by the clustered peaks the images), before this triggered activity spreads throughout the tissue (shown by the yellow region) as an ectopic propagation. When the same situation is simulated with

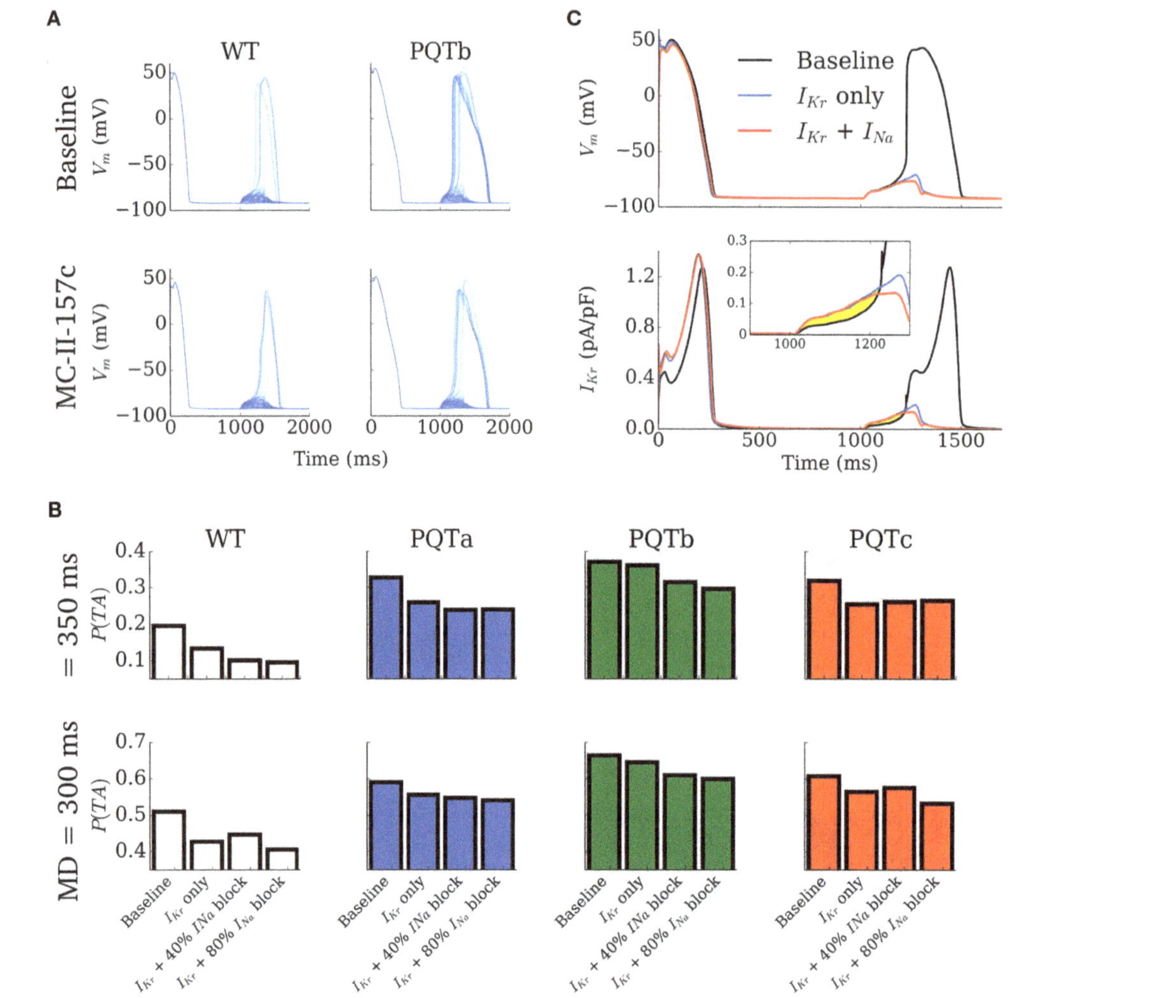

FIGURE 7 | Development of triggered action potentials in single cell. **(A)** 100 Action Potential traces for control (WT, left) and PQTb (right) under baseline (upper) and MC-II-157c (lower) conditions, associated with spontaneous Ca^{2+} release events. A proportion of the DADs manifest as triggered action potentials in all conditions. **(B)** Probability of DADs triggering full action potentials for control (WT) and PQTa-c under baseline and MC-II-157c conditions. The degree of I_{Na} block associated with MC-II-157c is varied between 0% (I_{Kr} only), 40 and 80%. The upper panel corresponds to a median RyR waveform duration of 350 ms; the lower panel to 300 ms. **(C)** Illustration of the mechanism by which MC-II-157c inhibits triggered activity, showing that the larger I_{Kr} (lower panel and inset) acts to oppose depolarising currents during the DAD. Yellow highlighted region clearly illustrates the differences between the conditions.

MC-II-157c (**Figure 8B**), triggered activity, and therefore ectopic propagation, is inhibited.

MC-II-157c Increases the Vulnerable Window in Tissue

An S1-S2 pacing protocol was applied to the 1D strand model in order to compute the vulnerability window: S2 stimuli were applied across a range of time intervals, centered on one in every five cells of the 100 comprising the model, from the tenth to the 90th.

Examples of propagation applied during the repolarisation phase in 1D tissue simulations are shown in **Figure 9A**: if the triggered activity occurs early (at 311 ms in this example), the resultant excitation is surrounded by refractory tissue and the triggered activity dies out without propagating; If the triggered activity occurs slightly later (e.g., 316 ms) then refractory tissue is encountered at only one side of the triggered activity site and unidirectional block (or unidirectional propagation) occurs, in the retrograde direction (back toward the endocardium) in this example; If triggered activity occurs later than this (321 ms in this example) then all surrounding tissue has recovered and the triggered activity propagates in both directions along the strand (i.e., ectopic propagation, analogous to the situation shown in 2D tissue in **Figure 8A**). It is the unidirectional block situation (i.e., when the triggered activity occurs in the VW) that can lead to re-entrant arrhythmias if this situation occurred in 2D or 3D tissue. The VW identifies occurrences of trigger and substrate interaction that may lead to arrhythmias, and so quantifying the size VW is a convenient method to examine effects of disease conditions and drugs on trigger and substrate interaction. The baseline VWs for WT and the PQTa condition are mapped out in **Figure 9B**, as well as VWs in

TABLE 1 | Incidence of ectopic activity in 2D tissue under WT and PQT ± MC-II-157c conditions.

t_i width	1,000				550				350			
Duration median	**300**	**250**	**200**	**150**	**300**	**250**	**200**	**150**	**300**	**250**	**200**	**150**
WT	0	0	0	0	0	0	0	0	0	0	10	10
PQTa	0	0	0	0	0	0	0	10	0	0	10	10
PQTa+C	0	0	0	0	0	0	0	0	0	0	10	10
PQTa+C_{Na}	0	0	0	0	0	0	0	0	0	0	10	10
PQTb	0	0	0	0	0	0	10	10	0	10	10	10
PQTb+C	0	0	0	0	0	0	10	10	0	10	10	10
PQTb+C_{Na}	0	0	0	0	0	0	10	10	0	10	10	10
PQTc	0	0	0	0	0	0	10	10	0	10	10	10
PQTc+C	0	0	0	0	0	0	6	5	0	9	10	10
PQTc+C_{Na}	0	0	0	0	0	0	0	0	0	1	10	10

The number of simulations where a premature excitation was observed is shown for each condition (out of a total of 10). The compound MC-II-157c is denoted by a "C" with I_{Kr} modification alone and "C_{Na}" with inclusion of 40% block of I_{Na}. Highlighted with red borders are the conditions in which MC-II-157c inhibits the development of ectopic activity.

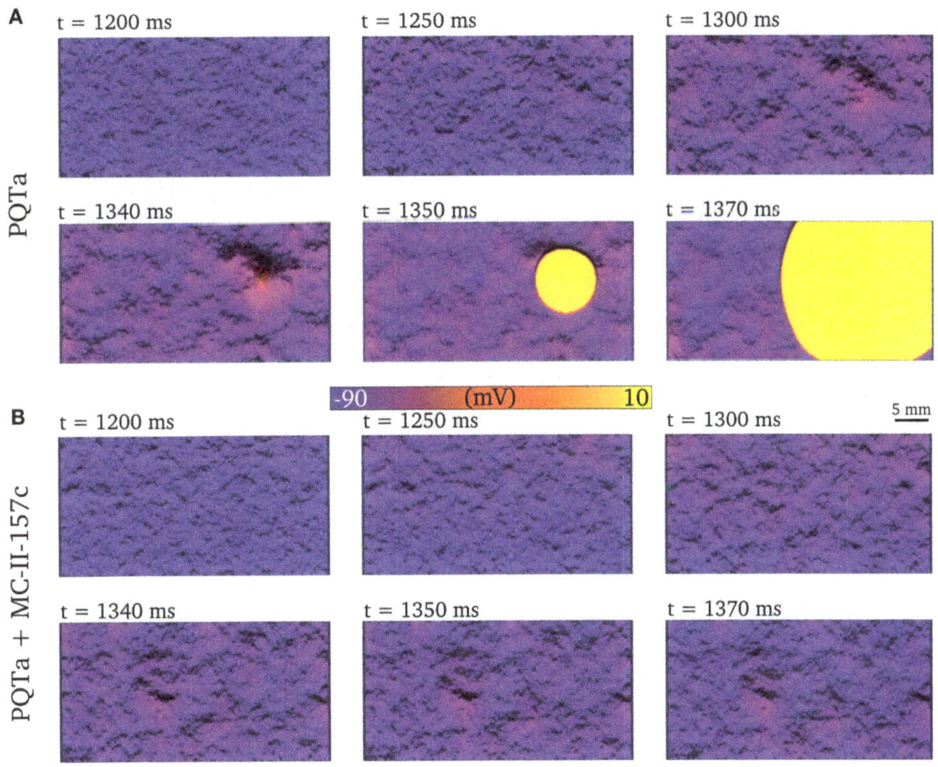

FIGURE 8 | Development of premature excitation in 2D tissue sheets. Temporal snapshots of the membrane voltage in a 2D slice of tissue during spontaneous Ca^{2+} release events for PQTa **(A)** and PQTa + MC-II-157c (I_{Kr} modification + 40% I_{Na} block, **(B)**. The color bar has been scaled to emphasize voltage differences in the DAD region and lighting has been added to further enhance local variation in voltage. Data corresponds to t_i width of 550 ms and duration median 150 ms.

these two situations with simulated addition of MC-II-157c (I_{Kr} modification plus 50% I_{Na} block), as well as with only the MC-II-157c I_{Kr} modification. These VWs are quantified by length (over which they occur in the 1D strand) and area (length × temporal width). In both WT and PQTa conditions, the drug increases both the length and the area of the VW (for example, length increases from 9 to 16 mm in the PQTa condition, and area increases from 78 to 101 mm.ms). Again, the influence of I_{Na} is different depending on the condition: including the effects of I_{Na} (i.e., the full MC-II-157c simulations compared to the I_{Kr} only simulations) increases the length of tissue over which the VW occurs in all conditions (e.g., from 12 to 16 mm in

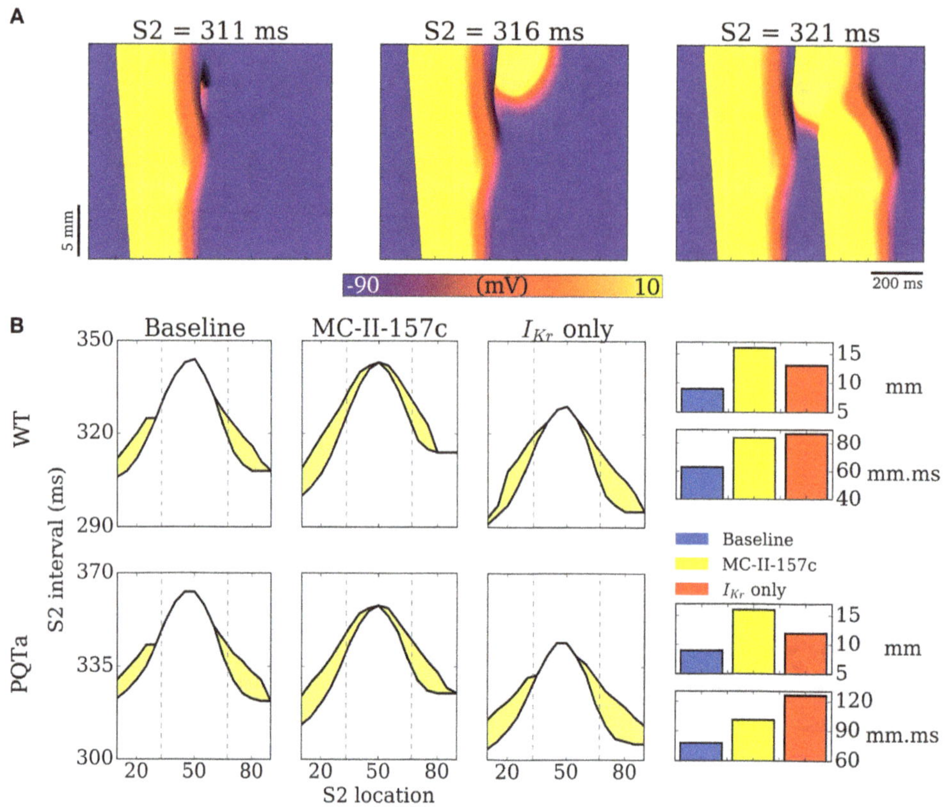

FIGURE 9 | Vulnerability windows to unidirectional conduction block. **(A)** Examples of propagation following applied S2 stimulus at different time intervals, illustrating conduction block (left), unidirectional conduction (middle) and full conduction (right). **(B)** Vulnerability windows for control (WT, upper) and PQTa (lower) under baseline, MC-II-157c (I_{Kr} modification + 40% I_{Na} block) and I_{Kr} modulation alone conditions. The lower line in each plot represents the refractory period (time below which no propagation occurs); the upper line represents the earliest time of bidirectional conduction; the area between the lines (shaded yellow) is the region within which unidirectional conduction occurs. Right panel is bar charts summarizing the length (mm) and area (mm.ms) of the vulnerability windows. Dotted lines illustrate the regions of the different cell types (ENDO, left; EPI, right).

PQTa), but reduces the overall area of the VW (e.g., from 126 to 101 mm.ms).

DISCUSSION

We used a multi-scale computational modeling approach to examine the interactions between cardiac arrhythmia trigger and substrate in general conditions associated with prolonged QT intervals, and their modulation by the hERG activator and sodium channel blocker MC-II-157c. Although we examined the effects of pharmacological modification on trigger and substrate interaction using a specific hERG activator, and gained novel insights into how modification of the depolarising (I_{Na}) and repolarising (I_{Kr}) membrane ionic currents targeted by the drug affects arrhythmia triggers and substrates, our findings also provide general insight into the role of ion-currents in controlling triggers and substrate at multiple scales which, along with insight from other *in silico* studies [see (Dutta et al., 2016; Mann et al., 2016) for recent examples], may be applicable to other pharmacological compounds that modify membrane ionic currents as well as pro-arrhythmic electrical remodeling.

Key Findings

Our key findings are that: (i) Despite the hERG activator MC-II-157c reducing the maximal conductance of I_{Kr} by 12% compared to WT, the drug's modifications to I_{Kr} activation, inactivation and deactivation kinetics result in an overall increase in I_{Kr} during the action potential, and a concomitantly reduced APD under all PQT conditions in all transmural cell types; (ii) Although MC-II-157c acts on membrane ionic currents carrying K^+ and Na^+, the drug has indirect effects on intracellular Ca^{2+} handling, particularly SR Ca^{2+} loading and related spontaneous SR Ca^{2+} release events and subsequent DADs, through modulation of the AP; (iii) Increased I_{Kr} (through its repolarising effects) and reduced I_{Na} (by decreasing cell excitability) act to reduce the probability of a DAD reaching threshold and developing into triggered activity at both cellular and tissue scales; and (iv) Despite MC-II-157c reducing triggered activity at the cell level, the drug can increase both the spatial region of tissue over which a VW for unidirectional conduction block occurs, as well as the temporal width of the VW at all points along the tissue, and in doing so increases the total spatiotemporal size of the VW. These results highlight the complex considerations which underlie overall vulnerability to arrhythmia at multiple scales.

Efficacy of MC-II-157c as an Anti-Arrhythmic Drug

At the isolated cell level, MC-II-157c reduces SR Ca^{2+} loading, reduces the occurrences of spontaneous SR Ca^{2+} release events, reduces DAD occurrences, and reduces the probability of a DAD developing into a triggered action potential. At the tissue level, the combination of these factors leads to a significantly reduced vulnerability to the development of ectopic beats; MC-II-157c reduces the probability of an ectopic beat development at given spontaneous release function distributions (i.e., synchronization degree) as well as inhibiting SR Ca^{2+} loading and thus reducing synchronization (which, itself, reduces the probability of ectopic beats). In relation to the development of Ca^{2+} induced triggers at single cell and tissue levels, therefore, our simulation results suggest that the drug has efficacy as an anti-arrhythmic.

However, even though arrhythmic triggered activity is reduced with the drug, the spatiotemporal area of the VW increased, and so the anti-arrhythmic effects of the reduced probability of an arrhythmia trigger occurring is opposed by the pro-arrhythmic effects of an increased arrhythmia substrate. This highlights the importance of examining the effects of pharmacological compounds on both the triggers *and* the substrates that underlie arrhythmia initiation: there is a delicate balance between increased/decreased trigger and increased/decreased substrate (i.e., trigger-substrate interaction) that determines whether any given trigger stimulus (e.g., a spontaneous SR Ca^{2+} release event) will result in unidirectional propagation and, potentially, initiation of a re-entrant arrhythmia. This is one potential reason that single cell studies showing efficacious effects of putative anti-arrhythmic drugs may not translate to the clinic.

The effects of MC-II-157c on the VW occur through two mechanisms due to the drug's action on both I_{Kr} and I_{Na}, both of which modify transmural dispersion of repolarisation. Activation of I_{Kr} causes heterogeneous changes to APD at the tissue level, the same mechanism as in our previous studies examining the effects of NS1643 (Peitersen et al., 2008). Block of I_{Na} results in slowed transmural conduction (Kléber and Rudy, 2004) and therefore delayed activation of epicardial (but not endocardial) tissue: this in turn modifies transmural dispersion of repolarisation, even though the change to APD is minimal with I_{Na} block. Block of I_{Na} also reduces excitability of the tissue, necessitating a larger trigger to initiate propagation, which also contributes to the change in the VW.

Varying Effects of Sodium Current Block

The role of I_{Na} loss of function in arrhythmogenesis has been examined in detail previously (see Clancy et al., 2015 for a review); however, one intriguing finding from our cell and tissue simulations was the varying effects that different magnitudes of I_{Na} block had on trigger development and substrate size. At the cell level, the probability of triggered activity developing from DADs did not follow a simple monotonic change with increasing I_{Na} block in all cases. Take, for example, the 350 ms Ca^{2+} release duration distribution results shown in the top panels of **Figure 7B**: In WT and the PQTb condition, I_{Na} block (in addition to the I_{Kr} modification) reduces the probability of DADs developing into triggered activity (relative to the I_{Kr} modification alone), with more block reducing this probability; that is to say, the greater the I_{Na} block, the more anti-arrhythmic (in terms of reducing triggered activity) the effects. However, in the PQTa condition, while 40% block of I_{Na} reduced the probability of triggered activity occurring, increasing block of the current to 80% slightly increased the probability of triggered activity; in this condition, a small amount of I_{Na} block has anti-arrhythmic effects, but increasing this small level of block is pro-arrhythmic. In the PQTc condition, I_{Na} block of any magnitude increased the probability of triggered activity (i.e., I_{Na} block is pro-arrhythmic), with the probability of triggered activity occurring increasing as I_{Na} block is increased. Similarly varied results were found for the 300 ms Ca^{2+} release duration distribution (lower panels in **Figure 7B**), although the anti-/pro-arrhythmic effects did not necessarily match those seen with the 350 ms distribution.

One further note of caution with regards to I_{Na} block comes from our tissue-level VW results in **Figure 9B**. Quantification of the length of tissue over which the VW occurs shows that 50% I_{Na} block (compare the full MC-II-157c effects to the effects with the I_{Kr} modification alone) increases this length, potentially due to an increase in transmural dispersion of repolarisation with I_{Na} block; analyses of these results alone would conclude that I_{Na} block is pro-arrhythmic. However, despite the spatial width of the VW increasing, block of I_{Na} results in the total spatiotemporal area of the VW decreasing (again, compare the full MC-II-157c effects to the effects with the I_{Kr} modification alone), i.e., an anti-arrhythmic result, likely due to the reduced excitability that results from I_{Na} block reducing the likelihood that any triggered activity would propagate.

Our tissue-level findings therefore indicate that I_{Na} block *per se* is an effective antiarrhythmic strategy (as seen with class I antiarrhythmic drugs; Camm, 2012), but our cell-level findings highlight that the magnitude of I_{Na} determines cell (and by extension, tissue) electrophysiological consequences in a manner that is not intuitive. The mechanisms underlying these varying effects of I_{Na} block on arrhythmogenesis, particularly on DAD initiation and their development into triggered activity, remain to be elucidated.

Modifying Abnormal Intracellular Calcium Handling through Membrane Current Modification

Although this study did not focus on the mechanisms of arrhythmia triggers (in that we prescribed SR Ca^{2+} release events under certain conditions), one interesting finding did emerge in relation to arrhythmia triggers that can result from abnormal intracellular Ca^{2+} handling: Modification of membrane ion channels carrying ions other than Ca^{2+} (K^+ and Na^+ in this case) can have beneficial effects in terms of restoring abnormal intracellular Ca^{2+} handling, through their actions in shortening APD. This was shown in **Figure 6**, where the increased SR Ca^{2+} loading (and resultant spontaneous SR Ca^{2+} release events) seen under PQT conditions was reversed by upregulating I_{Kr} and downregulating I_{Na}, which in turn shortened APD. This reduces the duration over which $I_{Ca,L}$ is activated, reduces the amount of Ca^{2+} crossing the cell membrane and entering the cell via that current, and thus reduces SR Ca^{2+} load. Furthermore, the combined action of both of these current modifications reduced the probability of DADs manifesting as triggered action potentials in single cell as well as triggered action potentials manifesting as fully propagating ectopic beats at the tissue scale. Targeting cell membrane ion channels carrying ions other than Ca^{2+} in order to restore abnormal intracellular Ca^{2+} handling (as seen in heart failure, for example; Lou et al., 2012) may be beneficial in cases where up/downregulation of Ca^{2+}-specific drug targets (ryanodine receptors or SERCA, for example) will alter the delicate homeostasis of an already-compromised system, yielding negative results (Ratner, 2015).

Development of Arrhythmic Conduction Patterns

One-dimensional models (other than 1D rings; e.g., Vinet and Roberge, 1994) cannot simulate re-entrant activity, and so it is necessary to use 2D and 3D models to examine how unidirectional propagation develops into re-entry. Although the quantitative characteristics of the VW examined in 1D tissues may change in 2D and 3D depending on the spatial locations of cell types (e.g., "base-apex" as well as transmural distributions), based on our previous work we would expect the qualitative characteristics to remain similar (Benson et al., 2007, 2008, 2011a). We show examples of 2D and 3D modeling in **Figure 10**: In **Figure 10A**, a trigger occurring in the VW (resulting in unidirectional conduction block) develops into re-entry in a simple 2D model; In **Figure 10B**, a trigger occurring outside the VW develops into ectopic propagation (i.e., not re-entrant) in a detailed 3D model of a human left ventricular wall slab, which manifests as significant differences in the body surface potential activation maps (**Figure 10C**). The advantages of using detailed 3D models (in this case, where the geometry is obtained from diffusion tensor MRI) lie in their ability to reproduce the orthotropic conduction velocities resulting from complicated tissue architecture (i.e., fiber and sheet structure; Benson et al., 2007; Smaill et al., 2013) and the boundary and curvature effects that can modulate electrotonic coupling and propagation (Walton et al., 2013; Campos et al., 2015): these effects are crucial in understanding the complex and chaotic propagation patterns underlying cardiac arrhythmias. Nevertheless, the 1D models used in this study allow us to examine arrhythmia trigger-substrate interaction in a simple and methodological manner.

Limitations

In this study, a general model of intracellular Ca^{2+} handling was integrated with a simplified formulation of a human ventricular AP model. Due to the general nature of the Ca^{2+} handling model, details of heterogeneity in Ca^{2+} handling were not included in order to avoid introducing artifacts. For this reason, and due to the multi-scale focus of the study, detailed investigation of the mechanisms of spontaneous release in single cell, and their regional dependencies, was not performed, and investigation was instead limited to the potential effect of MC-II-157c on reversing SR Ca^{2+} loading. There are many possible mechanisms of spontaneous release associated with diseases linked to prolonged QT interval (e.g., hyper phosphorylation of the RyRs; upregulation of SERCA; detubulation) which were not considered in the present study. However, the aim of this study was to investigate the multi-scale interaction between trigger and substrate, and the use of the simplified spontaneous release functions in single-cell and tissue simulations allowed this to be analyzed in a general manner and across a large range of conditions, independent of spontaneous release mechanism. In future, combining detailed single cell studies of the mechanisms of spontaneous release in disease conditions with tissue simulations of the same conditions would provide further mechanistic insight; a dynamic simplified spontaneous release model would furthermore allow the study of long-term interactions between trigger and substrate in tissue e.g., during re-entry.

The factors underlying the synchronization and propagation of ectopic activity are highly complex and it is therefore worth making explicit that our simplified approach (which does not consider, for example, heterogeneity in the distributions describing Ca^{2+} release) is primarily suitable for interpretation of general trends only, rather than as a quantitative analysis of the efficacy of MC-II-157c in modulating Ca^{2+} release dependent triggers; it is encouraging to note that our results are consistent with those of a previous study (Campos et al., 2015), with the emergence of premature excitation from independent stochastic events overcoming electrotonic load, and the steep, "all-or-nothing" relationship observed in tissue. This steep relationship also likely accounts for the lack of effect of MC-II-157c on PQTb (the condition exhibiting the highest vulnerability to ectopic activity), wherein the distributions selected were not close enough to the threshold region to reveal an effect.

The relative contribution of I_{Kr} to repolarisation is different in different models of the human ventricular action potential (Mirams et al., 2014): for example, I_{Kr} contributes more repolarising current in the ORd model (O'Hara et al., 2011) than in the ten Tusscher & Panfilov model (ten Tusscher and Panfilov, 2006), despite both models being validated against experimental data. It is therefore possible that our results overestimate the effects of the hERG activator MC-II-157c, although the identified pro- and anti-arrhythmic mechanisms will still be relevant.

The limitations of using 1D and 2D simplifications of 3D cardiac tissue have been discussed in detail previously (Clayton et al., 2011). Here we only note that the 1D strand model of the left ventricular wall allows us to examine mechanisms underlying how arrhythmia triggers and substrates interact to initiate unidirectional propagation, without the added complicating effects that geometrical (shape) and architectural (fiber, sheet etc.) considerations would bring. Nevertheless, it is anticipated that these geometrical and architectural effects will play a role not only in the transition from unidirectional propagation to re-entry, but on the initiation of the unidirectional propagation itself through, for example, electrotonic effects (Benson et al., 2007; Walton et al., 2013). Similarly, our 2D and 3D tissues were isotropic, i.e., no fiber or sheet structure, and so any conclusions drawn from these simulations should be interpreted with this in mind. Elucidating the roles that tissue geometry and architecture play in

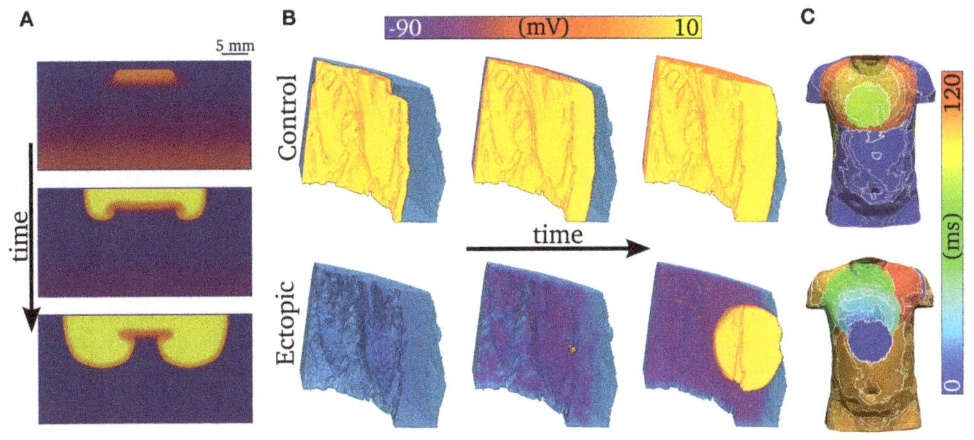

FIGURE 10 | Examples of abnormal electrical excitation. **(A)** Example of conduction block in a 2D sheet, analogous to that observed in the 1D strand for computation of the vulnerability windows. Three snapshots in time are shown to illustrate the potential of unidirectional conduction block to develop into asymmetric, re-entrant-like activity. **(B)** Propagation patterns in the 3D ventricular wedge, showing normal, control pacing (upper panel) and a spontaneous ectopic beat (lower panel). The propagation of DADs, preceding the ectopic beat, is clear by the purple colored regions in the lower center panel. The voltage color bar corresponds to both panels **(A,B)**. **(C)** Body-surface potential activation maps (time at which potential > 0.1 mV) associated with normal and ectopic propagation, highlighting the significant difference in spatial patterns between the two conditions.

arrhythmogenesis (Smaill et al., 2013) is an important next step in fully understanding arrhythmia trigger and substrate interaction.

The spatial distributions of endocardial, midmyocardial, and epicardial cell types across the human ventricular wall has still not been confirmed: some studies suggest that midmyocardial cells are found predominantly in isolated regions of the subendocardium (Glukhov et al., 2010), while others suggest a continuous population of midmyocardial cells in the subepicardial region (Drouin et al., 1995); these distributions may be dependent on species, location in the ventricular wall, and disease state (Antzelevitch, 2010; Strom et al., 2010). Because of this uncertainty, we set the spatial distribution of the three cell types to be equal in the transmural direction, but the effects of the electrotonic interactions of different regions of cell types are likely to be qualitatively similar if these distributions are altered.

The simulated model of MC-II-157c reproduced qualitatively the key features of the effect of the compound on I_{Kr} (i.e., an increased activity during a depolarising pulse), but it is important to note that there were significant differences between the simulation and experimental data (**Figure 5**): firstly, the formulation of I_{Kr} implemented does not have a time-dependent inactivation, which is observed in the experimental trace; secondly, the simulated data exhibited a larger difference in the magnitude of the current during the depolarisation step between baseline and MC-II-157c than observed experimentally. A more detailed model of I_{Kr} in both basal and MC-II-157c conditions would be essential for future and more detailed analysis of the compound specifically.

Furthermore, recent work, (e.g., Li et al., 2017), has highlighted that simple modulation of Hodgkin-Huxley current formulations, as used to simulate I_{Kr} in the ORd model, may not sufficiently capture complex drug-channel interaction dynamics, and that more complex Markov model formulations may be necessary to simulate such dynamics. However, until a full experimental characterisation of the dynamics of MC-II-157c effects on I_{Kr} under a range of conditions is carried out, allowing a validated Markov model of drug-channel interactions to be developed, we make use of the available data (Guo et al., 2014) to modify the Hodgkin-Huxley formulation used in the ORd model. The effects of MC-II-157c on I_{Na} are not as well characterized as its effects on I_{Kr} (Guo et al., 2014). We simulated the drug's action on I_{Na} by a simple reduction in the maximal conductance of the current. It is possible, however, that MC-II-157c also modifies the current's kinetics (i.e., shifts to the current's activation and inactivation curves, and/or a change to the time constants associated with these processes) in a similar manner to the way in which the kinetics of I_{Kr} are modified. Thus, further experimental characterisation of the drug's effects on both I_{Kr} and I_{Na} are required.

CONCLUSION

The relative balance of reduced trigger and increased substrate underlies a multi-dimensional role of MC-II-157c in modulation of arrhythmia vulnerability associated with prolonged QT interval. Our results highlight that studies examining the efficacy of putative anti-arrhythmic drugs need to assess the effects of the drug on both the triggers and the substrates involved in arrhythmogenesis, i.e., such studies should adopt a multiscale approach to examine both cell- and tissue-level effects.

AUTHOR CONTRIBUTIONS

All authors conceived and designed the study; MC, EP, and AB carried out simulations, and acquired and analyzed data; all authors interpreted the data; MC and AB prepared the first draft of the manuscript text; MC and EP prepared the figures;

all authors edited the manuscript; all authors approved the final version of the manuscript; all authors agree to be accountable for all aspects of the work in ensuring that questions related to the accuracy or integrity of any part of the work are appropriately investigated and resolved.

ACKNOWLEDGMENTS

Parts of this work were undertaken on ARC2, part of the High Performance Computing facilities at the University of Leeds, UK.

REFERENCES

Antzelevitch, C. (2005). Modulation of transmural repolarization. *Ann. N. Y. Acad. Sci.* 1047, 314–323. doi: 10.1196/annals.1341.028

Antzelevitch, C. (2010). M cells in the human heart. *Circ. Res.* 106, 815–817. doi: 10.1161/CIRCRESAHA.109.216226

Benson, A. P., Halley, G., Li, P., Tong, W. C., and Holden, A. V. (2007). Virtual cell and tissue dynamics of ectopic activation of the ventricles. *Chaos* 17:015105. doi: 10.1063/1.2404634

Benson, A. P., Aslanidi, O. V., Zhang, H., and Holden, A. V. (2008). The canine virtual ventricular wall: a platform for dissecting pharmacological effects on propagation and arrhythmogenesis. *Prog. Biophys. Mol. Biol.* 96, 187–208. doi: 10.1016/j.pbiomolbio.2007.08.002

Benson, A. P., Al-Owais, M., and Holden, A. V. (2011a). Quantitative prediction of the arrhythmogenic effects of *de novo* hERG mutations in computational models of human ventricular tissues. *Eur. Biophys. J. Biophys. Lett.* 40, 627–639. doi: 10.1007/s00249-010-0663-2

Benson, A. P., Bernus, O., Dierckx, H., Gilbert, S. H., Greenwood, J. P., Holden, A. V., et al. (2011b). Construction and validation of anisotropic and orthotropic ventricular geometries for quantitative predictive cardiac electrophysiology. *Interface Focus* 1, 101–116. doi: 10.1098/rsfs.2010.0005

Bezekci, B., Idris, I., Simitev, R. D., and Biktashev, V. N. (2015). Semianalytical approach to criteria for ignition of excitation waves. *Phys. Rev. E* 92:042917. doi: 10.1103/PhysRevE.92.042917

Bilet, A., and Bauer, C. K. (2012). Effects of the small molecule HERG activator NS1643 on Kv11.3 channels. *PLoS ONE* 7:e50886. doi: 10.1371/journal.pone.0050886

Bohnen, M. S., Peng, G., Robey, S. H., Terrenoire, C., Iyer, V., Sampson, K. J., et al. (2017). Molecular pathophysiology of congenital long QT syndrome. *Physiol. Rev.* 97, 89–134. doi: 10.1152/physrev.00008.2016

Camm, J. (2012). Antiarrhythmic drugs for the maintenance of sinus rhythm: risks and benefits. *Int. J. Cardiol.* 155, 362–371. doi: 10.1016/j.ijcard.2011.06.012

Campos, F. O., Shiferaw, Y., Prassl, A. J., Boyle, P. M., Vigmond, E. J., and Plank, G. (2015). Stochastic spontaneous calcium release events trigger premature ventricular complexes by overcoming electrotonic load. *Cardiovasc. Res.* 107, 175–183. doi: 10.1093/cvr/cvv149

Clancy, C. E., Chen-Izu, Y., Bers, D. M., Belardinelli, L., Boyden, P. A., Csernoch, L., et al. (2015). Deranged sodium to sudden death. *J. Physiol.* 593, 1331–1345. doi: 10.1113/jphysiol.2014.281204

Clayton, R. H., Bernus, O., Cherry, E. M., Dierckx, H., Fenton, F. H., Mirabella, L., et al. (2011). Models of cardiac tissue electrophysiology: progress, challenges and open questions. *Prog. Biophys. Mol. Biol.* 104, 22–48. doi: 10.1016/j.pbiomolbio.2010.05.008

Clusin, W. T. (2003). Calcium and cardiac arrhythmias: DADs, EADs, and alternans. *Crit. Rev. Clin. Lab. Sci.* 40, 337–375. doi: 10.1080/713609356

Colman, M. A., Parra-Rojas, C., and Perez-Alday, E. A. (2015). From microscopic calcium sparks to the ECG: model reduction approaches for multi-scale cardiac simulation. *Comput. Cardiol.* 42, 325–328. doi: 10.1109/CIC.2015.7408652

Colman, M. A., Pinali, C., Trafford, A. W., Zhang, H., and Kitmitto, A. (2017). A computational model of spatio-temporal cardiac intracellular calcium handling with realistic structure and spatial flux distribution from sarcoplasmic reticulum and t-tubule reconstructions. *PLOS Comput. Biol.* 13:e1005714. doi: 10.1371/journal.pcbi.1005714

Drouin, E., Charpentier, F., Gauthier, C., Laurent, K., and Le Marec, H. (1995). Electrophysiologic characteristics of cells spanning the left ventricular wall of human heart: evidence for presence of M cells. *J. Am. Coll. Cardiol.* 26, 185–192. doi: 10.1016/0735-1097(95)00167-X

Dutta, S., Mincholé, A., Zacur, E., Quinn, T. A., Taggart, P., and Rodriguez, B. (2016). Early afterdepolarizations promote transmural reentry in ischemic human ventricles with reduced repolarization reserve. *Prog. Biophys. Mol. Biol.* 120, 236–248. doi: 10.1016/j.pbiomolbio.2016.01.008

Glukhov, A. V., Fedorov, V. V., Lou, Q., Ravikumar, V. K., Kalish, P. W., Schuessler, R. B., et al. (2010). Transmural dispersion of repolarization in Failing and non-failing human ventricle. *Circ. Res.* 106, 981–991. doi: 10.1161/CIRCRESAHA.109.204891

Grunnet, M., Hansen, R. S., and Olesen, S.-P. (2008). hERG1 channel activators: a new anti-arrhythmic principle. *Prog. Biophys. Mol. Biol.* 98, 347–362. doi: 10.1016/j.pbiomolbio.2009.01.002

Guo, J., Durdagi, S., Changalov, M., Perissinotti, L. L., Hargreaves, J. M., Back, T. G., et al. (2014). Structure Driven design of novel human ether-a-go-go-related-gene channel (hERG1) activators. *PLoS ONE* 9:e105553. doi: 10.1371/journal.pone.0105553

Hansen, R. S., Diness, T. G., Christ, T., Demnitz, J., Ravens, U., Olesen, S.-P., et al. (2006). Activation of human ether-a-go-go-related gene potassium channels by the diphenylurea 1,3-bis-(2-hydroxy-5-trifluoromethyl-phenyl)-urea (NS1643). *Mol. Pharmacol.* 69, 266–277. doi: 10.1124/mol.105.015859

Hart, G. (1994). Cellular electrophysiology in cardiac hypertrophy and failure. *Cardiovasc. Res.* 28, 933–946. doi: 10.1093/cvr/28.7.933

Janse, M. J. (2004). Electrophysiological changes in heart failure and their relationship to arrhythmogenesis. *Cardiovasc. Res.* 61, 208–217. doi: 10.1016/j.cardiores.2003.11.018

Kalin, A., Usher-Smith, J., Jones, V. J., Huang, C. L., and Sabir, I. N. (2010). Cardiac Arrhythmia: a simple conceptual framework. *Trends Cardiovasc. Med.* 20, 103–107. doi: 10.1016/j.tcm.2010.09.003

Kléber, A. G., and Rudy, Y. (2004). Basic mechanisms of cardiac impulse propagation and associated arrhythmias. *Physiol. Rev.* 84, 431–488. doi: 10.1152/physrev.00025.2003

Kumar, K., and Zimetbaum, P. J. (2013). Antiarrhythmic drugs 2013: state of the art. *Curr. Cardiol. Rep.* 15:410. doi: 10.1007/s11886-013-0410-2

Lankipalli, R. S., Zhu, T., Guo, D., and Yan, G.-X. (2005). Mechanisms underlying arrhythmogenesis in long QT syndrome. *J. Electrocardiol.* 38, 69–73. doi: 10.1016/j.jelectrocard.2005.06.008

Li, Z., Dutta, S., Sheng, J., Tran, P. N., Wu, W., Chang, K., et al. (2017). Improving the *in silico* assessment of Proarrhythmia risk by combining hERG (Human Ether-à-go-go-Related Gene) channel-drug binding kinetics and multichannel pharmacology. *Circ. Arrhythm. Electrophysiol.* 10:e004628. doi: 10.1161/CIRCEP.116.004628

Lou, Q., Janardhan, A., and Efimov, I. R. (2012). Remodeling of calcium handling in human heart failure. *Adv. Exp. Med. Biol.* 740, 1145–1174. doi: 10.1007/978-94-007-2888-2_52

Mann, S. A., Imtiaz, M., Winbo, A., Rydberg, A., Perry, M. D., Couderc, J.-P., et al. (2016). Convergence of models of human ventricular myocyte electrophysiology after global optimization to recapitulate clinical long QT phenotypes. *J. Mol. Cell. Cardiol.* 100, 25–34. doi: 10.1016/j.yjmcc.2016.09.011

Mirams, G. R., Davies, M. R., Brough, S. J., Bridgland-Taylor, M. H., Cui, Y., Gavaghan, D. J., et al. (2014). Prediction of thorough QT study results using action potential simulations based on ion channel screens. *J. Pharmacol. Toxicol. Methods* 70, 246–254. doi: 10.1016/j.vascn.2014.07.002

Moss, A. J., and Kass, R. S. (2005). Long QT syndrome: from channels to cardiac arrhythmias. *J. Clin. Invest.* 115, 2018–2024. doi: 10.1172/JCI25537

Nachimuthu, S., Assar, M. D., and Schussler, J. M. (2012). Drug-induced QT interval prolongation: mechanisms and clinical management. *Ther. Adv. Drug Saf.* 3, 241–253. doi: 10.1177/2042098612454283

Němec, J., Kim, J. J., and Salama, G. (2016). The link between abnormal calcium handling and electrical instability in acquired long QT syndrome–does calcium precipitate arrhythmic storms? *Prog. Biophys. Mol. Biol.* 120, 210–221. doi: 10.1016/j.pbiomolbio.2015.11.003

Noble, D. (1972). The relation of Rushton's "liminal length" for excitation to the resting and active conductances of excitable cells. *J. Physiol.* 226, 573–591. doi: 10.1113/jphysiol.1972.sp009998

O'Hara, T., Virág, L., Varró, A., and Rudy, Y. (2011). Simulation of the undiseased human cardiac ventricular action potential: model formulation and experimental validation. *PLoS Comput. Biol.* 7:e1002061. doi: 10.1371/journal.pcbi.1002061

Pandit, S. V., and Jalife, J. (2013). Rotors and the dynamics of cardiac fibrillation. *Circ. Res.* 112, 849–862. doi: 10.1161/CIRCRESAHA.111.300158

Peitersen, T., Grunnet, M., Benson, A. P., Holden, A. V., Holstein-Rathlou, N.-H., and Olesen, S.-P. (2008). Computational analysis of the effects of the hERG channel opener NS1643 in a human ventricular cell model. *Heart Rhythm* 5, 734–741. doi: 10.1016/j.hrthm.2008.02.026

Perez Alday, E. A., Colman, M. A., Langley, P., Butters, T. D., Higham, J., Workman, A. J., et al. (2015). A new algorithm to diagnose Atrial ectopic origin from multi lead ECG systems-insights from 3D virtual human Atria and Torso. *PLoS Comput. Biol.* 11:e1004026. doi: 10.1371/journal.pcbi.1004026

Perez Alday, E. A., Ni, H., Zhang, C., Colman, M. A., Gan, Z., and Zhang, H. (2016). Comparison of electric- and magnetic-cardiograms produced by myocardial ischemia in models of the human ventricle and Torso. *PLoS ONE* 11:e0160999. doi: 10.1371/journal.pone.0160999

Perez Alday, E. A., Colman, M. A., Langley, P., and Zhang, H. (2017). Novel non-invasive algorithm to identify the origins of re-entry and ectopic foci in the atria from 64-lead ECGs: a computational study. *PLoS Comput. Biol.* 13:e1005270. doi: 10.1371/journal.pcbi.1005270

Ratner, M. (2015). Heart failure gene therapy disappoints but experts keep the faith. *Nat. Biotechnol.* 33, 573–574. doi: 10.1038/nbt0615-573a

Restrepo, J. G., Weiss, J. N., and Karma, A. (2008). Calsequestrin-mediated mechanism for cellular calcium transient alternans. *Biophys. J.* 95, 3767–3789. doi: 10.1529/biophysj.108.130419

Rush, S., and Larsen, H. (1978). A practical algorithm for solving dynamic membrane equations. *IEEE Trans. Biomed. Eng.* 25, 389–392. doi: 10.1109/TBME.1978.326270

Schwartz, P. J., Crotti, L., and Insolia, R. (2012). Long-QT syndrome: from genetics to management. *Circ. Arrhythm. Electrophysiol.* 5, 868–877. doi: 10.1161/CIRCEP.111.962019

Shaw, R. M., and Rudy, Y. (1995). The vulnerable window for unidirectional block in cardiac tissue: *J. Cardiovasc. Electrophysiol.* 6, 115–131. doi: 10.1111/j.1540-8167.1995.tb00763.x

Smaill, B. H., Zhao, J., and Trew, M. L. (2013). Three-dimensional impulse propagation in myocardium: arrhythmogenic mechanisms at the tissue level. *Circ. Res.* 112, 834–848. doi: 10.1161/CIRCRESAHA.111.300157

Starmer, C. F., Biktashev, V. N., Romashko, D. N., Stepanov, M. R., Makarova, O. N., and Krinsky, V. I. (1993). Vulnerability in an excitable medium: analytical and numerical studies of initiating unidirectional propagation. *Biophys. J.* 65, 1775–1787. doi: 10.1016/S0006-3495(93)81233-5

Strom, M., Wan, X., Poelzing, S., Ficker, E., and Rosenbaum, D. S. (2010). Gap junction heterogeneity as mechanism for electrophysiologically distinct properties across the ventricular wall. *Am. J. Physiol. Heart Circ. Physiol.* 298, H787–794. doi: 10.1152/ajpheart.00887.2009

ten Tusscher, K. H., and Panfilov, A. V. (2006). Alternans and spiral breakup in a human ventricular tissue model. *Am. J. Physiol. Heart Circ. Physiol.* 291, H1088–H1100. doi: 10.1152/ajpheart.00109.2006

Tomaselli, G. F., and Zipes, D. P. (2004). What causes sudden death in heart failure? *Circ. Res.* 95, 754–763. doi: 10.1161/01.RES.0000145047.14691.db

Tse, G. (2016). Mechanisms of cardiac arrhythmias. *J. Arrhythmia* 32, 75–81. doi: 10.1016/j.joa.2015.11.003

Venetucci, L. A., Trafford, A. W., and Eisner, D. A. (2007). Increasing ryanodine receptor open probability alone does not produce arrhythmogenic calcium waves: threshold sarcoplasmic reticulum calcium content is required. *Circ. Res.* 100, 105–111. doi: 10.1161/01.RES.0000252828.17939.00

Vinet, A., and Roberge, F. A. (1994). The dynamics of sustained reentry in a ring model of cardiac tissue. *Ann. Biomed. Eng.* 22, 568–591. doi: 10.1007/BF02368285

Wagner, S., Maier, L. S., and Bers, D. M. (2015). Role of sodium and calcium dysregulation in tachyarrhythmias in sudden cardiac death. *Circ. Res.* 116, 1956–1970. doi: 10.1161/CIRCRESAHA.116.304678

Walton, R. D., Benson, A. P., Hardy, M. E., White, E., and Bernus, O. (2013). Electrophysiological and structural determinants of electrotonic modulation of repolarization by the activation sequence. *Front. Physiol.* 4:281. doi: 10.3389/fphys.2013.00281

Wu, W., and Sanguinetti, M. C. (2016). Molecular basis of cardiac delayed rectifier potassium channel function and pharmacology. *Card. Electrophysiol. Clin.* 8, 275–284. doi: 10.1016/j.ccep.2016.01.002

Permissions

All chapters in this book were first published in SPRAQTIPB, by Frontiers; hereby published with permission under the Creative Commons Attribution License or equivalent. Every chapter published in this book has been scrutinized by our experts. Their significance has been extensively debated. The topics covered herein carry significant findings which will fuel the growth of the discipline. They may even be implemented as practical applications or may be referred to as a beginning point for another development.

The contributors of this book come from diverse backgrounds, making this book a truly international effort. This book will bring forth new frontiers with its revolutionizing research information and detailed analysis of the nascent developments around the world.

We would like to thank all the contributing authors for lending their expertise to make the book truly unique. They have played a crucial role in the development of this book. Without their invaluable contributions this book wouldn't have been possible. They have made vital efforts to compile up to date information on the varied aspects of this subject to make this book a valuable addition to the collection of many professionals and students.

This book was conceptualized with the vision of imparting up-to-date information and advanced data in this field. To ensure the same, a matchless editorial board was set up. Every individual on the board went through rigorous rounds of assessment to prove their worth. After which they invested a large part of their time researching and compiling the most relevant data for our readers.

The editorial board has been involved in producing this book since its inception. They have spent rigorous hours researching and exploring the diverse topics which have resulted in the successful publishing of this book. They have passed on their knowledge of decades through this book. To expedite this challenging task, the publisher supported the team at every step. A small team of assistant editors was also appointed to further simplify the editing procedure and attain best results for the readers.

Apart from the editorial board, the designing team has also invested a significant amount of their time inunderstanding the subject and creating the most relevant covers. They scrutinized every image to scout for the most suitable representation of the subject and create an appropriate cover for the book.

The publishing team has been an ardent support to the editorial, designing and production team. Their endless efforts to recruit the best for this project, has resulted in the accomplishment of this book. They are a veteran in the field of academics and their pool of knowledge is as vast as their experience in printing. Their expertise and guidance has proved useful at every step. Their uncompromising quality standards have made this book an exceptional effort. Their encouragement from time to time has been an inspiration for everyone.

The publisher and the editorial board hope that this book will prove to be a valuable piece of knowledge forresearchers, students, practitioners and scholars across the globe.

List of Contributors

Nicholas Ellinwood, Stefano Morotti and Eleonora Grandi
Department of Pharmacology, University of California, Davis, Davis, CA, United States

Dobromir Dobrev
West German Heart and Vascular Center, Institute of Pharmacology, University Duisburg-Essen, Essen, Germany

Kelly C. Chang, Sara Dutta, Kylie A. Beattie, Jiansong Sheng, Phu N. Tran, Min Wu, Wendy W. Wu, David G. Strauss and Zhihua Li
Division of Applied Regulatory Science, Center for Drug Evaluation and Research, Office of Translational Sciences, Office of Clinical Pharmacology, Food and Drug Administration, Silver Spring, MD, United States

Gary R. Mirams
Centre for Mathematical Medicine and Biology, School of Mathematical Sciences, University of Nottingham, Nottingham, United Kingdom

Thomas Colatsky
Marshview Life Science Advisors, Seabrook Island, SC, United States

Chunxiao Lv, Jia Liu, Ziqiang Li, Xi Du, Jinxia Sun, Yanfen Li, Ruihua Wang and Yuhong Huang
Department of Clinical Pharmacology, Second Affiliated Hospital of Tianjin University of Traditional Chinese Medicine, Tianjin, China

Changxiao Liu
State Key Laboratory of Drug Delivery Technology and Pharmacokinetics, Tianjin Institute of Pharmaceutical Research, Tianjin, China

Zhuhua Yao
Department of Cardiology, People's Hospital of Tianjin, Tianjin, China

Xiumei Gao
Engineering Research Center of Modern Chinese Medicine Discovery and Preparation Technique, Tianjin University of Traditional Chinese Medicine, Tianjin, China

Kui Ye
Department of Vascular Surgery, Tianjin 4th Center Hospital, Tianjin, China

Lanjun Sun
Department of Cardiology, Second Affiliated Hospital of Tianjin University of Traditional Chinese Medicine, Tianjin, China

Haibo Song
National Center for ADR Monitoring of China, Center for Drug Reevaluation of CFDA, Beijing, China

Laura L. Perissinotti, Pablo M. De Biase, Miranda C. Lee and Sergei Y. Noskov
Centre for Molecular Simulations, Department of Biological Sciences, Faculty of Science, University of Calgary, Calgary, AB, Canada

Jiqing Guo and Henry J. Duff
Libin Cardiovascular Institute of Alberta, Faculty of Medicine, University of Calgary, Calgary, AB, Canada

Pei-Chi Yang and Colleen E. Clancy
Department of Physiology and Membrane Biology, University of California, Davis, Davis, CA, United States

Haibo Ni
Biological Physics Group, University of Manchester, Manchester, United Kingdom Space Institute of Southern China, Shenzhen, China Key Laboratory of Medical Electrophysiology, Ministry of Education, Collaborative Innovation Center for Prevention and Treatment of Cardiovascular Disease/ Institute of Cardiovascular Research, Southwest Medical University, Luzhou, China

Dominic G. Whittaker and Wei Wang
Biological Physics Group, University of Manchester, Manchester, United Kingdom

Wayne R. Giles
Faculties of Kinesiology and Medicine, University of Calgary, Calgary, AB, Canada

Sanjiv M. Narayan
Department of Medicine, Stanford University School of Medicine, Stanford, CA, United States

Henggui Zhang
Biological Physics Group, University of Manchester, Manchester, United Kingdom Space Institute of Southern China, Shenzhen, China Key Laboratory of Medical Electrophysiology, Ministry of Education, Collaborative Innovation Center for Prevention and Treatment of Cardiovascular Disease/ Institute of Cardiovascular Research, Southwest Medical University, Luzhou, China School of Computer Science and Technology, Harbin Institute of Technology, Harbin, China

Pietro E. Lazzerini, Francesco Finizola, Mariarita Natale, Francesca Vanni, Beatrice Giabbani, Michele Caselli, Ilaria Lamberti, Franco Laghi-Pasini and Pier L. Capecchi
Department of Medical Sciences, Surgery and Neurosciences, University of Siena, Siena, Italy

Maurizio Acampa
Stroke Unit, University Hospital of Siena, Siena, Italy

Iacopo Bertolozzi
Cardiology Intensive Therapy Unit, Department of Internal Medicine, Hospital of Carrara, Carrara, Italy

Marco Rossi
Department of Medical Sciences, Surgery and Neurosciences, University of Siena, Siena, Italy Centre of Pharmacovigilance, University Hospital of Siena, Siena, Italy

Gabriele Cevenini
Department of Medical Biotechnologies, University of Siena, Siena, Italy

Rosella Fulceri and Alessandra Gamberucci
Department of Molecular and Developmental Medicine, University of Siena, Siena, Italy

Kevin R. DeMarco
Department of Physiology and Membrane Biology, University of California, Davis, Davis, CA, United States Department of Pharmacology, University of California, Davis, Davis, CA, United States Biophysics Graduate Group, University of California, Davis, Davis, CA, United States

Slava Bekker
Department of Physiology and Membrane Biology, University of California, Davis, Davis, CA, United States Hartnell College, Salinas, CA, United States

Igor Vorobyov
Department of Physiology and Membrane Biology, University of California, Davis, Davis, CA, United States Department of Pharmacology, University of California, Davis, Davis, CA, United States

Jaimit Parikh, Viatcheslav Gurev and John J. Rice
IBM T. J. Watson Research Center, Yorktown Heights, NY, United States

Jaehee V. Shim, Johan G. C. van Hasselt, Marc R. Birtwistle and Eric A. Sobie
Department of Pharmacological Sciences, Icahn School of Medicine at Mount Sinai, New York, NY, United States

Bryan Chun and Jeffrey J. Saucerman
Department of Biomedical Engineering, University of Virginia, Charlottesville, VA, United States

William Lee, Monique J. Windley, Jamie I. Vandenberg and Adam P. Hill
Molecular Cardiology and Biophysics Division, Victor Chang Cardiac Research Institute, Darlinghurst, NSW, Australia St. Vincent's Clinical School, University of New South Wales, Sydney, NSW, Australia

Ilija Uzelac, Yanyan C. Ji and Flavio H. Fenton
School of Physics, Georgia Institute of Technology, Atlanta, GA, United States

Daniel Hornung, Johannes Schröder-Scheteling and Stefan Luther
Max Planck Institute for Dynamics and Self-Organization, Gottingen, Germany

Richard A. Gray
Center for Device and Radiological Health, Food and Drug Administration, Silver Spring, MD, United States

Elizabeth M. Cherry
School of Mathematical Sciences, Rochester Institute of Technology, Rochester, NY, United States

Eliott Tixier, Fabien Raphel, Damiano Lombardi and Jean-Frédéric
Inria Paris, Paris, France, Sorbonne Universités, Université Pierre et Marie Curie—Paris 6, UMR 7598 LJLL, Paris

Trine Krogh-Madsen and David J. Christini
Greenberg Division of Cardiology, Department of Medicine, Weill Cornell Medicine, New York, NY, United States Institute for Computational Biomedicine, Weill Cornell Medicine, New York, NY, United States Cardiovascular Research Institute, Weill Cornell Medicine, New York, NY, United States

Anna F. Jacobson
Cardiovascular Research Institute, Weill Cornell Medicine, New York, NY, United States

Francis A. Ortega
Physiology, Biophysics and Systems Biology Graduate Program, Weill Cornell Graduate School, New York, NY, United States

Michael A. Colman, Arun V. Holden and Alan P. Benson
School of Biomedical Sciences and Multidisciplinary Cardiovascular Research Centre, University of Leeds, Leeds, United Kingdom

Erick A. Perez Alday
Division of Cardiovascular Medicine, Oregon Health and Science University, Portland, OR, United States

Index

www.ingramcontent.com/pod-product-compliance
Lightning Source LLC
LaVergne TN
LVHW082212200926
848484LV00008B/2244